MAXILLOFACIAL TRAUMA

MAXILLOFACIAL TRAUMA

CHARLES C. ALLING III, D.D.S.

Private Practice
Oral and Maxillofacial Surgery
Birmingham, Alabama

DONALD B. OSBON, D.D.S.

Late Professor and Chairman
Oral and Maxillofacial Surgery
University of Iowa
Iowa City, Iowa

LEA & FEBIGER

Philadelphia   1988

Lea & Febiger
600 Washington Square
Philadelphia, PA   19106-4198
U.S.A.
(215) 922-1330

Library of Congress Cataloging-in-Publication Data

Alling, Charles C., 1923–
  Maxillofacial trauma.

  Includes bibliographies and index.
  1. Maxilla—Wounds and injuries.   2. Face—Wounds
and injuries.   I. Osbon, Donald B., 1930–1986.
II. Title. [DNLM: 1. Maxillofacial Injuries—surgery.
WU 610 A437m]
RD526.A45   1987   617′.52   87-2732
ISBN 0-8121-1077-3

PRINTED IN THE UNITED STATES OF AMERICA

Print number: 5   4   3   2   1

DEDICATION

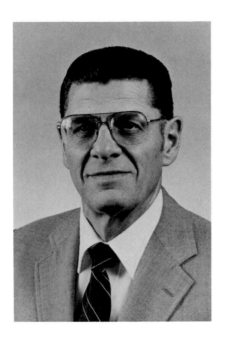

Donald B. Osbon, D.D.S.
Colonel, U.S. Army
Professor and Chairman
Oral and Maxillofacial Surgery
University of Iowa
10 March 1930–22 April 1986

Donald B. Osbon did not use the threescore and 10 years we are usually issued. What he did for the practices of thousands of physicians and dentists through his published works, lectures, and clinics; for tens of thousands of patients as their doctor; for hundreds of thousands of patients through his residents and students; and for the readers of this text through his influence in its development has seldom been exceeded—even by those who live fourscore and 20 years.

The attention to detail, the drive for perfection, and the intensity of purpose that characterized Don carried him to an international reputation in oral and maxillofacial surgery. He began as a first lieutenant and became a colonel in the Regular Army of the United States, which awarded him the highest rating possible in his surgical speciality. His second career, teaching at the University of Iowa, where he was a professor and chairman, furthered the development of one of the major teaching programs in this country.

Don's military career featured duties on three continents in everything from an Evacuation Hospital during the Vietnam War to Walter Reed General Hospital, Washington, D.C., where he received his clinical residency from then-Colonel Robert B. Shira. Eventually he was assigned to Letterman General Hospital, Presidio of San Francisco, where, as Chief of Oral and Maxillofacial Surgery, he conducted a top-notch clinical residency educational program. His post at Letterman had formerly been held by two of his teachers, General Shira and myself.

My wife Laura and I first met Don and his wife, Joan, in El Paso, Texas, at William Beaumont General Hospital, where Don was my first trainee in what today would be termed a general practice residency. He soaked up training so fast that I knew that someday this resident would be my peer and my teacher.

As the years went along, Don was, indeed, recognized as a leader among surgeons in the U.S. and was so cited in a national publication. He served on the editorial boards of the *Journal of Oral and Maxillofacial Surgery* and *Oral Surgery, Oral Medicine and Oral Pathology;* on numerous committees of the American Association of Oral and Maxillofacial Surgeons and the American Dental Association; and on the Advisory Committee of the American Board of Oral and Maxillofacial Surgery. The Advisory Committee several times selected him to be a potential director of the Board.

Don and I planned to be coauthors and coeditors of this textbook, and he maintained a lively and solid interest in and unfailing support for the project until his body was assaulted by a neoplasm that turned out to be an implacable enemy. He and I had planned to dedicate this volume to our wives. Now, Joannie and Laura join me in announcing, with great love and pride in Don, that this book is published for him.

Charles Alling III

FOREWORD

It is a great honor to be invited to write the Foreword for this book, which I know will be a valuable contribution to the professional literature. I have known Drs. Alling and Osbon for many years and have worked closely with them in various assignments: first in the U.S. Army and later in the academic community and civilian practice. From this close, intimate relationship I can attest to their superb qualifications to author this text on maxillofacial injuries.

While wars are regrettable, when they occur they provide a fertile field for experience in the management of maxillofacial injuries. Drs. Alling and Osbon, both of whom had distinguished careers in the Army Dental Corps, have assembled an outstanding group of contributors, many of whom have had extensive experience in the management of wartime and civilian casualties, and this book reflects their experiences and teachings in this important field.

In the Vietnam conflict, approximately 20% of the casualities were maxillofacial injuries. Because of the rapid evacuation system provided by helicopters and the presence in the combat zones of well-equipped and well-staffed hospitals, the patients with these injuries were usually on the operating tables receiving definitive treatment from superbly trained oral and maxillofacial surgeons within 1 to 2 hours following injury. Hence, the results were spectacular and the experience gained by the surgeons was incomparable.

One may ask, why a new book on maxillofacial injuries? The answer is simple. New developments are surfacing rapidly; in fact, it has been stated that dental and medical knowledge doubles every 5 years. The knowledge gained by oral and maxillofacial surgeons with vast practical experiences in the management of facial injuries must be made available to trainees in the specialty as well as to all practitioners who assume the responsibility for the management of these injuries. Hence, this book, authored by these outstanding authors and contributors, who unselfishly share their experiences with others, fills a role in the dissemination of the newest developments in this vital area of surgical practice. By following the tenets set forth in this text, the practitioner can be assured of bringing the latest and best therapy to his or her patients. The book covers the entire field of maxillofacial injuries and provides in-depth coverage of the problems encountered in this aspect of surgical practice.

I am confident that the vast majority of health professionals strive for perfection and work diligently to provide the best possible care. To accomplish this, they must be perpetual students and keep abreast of the developments and advancements in their fields of expertise. This book will be a valuable addition to the libraries of all who desire to provide the best possible care for the patients they serve.

I would be remiss if I did not add my personal tribute to one of the authors, Dr. Donald B. Osbon, whose untimely death in 1986 robbed us of one of our finest oral and maxillofacial surgeons. Don trained with me at

Walter Reed Army Medical Center and I have never known a finer surgeon or a finer individual. He was the epitome of what a health professional should be—honest, sincere, capable, caring, and dedicated to the well-being of his patients. He served in Vietnam during the most active period of the conflict, and the work he did and the experience he gained is almost beyond comprehension. We are deeply grateful for his contributions to oral and maxillofacial surgery and for his input into this important book.

Robert B. Shira, D.D.S., D. Sc. (Hon)
Professor of Oral Surgery, Tufts University
Major General, D.C., U.S.A., Ret.

PREFACE

The mission of this text is to present detailed information on concepts, methods, and techniques of treating maxillofacial trauma. It is necessary, I feel, to target an audience; in this text it is the surgical residents of medicine and dentistry. Because residency training is common for doctors in academic and private practices, the information in the text dealing with different aspects of maxillofacial injuries will be easily identified and useful in real-life situations of both teaching and practice. Fads in treatment are avoided, for the benefit of the patients, and the surgical care that is described is based on proven biotechnical applications of surgical anatomy and physiology.

The aim in treatment of traumatic injuries of the facial tissues is to preserve and restore the function and normality of facial features. This textbook is designed to be of immediate practical, clinical use for any doctor managing oral and maxillofacial injuries. The chapters are arranged in the usual order of managing maxillofacial injuries; the focal point of the text, however, is the patient, the total patient.

Because recognizing the extent of the injuries and appreciating the surgical anatomy are fundamental in planning rational treatment, a large part of this textbook is devoted to describing the making of the diagnoses. If the correct diagnoses are made, the correct treatments will follow; if the wrong diagnoses are made, faulty treatments may follow.

The patient who was subjected to acute trauma presents potential life-threatening challenges; further, the patient who has in-

curred maxillofacial trauma has potential long-range problems of great physical and social impact that may be minimized by correct management of the oral and maxillofacial injuries. This text delves deeply into the technical considerations of both early and intermediate care and describes the reconstruction of facial skeletal injuries. Logical analyses lead to appropriate treatment plans that are supported by details of surgical technique in the interest of the patient.

The background material for the text was accumulated from the authors' resources over the past three or four decades in the treatment of patients with oral and maxillofacial injuries.

Though all but one of the authors of this book are oral and maxillofacial surgeons, we felt no desire to establish territorial rights to patient care based on an academic degree, residency training, and Board certification. We have learned from other dentists, physicians, and, most importantly, from our practices, which have embraced hundreds of thousands of patients, and we wish to share our knowledge on behalf of other patients.

Interest and ability in managing maxillofacial injuries varies greatly among individual members of the specialties in oral and maxillofacial surgery, plastic and reconstructive surgery, otolaryngology, and ophthalmology. In most situations the interests of the patient are served best by a team appoach, when it is available.

For example, as DeFries, an otolaryngologist, wrote in a realistic assessment of one possible team approach, "Certainly the oral surgeon is pre-eminent in managing those injuries that result in derangement of the teeth and jaws. . . . The plastic surgeon is best known for his ability to deal with replacement of lost tissue, . . . the movement of skin flaps, . . . and the reconstruction of lost parts of the anatomy. The otolaryngologist is . . . most familiar with management of injuries to the nose, sinuses and orbital bones, . . . injuries to the larynx and with fractures of the temporal bone resulting in damage to the ear or facial nerve. The special skills of the ophthalmologist are self explanatory."[1]

DeFries accurately mentioned the controversy that may arise among specialists regarding who would treat the patient, a controversy frequently laced, in the words of DeFries, with ". . . pettiness, obliquity, pride, ignorance and downright prejudice (which) combine to obscure the real need, the need to provide to the patient all of those skills which are available . . ." There is neither thought nor intention in the writing of this text to garner patients for any special group of doctors. In fact, I believe arbitrary decisions regarding distribution of patients often produce inferior results.

The authors of this text have had and are involved in different treatment centers and situations of managing maxillofacial injuries in civilian and military centers. Thus, we were able to develop a text that gives a broad perspective of effective modern treatment methods.

Reference
1. DeFries, H.O.: Management of maxillofacial injuries: medical viewpoint. Milit Med 136:558–561, 1971.

Birmingham, Alabama　　Charles C. Alling III

CONTRIBUTORS

Charles C. Alling III, D.D.S, M.S., D.Sc. (Hon)

> Fellow, American College of Dentists, American Dental Society of
> Anesthesiology, American Association of Oral and Maxillofacial Surgeons
> (former officer of the Association)
> Diplomate and past-President, American Board of Oral and Maxillofacial
> Surgery
> Formerly:
>> Chief, Oral Surgery, Walter Reed, Letterman, and William Beaumont Army
>> General Hospitals
>> Chief, Professional Branch, U.S. Army Dental Corps, Office of The Surgeon
>> General
>> Professor, Chairman, and Oral and Maxillofacial Surgeon-in-Chief,
>> University of Alabama in Birmingham Medical Center
> Private practice, Birmingham, Alabama

Rocklin D. Alling, D.D.S.

> Fellow, American Association of Oral and Maxillofacial Surgeons
> Diplomate, American Board of Oral and Maxillofacial Surgery
> Chief, Oral and Maxillofacial Surgery Section
> Brookwood Medical Center
> Birmingham, Alabama

Hugh P. Brindley, D.M.D.

> Fellow, American Association of Oral and Maxillofacial Surgeons, American
> Dental Society of Anesthesiology
> Diplomate, American Board of Oral and Maxillofacial Surgery
> Chief, Oral and Maxillofacial Surgery Section
> Medical Center East
> Birmingham, Alabama

Guy A. Catone, D.M.D.

Fellow, American Association of Oral and Maxillofacial Surgeons
Diplomate, American Board of Oral and Maxillofacial Surgery
Director, Department of Dentistry
Head, Division of Oral and Maxillofacial Surgery
Allegheny General Hospital
Pittsburgh, Pennsylvania

Kenneth Dolan, M.D.

Fellow, American College of Radiology
Professor of Radiology
Diagnostic Radiologist, Head and Neck Division
University of Iowa Department of Radiology
Iowa City, Iowa

T. William Evans, D.D.S., M.D.

Fellow, American College of Dentists, International College of Dentists,
    American Association of Oral and Maxillofacial Surgeons, American Dental
    Society of Anesthesiology
Diplomate, American Board of Oral and Maxillofacial Surgery, former Advisory
    Committeeman of the Board
Associate Professor, Oral and Maxillofacial Surgery
College of Dentistry
Assistant Professor, Emergency Medicine
College of Medicine
Ohio State University
Columbus, Ohio

Kenneth K. Kempf, D.D.S.

Fellow, American Association of Oral and Maxillofacial Surgeons
Diplomate, American Board of Oral and Maxillofacial Surgery
Former Assistant Professor, Department of Surgery
Uniformed Services University of Health Sciences
Bethesda, Maryland
Former Director, Division of Oral and Maxillofacial Surgery
Department of Hospital Dentistry
University of Iowa Hospitals and Clinics
Iowa City, Iowa
Private Practice
Staff, St. Francis Medical Center
La Crosse, Wisconsin

Robert A.J. Olson, D.M.D.

Fellow, American Association of Oral and Maxillofacial Surgeons
Diplomate, American Board of Oral and Maxillofacial Surgery
Associate Professor and Chairman, Department of Oral and Maxillofacial
    Surgery
College of Dentistry
University of Iowa
Iowa City, Iowa

David W. Shelton, D.M.D.

Fellow, International College of Dentists, American Association of Oral and
    Maxillofacial Surgeons
Diplomate, American Board of Oral and Maxillofacial Surgery
Professor, Department of Oral and Maxillofacial Surgery
School of Dentistry
Professor, Department of Surgery
School of Medicine
Medical College of Georgia
Augusta, Georgia

ACKNOWLEDGMENTS

IN APPRECIATION

To Those Who Went Before

In the 1960s, U.S. Army officers accepted invitations by Major General Robert B. Shira and me to produce a textbook on maxillofacial injuries, and the book was completed through the first draft. The demands that the Vietnam War put on oral surgeons involved in the Army chains of medical evacuation of the wounded forestalled the completion of the textbook. The authors in the initial project included a civilian consultant, Dr. James. R. Hayward, and U.S. Army oral surgeons Colonels Cecil R. Albright, James E. Chipps, David C. Hazard, E. Eugene Hunsuck, W. Benjamin Irby, Leo Korchin, Robert H. Marlette, Donald B. Osbon, Martin Steiner, and Edward H. Stiesmeyer. Included in the initial group of authors were Colonel Jack J. Kovaric, general surgeon; Colonel Gilbert Lilly, oral pathologist; and Peter M. Margetis, biomaterials researcher. Generous contributions of illustrations, some of which are used in this text, were given by Colonels Jack B. Caldwell, Leon D. Fiedler, Roy C. Gerhard, Kenneth W. Hughes, Roderick L. Lister, Paul H. McFarland, Calvin W. Thompson, Henry C. Thompson, and Robert D. Youmans, and by Dr. Samford Moose, a civilian consultant.

The authors in the original project agreed to the following dedication of their textbook:

The care of the complex of structures and functions that compose the face call for the highest dedication of talents by medical and dental specialists. To these colleagues, who care for the injuries of others, we dedicate this text.

In the late 1970s, Dr. Donald B. Osbon joined me in revitalizing the text in the spirit of the above dedication. In 1986, Don, richly graced with integrity and professionalism, moved on to the rewards of eternity.

To Those Behind the Lines

To Dr. Charles Porter, Director of Medical Education/Research, and to Medical Librarian, Miss Lucy Moor, of A.M.I. Brookwood Medical Center, Birmingham, Alabama, special thanks for your steady support.

Very special gratitude is due to friends at Lea & Febiger, the oldest publishing house in the United States. Mr. Christian "Kit" Spahr, a partner at Lea & Febiger, has been a continuing force in my literary life since the mid-1960s, and his friendship is treasured. I have been fortunate to have had an empathetic and superb editor, Mr. Raymond Kersey. Copy editor, Ms. Amy Norwitz, has been a guardian tigress of the accuracy of the written word, and I claim as my own all mutant grammar! It is a pleasure to be in the company of all the members of the Lea & Febiger firm, with their sense of excellence in nurturing and producing a book.

"What is the use of a book," thought Alice,

"without pictures . . . ?" Teaching surgical techniques requires pictures, and the pictorial content of this book is credited to a host of medical illustrators and audiovisual specialists. A few of these friends are Mr. John Roll, formerly a Department of the Army employee; Mr. Harry Jermazjian, of the Veterans' Administration Hospital, Birmingham, Alabama; and the wife and husband team of Amy and Sam Collins, of Birmingham, Alabama. Mr. William F. Davis, Supervisor, Instructional Resources, at Brookwood Medical Center typified the support given by the all members of the Center's staff as he provided for production of key photographs.

My respected colleague and esteemed friend, Dr. Hugh Brindley, besides writing a chapter, also did the artwork for many illustrations.

To Those on the Line

For learning beyond knowledge, I am especially beholden to two doctors' doctors, John J. Lytle and Bill C. Terry. In the area of oral and maxillofacial trauma, my grateful respects are extended to Drs. James R. Hayward, Robert B. Shira, and Charles A. McCallum; to the neurosurgeon, Dr. Harold Murphree, and the orthopedic surgeon, Dr. George Omer, at the 121st Evacuation Hospital in Korea; to the orthopedic surgeon, Dr. Benjamin Rutledge, at the 387th Station Hospital and the 5th Field Hospital in Germany; and to the oral and maxillofacial surgery, the plastic and reconstructive surgery, the oto-

laryngology, and the anesthesiology community of doctors of Birmingham, Alabama.

Many of us have been fortunate enough to have friendships with oral and maxillofacial surgeons of other nations. These surgeons often have been celebrated international leaders, often representative of the solid core of practicing doctors who, with great nobility, care for their patients and our profession. With our mutual learning in the management of traumatized patients, my collegial greetings are passed from the East to the West to Doctors and Misters Kim Hong Ki and Chung Soon Kyung of the Republic of Korea; Matthew Chao and Richard Chang, the Republic of China; Chuachote Hansasuta and Vacheree Chang, Thailand; Saud Ahmed Mortazavi, Iran; Hashim Hassan and Raja K. Kummoona, Iraq; Angelos Angelopoulos, Greece; the considerate and rightfully renowned Norman L. Rowe, England; Sigurjon H. Olafsson, Iceland; Manuel Silbiger and J.J. Barros, Brazil; and, in Canada, Simon Weinberg, Alva E. Swanson, and my housestaff mentors, R. Keith Lindsay and Robert S. Van Alstine.

Words written here are not appropriate to express all of the whys; therefore, suffice it to write that a special hug is reserved for my wife, Laura. Rocklin, one of our children and the senior (but not the eldest!) member of our private practice, has made available the time and resources necessary for this and similar projects. Thanks, Rocky!

Birmingham, Alabama   C.C.A.
                                          1988

CONTENTS

xvii

1

INFLUENCE OF LAND WARFARE ON THE MANAGEMENT OF MAXILLOFACIAL INJURIES IN THE U.S.

CHARLES C. ALLING III

After millennia of men's hacking away at each other with sharp and blunt objects, the effect of the Industrial Revolution on the profession of arms in the mid-nineteenth century changed the character of battlefields. The production of improved armaments of rifling, fixed ammunition with conoidal bullets, exploding artillery, and grenade projectiles, in addition to improved transport and rapid communication by telegraph, made the Crimean War and the American Civil War radically different from previous wars. New methods of transport and communication permitted armies to be measured in the hundreds of thousands of men; men who were, for the most part, conscripted civilians, not mercenaries. War thus became both vast in scale and very personal to family and friends.

THE AMERICAN CIVIL WAR

By the time the Civil War began, the published experiences of the Crimean War were used by J. J. Chisholm in *A Manual for Military Surgery for Use of the Surgeons of the Confederate Army*:

> "Wounds of the face from gunshot . . . were usually more distressing from the deformity they occasion, than dangerous to life . . . in the treatment of gunshot wounds in the face where bones are splintered and torn, the surgeons should always retain and replace as many of the broken portions as possible. It is often surprising how small connexions (sic) with neighboring soft parts will suffice to maintain vitality and lead to restoring unions in this region . . ."[1]

The Surgeon General of the Confederate States Army, Dr. Samuel G. Moore, recognized the demand for oral surgery to treat soldiers and encouraged its use in hospitals of the South. He wrote,

> A study of the available statistics revealed that the average Confederate soldier was wounded about six times . . . and each time seriously enough to receive treatment . . . and it is inevitable that a large portion of these wounds affected the face and jaws.[2]

Following interaction between the Confederate Congress and the Bureau of Conscription, dentists were assigned to hospitals in the Southern states and received extra remuneration for extraordinary skills. To this evolving position of specialized care for the wounded, come the contributions of Dr. James B. Bean, a civilian dentist.

As is often the case during warfare, when clinical material is distressingly abundant and the need for effective and efficient management concepts is desperate, the emergence of skilled specialists influences the evolution of surgical and medical advances. Of course, at any one time, similar original observations are probably being made independently by practitioners in different areas of the world. However, Bean's background in dentistry and his special interest in articulation of teeth led to his unique visualization and development of intraoral splints to reduce and stabilize fractures of the maxillofacial skeleton. The Medical Inspector of the Confederate Army, Dr. C. N. Covey, described Bean's work:[2]

> The history of this class of fractures has brought heretofore as little honor to the profession as it has benefit to the patient; . . . I desire to call attention to the treatment of fractures of maxillary bones, according to the method originated by J. B. Bean of Atlanta, Georgia . . . The frequency of this class of fractures in military surgery, the almost total want of success among surgeons, with a treatment usually adopted, rendered this plan (perfect as it is, and attended with such happy results), one of special interest . . . I directed that a ward should be opened in one of the hospitals at Macon, Georgia, to which all cases in the hospital department of that section should be sent. Very soon over 40 cases were collected, and were treated with the most perfect success.
> The Confederate States' Surgeon General, Dr. Moore, directed that . . . all cases of fractures of superior and inferior maxillary bones now in the hospital, or that may hereafter be admitted . . . be placed in a special ward and that Dr. Bean's techniques be employed.[2]

Until the time of Bean's splints, the treatment of maxillofacial skeletal injuries consisted, as it had since the time of Hippocrates, of the use of facial and cranial bandages.

Independent of the contributions by Dr. Bean of the Confederate States, Dr. Thomas B. Gunning, a dentist from New York, NY, devised a series of splints that would orient fractures of the mandible against the maxilla. These splints, like those of Dr. Bean, relied on impressions of the dentition, and throughout the next century certain intraoral splints were frequently referred to as Gunning's splints. The leading surgeons of that time, although recognizing the ingenuity of Gunning's contributions, felt that they, the surgeons, were " . . . neither skilled in mechanics nor ingenious" enough to use the devices.[2] Therefore, physicians continued to use head bandages. Interestingly, when Gunning was asked to treat bilateral mandibular fractures incurred by William H. Seward, Secretary of State, when he fell from a carriage, the physicians attending Secretary Seward refused to have Dr. Gunning treat their patient for nearly a month following the injury. Eventually, the splints were placed and bony union was achieved.

Most importantly, as Schwartz emphasized, the positive recognition given to the dentists of the times played an important part in establishing the relationship of dentistry to the new specialty of oral surgery.[2] This relationship was described by Cryer toward the close of the century, when he pointed out that oral surgery

> . . . is perhaps unique in that while really a department of surgery, educational approach to it is through dentistry and not through medicine.[3]

Lest, from the way the Civil War is sanitized for television, we regard it as a romantic interlude, we must recall that the field conditions in which both forces lived and fought were extremely crude. For example, in the South, which faced superior military forces for most of the war and which was isolated from the rest of the world's supplies by blockades, the lot of the soldiers and civilians was often one of grim and determined survival. For an individual with an oral and maxillofacial wound, the liquid and soft diets were mixtures of corn bread and sorghum. Nevertheless, the surviving records (most of the reports were lost when Richmond was burned and evacuated on April 2, 1865) describe treatment that matched treatment of a century or more later. The U.S. government–sponsored

History of the Civil War included hundreds of case reports.[4] For example, a sergeant wounded in 1864 was described with an entrance wound in the right cheek, complex and compound fractures of the entire maxilla, and bilateral fractures of the mandible. Having severe swelling of his tongue, he was fed by tube and funnel until he stabilized 3 weeks later. By that time an interdental splint had been fashioned and was placed and stabilized with occipitofrontal bandages. Within weeks the patient had a safe airway, was ingesting liquids, and was comfortable. Two months postoperative, his condition was described as " . . . bone united; antagonism of the teeth perfect; no deformity; . . ."[4]

WORLD WAR I

The *Journal of the American Medical Association's* section on stomatology contained a report in 1910 pertaining to the management of mandibular fractures written by Colonel Robert T. Oliver, D.D.S., the Supervising Dental Surgeon of the U.S. Army, stationed at West Point, NY.[5] Colonel Oliver was later to become chief of the U.S. Army Dental Corps and was elected president of the American Dental Association. Dr. Oliver prefaced his 1910 remarks by noting that the dental profession had originated and championed the application of interdental splints. In the report, he proposed itermaxillary and intradental wiring for immobilizing the mandible to the maxilla. Beginning in 1903, Dr. Oliver had begun using copper wire instead of silver wire to fashion loops in the various locations of the mouth. Between these loops, he placed traction wires to immobilize the mandible and fix it to the maxilla. He noted that in some instances a general anesthetic would be required and that the interdental immobilizing wires " . . . should not be introduced until the next day, after the fear of nausea and vomiting has passed. Even then it is well to leave a small pair of wire-cutting shears with the attendant, with instructions how and when to use them should such interference be necessary." Dr. Oliver described the use of liquid diets and " . . . hot antiseptic mouth washes."

I want . . . to say most emphatically that the most important thing in treating jaw fractures, is to restore occlusion and reproduce the function of mastication . . . This is especially true in the Army for the soldier's physical fitness in military efficiency is to a great extent dependent upon his ability to masticate his foods . . . his personal appearance counts for nought. . . . The method I have described was developed during my service in the Phillipine Islands and is a result of the gradual evolution of experimental wiring in these cases . . . Previously I had always used silver wire—fleurs sutures—but there were none available at that hospital and as an expedient an orderly was sent with a note to a nearby Signal Corps station requesting some 20 gauge wire. He returned with a big roll of copper field telephone wire, from which I burned the insulation. After annealing and sterlizing, this was used and proved so efficacious and superior to the silver wire in being tougher, less ductile and possessing greater stability of the twist, that it has been used ever since.

Converse reports with great respect and affection on the wartime contributions of Dr. Varaztad H. Kazanjian.[6] During the First World War, Kazanjian, a dentist, traveled to England as a member of the Harvard unit. As Dr. Converse noted, "Curiously enough, there was no dental corps in the British Army and only 15 dentists." Dr. Kazanjian's contributions were very similar to those earlier recorded by Drs. Bean, Gunning, and Oliver; "He devised a technique of holding the ramus of the jaws in proper position by means of wires. In the cases of patients who had no teeth, he made special splints to hold the fragments together . . . and over which the soft tissues of the face were sutured." The British Army established its first maxillofacial treatment center in France with Dr. Kazanjian as the chief. He received much publicity, and King George V invested him as a Companion of the Most Distinguished Order of St. Michael and St. George. When Dr. Kazanjian returned to the U.S. in 1919, he obtained a doctorate in medicine after two years of study. Dr. Converse noted that there was a general lack of appreciation of Dr. Kazanjian and of his contributions by the surgeons in the Boston area. However, Kazanjian was, in the words of his friend Dr. Converse, " . . . content to perform his work and enjoyed the tremendous satisfaction he derived from what he was able to do for his patients."

Among the others who applied the principles and techniques enunciated by Drs. Bean, Gunning, and Oliver in the decades between the Civil War and World War I were Lt. Colonel Robert H. Ivy, M.C., U.S. Army, and Major Joseph D. Eby, D.C., U.S. Army. Major Eby, stationed at Walter Reed U.S. Army General Hospital, published a paper in 1920 that was replete with case reports describing devices whose objective was to return shattered facial skeletons to normal anatomic relationships using cast metal splints carried on the remaining dentition (Fig. 1–1A).[7] Based on the management of war injuries, Major Eby remarked, [Our accomplishments have] . . . shown those who in former years who have tried to belittle a dental surgeon in the Army by refusing him equal right with the medical man, that dentistry is a profession; and fully deserves the recognition it now enjoys." Major Eby published the eyelet wiring technique, usually referred to as Ivy loops, in 1921.[8] Ivy, who time and again demonstrated his personal and professional integrity in matters dealing with oral surgery, wrote in 1938 that the technique was "by no means original" with him but was "a modi-

fication of that described by Colonel Robert T. Oliver, D.C., U.S. Army."[9] Ivy further commented that the technique was first called to his attention by Eby in 1918.

Lt. Colonel Rea P. McGee, D.C., U.S. Army read a paper to the Section on Stomatology at the Tenth Annual Session of the AMA in Atlantic City, in 1919 about his World War I experiences in a mobile hospital (Fig. 1–2).[10]

It was my good fortune to be detailed as a maxillofacial surgeon to the U.S. Mobile Hospital No. 1, American Expeditionary Forces, and it is from experiences gained there that I speak. The Mobile Hospital was always in the area between the 75s and the 6-inch guns. Mobile Hospital No. 1 was essentially a front-line organizaton, moving as many as 14 times during the period of hostilities . . . with a bed capacity of 200 (we) performed in all 6048 major operations. The conditions for maxillofacial work at Mobile Hospital No. 1 were extremely favorable, because we moved so frequently that we were not hampered with orders.

Our advanced position made it possible for us to receive many patients as early as 2 hours after they were hit . . . we received only the most desperately wounded men . . . covered with blood and dirt, . . . extreme exhaustion, . . . labored respiration . . . examined with the fluoroscope. (We used) gasoline to wash the

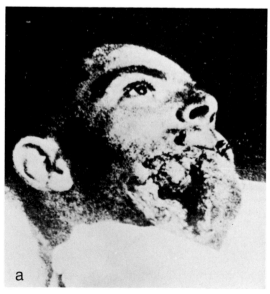 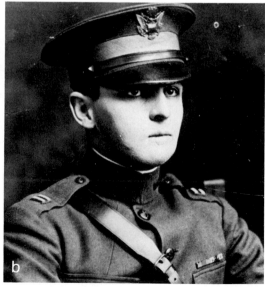

FIG. 1–1. **a,** Before and **b,** after treatment of a casualty who received definitive care at Walter Reed Army Hospital during the time of service by Colonels Robert H. Ivy, Robert T. Oliver, and Joseph D. Eby. (Courtesy of the U.S. Armed Forces Institute of Pathology.)

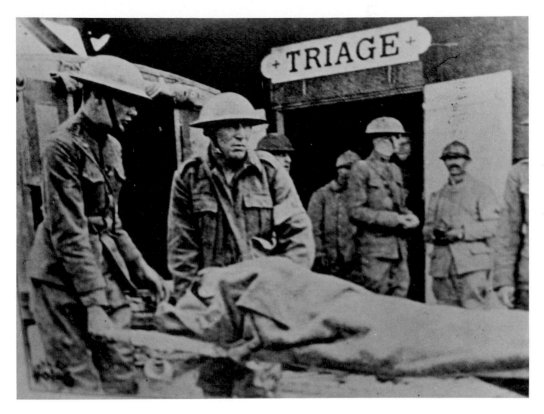

FIG. 1–2.   World War I triage and early surgery station on the Western Front.

faces . . . Fortunately for us, the American habit of taking care of the mouth and teeth and the service of the Dental Corps of the Army rendered septic mouths a rarity . . . the mucous membrane (is repaired) before the cutaneous surface is sutured . . . tension sutures were used . . . live tissues and all bruised tissues must be preserved . . . The great points to observe in the front-line work are conservation of bone, mucous membrane and skin. . . . All bone fragments that have live periosteum must be preserved . . .

This work absolutely demands both a surgical and dental training . . . (There was a precedent set in) the establishment of the specialty of surgery of the face and jaws, (and the) . . . arrangement of placing a dental officer in charge of a surgical department, to handle all cases of the maxillofacial type. Those who follow us in the next war should have comparatively little difficulty in beginning where we leave off.

WORLD WAR II

World War II descended upon a U.S. that still had occasional horse and buggies on the road and only a few hundred miles of interstate highways. At a time when transport of personnel and material by air was a rarity, the nation entered into global conflicts embracing every climate and continent on earth and involving millions of servicemen and -women.

The U.S. Army Dental Corps expanded from approximately 250 dental officers to over 15,000 during the World War II period of hostilities.[11] As with the U.S. Navy, there were Herculean complexities of procurement, training, assignment, and utilization of civilian dentists wearing uniforms. In terms of the oral and maxillofacial surgery needs, the Army Dental School cooperated with the Army Medical School and Walter Reed General Hospital in amalgamating oral and maxillofacial surgeons and plastic surgeons into teams. Training for these teams was also supplied by Columbia University, Harvard University, University of Pennsylvania, St. Louis University, Mayo Foundation, and Tulane University.

At Columbia University, the teaching was directed by Henry S. Dunning, D.D.S., M.D., who organized the first oral surgery clinic in New York, NY in 1906 and then chaired the committee that founded the first university dental school in New York at Columbia University in 1916.[12] He served with the Presbyterian Hospital unit of World War I in France and came under the influence of Sir Harold D. Gillies and Colonel Vilroy P. Blair. His teachings live on in the brains and hands of surgeons as each generation transfers knowledge to the next.

The vast differences in combat situations prevented a single system for evacuation of wounded servicemen; however, a prototypic maxillofacially injured patient could have been handled in the following manner (Fig. 1–3). Within minutes after being wounded, the injured man would have been treated by basic first aid by a Medical Department soldier assigned to the combat unit; the principal objective was to move the casualty away from the combat area to the supporting battalion aid station and thence to a division collecting station. The collecting stations, within range of hostile mortar fire, accumulated casualties to be transported to clearing stations. Several miles behind the front lines, the clearing stations to which a dentist was usually assigned, would manage hemorrhage, treat shock, and possibly provide temporary immobilization of facial skeletal fractures. Next, the injured serviceman was taken to an evacuation hospital, which was usually behind the range of ordinary artillery fire. When the influx of casualties was heavy, a maxillofacial surgical team might be assigned. This team would perform conservative debridement, immobilization of fractures, and placement of drains. As soon as it was safe for a patient to travel, he was transferred to a general hospital in the combat area and a maxillofacial surgical team would perform final fixation of fractures and definitive care of the soft-tissue injuries. The facilities used and the placement of medical units varied greatly, depending on the terrain and situation in the combat zone. In most instances, the maxillofacially injured soldier was then transferred to the U.S. In a 5-month period in 1945, 5000 casualties with head and neck and related injuries were returned by air from overseas areas. Eight military hospitals in the U.S. were designated to receive cas-

ualties with the most complex maxillofacial injuries. Other general hospitals had oral surgeons and managed similar maxillofacially injured troops well.

One of the most distinguished military oral surgeons of the first part of this century was Colonel Roy A. Stout. During World War II he was the Senior Consultant in Maxillofacial Surgery in the European Theater of Operations. Prior to Wold War II, he served in the Phillipine Islands and Hawaii and was the personal dentist to Generals Douglas MacArthur and Dwight D. Eisenhower. During his second tour of duty at Walter Reed General Hospital and in Europe, he taught refresher courses in the treatment of war injuries to oral and plastic surgeons. He was active in oral surgery throughout his postmilitary years, serving on the faculty of the University of Texas Medical Branch in Galveston, Tex. Thousands of maxillofacial injuries were treated with the Stout's continuous loop wiring technique, which Colonel Stout insisted was done better with brass than stainless steel wires.

Dentists who were surgeons or were to become surgeons as a result of their World War II experience include Colonel Jack Caldwell, famed for his pioneering and farsighted development of the vertical osteotomy of the mandibular rami for correction of mandibular deformities; Colonels Charles Cashman and Arthur Hemberger, protégés of Colonel Stout and among the first military men to be certified by the American Board of Oral and Maxillofacial Surgeons (ABOMS); Colonel W."Ben" Irby,[13] author, teacher, consultant to both the European and Pacific Theaters of Operations who operated on over 5000 trauma patients in his career; Lowell McKelvey, later to be dean of the Dental School of Puerto Rico; Colonel James E. Chipps, who was later to distinguish himself in the Korean War; and Major General Robert B. Shira.

World War II brought about a great expansion in the U.S. Navy Dental Corps.[14] The number of officers on duty increased from 234 to a peak of over 7000 during the hostilities. During this time, some 8000 maxillofacially injured servicemen were treated by the U.S. Navy Dental Corps. Among the honors accorded to the U.S. Navy Dental Corps during

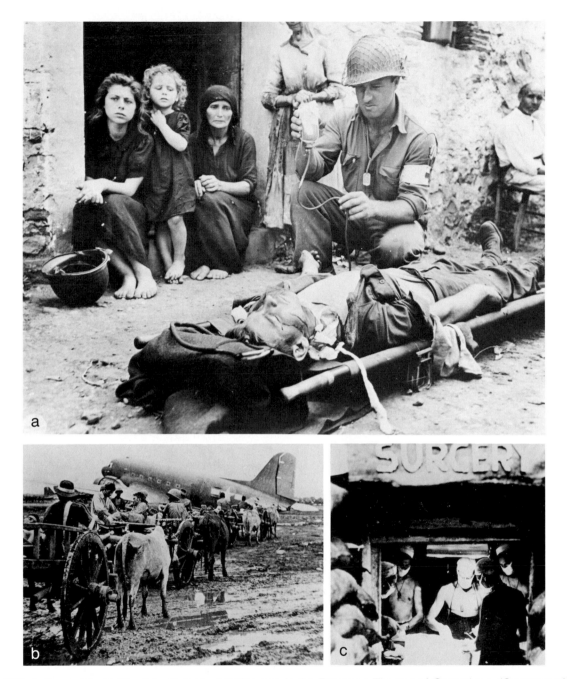

FIG. 1–3.　**a,** World War II battlefield casualty care in the European Theater of Operations. (Courtesy of U.S. Army Signal Corps.) **b,** Evacuation of casualties from southern Europe; often, local resources were used. **c,** Surgery in the combat zone in the Pacific Theater of Operations. (Courtesy of the Department of the Army.)

World War II was the naming of three naval vessels for dental officers: *U.S.S. Crowley, U.S.S. Tatum,* and *U.S.S. O'Reilly.*

Since prehistoric times, throughout the histories in the Bible, and in countless conflicts across our planet for the past 2000 years, young men thrust into battle adapt and serve, as expressed in the informal words of Captain Donald E. Cooksey, U.S.N., Ret.

> I went to Midway in June 1941, 1 year out of school, as the Dental Officer of the Sixth Defense Battalion, U.S. Marine Corps. Things were quiet, the fishing good, skin diving excellent and only rumblings of Pacific War. Saturday, December 6, (1941) I went diving for lobster and got a big one. Bob, the executive officer, and I ate it after the poker game and retired at about 0130. The adjutant came through the quarters at 0700 screaming, "Get up, get up, the Japs have bombed Pearl Harbor." During the day, I had to go to the Pan Am Hotel to inventory and accept their liquor supply since the hotel personnel planned to depart on the Clipper returning from Wake Island. I was in the process of doing this when destroyers hit us with shell fire about 2130, and we suffered the first casualties of the war on Midway. On June 4 (1942) we were hit (the Battle of Midway). Our medical facilities remained intact. We treated island casualties and aviators from the carriers which were picked up by our patrols. By the 10th we had buried our and the [Japanese] dead, evacuated most of the ambulatory casualties who would not be returned to duty. About June 15th, I decided that surgery was for me . . .

Dr. Cooksey went on during World War II to serve on the U.S.S. Wisconsin, which, as a part of a fast-carrier task force, acted as a hospital ship, receiving casualties transferred at sea from smaller ships to the more extensive medical facilities of the capital ship. He was a teacher throughout his Navy career and, among other tributes by his peers, became president of the American Board of Oral and Maxillofacial Surgery.

Recalling the raw numbers of naval and army dental officers on duty and the treatment of thousands of maxillofacial injuries does not recount the acts of sacrifice, ingenuity, and heroism. From Dr. Thomas Cook's[15] duties in the isolation of the Burma road area in Asia, to Dr. Cooksey's direct involvement in the East Pacific Ocean in battle-

ships and on a bull's-eye of an island, to Colonel Roy Stout's contributions in the European Theater and his embracing duties in the Sahara desert at one extreme and the Arctic tundra on the other, hundreds of dental officers provided the highest standards of oral and maxillofacial care.

1946 TO 1950

Following World War II, demobilization left the battle-torn but liberated lands of Western Europe nearly naked of Allied armed forces. The vacuum of effective military power held less than ten Allied divisions, none at fighting strength. At one point, the manpower equivalent of about two U.S. divisions was all there was of U.S. military power in Western Europe, and the European Command had only two oral surgeons; one, Lt. Colonel Arthur Hemberger, was experienced and certified; the other was a recent dental school graduate with only a few weeks of preceptor training by Colonel Cashman. There were relatively few troops to care for, but these were spread across terrain torn and were in cities crumbled by war. There was no effective professional communications with German colleagues. The undermanned medical facilities in Japan and Korea were very similar to those of the European Command and were abruptly challenged by the Korean War.

When the U.S. Army Air Corps matured into the U.S. Air Force in 1949, transfers were available within the Armed Forces to join the new service. In addition to providing direct care to the airmen, the Air Force used specialists in air evacuation of casualties, which was soon to be tested in the Korean War and which was well established during the Vietnam War. During the next three decades, the Air Force established training and consultant programs in oral and maxillofacial surgery that took their place alongside those of the Army and Navy.

KOREAN WAR

The uneasy peace following World War II was shattered when North Korea attacked

South Korea in 1950 and the U.N. entered the fray. The Korean War proved to be a watershed for military maxillofacial surgery. Tokyo Army Hospital, thanks to growing capabilities of air evacuation, was often the first major treatment facility for the battle-injured. Dr. Bruno Kwapis[16] and a few other oral surgeons provided early care of maxillofacially injured patients in the Mobile Army Surgical Hospitals (MASH) and the 121st Evacuation Hospital in the combat zone, and the soldiers were then evacuated to Tokyo Army Hospital (Fig. 1–4). The press of casualties was so heavy at one time that a circus tent was placed in front of the Tokyo Army Hospital to house incoming casualties; Colonel Chipps treated over 2000 maxillofacially injured soldiers during the conflict.[17] Serendipitously, the confluence of the assignment to Chipps' maxillofacial surgical team of a splendidly trained and talented plastic and reconstructive surgeon, Dr. Marvin Cullen, the availability of antibiotics, the liberal use of nasogastric tubes and tracheostomies, and the provision of talents and resources to men newly injured produced superior results, shorter hospitalizations, and a decreased need for definitive reconstructive surgery.

The U.S. Navy hospital ships, *U.S.S. Repose* and *U.S.S. Haven*, shared duties in the Korean War along with the Danish ship, *Jutlandia*. These three ships were in the area of Pusan during the time the U.N. clung to a perimeter area on the southern tip of the Korean pen-

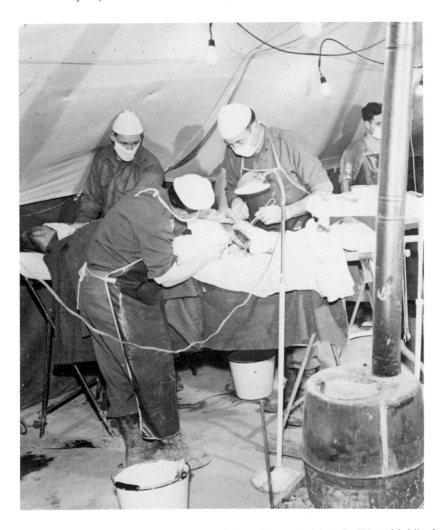

FIG. 1–4. Korean War surgical teams provide care in hastily erected tent facilities, Mobile Army Surgical Hospitals, that kept pace with a rapidly changing battlefront. (Courtesy of U.S. Army Signal Corps.)

insula. The *Repose* and *Haven* moved from the Pusan perimeter to support the famous and end-run invasion at Inchon, and they received casualties that were " . . . hot and dirty by chopper and Mike boat, as the MLR was very close . . . " Those were the words of junior officer Donald Cooksey, who had gained valuable experience at the Battle of Midway and at sea on a battleship in World War II. He mentioned that the *Haven* had the first helicopter flight deck; at that time, the *Repose* had two barges tied alongside upon which the choppers landed. The oral surgeons aboard the *Repose*, in addition to providing oral and facial reconstructive surgical care, also served on orthopedic and general surgical teams. Another junior naval oral surgeon, Edward Raffetto, later to be an admiral, replaced Cooksey and continued the tradition of service beyond the call of duty for the wounded of the U. N. and the Republic of Korea Army, as well as civilians evacuated to the U.S. Navy hospital ships.

1954 TO 1960

Following the Korean War, came a surge of research and training in the Armed Forces. Much is owed to chiefs of the U.S. Army Dental Corps, Major General Robert H. Mills, one of the original 14 Dental Corps officers in the U.S. Army and the first to be a major general; Major General Walter D. Love; and Major General Thomas L. Smith, who had been the Dental Surgeon of the European Theater of Operations. These officers saw the need for advanced education in the specialties of dentistry and made training available in civilian and U.S. Army general hospitals. Coming from these training programs were many individuals who made important contributions to oral and maxillofacial surgery and the other dental specialties in the decades that followed in the military in second and third careers in teaching and administration in civilian universities, and as leaders in the private sector.

During the decade between the Korean and the Vietnam Wars, hundreds of civilian and military oral and maxillofacial surgeons developed and learned advanced skills in managing facial bones through open procedures

to correct developmental and acquired defects of the face. These extraoral experiences with facial skeletal surgery helped lay the foundation for the sophisticated and brilliant contributions of oral and maxillofacial surgeons in Vietnam.

During this time, a remarkable individual became one of the most renowned oral surgeons in history. Major General Robert Shira was president of the American Dental Association, the American Association of Oral and Maxillofacial Surgeons, and the American Board of Oral and Maxillofacial Surgery, to name but a few of his leadership accomplishments. In 1966, General Shira was responsible for bringing Professor Hugo Obwegeser from Switzerland to lecture at Walter Reed Army Medical Center (Fig. 1–5). The information brought by Professor Obwegeser regarding advances that could be obtained through advance orthognathic and preprosthodontic surgery helped stimulate the dental profession in this country and set the stage for the rapid development of facial skeletal surgery in the U.S.

VIETNAM WAR, 1964 TO 1973

In the Vietnam War, oral and maxillofacial surgery was brought to the battlefield, where the initial surgical treatment was often also the intermediate and definitive care by oral and maxillofacial surgeons close to the Army and Marine troops. Helicopter evacuation brought the casualties from the point of injury directly to the specialists; the "choppers" frequently received communications regarding the delivery site of the casualties on board en route to the specialty treatment center that best suited the needs of the individual patients. The choppers evacuated wounded patients to specialty surgeons often within minutes of the infliction of the wound, which decreased morbidity.

At the initiative of the U.S. Army Research and Development Command, the U.S. Army established the oral and maxillofacial research activity of The Letterman Hospital Research Center with a major mission for research in maxillofacial injuries. In addition to working on alloplastic devices for immediate recon-

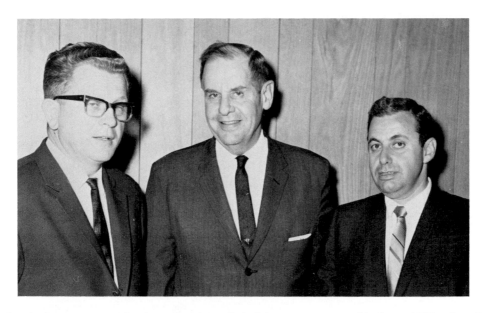

FIG. 1–5.   An important meeting in oral and maxillofacial surgery occurred in June, 1966, when Professor Hugo Obwegeser (left) presented a series of lectures at Walter Reed Army Medical Center, Washington, D.C. General Robert Shira (center) and Dr. Howard Adilman (right) were instrumental in organizing this event. (U.S. Army Signal photograph by Irwin J. Halpern.)

struction of maxillofacial injuries, pulsating water debridement of wounds, and other studies, this unit accumulated definitive statistics on combat-area maxillofacial injuries. Lt. Colonel Gilbert Lilly, an oral pathologist, and Lt. Colonel Martin Steiner, an oral surgeon, headed this special research unit. The major U.S. Army research unit was the U.S. Army Institute of Dental Research, which has broader missions in research. During the Vietnam War, its roster included Lt. Colonel E. Eugene Hunsuck, who devised the Hunsuck modification of the sagittal split of the mandibular rami for orthognathic surgery and who field-tested pulsating water debridement of injuries in Vietnam as well as the use of cyanoacrylates for dressing soft-tissue injuries.

Lt. Colonel Donald B. Osbon reported on the early treatment of 1600 patients with maxillofacial injuries during a 12-month period in the 24th Evacuation Hospital;[18] Lt. Colonel James Andrews reported on his surgical experience with 119 patients in the Vietnamese Military Maxillofacial Center;[19] Lt. Colonel L. Thomas Gallegos managed 639 oral and maxillofacial surgical cases; the farsighted statistical report by Tinder and others and by Lt.

Colonel Gibert E. Lilly of nearly 3000 maxillofacially injured patients highlighted the benefits of having rapid evacuation in the field of combat to oral and maxillofacial surgeons.[20,21] The Armed Forces Services Commission of the Federal Dentaire Internationale requested the U.S. Army Dental Corps to prepare a report as a guide for dental officers in the early management of maxillofacial war injuries; this was done under the editorship of Colonel Paul H. McFarland and contained excellently detailed chapters by Lt. Colonels Lee Getter, Gilbert E. Lilly, Donald B. Osbon, and Calvin W. Thompson.[21]

Because the contested land in Vietnam was circumscribed, there was a confluence of high-technology transportation and surgical specialists in the combat zone (Fig. 1–6). In a personal communication, Colonel David W. Shelton said:

> . . . throughout the war we enjoyed total and complete freedom of the air, a situation which had considerable influence on our ability to move casualties by air. It was a war in which there were no [front lines] behind which were secure "rear areas." The whole of South Vietnam was a combat zone. We . . . occupied the ground on which we stood; the rest was theirs,

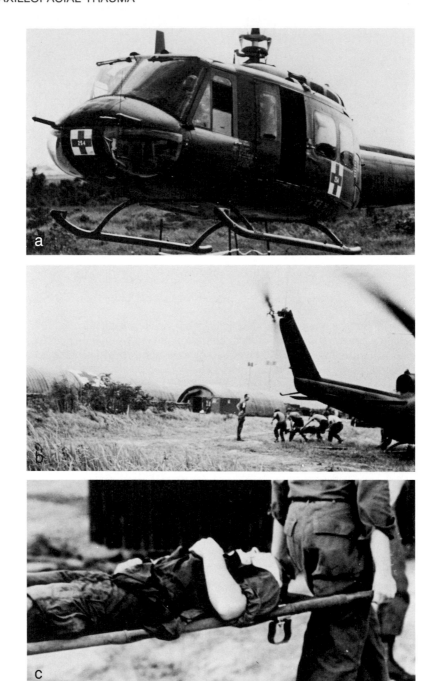

FIG. 1–6.   **a,** U.S. Army chopper pickup of a casualty from the battlefield. **b** and **c,** Arrival of chopper and casualty at an evacuation hospital in the combat zone. (Courtesy of the U.S. Armed Forces Institute of Pathology.)

especially at night. It was a war that started in a trickle, escalated to a thunderclap, and receded into an uneasy interlude during which we, the American military presence, took our leave. Accordingly, weapons, tactics, types of wounds and injuries . . . changed, and the number of casualties ebbed and then flowed, at times torrentially, and then ebbed again, from the beginning to the end of our involvement. Those who served early in the war faced a different situation than those who served at its height. Those who served late in our involvement had yet another experience.

The first trained Army OMS [oral and maxillofacial surgeon][in Vietnam], Captain John E. Salem, . . . assigned to the 8th Field Hospital located at Nha Trang [from] February 1964 [to] February 1965]. Major Calvin W. Thompson arrived at the 8th Field Hospital in April 1965, 2 months after the departure of Salem. This brief hiatus dramatically underscored the importance of having an OMS present in Vietnam [because] maxillofacial casualties were being generated at an accelerating rate [and] maxillofacial cases [needed to be] evacuated to Clark Air Force Base in the Phillipines.

Under these conditions, Colonel Shelton, as typical of other Army OMSs, operated on 230 OMS patients and performed a number of procedures usually classified as general orthopedic or neurosurgical, administered general anesthesia when the need arose, and, for half of his tour, was the Chief of Professional Services. One of the most unusual OMS experiences in the Vietnam War was described by Shelton as follows:

The last Army OMS (in Vietnam) was Major Alfred E. Tortorelli. His experience was rather unique. Arriving in-country on August 12, 1972, the same day as the last U.S. combat troops left Vietnam, he was assigned to the U.S. Army Hospital Saigon (formerly the 3rd Field Hospital). He operated on maxillofacial battle casualties when required; almost exclusively Vietnamese soldiers and Cambodian and Montagnard mercenaries . . . at the USAH Saigon until it was turned over to the Seventh Day Adventists Organization in mid-March, 1973. On March 22, 1973, Major Tortorelli received orders assigning him to the Four Party Joint Military Commission, whose task it was to implement the terms of the Paris Peace Accords. . . . The Commission was disbanded on March 30, 1973. The following day, at 1700 hours, the last charter flight to de-

part Vietnam lifted off the runway of Saigon's Ton Son Nhut Airbase bound for Travis AFB, California. Aboard that aircraft was the last U.S. military OMS, as well as the last dental officer to leave Vietnam, and that was Major Tortorelli.

Helicopter evacuation brought injured U.S. Marines and Army troops to oral and maxillofacial surgeons just over the horizons in the hospital ships, the *U.S.S. Repose* and the *U.S.S. Sanctuary*, floating marvels of the best Western medical technology, for definitive care. As documented and reported by Commander Bill C. Terry, in a series of 110 patients, 41% were able to return to duty in the combat zone as a result of the professional and physical capabilities represented by the hospital ships.[22]

The U.S. Air Force had oral and maxillofacial surgeons on islands and land-masses adjacent to the battle zone, and hence the casualties were seen within hours following injury. Colonels Howard Morgan and Lucien Szymd reported on 1000 patients in 33 months who went through their installation in the Phillipine Islands.[23] They were able to perform advanced procedures, including bone grafts, and thus to reduce the overall hospitalization time.

This complex of military oral and maxillofacial surgeons serving on the embattled land and hospital ships and in nearby lands allowed definitive care to be given at several points in the chain of evacuation of casualties. If the medical facilities in the battle zone were full, as happened during the Tet offensive, the intermediate and definitive care were often provided halfway around the world following jet aircraft evacuation (Fig. 1–7). In fact, those of us serving in the continental U.S. military hospitals could tell by observing the techniques used in the surgical care whether an oral and maxillofacial surgeon had initially treated the patient prior to evacuation; often it was possible to tell which oral and maxillofacial surgeon had treated the patient by the special way that he handled surgical details.

Among the valued spin-offs of the Vietnam War is the research of Captain Philip Boyne of the U.S. Navy.[24] He performed biomedical research with cancellous bone grafting techniques that was the basis for repair of ac-

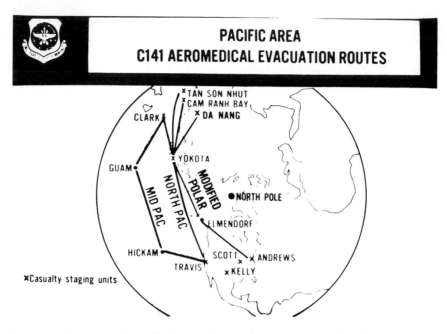

FIG. 1–7.   Air evacuation routes from Southeast Asia to the continental U.S. (Courtesy of the U.S. Armed Forces Institute of Pathology.)

quired skeletal defects, prosthodontic applications, and management of congenital facial clefts. Dr. M.D. Curley and his U.S. Navy colleagues reported on the thought-provoking long-term psychological effects felt by patients with maxillofacial casualties; they noted that the patient usually had clear recall of comments made by those attending him at the time of injury and during the immediate phases of treatment; hence, off-hand remarks by medical personnel desensitized by a flow of casualties would dash the morale of an injured trooper. From these sophisticated laboratory and psychological studies to Major James E. Salem's practical report on airway management of Army casualties,[26] the Vietnam warfare performance by the military oral and maxillofacial surgeons, who are represented in the excellent textbook on war injuries edited by Captain James Kelly of the U.S. Navy,[27] deserves the approbation of all dentists who are surgeons, those dentists who preceded them, and those who will follow them in emergency rooms in civilian and military settings.

The 60 U.S. Army OMS served for approximately 12 months in Vietnam in field hospitals, evacuation hospitals, and specially designated hospitals such as the Cong Hoad

Military Hospital in Saigon. These hospitals were spread across the peninsula; for example, the 24th and the 93rd Evacuation Hospitals were at Long Binh, the 71st Evac was at Pleiku; the 37th Evac was at Vung Tau; and the 95th Evac Hosp was at Da Nang. The 20 or so U.S. Navy OMS served either on the hospital ships *Repose* or *Sanctuary* for approximately 2 years or in the naval hospital at Da Nang for 1 year. The U.S. Air Force OMS served in the Phillipine Islands at Clark Air Force Base for 3-year tours of duty.

Military oral and maxillofacial surgeons learned, relearned, refined, and reported in the wars of the twentieth century the lessons learned earlier for management of facial injuries.[28,29,30] They shared information on the details of care based on the principles of restoring the integrity of the oral cavity with the early use of intraoral splints and then caring for the overlying soft tissues. They recognized the need for very conservative debridement of facial tissues, the need for generous irrigations, and the benefit of intermaxillary fixation. In the Korean and Vietnam Wars, early evacuation to specialty surgeons became a touchstone of the best way to decrease morbidity and death rates, to conserve tissues, and to decrease the length of hospitalizations.

In this effort Captain Donald Cooksey observed that oral and maxillofacial surgery, ". . . a tiresome sideline of medicine in past centuries, became a thriving and driving force for dentistry."[31]

REFERENCES

1. Tebo, H.G.: Oral surgery in the Confederate Army. Bull Hist Dent 24:28–35, 1976.
2. Schwartz, L.L.: The development of the treatment of jaw fractures. Oral Surg 2:193–221, 1944.
3. Cryer, M.H.: Contributions of dentistry in surgery. Dent Cosmos 39:102, 1897.
4. Otis, G.A. and Barnes, J.K.: The Medical and Surgical History of the War of the Rebellion (1861–65). The Government Printing Office, Washington, D.C., 1875.
5. Oliver, R.T.: A method of treating mandibular fractures. JAMA 54:1187–1191, 1910.
6. Converse, J.M.: The extraordinary career of Doctor Varaztad Hovhannes Kazanjian. Plast Reconstr Surg 71:138–142, 1983.
7. Eby, J.D.: Principles of orthodontia in the treatment of maxillofacial injuries. Int J Orthod and Oral Surg 6:273–310, 1920.
8. Eby, J.D.: Intermaxillary wiring. J Natl Dent Assoc 8:771–782, 1921.
9. Ivy, R.H. and Curtis, L.: Fractures of the Jaws. Philadelphia, Lea & Febiger, 1938, p.60.
10. McGee, R.P.: Maxillofacial surgeon in mobile hospital. JAMA 73:1114–1118, 1919.
11. Jeffcott, G.F.: United States Army Dental Service in World War II. Washington, D.C., Dept. of the Army, Office of the Surgeon General, 1955.
12. Kurtz, M.D.: Columbia University and those who made it the mecca of dental education. Bull Hist Dent 26:86–102, 1978.
13. Irby, W.B.: Facial injuries in military combat: intermediate care. J Oral Surg 27:548–550, 1969.
14. Taylor, R.W.: History of Naval Dentistry. J Am Coll Dent 26:195–208, 1958.
15. Cook, T.J.: The role of the oral surgeon in a general hospital in war. J Oral Surg 9:3–17, 1951.
16. Kwapis, B.W.: Early management of maxillofacial war injuries. J Oral Surg 12:293–309, 1954.
17. Chipps, J.E., et al.: Intermediate treatment of maxillofacial injuries. U.S. Armed Forces Med J 4:951–976, 1953.
18. Osbon, D.B.: Early treatment of soft tissue injuries of the face. J Oral Surg 27:480–487, 1969.
19. Andrews, J.L.: Maxillofacial trauma in Viet Nam. J Oral Surg 26:457–462, 1968.
20. Tinder, L.E., Osbon, D.B., Lilly, G.E., and Cutcher, J.L.: Maxillofacial injuries sustained in the Viet Nam Conflict. Milit Med 134:668–672, 1969.
21. McFarland, P.H. (ed.): A Guide for Dental Officers in Early Management of Maxillofacial War Injuries. Washington, D.C., Dept. of Army, Surg. General's Office, 1972.
22. Terry, B.C.: Facial injuries in military combat: definitive care. J Oral Surg 27:551–556, 1967.
23. Morgan, H.M., and Szmyd, L.: Maxillofacial war injuries. J Oral Surg 26:727–730, 1968.
24. Boyne, P.J.: Restoration of osseous defects in maxillofacial casualties. J Am Dent Assoc 78:767, 776, 1969.
25. Curley, M.D., Walsh, J.M., and Triplett, R.G.: Wartime management of oral and maxillofacial wounds: the casualty's point of view. Milit Med 148:723–726, 1983.
26. Salem, J.E.: Intubation of conscious patients with combat wounds of upper respiratory passageway in Viet Nam. Oral Surg 24:701–702, 1967.
27. Kelly, J.F. (ed.): Management of War Injuries to the Jaws and Related Structures. Washington, D.C., Government Printing Office, 1977.
28. Prosser, A.M.: A dental officer with 40 Commando. J R Nav Med Serv 69:40–41, 1983.
29. Shukers, S.: Immediate management of severe facial war-injuries. J Maxillofac Surg 11:30–36, 1983.
30. Awty, M.D., and Banks, P.: Treatment of maxillofacial casualties in the Nigerian civil war. Oral Surg 31:4–18, 1971.
31. Cooksey, D.E.: History of oral surgery in the United States Navy. J Oral Surg 20:365–374, 1962.

This chapter was written for this textbook and for the American Association of Oral and Maxillofacial Surgery (AAOMS). The AAOMS document embraces all of the Federal Services oral and maxillofacial surgery, in addition to the Armed Forces. Special appreciation is extended to the following who shared personal experiences, proofread sections when requested, and always gave encouragement to this project.

Major General Robert B. Shira, D.C., U.S.A., Retired
Colonel James E. Chipps, D.C., U.S.A., Retired
Colonel David W. Shelton, D.C., U.S.A., Retired
Captain Donald Cooksey, D.C., U.S.N., Retired
Dr. Carl E. Schow, Jr.

2

GENERAL MANAGEMENT OF ACUTELY INJURED PATIENTS

T. WILLIAM EVANS

Trauma is the principal cause of death in individuals in the first four decades of life in the U.S. More than 100,000 fatal accidents occur each year, most of the deaths occurring during the first 3 hours after the accident. Many of these fatalities can be prevented by more effective management of the trauma patient either during the first hour at the scene of the accident (prehospital phase) or later in the emergency room (emergency phase).

Two different sets of professional personnel are responsible for the treatment of the traumatized patient during these two critical periods. The initial management of the trauma patient at the scene of the accident is usually provided by trained paramedic personnel. The secondary emergency management is provided in the emergency room by trained medical personnel. It is incumbent upon maxillofacial surgeons, as important members of the trauma team, to become familiar with both areas of management.

The maxillofacial surgeon, being an expert in assessing, establishing, and maintaining an airway in a patient, particularly the trauma patient with facial injuries, should be intimately involved with the initial and continuing education of paramedic personnel be-

cause an obstructed airway from facial injuries is often the cause of death during the first important hour after the traumatic incident, before the patient is brought to the emergency room. Only well-trained paramedics can control facial, intraoral, intranasal, or pharyngeal hemorrhage, which can often lead to airway obstruction and death immediately after the accident.

If the initial management of the trauma patient with facial injuries has been successful, the patient should arrive for secondary management at the emergency room in a relatively stabilized condition. Usually, the acutely injured patient with facial injuries is examined briefly by the emergency physician, who may determine that the patient's only problems are facial injuries. The maxillofacial surgeon is then given full responsibility for the patient. It is vitally important, however, that the *entire* patient be completely evaluated and reevaluated and the appropriate treatment initiated. Often the emergency personnel react to only the dramatic facial injury, and more occult or life-threatening injuries go unnoticed.

The maxillofacial surgeon must be expert in assessing all systems in the acutely injured patient. An abnormality that has been discovered by examination and re-examination usually is managed by the appropriate medical specialist following consultation by the maxillofacial surgeon. Evaluation and management of the acutely injured patient continues after the patient is admitted to the hospital, during the intraoperative period, and postoperatively until discharge.

INITIAL MANAGEMENT (PREHOSPITAL PHASE)

The primary responsibilities of the trained paramedic personnel are to establish and maintain an airway, resuscitate if required, control excessive hemorrhage, and safely transport the patient. Secondary responsibilities are intravenous therapy, application of a pneumatic antishock garment, if required, and temporary stabilization of fractures.

Many accident victims with facial trauma are dead on arrival (DOA) at the hospital emergency room because a patent airway was not immediately established. This failure usually occurs either because the personnel were not trained in establishing a patent airway in a person with facial trauma or because they were not trained to control intraoral or pharyngeal hemorrhage, which will obstruct the airway.

AIRWAY

Establishing and maintaining a patent airway is the primary concern in the initial management of an acutely injured patient, especially one with facial trauma. If the patient has an adequate airway and is in no danger of losing it, no further airway management should be performed until the cervical spine is evaluated. If the patient does not have a patent airway, the least-manipulative procedure to establish the airway should be executed. In the patient with severe facial trauma, a cervical fracture should be assumed until ruled out, since excessive movement of a fractured cervical spine can cause a fracture-dislocation with neurologic injury. In the majority of cases, an adequate airway can be established without excessive manipulation.

Often the simplest procedures obtain the best results. Obstructive airway problems can be solved by a simple examination of the mouth and oropharynx with an index finger. Many times, removal of foreign bodies, e.g., dentures (Fig. 2–1), teeth, or blood clots, is the only treatment required. Tongue obstruction of the oropharynx from either lack of anterior support of the tongue from a comminuted fracture of the mandible or from a swollen tongue may cause airway obstruction. Immediate control of the tongue is accomplished by anterior traction on the tongue by placing a towel clip, wire, heavy suture, or even a safety pin through the anterior portion of the tongue and pulling and fixing the tongue forward. This fixation can be done without undue manipulation of the cervical spine.

Introduction of an oral or nasopharyngeal airway is often sufficient to maintain an airway in a patient who is breathing spontaneously. If oral or nasoendotracheal intubation is required, manipulation with a laryngoscope should be kept to a minimum; a nasoendotracheal tube blind insertion can be performed with minimal manipulation. If this procedure is unsuccessful, an oral endotracheal tube can sometimes be introduced by inserting an index finger through the mouth into the vallecula epiglottica or posterior to the epiglottis and inserting the tube along the index finger into the glottis (Fig. 2–2). This technique can be used also when a laryngoscope or endotracheal tube is not available; stethoscope tubing can be substituted for an endotracheal tube. If none of the above methods is successful immediately and the patient does not have an airway, oral endotracheal intubation with a laryngoscope or transtracheal ventilation is mandatory.

Transtracheal ventilation by cricothyroidotomy or tracheostomy is indicated when the above procedures have been unsuccessful or when the glottis is completely obstructed. Tracheostomy should be performed in a controlled situation as an elective procedure.

Cricothyroidotomy (also known as coniotomy) through the cricothyroid membrane is an effective, safe emergency procedure to establish transtracheal ventilation. It can be performed with one of the commercial cri-

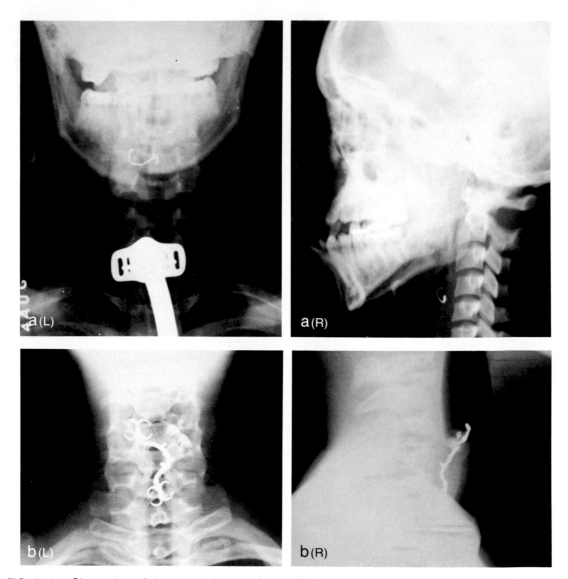

FIG. 2–1.   Obstruction of the upper airway. **a L** and **R**, Fragment of an acrylic denture, identified by the radiopaque wire, displaced into the laryngeal portion of the pharynx following facial trauma; note that the anterior mandible was fractured and that a tracheostomy has been performed. (The patient was managed at Ft. Campbell, Ky, by Dr. Donald B. Osbon.) **b L** and **R**, Partial denture caused great airway distress as it passed the aperture of the larynx. It was retrieved with an anesthetic tube forceps from its lodgement in the superior esophagus under direct vision using a laryngoscope. (The patient was managed at Ft. Knox, Ky.)

cothyroidotomy instruments or with a scalpel or any knife. A 1- to 2-cm-wide horizontal incision extending deep through the membrane between the thyroid cartilage and the cricoid cartilage is made with one stroke. If the knife is inserted too deeply, it will strike the broad lamina of the cricoid cartilage without harm. Any hollow tube to maintain the orifice is inserted into the trachea. A small

endotracheal tube is advantageous because of its flexibility and the ease with which a self-inflating resuscitation bag (ambu bag) can be connected if necessary. A tracheostomy tube can be utilized. In the absence of an endotracheal or tracheostomy tube, the hollow barrel of a disassembled ball-point pen or stethoscope tubing is sufficient.

Insufflation is a safe, effective means to

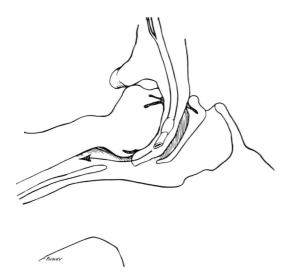

FIG. 2–2. Inserting an oral endotracheal tube. A finger may be used for retraction and stabilization of the tongue and mandible and as a guide for the passage of an oral endotracheal tube.

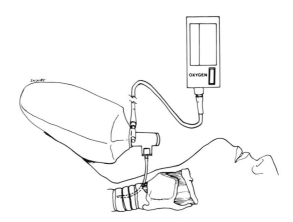

FIG. 2–3. Insufflation for basal oxygen requirements. A vascular catheter can be placed through the cricothyroid membrane and, after being connected to a positive flow of oxygen, can provide the route for basal oxygen requirements for 30 to 45 min.

meet the basal oxygen requirements of 150 ml/m²/ min for a short period of time (30 to 45 min) until an elective tracheostomy can be performed. A vascular intracatheter needle (intracath) with a 14-gauge catheter is inserted into the trachea through the cricothyroid membrane. The needle is removed, leaving the catheter in place. A no. 7 anesthesia connector can be placed in the catheter connector for attachment to an ambu bag and oxygen (Fig. 2–3). A Y connector may be utilized or another catheter may be placed for expiration. Ventilation at a rate of 30 to 40 times/min is required.

After a patent airway has been established, by whatever means, 100% oxygen should be administered.

HEMORRHAGE

Exsanguinating hemorrhage should be identified and controlled immediately after the airway is established. Direct pressure is the best method for controlling rapid blood loss. Neither hemostats nor tourniquets should be used by paramedic personnel. Pneumatic splints are helpful on the extremities.

Unrecognized intraoral, nasal, or pharyngeal hemorrhage secondary to facial trauma

can often cause fatal airway obstruction. The first step, which is to recognize the problem, can be accomplished only by inspecting the mouth. Immediate control of this excessive hemorrhage may be the lifesaving treatment in an accident victim who has no problems other than facial trauma.

Direct pressure is the best way to control this type of hemorrhage. If this measure is unsuccessful, constant intraoral suction should be maintained until the patient arrives at the hospital emergency room. Supporting the facial fractures against an intact cranium by establishing a satisfactory occlusion and placing an extraoral pressure dressing will sometimes control intraoral, intranasal, or pharyngeal hemorrhage.

Anterior nasal hemorrhage is managed by packing the anterior nose; concurrent use of a topical vasoconstrictor is optional (see Chapter 11). Posterior nasal hemorrhage is tamponaded by applying pressure with a posterior nasal pack (Fig. 2–4), either the typical gauze posterior nasal packs or one or two small Foley catheters and inflating the balloons with air. The latter method is much easier for paramedic personnel to perform.

In the facial trauma patient, an excessive amount of hemorrhage that can compromise the airway can occur from the palatal area. Palatal hemorrhage can be controlled by placing a gauze palatal pack. Pressure may be

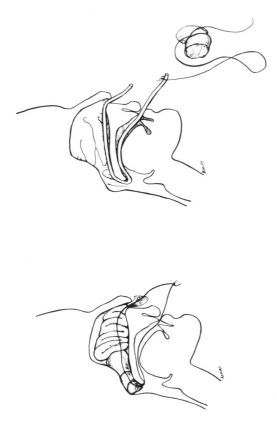

FIG. 2–4. Anterior and posterior nasal packing. Nasal packs, either with gauzes or with air-inflated Foley catheters for posterior pressure and support, are placed to tamponade hemorrhages originating in the intranasal area.

maintained against the palatal pack by suspending the pack with a wire or wires brought out through both cheeks and tied over the top of the head. Most intraoral hemorrhages may be controlled by placing 4 x 4–inch gauze packs (see Chapter 4).

TRANSPORTATION

The primary responsibilities of paramedic personnel are to initially stabilize the trauma patient and safely transport the patient to a hospital emergency room for definitive treatment. In the past, severe trauma patients, particularly those with facial injuries, were brought DOA to emergency rooms because paramedic personnel did not have the knowledge or ability to establish and maintain an airway or control excessive hemorrhage, especially in the head and neck area. Today,

paramedics are well-trained to stabilize and transport the multiple trauma patient.

Although establishing and maintaining an airway, controlling excessive hemorrhage, and resuscitating the patient if necessary are the most important procedures performed by paramedic personnel during the immediate prehospital phase of treatment, most paramedics are capable of performing other important tasks. These tasks can be accomplished during the transportation phase.

An intravenous (IV) line can be established and a balanced salt solution administered. Rate of administration should be as rapid as possible unless the time for transportation is to be long. If signs of shock are present, two IV lines should be established and fluid given rapidly.

Most paramedic teams today are capable of applying Medical Anti-Shock Trousers (MAST) if required. The clearest indication for the use of a MAST suit is hypotension resulting from major bleeding, especially from abdominal or lower extremity trauma. The pneumatic trousers can be inflated to tamponade bleeding and to replete the central circulation. The use of a MAST suit is indicated in all cases of severe hypotension, even in the presence of head and thoracic trauma. Restoration of adequate perfusion pressure is the most important element in severe hypotension. In a patient with significant head trauma and hypotension, initial efforts must be directed toward restoring adequate cerebral perfusion, not toward reducing intracranial (ICP) pressure. Because decreased cerebral blood flow may increase cerebral edema, restoring adequate perfusion is even more significant. While the MAST suit may increase blood volume in a thorax containing a bleeding vessel and therefore may slightly increase the total blood loss, its use is still beneficial to increase the perfusion of the brain until definitive resuscitation takes place. The MAST suit should not be removed until the patient is safely under the direct care of medical personnel who are knowledgeable in the deflation procedure and who have the shock under control. In many instances, the MAST suit should be left in place until the patient is in the operating room.

A brief neurologic evaluation to establish

the patient's level of consciousness is valuable if the other important tasks have been accomplished. A good method is to describe the level of consciousness by the AVPU method:

A—*A*lert
V—Responds to *V*ocal stimuli
P—Responds to *P*ainful stimuli
U—*U*nresponsive

The patient's pupillary size and responsiveness is also helpful in establishing neurologic baseline information, which is valuable to the clinician who will evaluate the patient's neurologic status in the emergency room.

EMERGENCY MANAGEMENT (EMERGENCY ROOM PHASE)

The hospital emergency room managment of the acute trauma patient is conducted by the emergency physician and the trauma team. The maxillofacial surgeon is an important member of the trauma team and should be well versed in the total management of the acutely injured patient. This management is performed in a logical sequential manner.

INITIAL EVALUATION

The initial evaluation of the acutely injured patient is similar to that assessment performed by the paramedics at the scene of the accident; the priorities are *airway, breathing,* and *circulation.* This is a brief evaluation of the patient's immediate vital status. All clothing should be completely removed from the patient.

The airway should be checked for patency and volume. Breathing should be evaluated. Is the breathing spontaneous? Is the tidal volume adequate? Will breathing assistance be required? Are the breath sounds adequate bilaterally? Circulation is evaluated in this initial assessment by estimating cardiac output by palpating the pulse. The patient's pulse should be assessed for quality, rate, regularity, and site. The strength of the pulse, the estimated filling effectiveness of the artery being palpated, provides an indirect measurement of the systolic pressure. Generally,

if a radial pulse is palpable, the systolic pressure will be above 80 mm Hg. If the femoral pulse is palpable, the systolic pressure will be above 70 mm Hg. If the carotid pulse is palpable, the systolic pressure can be assumed to be above 60 mm Hg.

If the airway and breathing are adequate, the next step is to insert bilateral large-bore (10- to 14-gauge) IV catheters if not previously done. One of the IV catheters should be placed centrally through the subclavian or jugular vein. Venous blood should be collected for type and crossmatching and basic chemistries (hemoglobin, hematocrit, electrolytes, and blood urea nitrogen [BUN]). Arterial blood should be obtained for baseline arterial blood gases. The placement of a Foley catheter and a nasogastric tube can now be considered if not contraindicated by urethral transection or severe midfacial trauma.

SHOCK

Management of the acutely injured patient requires a working knowledge of the clinical entity known as shock. Although there are several types of shock, the maxillofacial surgeon will usually be confronted with only traumatic or hypovolemic shock. Hypovolemic shock is a syndrome caused by a derangement of cellular metabolism due to a lack of tissue perfusion (microcirculation) caused by a relative decrease in blood volume.

Obvious shock in the acutely injured patient presenting to the emergency room will be managed immediately by the emergency physician and the trauma team. Often, however, the patient presents with adequate vital signs but is actually in unrecognized compensated or impending shock. This state must be recognized and treated promptly.

There may be several inapparent reasons for a traumatic loss of blood volume. A large amount of blood loss at the scene of the accident may not be recognized or reported by paramedic personnel. Bleeding in the retroperitoneal spaces may not be immediately apparent. Also, a fractured femur may hide up to 1500 ml of blood unless the thighs are measured and compared. A fractured pelvis can result in a local internal loss of more than 2000 ml of blood. Loss of blood volume for any apparent or inapparent reason will cause different degrees of impending shock. The degree is usually related to both volume of blood loss and rate of blood loss.

Clinical Picture

The well-informed clinician should immediately recognize the subtle clinical symptoms and signs of impending shock. These are listed in the order in which they might appear in impending shock.

Sensorium. Early symptoms and signs of impending shock are agitation, restlessness, and anxiousness. According to many clinicians, one of the first symptoms of impending shock is thirst. Cellular dehydration causes dryness of the oral and pharyngeal mucous membrane. Adrenergic stimulation is the major reason for the altered sensorium. As shock progresses, the sensorium becomes depressed because of decreased cerebral perfusion. This sensorial depression from shock is often mistaken for an intracranial injury.

Skin and Mucous Membrane. Skin and mucous membrane will be cool and pale. They may or may not be clammy and moist. These signs are secondary to decreased peripheral blood flow from shunting, secondary to the adrenergic response.

Capillary Refill. Pressure on a fingernail or hypothenar eminence results in prolonged blanching. Normal capillary refill time is usually about 2 sec, or the time it takes to say "capillary refill." Slow capillary refill is secondary to low peripheral blood flow.

Pulse. Typically the pulse is weak and rapid, although this sign may be the most variable in early impending shock. As the shock state progresses, the pulse is weak and rapid because of increased sympathetic activity, lowered stroke volume, and decreased pulse pressure.

Veins. Peripheral veins are collapsed if the patient's cardiac status is normal. This state is secondary to low peripheral venous pressure.

Respiration. Respiration in early shock tends to be rapid because of anxiety and stimulation of the respiratory center by catecholamines.

Pulse Pressure. Pulse pressure is a very reliable indicator of impending shock. The lowered stroke volume lowers the systolic pressure while the adrenergic response elevates the diastolic pressure, giving a predictable decreased pulse pressure.

Blood Pressure. The blood pressure is usually not a reliable measure of early impending shock. Many variables are involved, such as the amount of blood volume, preload, afterload, stroke volume, and adrenergic response. The blood pressure in a patient with impending shock may be normal or high. Because of decreased pulse pressure, the blood pressure may be unobtainable by conventional means but can be found to be adequate when measured directly an an intra-arterial line.

Urine Output. Urine output is a very reliable measurement of shock. The adrenergic response is selective initially and affects those organs such as the skin, kidneys, and liver that are most resistant to hypoxia in order to divert blood flow to the more vital organs such as the brain and heart. Urine output is directly proportional to renal cellular perfusion. The relative oligemia suffered by the kidneys in response to shock is usually immediate. If the kidneys are excreting less than 30 ml of urine/hr, it can be assumed that perfusion is inadequate.

Central Venous Pressure (CVP). Although pulmonary wedge pressure obtained with a balloon catheter may give more information about the preload on the left side of the heart, in the majority of cases of acute trauma this same information can be obtained indirectly from a CVP line in the superior vena cava. In the typical trauma patient without pre-existing cardiac disease, a CVP of less than 10 cm of water indicates impending or frank shock. However, a normal CVP of 10 to 15 cm does not rule out shock. The CVP is an accurate sign but must be interpreted correctly. Obtaining a baseline CVP is important for monitoring therapy.

Hematocrit. A low hematocrit can be indicative of hemodilution from extravascular extracellular fluid moving intravascularly in an attempt to replace the lost intravascular fluid. Although this condition is indicative of shock, however, it usually is not apparent for at least 3 hrs post-trauma; during the first 3 hrs after a traumatic incident and acute blood loss, the hematocrit may be deceptively normal.

When the patient's signs and symptoms indicate shock or impending shock, treatment should be initiated immediately. The more aware the clinician is to the early subtle signs and symptoms of impending shock, the earlier the treatment will be started and the better the chance will be of reversing the problem.

Pathophysiology

A thorough knowledge of the pathophysiology of shock is imperative. Not only does this knowledge aid in the treatment of traumatic shock, but it is useful in understanding the management of the patient preoperatively, intraoperatively, and postoperatively. The same principles of pathophysiology are involved whether the patient suffers from traumatic hemorrhage or surgical hemorrhage.

The pathophysiology of traumatic or hypovolemic shock is dynamic; many events occur at the same time. The initial event is the acute loss of blood volume. Several responses of the body to this loss of blood, if not interrupted by treatment, ultimately lead to the final state of shock. Continuing events lead to irreversible shock and, ultimately, death. The underlying pathophysiologic problem in shock is inadequate tissue oxygenation.

The first response to acute hemorrhage is baroreceptor and other activity that ultimately stimulates an adrenergic response. This compensating mechanism is designed to maintain an adequate blood flow to the brain and heart. Because of this divergence of blood flow, the heart may receive 25% of the cardiac output instead of the normal 5% and the brain may receive 75% of the cardiac output instead of the normal 20%. This selective vasoconstriction will also reduce total vascular capacity by as much as 20%, which accounts for the body's ability to tolerate a blood loss of up to 20% of the blood volume with minimal effects. This adrenergic response is also responsible for many of the previously described signs and symptoms present in impending shock.

If treatment is not initiated during the early compensatory adrenergic phase of shock, certain cardiovascular events lead to a decreased cardiac output. The decreased blood volume decreases the end-diastolic volume or preload of the heart. The tachycardia decreases diastole, which also decreases the end-diastolic volume and decreases coronary artery filling, which occurs during diastole. The decreased blood pressure causes similar cardiac events. All of these abnormal cardiovascular events occur concurrently and a vicious cycle is established that ultimately lowers the cardiac output.

Aggregation and stagnation of the blood causes an increased blood viscosity. A combination of this increased blood viscosity, the increased peripheral resistance, the lowered cardiac output, and shunting leads to decreased peripheral flow. Other compensatory mechanisms occur continuously, such as movement of the extracellular fluid into the intravascular and intracellular spaces but over hours of time. The balance of all of these events in this cycle, in the absence of treatment, progresses to decreased peripheral flow or decreased tissue perfusion. The microcirculation involved is approximately 90% of the total body vasculature, about 60,000 miles of blood vessels.

The foregoing events lead to tissue hypoxia in the organs not adequately perfused. This hypoxia causes several metabolic derangements at the cellular level. Because the cell is unable to metabolize glucose aerobically through the citric acid cycle (Krebs cycle), anaerobic metabolism must be used by the cell through the Embden-Meyerhof pathway and pyruvate is metabolized to lactic acid, causing a metabolic acidosis. The membrane potential of the cell is disturbed through interference with the sodium pump, probably by an endorphin secreted by the hypothalamus. Sodium chloride and extracellular water enter the cell and potassium leaves the cell. This increased extracellular potassium cannot be measured in the usual way because it is bound to collagen in the interstitial fluid. Regulation of calcium is compromised. The adenosine triphosphatase (ATP) system is altered and, ultimately, cellular organelles are destroyed, releasing enzymes that cause cellular destruction.

This metabolic chain of events leads to a complete loss of vascular tone, which causes pooling and stagnation of blood, lowering the blood volume further; the vicious cycle continues until the shock is refractory to treatment. Usually, the metabolic derangements and complete renal failure lead to the patient's death.

Treatment

It is obvious from a knowledge of the pathophysiology of traumatic shock that morbidity is decreased the sooner treatment is started, and hence early recognition and management during the reversible stages of hypovolemic shock is mandatory. Treatment must be aimed at maintaining flow and tissue perfusion, not at elevating blood pressure. The clinician must turn a "swamp" into a "running brook."

A relatively intact circulatory system is required to maintain life. Whereas one can survive with 20% of the liver, 25% of the kidney mass, 50% of the lung capacity, and 30% of the red blood cell mass, one must have at least 75% of the circulating volume to survive. An adult's whole-blood volume is approximately 7% of the ideal body weight, approximately 5 L in a 70-kg adult, or 70 ml/kg of body weight. In a child the blood volume is 9% of the ideal body weight, or 90 ml/kg of body weight. Compensatory mechanisms will initially protect a 70-kg adult after a 750-ml blood loss. A hemorrhage of up to 750 ml should be closely monitored, however, and a blood loss of more than 750 ml should be aggressively treated.

The ultimate goals for treatment are to improve flow, prevent renal failure, and shift the oxygen dissociation curve to the right. Assuming that the cause of the acute blood loss has been or is being corrected, recognition of impending shock should precipitate immediate therapeutic measures.

Oxygen. Oxygen 100% should be administered via the airway obtained previously. If there is any doubt about the respiratory exchange before the results of the arterial blood gases are obtained, ventilatory support should be provided. Avoid hyperventilation, which induces respiratory alkalosis; which in turn will shift the oxygen dissociation curve to the left.

Shock Position. The legs should be elevated 30° and the head elevated 20° immediately (Fig. 2–5). Trendelenburg's position should be avoided because a lowered head interferes with diaphragmatic excursion. If a spine injury is suspected, however, the Trendelenburg position is used to keep the spine straight and immobilized.

Intravenous Catheters. In shock, the peripheral veins are collapsed and large-bore IV lines should be placed in ports such as the subclavian or jugular vein. The subclavian vein is an ideal vein to be cannulated during shock because a fascial sling prevents the vein from collapsing during hypotension. The tip of one catheter should be in the superior vena cava for CVP measurement. CVP is a valuable tool for monitoring fluid administration and has been found to be equal in value to the pulmonary wedge pressure in a previously healthy acutely injured patient.

Urinary Catheter. Measurement of urinary output is one of the easiest and most accurate measurements of tissue perfusion. Collection of urine is important also for obtaining a urine urea nitrogen (UUN) for another accurate indicator of renal failure, the BUN:UUN ratio.

Laboratory Tests. Venous blood should have been obtained for type and crossmatch, hemoglobin/hematocrit, electrolytes, glucose, and BUN. Blood can be drawn when one of the venous lines is placed. The arterial blood for baseline blood gases should be drawn from the radial or femoral artery with a polytef catheter, and this catheter should be left in place to monitor arterial pressure. Urine should be collected for a routine urinalysis and a baseline urine urea nitrogen level.

Fluid Replacement. The essential element for treatment of impending or frank shock is adequate volume replacement. Because cold fluids will lower the body temperature and shift the oxygen dissociation curve to the left, solutions should be relatively warm. Blood taken directly from a refrigerator should be warmed before administration, if possible.

A blood loss of 10% (500 ml) in the average 70-kg adult will elicit no clinical signs or symptoms. Replacement of this loss with twice the amount (1000 ml) of the estimated

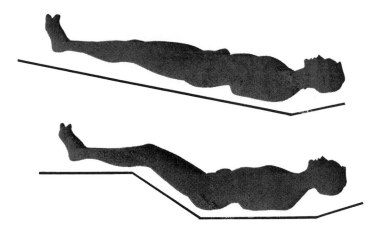

FIG. 2–5.   Shock position. **a,** The dependent head position, as with Trendelenburg's position, should be avoided unless a spinal injury is suspected. **b,** The shock position of about a 30° elevation of the upper legs and 20° elevation of the head will assist in diaphragmatic excursions and will decrease intracranial pressures.

blood lost and with a balanced salt solution such as lactated Ringer's solution is adequate.

A blood loss of 20% (1000 ml) will elicit the early clinical signs and symptoms of impending shock. If the blood loss is greater than 20%, frank shock is present. An estimated blood loss of 15% or greater should be aggressively treated with fluid replacement. The actual fluid loss is really greater than the measured loss because of translocation of extracellular fluid.

The fluid of choice for initial volume replacement is lactated Ringer's solution. This is a balanced isotonic salt solution that is very close to the composition of extracellular fluid and, after passing once through the liver, where the lactate is converted to bicarbonate, is almost exactly like extracellular fluid. It is a safe solution that can be given in large quantities and in the absence of pulmonary injury or sepsis will not cause pulmonary edema.

The lactated Ringer's solution will provide a transient fluid volume for the intravascular space and will replace the functional extracellular fluid. As volume replacement, it improves peripheral flow by increasing cardiac ability to pump blood and by diluting viscous blood in the microcirculation. It helps correct the metabolic acidosis by producing bicarbonate from lactate. The 44 mEq of lactate in 1 L of lactated Ringer's solution is converted to 28 mmol of bicarbonate after one passage through the liver. This function of the liver is

apparently one of the last liver functions to deteriorate, occasionally functioning even for a short period after somatic death.

In the presence of impending or frank shock, the amount of fluid to be replaced is critical. Usually, this amount is difficult to estimate because it depends on an accurate estimate of blood loss, which is difficult to assess and because there are many rules based on the estimated blood loss. One rule is to replace twice the volume lost; another, to replace the volume in milliliters that is equal to the patient's weight in kilograms multiplied by the percentage of the estimated loss.

An excellent method of volume replacement for both the healthy heart and the unhealthy heart is the fluid challenge–CVP response method, which measures the ability of the heart to accept a fluid challenge. If the patient is exhibiting signs and symptoms of impending or frank shock, at least 2000 cc of balanced salt solution should have been given since the traumatic incident. Subsequently, a challenge of 200 cc of solution should be administered over a 5-min period. The response of the CVP is monitored. If the CVP does not increase over 2 cm, another 200 cc is infused immediately. If the CVP does increase over 2 cm, another 200 cc of fluid is rapidly infused after a 5-min delay. If the CVP increases more than 5 cm, the rapid infusion of fluid is stopped and the cardiac status and clinical signs are evaluated. If the CVP increases 5 cm or more and stabilizes and the cardiac status is physiologic, fluid infusion can be slowed. This method is also known as the 5:2 method. After the patient's clinical signs return to normal, another 10% of fluid will be required.

A patient who has lost more than 30% of the blood volume requires immediate aggressive fluid replacement. In these cases, a no. 8 French catheter can be placed intravenously by cutdown and the IV tubing can be replaced with genitourinary (GU) tubing for rapid administration of warm crystalloid solution and fresh whole blood. By this method, it is possible to administer 1500 ml of warm solution or 500 ml of warm fresh whole blood per minute.

An intravascular space volume expander is sometimes helpful. One unit of low–molecular-weight dextran or hetastarch may be given to provide a more permanent expansion of intravascular volume. More than one unit substantially increases the chances of side effects such as an anaphylactoid reaction or a hemorrhagic diathesis. Because intravascular volume expansion interferes with blood typing, blood should be drawn for type and crossmatching before the low-molecular weight dextran or hetastarch is administered.

Dracula's slogan "A little blood is good . . . a lot of blood is better" is not necessarily the best way to treat impending or early shock!

In most acutely injured young adults who have lost less than 20% of their blood volume, lactated Ringer's solution may be the only solution required in treatment. If more oxygen-carrying capacity is required, packed red blood cells may also be administered.

Warm, type-specific, crossmatched, fresh whole blood is the ideal replacement fluid for a patient in frank shock. Administration of any other type of whole blood is often accompanied by sometimes severe complications. It is rare for a patient not to be stabilized sufficiently with lactated Ringer's to allow time for complete crossmatching. If warm, type-specific, crossmatched, fresh whole blood is not available, warm, type-specific, cross-matched, packed red blood cells, packed platelets, and lactated Ringer's solution are usually sufficient except for patients with severe problems. Uncrossmatched O-negative universal donor blood should be considered only in treating massive exsanguinating injuries.

Whole blood or packed red cell administration can be monitored with the hemoglobin and hematocrit. One unit (500 cc) of whole blood or one unit (250 cc) of packed red cells should increase the hemoglobin by 1 g and the hematocrit by 3% after hemodynamic equilibrium has taken place. An ideal hematocrit should be 35% in a patient who has been in shock. Greater than 35% will decrease peripheral flow because of increased viscosity, and less than 35% will decrease the oxygen-carrying capacity of the blood.

Drugs. If volume replacement has been adequate, drug therapy in early shock is usually not indicated and may be of small benefit in frank shock.

Sodium Bicarbonate. Sodium bicarbonate should *not* be given in shock until the results of the blood gases are reviewed unless large amounts of whole blood have been given. Stored bank blood can cause an acidosis in a patient with poor tissue perfusion if given in large amounts. If acidosis has occurred, one ampule (44.6 mEq) of sodium bicarbonate should be given for every five units of blood.

Although it is assumed that a patient in impending shock or frank shock is in metabolic acidosis, such is not always the case. Rather, respiratory alkalosis is a more common and more severe problem in early shock, and bicarbonate will worsen this condition. A mild acidosis is actually beneficial to the shock patient. Cardiac output is higher during a mild acidosis and the incidence of arrhythmias is less.

Steroids. Steroids decrease the peripheral resistance, increase tissue perfusion, prevent lysozomal enzyme release, and protect the cell membrane. A pharmacologic dose of 1000 mg of methylprednisolone is given intravenously every 6 hrs for four doses.

Antibiotics. Prophylactic antibiotics are indicated in an acutely injured patient with open wounds. A broad spectrum antibiotic such as ampicillin or a cephalosporin is useful. Prophylaxis against gram-negative enteric organisms may be indicated in prolonged shock if intestinal tract barriers are suspected to have been impaired. Cefoxitin is an effective antibiotic against the aerobic coliforms and the anaerobic gastrointestinal tract bacteria including Bacteroides fragilis.

Digitalis. If cardiac function is reduced for any reason, an inotropic drug is indicated. Evidence of congestive heart failure or an abnormally elevated CVP may indicate digitalis therapy. Digoxin 0.5 mg should be given intravenously immmediately. Every 3 hrs, 0.25 mg should be given for four doses. An electrocardiogram (ECG) should be monitored for digitalis effect. Another easily titratable inotropic drug is dolbutamine. The use of inotropic drugs after trauma is a matter of controversy.

Diuretics. Decreased urinary output is usually an indication of inadequate fluid volume. Oliguria with low urine specific gravity and low osmolarity and high urine sodium may indicate the need for a diuretic to help prevent renal failure. An osmotic diuretic such as mannitol (1 gm/kg of 20% solution over 1 hr) or furosemide (40 mg) are the diuretics of choice.

Other Drugs. Many other drugs have been used with mixed results in frank traumatic shock. Isoproterenol, a beta adrenergic drug, has an inotropic effect on the heart and is a peripheral vasodilator: however, it may make the heart work too hard and increase the heart's oxygen consumption. Dolbutamine is a selective cardiac beta agonist. Inotropin, in correct doses, has a beta adrenergic effect on the heart without increasing heart rate, and it increases renal and splanchnic blood flow. Nitroprusside is a smooth-muscle vasodilator and reduces the afterload on the heart and should be used with an inotropic agent. Most of the aforementioned drugs have no place in traumatic shock therapy and may, in fact, cause iatrogenic problems. These drugs are more useful in the treatment of cardiogenic shock.

Several drugs are currently in the experimental stage and may prove to be beneficial in the treatment of traumatic shock. ATP-magnesium chloride has been helpful in experimental low-flow states, with an improvement in cell function mediated by microcirculatory, cell membrane, or energy recycling effects. Naloxone improves survival in experimental shock, possibly by blocking endogenous opiates.

MONITORING

After appropriate therapeutic measures have been taken, the patient must be monitored to evaluate treatment and direct future decisions.

Blood Pressure. Because flow is a function of both pressure and resistance, pressure and flow often are not parallel. While arterial blood pressure is often not an indicator of adequate blood flow, an adequate arterial pressure is necessary for adequate tissue blood flow (tissue perfusion). The ideal mean arterial pressure (diastolic pressure plus 30% of the pulse pressure) should be between 80 and 90 mm Hg. A mean arterial pressure of greater than 90 mm Hg decreases peripheral flow because of increased resistance. A mean arterial pressure of less than 80 mm Hg is inadequate to perfuse the coronary arteries.

Monitoring blood pressure using a sphygmomanometer may be unsatisfactory in a patient in impending or frank shock because the Korotkoff sounds depend on the pulse pressure, which is usually low in these patients. The vibrations produced within the artery may be too low in amplitude to be audible with a stethoscope, and the expansion of the artery may be too small to produce a palpable pulse.

Blood pressure should be monitored by a direct continuous method from an arterial catheter. The initial arterial blood gases are easily drawn from the radial artery using a polytef catheter. This catheter can be left in place and connected to a transducer for direct measurement.

Pulse. Intermittent digital monitoring of the pulse is an accurate empirical method to assess a patient's condition. (The value of checking the pulse in monitoring a patient is directly proportional to the experience of the clinician.)

Central Venous Pressure. In the previously healthy acutely injured patient, the CVP response is an invaluable guide to therapy. It is a reliable approximation of the efficacy of venous return and, indirectly, of the efficiency of the cardiovascular mechanism.

Its use as a guide to fluid replacment has already been described. The relative increase or decrease of the CVP is more important than the actual value. However, in patients who have a normal cardiovascular mechanism and adequate fluid volume, the CVP should remain between 10 and 15 cm of water. Rarely in acute trauma is a balloon flotation (Swan-Ganz) catheter required.

Urine Output. In the previously healthy acutely injured patient, the most reliable measurement to evaluate therapy and tissue perfusion is the urine output. If the urine output is greater than 30 ml/hr without diuretics, the renal blood flow is adequate, which indicates that other organ perfusion is adequate also. In children, the urine output should be 0.5 ml/kg of body weight, and in infants it should be 1 ml/kg of body weight.

Blood Urea Nitrogen/Urine Urea Nitrogen Ratio. The BUN/UUN ratio is an excellent test to evaluate and monitor renal function in an acutely injured patient. Usually the reason for the ultimate demise of an acutely injured patient 3 or more hours after the injury is acute renal failure. A BUN/UUN ratio of less than 1:20 is indicative of either prerenal failure or renal failure and should be aggressively treated with volume replacement. Dialysis is sometimes required.

Blood Gases. Intermittent arterial blood gas determination is an important adjunct in treating and monitoring the acutely injured patient. Blood gases are used in evaluating the patient's respiratory status and acid-base balance. (Acid-base balance will be discussed with postsurgical management of the patient.)

The P_{O_2} reflects not only the function of the lungs, but also the potential amount of oxygen available to the tissues. The P_{O_2} tells how much oxygen is in physical solution, a figure that in turn reflects the degree of hemoglobin saturation. Normal P_{O_2} is 75 to 100 mm Hg. In evaluating the blood gases it is assumed that the patient's cardiac status is functional and the hemoglobin concentration is adequate. The percentage of oxygen being inspired must also be taken into consideration. A P_{O_2} of less than 75 mm Hg is indicative of poorly ventilating alveoli from pulmonary edema, atelectasis, or obstruction.

The P_{CO_2} measures the function of the pulmonary alveolar membrane. Normal P_{CO_2} is 35 to 45 mm Hg. In the presence of a normal pH, a P_{CO_2} of more than 45 mm Hg may indicate hypoventilation, obstruction, or emphysema.

Hematocrit. After hemodynamic equilibrium has been established, the hematocrit is an accurate guide to red blood cell replacement therapy, as previously described.

EMERGENCY PHYSICAL EVALUATION

The initial evaluation in the emergency room may reveal acute life-threatening problems that must be addressed immediately. After the appropriate emergency treatment has been finalized and the patient is in a stable condition, the next step is to evaluate the patient systematically for occult injuries. This brief evaluation performed in the emergency room does not take the place of the complete history and physical examination the patient will undergo after admission to the hospital; its purpose is to disclose any significant defects or injuries that will require that the maxillofacial surgeon consult an appropriate medical specialist.

The emergency physical examination is followed by other similar brief evaluations during the first 24 hrs of admission. Often the first examination is relatively unremarkable and treatment of the facial injuries is initiated by the maxillofacial surgeon. Many times occult problems do not become apparent for 12 to 24 hrs after the traumatic incident and the maxillofacial surgeon has the responsibility of diagnosis and appropriate consultation.

History

As in all patient evaluations, the past history is important. The history taken during the emergency physical examination is brief and provides baseline information for further evaluation and treatment.

Loss of Consciousness or Amnesia. Interrogation regarding loss of consciousness or amnesia is an important element in the neurologic baseline that was established by the paramedics. This documented information is particularly important to the appropriate specialist who might subsequently evaluate the patient.

A loss of consciousness is basically a disturbance of neurotransmission activity secondary to pressure on or a blow to the reticular activating system in the midbrain (pons). Any loss of consciousness is indicative of a cerebral concussion. A loss of consciousness of greater than 15 min may indicate a cerebral contusion or a more severe injury.

Amnesia for the accident or a short period before the accident is the hallmark of a cerebral concussion. Post-traumatic amnesia is a valuable index of cerebral injury, particularly if the length of time can be documented.

Previous Serious Illnesses. A positive past medical history may dictate or change the treatment plan.

Allergies. A knowledge of known allergies is important before definitive treatment is initiated.

Medicatons. Medications the patient was taking previous to the accident may give information about past medical history.

Pain. A traumatized patient usually has generalized pain. It is important to isolate specific areas of severe pain that may be the first symptom of an occult problem. For example, a specific localized headache may be important.

General Appearance

The patient should be completely undressed for a complete evaluation. *Any* contusions or swelling should be noted. A bent leg or laceration should be completely examined.

Four body areas should be included in the *emergency* physical examination to rule out immediate occult problems: thorax, lungs, and heart; abdomen (pelvis, kidneys); neck and head; and eyes.

Thorax, Lungs, Heart

The thorax, lungs, and heart are evaluated first and at the same time. This evaluation is conducted by utilizing the following methods: inspection, palpation, auscultation of both heart and lungs, radiography (PA and lateral chest, rib detail), CT scan (experimental), ECG (12-lead) (serial—q12h × 3), and blood gases.

Problems suspected in multiple trauma patients are as follows, in order of frequency of occurence:
1. Rib fractures
2. Lung contusion
3. Pneumothorax
4. Hemothorax
5. Cardiac contusion
6. Cardiac tamponade
7. Larynx fracture
8. Aortic disruption
9. Tracheal bronchial disruption

Abdomen (Pelvis, Kidneys)

Of patients who have intra-abdominal injury, 75% have no marks on the skin and 75% have pain. This means that 25% of patients with intra-abdominal injury have no abdominal pain! The abdomen is evaluated by using the following methods: inspection, palpation, auscultaton, radiography (flat and upright, IVP, possible cystogram), CT scan, and diagnostic peritoneal lavage. Peritoneal lavage should be performed by an experienced clinician. The standard site for entry into the peritoneal cavity is in the midline at a point approximately one third to one half the distance from the umbilicus to the symphysis pubis. A catheter is introduced and approximately 1000 ml of normal saline is introduced in the adult and resiphoned. In a child, 10 ml/kg is introduced. A rapid bedside method of interpreting the lavage fluid for intraperitoneal bleeding is to attempt to read newsprint through the intravenous tubing attached to the catheter as the fluid returns from the abdomen. An inability to do this may indicate a positive lavage. A more accurate method is laboratory analysis. A cell count of greater than 100,000 red cells/mm^3 or 500 white cells/mm^3, an amylase level over 400 units, and the presence of bacteria, feces, or bile all may indicate a positive lavage.

Problems suspected in multiple trauma patients are as follows, in order of frequency of occurrence:
1. Ileus
2. Ruptured spleen
3. Contused liver

4. Contused kidney
5. Ruptured bladder
6. Contused pancreas
7. Ruptured bowel

Neck

Facial injuries are associated with a 7 to 15% incidence of occult neck injury. The primary injury to the neck is a fractured cervical spine including a fracture of the odontoid process. Often the first symptom elicited is a complaint of a stiff neck. Altered sensation of the neck and arms may indicate a cervical fracture. The most definitive diagnostic aid is cervical radiographs including a swimmer's view and an open-mouth Waters view. The interpretation of cervical radiographs is difficult for most clinicians, and a radiologist's interpretation is advisable. A helpful memory aid in evaluating cervical radiographs is to use the letters of the word "CERVICAL."

C—Cord (lateral)—The sagittal diameter of the spinal cord should not be less than 12 mm anywhere. Two smooth continuous lines should run from the boundaries of the canal, one along the backs of the vertebral bodies, another connecting the bases of the spinous processes.

E—Exits (oblique)—The exits or foramina for the spinal nerves should be round, fairly smooth, and of similar dimensions, becoming slightly larger in the lower vertebrae.

R—Retropharyngeal (lateral)—The retropharyngeal soft tissue should be less than one third the AP diameter of the corresponding vertebrae and no more than 5 mm thick in the C1-C4 area. This thickness may be wider in the lower area but never more than 70% of C4's width. The prevertebral fat stripe should be no more than 3 mm from the margin of the vertebral body.

V—Vertebrae (lateral and AP)—Each vertebra must be clearly outlined and evaluated. No vertebral body height should be less than the one immediately above it. The apophyseal joint spaces should be regular with the joint surfaces parallel.

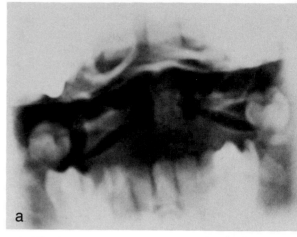

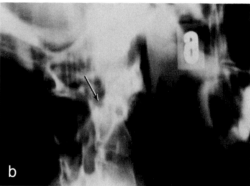

FIG. 2–6. **a** and **b**, Open-mouth view for evaluation of C1 is indicative of a fracture of the odontoid process. The fracture is confirmed in the lateral view. (Courtesy of Dr. Adam Robertson, Cooper Green Hospital, Birmingham, Ala.)

I—C1 (open mouth)—The relationship of C1 to the odontoid process should be assessed. The odontoid should be vertical and have an equal relationship to the lateral masses of C1 (Fig. 2–6).

C—Cranium—Although the radiographs are of the cervical spine, the base of the skull is readily apparent and can be evaluated radiographically.

A—Alignment—Any abrupt change in the alignment of the vertebral bodies and spinous processes or in the uniformity of the spaces between should be regarded with suspicion.

L—Last—The last cervical vertebra (C7) should be carefully evaluated and often requires a special view, the swimmer's projection.

Head

Evaluation of the head is important because of the underlying possibility of brain injury, which has a high incidence of morbidity and mortality. This evaluation is conducted to utilize the following methods: inspection (neurologic exam), palpation, radiography (skull, angiography?), CT scan, serial EEGs. Skull radiographs can be interpreted using the eight "S's," as follows:

S—Soft tissue—note swelling of soft tissue, which may indicate underlying abnormalities.

S—Skull—outline the cranial cortex, looking for abnormalities.

S—Sutures—compare the cranial sutures of both sides for laceration and position.

S—Symmetry—evaluate symmetry; benign structures are usually bilateral and symmetric. In 50% of adults, the pineal gland is calcified. A shift of more than 3 mm from the midline in the pineal gland may indicate a space-occupying lesion.

S—Spine—the upper portion of the cervical spine is usually seen on lateral skull radiographs, and C1—C2 and the odontoid process can be evaluated.

S—Sinuses—Check for fluid in the sphenoidal or frontal sinuses, which suggests fracture.

S—Sella—evaluate the sella turcica for normality.

S—Sound—evaluate the petrous pyramids of the temporal bones for fractures on the AP projection.

The CT scan provides superior evaluation for intracranial injuries including hematoma and midline shift (Fig. 2–7). It enables identification of skull fractures, facial bone fractures, and cervical spine fractures not identifiable by plain radiographs, and it helps assess soft tissues. CT of facial bones gives the complete position of all bone structures, as well as soft-tissue structures, including the eyes.

Essentially, the trauma patient's head is evaluated to diagnose four conditions: fractured skull (especially basilar), cerebral contusion, cerebral edema, and intracranial hemorrhage. A fractured skull other than a basilar

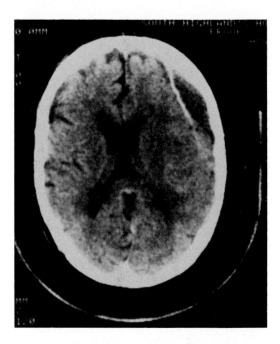

FIG. 2–7. CT scan demonstrates a hematoma with a midline shift of the brain. (Courtesy of Dr. Robert Ryan, Brookwood Medical Center, Birmingham, Ala.)

skull fracture with cerebrospinal fluid leak is important only if the brain or intracerebral blood vessels are injured.

All four conditions will give basically the same neurologic signs. The maxillofacial surgeon's responsibility is to evaluate the patient to determine if any of these conditions exist, rather than to specify the problem. The appropriate neurologic specialist will determine the pathologic entity.

A basilar skull fracture is a relatively frequent fracture associated with severe facial trauma. It is often difficult to diagnose. The following signs may be an indication of a basilar skull fracture: cerebrospinal fluid rhinorrhea or otorrhea; Battle's sign (mastoid ecchymosis), which usually occurs 6 to 12 hrs after trauma; Pandy bear sign (orbital bleed), which usually occurs 1 to 6 hrs after trauma; bulging blue tympanic membrane; and no posterior limit to subconjunctival ecchymosis (orbital roof).

A contused brain, cerebral edema, or intracranial hemorrhage may present with similar signs and symptoms. These clinical signs and symptoms are secondary to either increased intracranial pressure or direct brain injury. As with shock syndrome, it is important to diagnose the problem during the early stages to decrease morbidity. The early neurologic signs and symptoms of brain injury are focal headache; disorientation, i.e., a change in the level of awareness or alertness, restlessness (an excellent early sign); drift or pronator sign in which, with the arms outstretched and the hands in a supine position, one arm will drift and the hand will start to pronate (an earlier sign than decreased strength in one hand); and vomiting.

Later neurologic signs that become apparent after the intracranial problem increases are alteration of consciousness; change in vital signs (pulse decreases, respiration decreases, and blood pressure increases); and lateralizing signs. These include CNIII, motor, sensory, and reflex aberrations such as dilated pupil on ipsilateral side, decreased strength or a drifting on the contralateral side, aberrant sensation on the contralateral side, and increased deep tendon reflexes on the contralateral side and a positive Babinski's reflex on the contralateral side.

When these neurologic signs and symptoms present rapdily over a short period of time, usually immediate neurosurgical intervention is indicated. Usually these signs and symptoms appear gradually, and medical therapy is directed toward decreasing the intracranial pressure with fluid restriction, diuretics, and hyperventilation.

Eyes

The eyes of all patients with facial trauma should be evaluated immediately. Often, serious eye injury is present but is unnoticed because of attention to more dramatic injuries. The sclera should be examined for lacerations and the cornea for abrasions. The visual acuity and color vision should be evaluated. The fundus should be examined with an ophthalmoscope for hemorrhage and disc swelling or ischemia.

After the emergency physical examination has been completed and appropriate consultation obtained and before admission of the patient to the intensive care unit (ICU), the airway should be re-evaluated. If indicated, an elective tracheostomy can be performed at this time.

Tetanus prophylaxis should be administered according to the following schedule: If the patient's immunization record is uncertain, if the patient was not previously immunized, or if immunization occurred more than 10 years ago:
  a. clean wounds—0.5 ml tetanus toxoid
  b. dirty wounds—0.5 ml tetanus toxoid + 250 cc tetanus immune globulin (TIG) + penicillin (or other appropriate antibiotic)

If the patient was immunized in the past 10 years:
  a. clean and dirty wounds—0.5 ml tetanus toxoid + penicillin (or other appropriate antibotic)

ADMISSION ORDERS

The following are typical admission orders for a multiply injured patient with facial injuries who is admitted to the ICU. If some of the radiographic or laboratory tests have been accomplished in the emergency room, they can be omitted. Some tests, like the ECG and chest radiograph, should be repeated, because cardiac or lung contusions often may not become apparent for 12 to 24 hrs after the traumatic incident.

1. Admit to ICU
2. VS q15 min × 4h, then qh
3. Notify Dr. _____ for systolic BP greater than 200 or less than 90, pulse greater than 120 or less than 50, respirations greater than 30 or less than 16, rectal temperature greater than 102°, and urine output less than 30 ml/h
4. I & O
5. Craniotomy checks q2h (Evaluate neurologic decompensation—level of consciousness, pupil size and reaction, strength or drift, reflexes)
6. ECG qd × 3h (Evaluate cardiac contusion)
7. Abdominal girth q4h
8. Notify Dr. _____ if patient complains of left shoulder pain (spleen)
9. Hbg and hct q4h
10. Blood gases q6h (lungs, acid-base balance)

11. CBC (WBCs increase more than 15,000, suspect liver or spleen problem)
12. Blood sugar
13. Electrolytes
14. U/A, Creatine, BUN, UUN (kidneys)
15. Amylase (pancreas)
16. Total bilirubin, alkaline phosphatase, SGOT, LDH, PT, PTT (liver, clotting mechanism)
17. CPK-MB isoenzyme (heart)
18. Type and cross match for 2 units of whole blood or packed RBCs
19. X-rays or CT scans (that have not been ordered in ER)
20. IV orders: Through arm catheter —5% D/RL—1000 ml q12h - add 10-ml units crystalline penicillin to each IV (*Antibotic* and fluid may change depending on situation)
21. Sulfadiazine 1 g piggyback IV q8h (CSF leak) (or *cefazolin*)
22. Pentazocine 30 mg IM q4h prn: pain (minimal neurodepressant)
23. Dexamethasone 4 mg IVC q6h (cerebral edema)
24. Complete bed rest in semi-Fowler's position (best position if a basilar skull fracture is present with CSF leak)
25. Ice chips only PO
26. Nasogastric tube to intermittent low suction—irrigate q4h with 50 ml saline
27. Monitor CVP, notify Dr. _____of CVP greater than 15 or less than 10
28. Tracheostomy care
    a. Aerosol O_2
    b. Remove and clean inner cannula qh
    c. Deep rapid suction qh
    d. If secretions are thick, instill 5 gtts of sterile saline into trach tube
    e. Change dressing bid.
    f. No. 16 sterile French catheter at bedside (for changing tube)
    g. Ventilation orders as indicated

Although this example of admission orders is fairly complete, many other different orders could be added depending on the situation. For example, if inappropriate antidiuretic hormone syndrome (hyponatremic natriuresis) or diabetes insipidus (polydipsia, polyurea, urine hypo-osmolality) is suspected because of head injury, serum and urine osmolalities and serum and urine sodiums should be included.

If all systems are stable and the only apparent severe injuries are facial, a decision must be made about when to take the patient to surgery for the repair of the facial fractures and lacerations. Facial lacerations can be covered with sterile saline gauze and, if kept moist with saline, can be repaired in 12 to 24 hours without compromising the cosmetic result. Because of the possibility of an occult injury that may not manifest itself for 12 hours or more, observing the patient for at least 12 hours before the definitive maxillofacial surgery is often recommended.

PREOPERATIVE, INTRAOPERATIVE, AND POSTOPERATIVE MANAGEMENT

After the severely traumatized patient has been stabilized physiologically, the definitive surgery can be planned. Knowledge of the pathophysiology of shock is invaluable in management of the preoperative, intraoperative, and postoperative phases of the patient's treatment course.

At this stage, the management of the patient is concerned with control of metabolic requirements. The clinician must have a thorough knowledge of the patient's metabolic requirements including fluid balance, electrolyte balance, acid-base balance, and nutrition. Proper kidney function greatly simplifies maintenance; the goal of patient management becomes one of prevention of metabolic derangements, rather than treatment. If the clinician supplies the patient with sufficient metabolic raw materials, the patient's normal renal function will fulfill the metabolic requirements and correct derangements. The patients's kidneys will selectively retain and excrete individual metabolites and ions and thereby maintain balance.

The body's metabolic response to trauma, whether it is accidental trauma or surgical trauma, is the same. The patient loses body protein and goes into negative nitrogen balance, sodium and water (from increased ADH secretion) are retained, potassium is excreted, and depending on the circumstances, either acidosis or alkalosis can occur. These responses to trauma or surgery must be treated and further prevented.

FLUID BALANCE

Of body weight, 50% is water. After severe trauma or long surgery, this water is mobilized and immobilized by several different mechanisms. Formulating a specific regimen for fluid replacement after trauma and before, during, and after surgery is difficult. Awareness of the basic principles of fluid therapy and constant monitoring of results are important. The CVP, urine output, and daily weight must be closely monitored to determine whether to correct a fluid deficit preoperatively, determine how much to replace for new losses during surgery, and determine postoperative maintenance replacement.

The most consistent problem presurgically is to determine whether the patient's fluid volume is sufficient. The trauma patient may have adrenergic-compensated dehydration while all of the vital signs are normal. A general anesthetic will alter the compensatory mechanisms, and hypotension and other problems will follow. A simple preoperative test to unmask these compensatory mechanisms to determine if preoperative fluid should be administered is the chlorpromazine (CPZ) test. A dose of 0.2 mg/kg is administered IV. A 25% drop in systolic pressure indicates hypovolemia, whereas normovolemic patients do not become hypotensive after administration of a small dose of chlorpromazine.

Intraoperatively, the best indicator of volume replacement is the urine output from an indwelling catheter. Urine output should be at lease 30 ml/hr, or 60% of the fluid volume administered. Hints of volume depletion during general anesthesia are diastolic hypertension and tachycardia. These signs usually occur before hypotension.

Normal fluid requirements are 1500 ml of fluid for the first 20 kg of body weight/24 hrs, plus 20 ml fluid for each remaining kilogram of body weight/24 hrs (approximately 2500 ml in a 70-kg person). Volume replacement during surgery and immediately postoperatively can be estimated by administering ½ of the

normal requirement plus 1½ times the estimated blood loss during the operation.

Although what type of fluid to administer intraoperatively is a matter of controversy, an effective regimen is to initially administer 1000 ml 5% dextrose in lactated Ringer's solution followed by lactated Ringer's solution. The initial dextrose will supress ADH and allow the kidneys to function properly to give appropriate urine output. The dextrose also protects the liver from the hepatotoxic effects of the inhalation anesthetic agent by preventing breakdown of liver enzymes that are used to metabolize the anesthetic agent. Dextrose should be used only initially because an excessive amount will cause an osmotic diuresis. The Ringer's lactate solution closely approximates extracellular fluid, provides a transient intravascular volume, corrects any translocation or functional space problems, and suppresses aldosterone secretion. The suppression of aldosterone will allow the kidney to excrete sodium, retain potassium, and maintain the urine output. The Ringer's lactate solution must be given immediately after the blood loss in order to suppress aldosterone.

Blood replacement is seldom indicated in a stable patient until at least 750 ml of blood is lost unless the hemoglobin and hematocrit were low at the start of surgery. The best blood product for excessive rapid hemorrhage is warm, type-specific, crossmatched, fresh whole blood. Usually, the component of choice is packed red blood cells. One unit of red cells will usually raise the hematocrit by two to three points.

Postoperatively, the remaining 50% of the calculated normal metabolic requirement, in addition to the insensible gastrointestinal fluid loss should be administered over the remainder of the 24 hrs. In the typical patient with facial trauma and intermaxillary fixation, oral intake for the first few days is minimal, particularly if post-operative ileus is present and fluid by nasogastric tube cannot be administered. Administration of 3000 ml of IV fluids/day is typical, and a regimen of 1000 ml of 5% dextrose in lactated Ringer's alternated with 5% dextrose in water is desirable. The dextrose provides at least 200 cal (equal to one cup of coffee with sugar and toast)/L, prevents ketoacidosis, and prevents protein catabolism. Normal saline would provide too much sodium (and particularly chloride) and is hyperosmolar. Hence, if saline is to be used, one half normal saline is appropriate.

If the patient has a fever postoperatively, add to the postoperative fluid regimen 250 ml of fluid/day/degree.

Postoperative fluid therapy in infants and small children is extremely precise and should be monitored by a pediatric expert. A good rule that may be used in small children is a maintenance level of 1200 ml/m²/day. Body surface in square meters can be estimated by body weight (3 lbs of body weight = 0.1 m²).

ELECTROLYTE BALANCE

In the majority of cases, treatment of electrolyte imbalances after trauma or surgery should not be given priority—the immediate concern is restoration of fluid volume and, possibly, of acid-base balance. Electrolyte measurements immediately after trauma or surgery usually do not give a true picture of the useful concentration of electrolytes, since electrolyte homeostasis usually does not occur for 24 to 48 hrs after the traumatic incident in the appropriately treated patient. Therefore, the immediate electrolyte determination after trauma or surgery should be used only to obtain baseline information. Aggressive treatment of disorders should be delayed unless other information, such as large gastrointestinal fluid loss or a measured hyperkalemia associated with a bradycardia and/or peaked T wave, dictates treatment.

Potassium. The most critical electrolyte is potassium. Whereas patients will tolerate an imbalance of sodium and chloride reasonably well, a small imbalance of potassium may be detrimental. Normal serum potassium is 3.5 to 5 mEq/L. The maintenance requirement for potassium is 60 mEq/day.

Hyperkalemia after trauma or extensive surgery is due either to release of potassium from the cell into the extracellular fluid or to iatrogenic causes. Treatment, if indicated, should be directed toward driving the potassium back into the cells with insulin, calcium gluconate, and sodium bicarbonate. Hypokalemia is treated by intravenous potassium chloride. Potassium from gastrointestinal fluid drained by a nasogastric tube should be replaced at the rate of 40 mEq of potassium/L of nasogastric drainage/day. If intravenous penicillin is being administered, each 5 million units of crystalline penicillin has 10 mEq of potassium. Approximately 100 mEq of potassium is required to raise the serum potassium concentration by 1 mEq/L. Potassium administration in the presence of low urine output is dangerous.

Sodium. Losses of sodium from the body are always combined with water losses. The result of sodium depletion is extracellular volume depletion. Normal serum sodium is 135 to 145 mEq/L, and the maintenance requirement for sodium is 80 mEq/day. Hyponatremia is treated with intravenous saline, and hypernatremia is treated with intravenous dextrose in water.

ACID-BASE BALANCE

Disturbances in acid-base metabolism are not uncommon in the multiple trauma or postsurgical patient. These problems are usually self-limiting in the previously healthy patient and are corrected by treatment of the primary problem causing the acid-base discrepancy. Aggressive treatment of the acid-base problem itself is usually not warranted and may in fact cause further problems. However, a basic knowledge of acid-base metabolism is important.

Normally, the extracellular fluids have a pH between 7.35 and 7.45. This value is determined by the ratio of paired acid and base buffers. The most important of these are bicarbonate and carbonic acid (normal ratio, 20:1). Plasma bicarbonate and carbonic acid constitute the total plasma carbon dioxide (normal, 20 to 30 mEq/L).

The carbonic acid concentration is regulated by the respiratory minute volume. An increase in expired carbon dioxide tends to reduce the plasma carbonic acid concentration, raising pH and causing an alkalosis. Conversely, reduced expiration of carbon dioxide decreases pH and causes an acidosis.

Concentration of bicarbonate is regulated by the kidney. An increase in renal tubular secretion of H^+ ions leads to a rise in plasma

Table 2–1.   Acid-Base Disturbance as
Determined by P_{CO_2} and pH

	P_{CO_2}	pH
Metabolic alkalosis	Increased	Increased
Respiratory alkalosis	Decreased	Increased
Metabolic acidosis	Decreased	Decreased
Respiratory acidosis	Increased	Decreased

bicarbonate concentration, an elevated pH, and a resultant alkalosis. Conversely, a decrease in renal tubular secretion of H^+ ions results in decreased plasma bicarbonate, a decreased pH, and a resultant acidosis.

The minimum for diagnosis of an acid-base disturbance is the determination of plasma total carbon dioxide content and an accurate assessment of the clinical situation for possible metabolic or respiratory disorders. A more accurate and easily determined method is through understanding and interpreting the patient's arterial blood gases and pH. Diagnosis of an acid-base disturbance is determined by the results of the pH and P_{CO_2} (Table 2–1)

The common acid-base disturbance in the trauma patient, especially associated with shock, is usually assumed to be metabolic acidosis. Often, however, the primary acid-base disturbance is a respiratory alkalosis or a mixed acid-base disturbance. The indiscriminate administration of sodium bicarbonate to a patient with an already high pH may lead to a cardiac arrhythmia or cardiac arrest. Careful evaluation of the patient and the patient's arterial blood gases and pH is indicated before any treatment is started.

NUTRITION

All trauma patients or patients who have had extensive surgery have a significant metabolic requirement. The overall response of a patient to treatment is directly proportional to how this requirement is satisfied.

After trauma or surgery, the patient requires a great amount of energy (500 calories/day) to maintain metabolism and support repair. Approximately enough carbohydrate is present in the body to supply 1200 cal at a time when the body needs 5000 calories/day. After the 1200 carbohydrate calories are used, the body starts to break down protein for uti-

lization, putting the patient in a negative nitrogen balance. The body has approximately 166,000 total calories; the use of 50,000 of these calories without replacement leads to death. Sufficient nutrient substance must be administered to the patient at the earliest possible time.

The metabolic response to trauma increases the patient's requirements for nutritional substances at a time when it is difficult to supply them. If the patient has had facial trauma and subsequent maxillofacial surgery, oral intake may be compromised for an extended length of time because of the intermaxillary fixation.

If an ileus is not present, as it often is after trauma or extensive surgery, tube feedings of elemental diets are the best method to supply the necessary nutrients. If tube feedings are not possible, hyperalimentation or total parenteral nutrition must be utilized.

POSTOPERATIVE MANAGEMENT

Generally, postoperative management of the trauma patient who had no previous medical problems is only supportive. The major mistake in management is usually aggressive overtreatment. If all previously discussed parameters are carefully monitored and sufficient nutrient substance is provided, the patient will usually have an uncomplicated postoperative course.

Postoperative orders for the maxillofacial trauma patient are as follows:
1. VS q15min until stable, then qid × 2d, then bid
2. I & O
3. Notify Dr. _____for systolic BP > 200 or < 90, P > 120 or < 50, R > 30, Rectal temp >102° or if pt. hasn't voided by 6 PM
4. Hold blood for 24 hrs then release
5. CBC in AM
6. NG tube to intermittent low suction, irrigate /c 50 cc N/S q4h
7. Oxymorphone 0.3 mg IV q 30 min prn pain in RR
8. Meperidine 50 mg and promethazine 25 mg IM q4h prn pain
9. IV orders: 1000 cc 5% D/RL /c 5 mil units crystalline pcn and 20 mEq KCl alternat-

ing /c 1000 cc 5% D/w /c 5 mil units crystalline pcn IV q8h

10. Dibucaine ointment to lips prn (at bedside)
11. Cepacol—H_2O_2 (½-½) mouthwash at bedside
12. Oxymetazoline nose spray—spray twice in each nostril q4h × 48 h
13. Complete bed rest in semi-Fowler's position—encourage pt. to move legs
14. Scissors and suction at bedside
15. Encourage pt. to cough and deep-breathe qh
16. Gently suction pharynx through nose prn
17. Clear liquid diet postnausea, progress to full liquid diet with high-protein supplement

These postoperative orders must be modified according to the patient's condition. Other orders may be indicated, such as serial laboratory studies, tracheostomy care, wound care, other medications, CVP monitoring, and total parenteral nutrition. Postoperative respiratory assistance is often helpful to prevent atelectasis.

The simplest and most important parameters to be monitored during the immediate postoperative period are the vital signs. Respiratory rate and pulse rate offer a wealth of useful information about a postoperative patient. Temperature is also very important; an elevated temperature during the first 24 hrs after surgery may indicate atelectasis, although an elevated temperature during the first 24 hours after maxillofacial surgery that involves the mouth or nose is common. Therefore, auscultating the lungs postoperatively is particularly important; auscultation reveals atelectasis earlier and more consistently than chest radiographs. Rales often precede decreased or absent breath sounds over areas of atelectasis.

If the appropriate preventive and therapeutic measures were taken preoperatively, the postoperative management of the trauma patient who had no previous medical problems consists mainly of monitoring. If there has been no overaggressive treatment and there is no complicating pathology, the patient should have an uneventful postoperative course.

3

IMAGING

Part 1
Medical Radiography
Kenneth Dolan

A number of examination imaging methods are available to the practitioner who treats maxillofacial injuries. The array of plain radiographic studies, panoramic radiographs, linear or hypocycloidal tomography, and computed tomography presents so many examination choices that gaining perspective in the use of available modalities may be difficult.

The initial evaluation of a patient with a facial injury is best supplemented with plain radiographic evaluation. Further examination with conventional tomography or computed tomography may then be used to answer specific questions arising from the plain film evaluation.

Panoramic radiographic examination may be used to evaluate mandibular or maxillofacial structures but is limited to use in the cooperative patient who is able to sit upright; few centers are equipped with horizontal panoramic machines. Panoramic radiography is also limited in that it is only a two-dimensional means of study. With significant fragment injury, three-dimensional evaluation is necessary.

Conventional tomography makes use of a moving radiographic tube and film. The mo-

tion may either be linear or make use of a complex geometric figure. In linear tomography a movable axis is positioned along a rod that connects the radiographic tube and film holder. The position (axis) through which tube and film rotate may be adjusted (raised or lowered) to match the plane of the body being examined. Multiple tomographic "cuts" are then obtained through the anatomic area of interest.

The radiographic tube and film holder move in opposite directions during the exposure blurring everything but the radiographic information in the plane of the axis of rotation. This opposite movement gives a layer effect to the part being studied, so that the sharp layer can be seen and analyzed without any interference by overlying structures. However, the inadvertent imaging of other linear structures lying in the direction of tube travel produces so-called parasite lines that may partly obscure the structures in focus. Another limiting feature in tomography is that the thickness of the layer of tissue in "focus" is directly proportional to the distance of travel of the radiographic tube. Because maximum movement permitted with linear tomography is about 75 cm, the slice produced is about 0.5 cm thick, which is relatively thick for facial anatomy evaluation. In order to lengthen tube and film travel to produce thinner anatomic slices, manufacturers have produced machines that use complex motions. These complex motions also reduce or exclude parasite lines, so that only information lying in the anatomic plane being studied is represented by the film image.

Several geometric figures are used in complex-motion tomography. Circular, elliptical, hypocycloidal, or trispiral tube and film motion are now available. With the hypocycloidal mode, the radiographer may obtain a layer thickness of 1 mm with maximal blurring of overlying structures. Serial sections are routinely obtained beginning on the orbital-maxillary surface plane. These views represent a 1-mm-thick layer. Sections are then made at 5-mm intervals through the face in coronal and lateral planes for a complete evaluation.

While very detailed anatomic information is available with this technique, most of the information relates to bony structures, as is the case with a plain radiograph, and very little information about soft tissue is obtained. Also, whereas information regarding only a thin slice is obtained, the entire volume of the face and head are being exposed to x rays and may receive up to 30 or 40 rads during a complete examination. (Further information about tomography may be obtained from the study by Littleton.[1])

Computered tomography (CT) makes use of an x ray beam and does produce an anatomic layer section, but there the similarity to conventional tomography ends. Several generations of CT equipment have been produced since the single detector and radiographic tube machine that required 1 min for a low-resolution view became available in the early 1970s.

The current fourth-generation equipment makes use of an array of detectors that are arranged in a circular fashion within the gantry of the detector. The equipment available to us has a 1200-detector array. These encircle an aperture within the center of the gantry into which the part to be examined is placed. The radiographic tube is mounted on circular rails and aligned with each detector.

During an exposure the radiographic tube passes through a circular track around the body part being examined. Each detector measures the amount of radiation absorbed by that anatomic portion and compares this amount to the amount of radiation detected when only air is present in the examining area. From this difference, the computer can calculate the linear absorption number for each region of a rectangular (x-y axis) matrix that includes the body part being studied.

The computer further calculates a density number for each pixel (point) within the matrix. From this calculation, by means of a complex software program ("backpointing"), an image can be formed on a cathode-ray tube screen. This image is a composite of all densities within the part being studied, clearly demonstrating bone, blood, soft tissue, fat, and air densities. The image represents the axial section of the body part. In the case of facial injury, examination consists of taking sections 1 mm thick at 3-cm intervals through the area of interest.

In CT, unlike in other radiography, only the layer being examined is exposed to x rays. Therefore, if each exposure requires 2 rads of radiation, the whole part being examined receives only this amount. Also, radiographic images require a tenfold tissue density difference for detection, whereas CT differentiates minor tissue density differences. (Further information can be obtained from any basic CT text.[2])

In this era of price-consciousness in patient care it is of interest to note that, if the plain radiographic examination can be considered as costing 1 unit, conventional tomography costs 1.5 to 2.0 units and CT costs 2.5 to 5.0 units. The main consideration, however, is to obtain the principal information required to properly evaluate the patient's condition and to obtain information needed for surgical repair.

RADIOGRAPHIC ANATOMY OF MAXILLOFACIAL STRUCTURES

PLAIN FILMS

A usual combination of views for facial injury includes the Waters projection, Caldwell projection, and lateral view. The basal view (submentovertex projection) may be obtained as an underexposed view for the zygomatic arches, or as a conventional exposure for mandibular and facial features. The panoramic radiograph is used for evaluation of the mandible and maxillary features but is not advocated for evaluation of other facial features.

Waters View

The Waters view is obtained as a posteroanterior (PA) projection if the patient can sit or stand upright or can assume a prone position with the head and neck hyperextended. This projection places the facial bones closest to the film for best detail, with the nose and chin in contact with the film holder. Because the orbital and maxillary borders as well as the zygomatic arches diverge from back to front, the PA projection gives the best representation of these parts. Ideally, the patient is positioned so that the maxillary sinus alveolar border lies just above the petrous surface of the temporal bone.

Figure 3–1a is a standard Waters view. Both maxillary sinuses are clear. If one identifies the glenoid fossas on each side and the upper margin of the zygomatic arches, then the outer border of the orbital processes of the zygoma and the frontal bones may be followed to the lesser temporal fossas (line 1). Just above the glenoid fossas is the temporal component of the zygomatic arch under-surface, which one may follow in continuity with the lateral maxillary sinus walls down to the alveolar borders (line 2). These two lines form the outline of an elephant head and trunk. The trunk is the zygomatic arch.

The other major line of continuity follows the outline of the orbital borders and the nasal arch. Beginning at the frontal sinus lateral border, a cortical line representing the upper palpable orbital rim is seen. This line continues downward along the inner margin of the orbital process of the frontal bone and zygoma and is continuous with the inferior palpable border of the orbit. Medially this cortex is continuous with the frontal process of the maxilla, continues with the arch formed by the two nasal bones, and merges with the

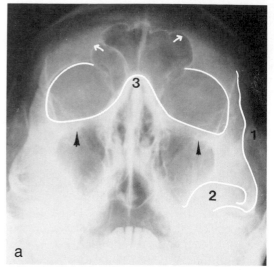

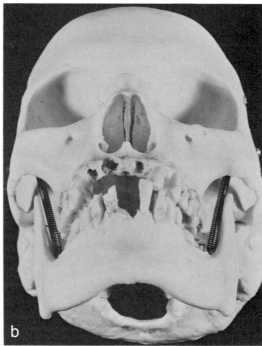

FIG. 3–1.   The Waters view. **a,** Waters radiograph with the three lines of continuity. Infraorbital canals (arrowheads). Frontal sinus borders (arrows). **b,** Skull in Waters position.

inferior, lateral, and superior orbital borders on the opposite side (line 3).

Figure 3–1b is a view of the facial skeleton in Waters position. Other features evident on this view are the frontal sinuses and their margins, the maxillary alveolar arch, and the infraorbital neural-vascular canals. Portions of the frontal bone surrounding the sinuses and orbits can also be seen.

Caldwell View

Periorbital features and the inferior maxillary margins are best visualized in the Caldwell projection. This is obtained as a PA view with the nose and forehead in contact with the film holder. Ideally the orbital floor lies just above the petrous surface of the temporal bone, as seen in Figure 3–2a. Line 1 from the Waters view is foreshortened but can also be seen along the outer oribital margin on the Caldwell view. About 1.5 cm below the place where line 1 ends in the temporal fossa, the zygomaticofrontal (ZMF) suture is evident as a transverse line. The inner orbital border should be identified at this level.

The upper orbital border consists of two parts. The palpable portion is the lower edge of the upper orbital margin. The cortical line paralleling this edge is the anterior orbital roof. The posterior orbital roof extends obliquely downward to reach the superior orbital fissure. Medially, the orbital margin of the frontal sinus is continuous with the medial orbital border until this border divides into two lines. The outer line represents the lamina papyracea surface of the ethmoidal sinus. The more medial cortical line is the posterior lacrimal crest.

The orbital floor is continuous with the two medial cortical lines of the orbit. The lamina papyracea is continuous with the posterior floor of the orbit (posterior maxillary sinus roof) near the inferior orbital fissure. The posterior lacrimal crest line is continuous with the anterior orbital floor (anterior maxillary sinus roof). Peripheral to the floor lines, a short part of the inferior palpable orbital border completes the inferior orbital detail and is continuous with the inner margin of the orbital process of the zygoma, which continues upward to the ZMF suture. The superior orbital fissure lies obliquely in the medial portion of the orbit.

The inferior maxillary (alveolar) surface can be seen below the density of the petrous bone. Medial to this the horizontal hard palate and perpendicular nasal bony septum are visualized.

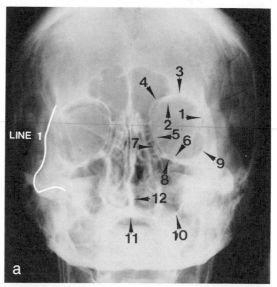

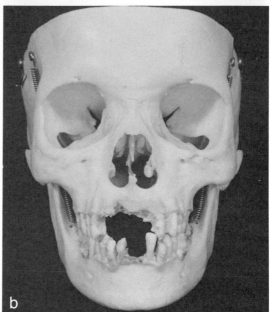

FIG. 3–2. The Caldwell view. **a,** Caldwell radiograph. Line one drawn. Zygomaticofrontal suture (1). Upper palpable border (2). Anterior orbital roof (3). Frontal sinus margin (4). Lamina papyracea (5). Posterior orbital floor (6). Anterior lacrimal crest (7). Anterior orbital floor (8). Orbital process of zygoma (9). Inferior alveolar margin of maxilla (10). Hard palate (11). Bony nasal septum (12). **b,** Facial skeleton in Caldwell position.

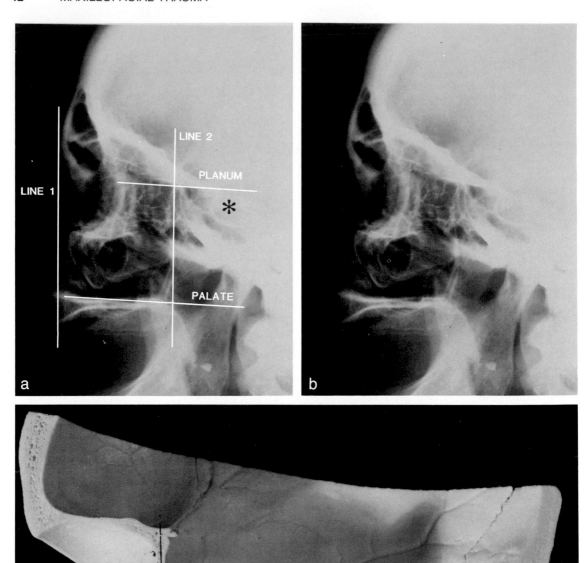

FIG. 3–3.   The lateral view. **a,** A lateral radiograph with perpendicular and horizontal orientation lines. Sella turcica (*). **b,** A lateral radiograph without orientation lines. **c,** A lateral skull preparation showing the perpendicular orientation lines. **d,** A central lateral skull preparation showing the horizontal orientation lines. Sella turcica (*).

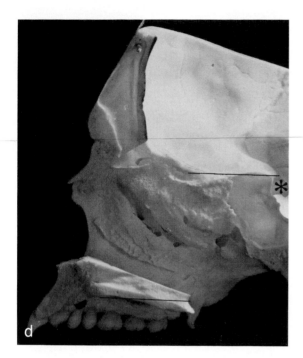

FIG. 3–3 (continued).

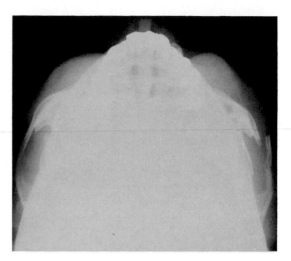

FIG. 3–4. The underexposed basal view. Normal right and fractured left zygomatic arch.

Figure 3–2b is a view of the facial skeleton in the Caldwell position.

Lateral View

The lateral view is used essentially for anatomic orientation of the facial skeleton (Fig. 3–3). Line 1 is a perpendicular plane tangential to the frontal sinus surface above and tangential to the anterior nasal spine of the hard palate below. Paralleling line 1 in normal patients, line 2 is a perpendicular plane tangential to the greater sphenoidal wings above and tangential to the posterior maxillary sinus walls below.

The planum sphenoidale is the horizontal roof of the sphenoidal sinus and lies just in front of the sella turcica. Another horizontal line is formed by the nasal surface of the hard palate. These lines should parallel one another in the normal patient. Using these perpendicular and horizontal lines the examiner can evaluate a shift in position of large fracture fragments.

Basal View

The basal view may be done as a submentovertex projection with the patient in a sitting position, or as a verticosubmental projection with the patient in the prone position. Figure 3–4 shows an example of the use of an underexposed basal view to demonstrate the normal right zygomatic arch and a fracture of the left arch (see below). A conventionally exposed basal view may help with analysis of the facial anatomy. CT axial views show details of the facial skeleton to much better advantage than conventional basal radiographs.

Panoramic View

The panoramic radiograph permits evaluation of the entire mandible on one film. The technique is equivalent to a thick-section tomograph and allows visualization of fractures that may be obscured by overlying structures on plain radiographs. Features of the maxillary sinus margin and pterygoid processes may also be demonstrated with this system of examination. Figure 3–5 is a panoramic view made with an Orthopantomograph unit. In this view the alveolar, zygomatic, and posterior maxillary sinus borders are evident. The pterygoid plate and pterygopalatine fossa can also be evaluated. The inferior zygomatic arch margin can be traced from the glenoid fossa to the zygomatic recess.

TOMOGRAPHY

Tomographs can be used to supplement plain film information in various fractures.

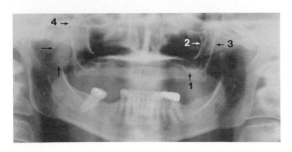

FIG. 3–5. The panoramic radiograph. Alveolar margin of maxilla (1). The zygomatic recess (2). The posterior wall (3). The pterygopalatine fossa (4). Pterygoid plate (arrows).

We used 1-mm-thick taken at 5-mm separation in either the coronal or lateral projection when indicated. Detail companion normal views will be demonstrated when needed in the following examples of injury.

COMPUTED TOMOGRAPHY

Although serial contiguous axial sections are obtained between the planes of the palate and orbital roof when a patient with a facial injury is examined, the normal anatomy of only a few representative axial views will be used for orientation purposes in this section.

The hard palate CT plane is represented by Figure 3–6a. In this view the entire palate is visualized. Posteriorly the medial and lateral pterygoid plates are evident. The alveolar recesses of the maxillary sinuses can be seen along the lateral palatal borders. The mandible is sectioned in an intercondylar plane. Masseter muscles overlie the mandible, and the pterygoid muscles can be followed medially to the pterygoid plates.

The midmaxillary CT plane is represented by Figure 3–6b. Zygomatic arches curve posteriorly from the lateral border of the maxillary sinus borders to reach the temporal bone. The arches enclose the tip of the mandibular coronoid process. Anterior to this a portion of the temporalis tendon is outlined by retromaxillary fat. The bony septum and portions of the nasal turbinates are evident centrally in the nasal fossa.

The midorbital CT plane is illustrated in Figure 3–6c. The globe, lens, and optic nerve are seen in each orbital space. Both medial and lateral rectus muscles are evident. An-

teriorly, the curved nasal arch joins the lamina papyracea surface of the ethmoidal sinuses and can be traced back to the sphenoid bone near the superior orbital fissure. Laterally, the zygomatic orbital process and sphenoid surface form the outer orbital wall. The sphenoid bone and squamous portion of the temporal bone enclose the temporal lobe of the brain.

The upper CT section demonstrated in Figure 3–6d is on the plane of the frontal sinuses and shows how the frontal bone and orbital roof join. The diamond-shaped suprasellar cistern lies in the center of the brain portion of this view.

The preceding views were obtained with a soft-tissue mode. Figures 3–7a and 3–7b were obtained with a bone mode setting on the CT console. They are equivalent to Figure 3–6b and 3–6c in position and show the excellent bone detail in this mode of viewing.

Upper sections are important in evaluating brain injury or intracerebral blood (Chapter 2).

Fourth generation scanners can be used to produce oblique direct coronal maxillofacial projections or may be used to provide computed reconstructions in the axial or coronal plane.

Figures 3–8a through 3–8c are representations of direct coronal CT views in a patient with left maxillary sinus hypoplasia. The plane of Figure 3–8a extends through the orbital roof on both sides. The ethmoid sinuses, crista galli, and perpendicular plate are in the midline. Below the orbit, the plane is anterior to the maxilla.

The view in Figure 3–8b is 1 cm posterior to that in Figure 3–8a, in Figure 3–8b, the entire oribital rim is evident. Ethmoidal cells and the nasal turbinates are visualized centrally. On the right are the anterior margins of the maxillary sinus. On the left, the plane passes tangentially to the anterior maxillary sinus wall. The infraorbital neurovascular canal is seen as a perpendicular line. The image in Figure 3–8c lies 3 cm behind that of Figure 3–8b. This view shows the posterior ethmoid air cells and the superior orbital fissures above. The midmaxillary sinus plane is evident. The right maxillary sinus is normal. The left is hypoplastic and filled with an une-

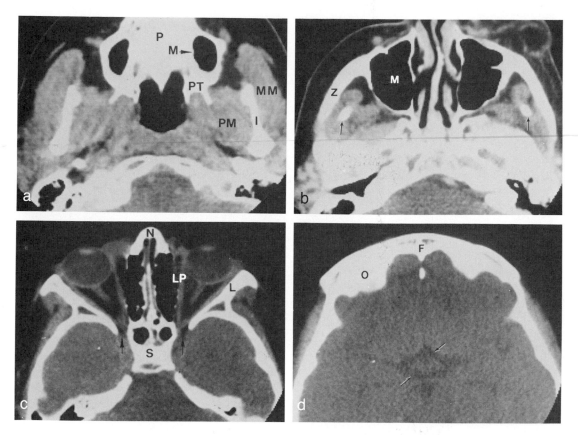

FIG. 3–6.   Maxillofacial axial CT examination. **a,** Axial CT through the hard palate plane. Palate (P). Maxillary alveolar recess (M). Pterygoid plates (PT). Intercondylar plane of mandible (I). Masseter muscle (MM). Pterygoid muscles (PM). **b,** Axial CT through the midmaxillary plane. Maxillary sinus (M). Zygomatic arch (Z). Coronoid process of mandible (arrowheads). **c,** Midorbital axial CT plane. Nasal arch (N). Lamina papyracea (LP). Lateral orbital border (L). Superior orbital fissures (arrows). Sphenoid bone (S). **d,** Frontal sinus axial CT plane. Frontal bone (F). Orbital roof (O). Suprasellar cistern (arrows).

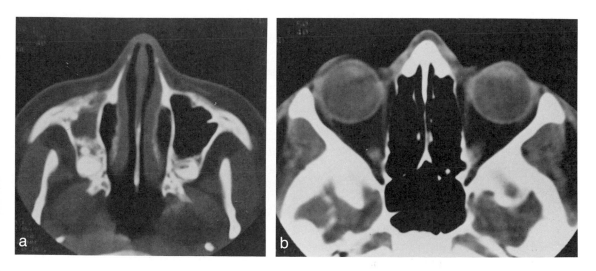

FIG. 3–7.   Maxillofacial axial CT examination (bone mode). **a,** Midmaxillary CT with same features as Fig. 5–6b. **b,** Midorbital CT with same features as Fig. 3–6c.

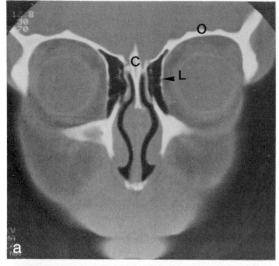

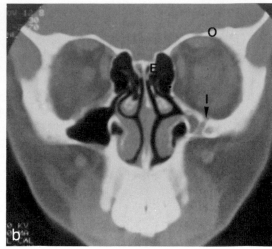

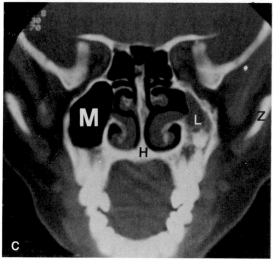

FIG. 3–8. Direct coronal facial CT. **a,** Anterior orbital plane. Orbital roof (O). Lamina papyracea and ethmoid sinus (L). Crista galli and perpendicular plate (C). **b,** Coronal section through orbit and anterior maxilla. Orbital roof (O). Ethmoid sinus (E). Infraorbital neurovascular canal (I). **c,** Coronal section through superior orbital fissure and maxillary sinuses (M). Hypoplasia and uninterrupted tooth (L). Hard palate (H). Zygomatic arch (Z).

rupted tooth and soft tissue. A portion of the zygomatic arch is present laterally on both sides.

PRINCIPLES OF RADIOGRAPHIC EVALUATION OF MAXILLOFACIAL INJURY

INDIRECT SIGNS

Indirect signs of injury evident on radiographic studies should alert the examiner to the possibility of skeletal injury. Because most of the indirect signs of injury may also be found in association with sinus inflammatory disease, these findings only suggest the presence of possible injury.

If blood fills a maxillary sinus after injury, the sinus will become opaque on radiographic examination. Incomplete filling of the sinus results in an air-fluid level between the blood accumulation and residual air. If blood is trapped under a sinus mucosal surface it may produce a dome-shaped density similar to that produced by intrasinus cysts or polyps. Soft-tissue swelling produced by edema or hematoma may produce an area of increased density on plain films. CT is especially helpful in locating soft-tissue changes, especially in the periorbital and retrobulbar area.

DIRECT SIGNS

Direct signs are changes in bone on either plain films or CT that specifically indicate bone interruption. Most commonly a separation of bone edges occurs in association with a fracture. This separation interrupts the expected continuity of a cortical line in radiographic studies. If a compressive rather than a shearing force affects the involved bone, the bone may be "buckled" or comminuted in appearance. The same compressive force may produce separation and subsequent overlap, producing a "thickening" in appearance of the involved area. In some fractures only displacement in position of the involved bony area will indicate the presence of a fracture. Air present in the orbital or intracranial regions strongly indicates a fracture extending through a nearby sinus.[3]

RADIOGRAPHIC PATTERNS OF MIDFACIAL INJURIES

Two broad categories typify the forms of midfacial injuries. Local fractures apply to injuries that produce a limited area of involvement in the facial area over which a blow lands. Only local injury results because the injuring object travels with relatively low velocity. Usually these fractures consist of small fragments and require only local repositioning and fixation. Local fracture varieties include orbital margin fracture, orbital blow-out fracture, nasal fracture, zygomatic arch fracture, ZMC fracture, frontal process of maxilla fracture, and mixed midfacial fractures.

Complex injuries result from application to facial structures of much stronger force such as that produced by an auto accident. In these injuries, local comminution is present at the site of contact. In addition, strong shearing forces produce interruption throughout a large facial area and result in a much larger free fragment, or sometimes, several large separated facial bone fragments. Complex facial fractures include Le Fort I fracture, Le Fort II fracture, Le Fort III fracture, mixed Le Fort fractures, and "burst" fracture.

Local Midfacial Fractures

Orbital Margin Fractures
The upper and lower orbital borders curve into a perpendicular position and represent

promontories that may be fractured by a local blow.

The right outer orbital rim in Figure 3–9a has been struck and divided into two small fragments overlying the lacrimal gland area.

Similarly a local blow has interrupted the left inferior orbital rim in the patient illustrated by Figure 3–9b. In this Waters view the infraorbital canal on the right is intact, as is the inferior orbital rim. An oval soft-tissue density is present in the upper left maxilla. The infraorbital canal is rotated into the sinus and a defect in the inferior orbital rim is present.

Orbital Blow-out Fracture
The first description of the orbital blow-out fracture was by King and Samuel.[4] They described downward displacement of the orbital floor without damage to the orbital margin surrounding the facial bones. That the orbital margin is intact is the most significant radiologic feature. The orbital floor fracture and displacement are posterior to the inferior orbital margins.

Because the best view for the inferior orbital border is the Waters projection, this view is used as an initial means of evaluating orbital integrity. In Figure 3–10a, the examination shows an intact orbital margin on both sides. However, the right maxillary sinus is opaque because the patient had received a blow to his eye on this side.

The Caldwell view best defines the orbital floor, as seen in Figure 3–10b, in which both anterior and posterior cortical borders of the floor are evident on the left side. Similarly, in the Waters view (Fig. 3–10a), the posterior orbital floor line is visible on the left. This line projects across the upper maxillary sinus cell. The orbital floor is markedly displaced downward on the right side in both views.

Coronal and lateral polytomographic examination, used for further evaluation previously, has largely been replaced by CT evaluation to diminish the x ray exposure needed for the examination. Figure 3–10c illustrates the CT appearance of an orbital blow-out fracture.

Similar blow-out change in the ethmoid area occurs in about 40% of patients with an orbital floor fracture.

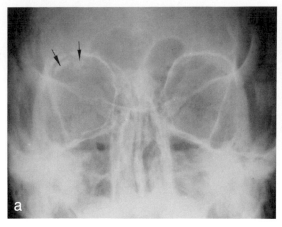 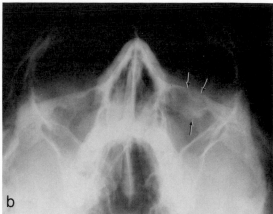

FIG. 3–9. Orbital margin fractures. **a,** Two fragments (arrows) resulting from an upper right orbital rim injury. **b,** Left inferior orbital rim fracture. A soft-tissue mass is present in the upper sinus (arrows), and the infraorbital canal is no longer evident.

Nasal Fracture

An underexposed lateral view best shows the nasal bones and is used to illustrate any transverse nasal fracture. Figure 3–11a illustrates a nasal tip fracture on an underexposed lateral view of the nose.

A more extensive nasal injury is evident in Figure 3–11b in which a tip fragment and a transverse fracture are illustrated.

Though seldom used to define local nasal injury, CT shows such injury to good advantage. Figures 3–11c and 3–11d are two frames of a CT exam showing distortion in the shape of the nasal arch caused by fracture and separation of the nasal bones from their maxillary attachments.

Longitudinally oriented nasal fractures are best demonstrated using the Waters view.

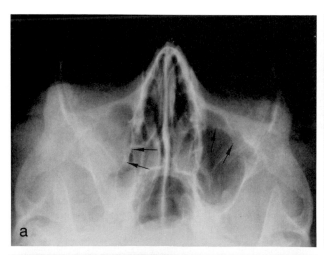 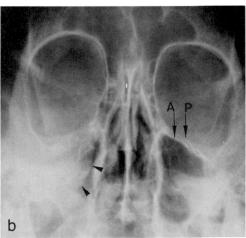

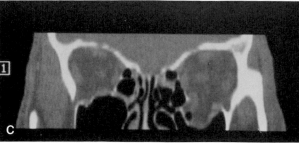

FIG. 3–10. Right orbital blow-out fracture. **a,** Waters view with intact orbital rims. The right maxillary sinus is opaque. Posterior orbital floor (vertical arrows). Blow-out fracture (horizontal arrows). **b,** Caldwell view with intact anterior (A) and posterior (P) orbital floor surfaces. Markedly displaced orbital floor (arrowheads). **c,** Coronal CT of a right-sided blow-out fracture.

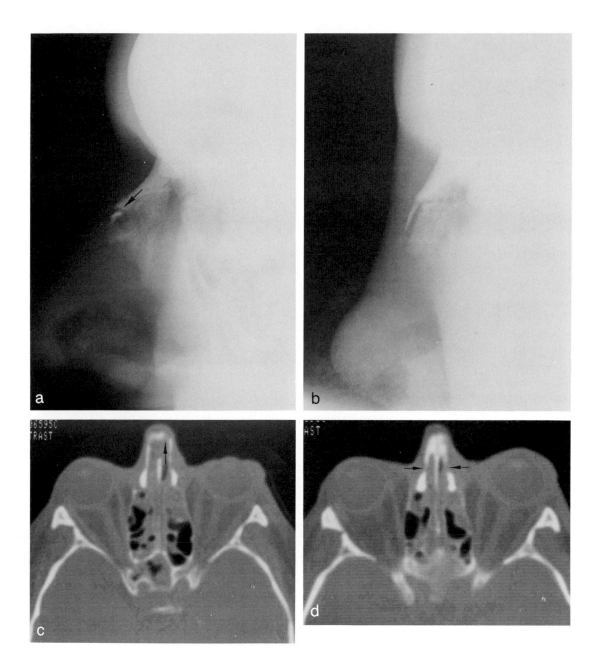

FIG. 3–11.   Nasal fractures. **a,** Underexposed lateral view to show a nasal tip fracture (arrow). **b,** Under-exposed lateral view with more extensive tip injury and an associated transverse fracture. **c,** Axial CT showing a left nasal fracture (arrow). **d,** Axial CT at higher level with separation of the nasal bones from the maxillary process (arrows).

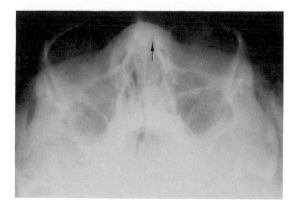

FIG. 3–12.   Waters view revealing a severely comminuted nasal arch fracture. A longitudinal fracture is evident on the left (arrow).

The nasal bones may be so comminuted by injury that the nasal arch is no longer recognizable as such. Figure 3–12 illustrates such an extensive local injury. A separated longitudinal fracture is present on the left. Injury such as this may imply a combination injury of the nose and an adjacent skeletal portion such as the frontal bone or orbital process of the maxilla. These fractures will be considered below with mixed injuries.

Zygomatic Arch Fracture

The typical zygomatic arch fracture is best illustrated in the underexposed basal projection. Some radiographers use a basal projection in which the head is slightly tilted away from the injured side. This position helps avoid superimposition in the skull and is termed the bucket-handle view. Because only one zygomatic arch can be demonstrated this way, a view of each side is usually needed for comparison purposes. Figure 3–13a is a bucket-handle view of one side and shows an example of the "typical" zygomatic arch fracture in which a central "inbending" fracture is present and two "outbending" fractures are also found. One outbent fracture lies in front of and one lies behind the area of inbending.

Distortion in position of the arch characterizes the appearance of a zygomatic arch fracture in Waters postion. As seen in Figure 3–13b, the right zygomatic arch is depressed in the center compared to the left. An abnormal linear density is present where the an-

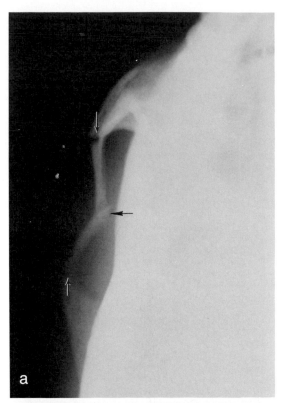

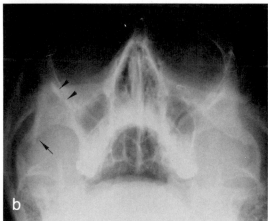

FIG. 3–13.   Right zygomatic arch fracture. **a,** Underexposed basal (bucket-handle) view with a central depressed fracture (arrow) and an anterior and posterior outbending fracture (vertical arrows). **b,** Waters view of same patient. The central depression is evident (arrow). An abnormal linear density is present at the overlapping anterior fracture edge (arrowheads). (A repaired left tripod fracture is present.)

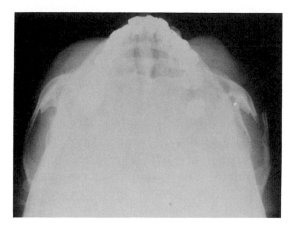

FIG. 3–14.   Zygomatic arch fracture variation. Note that the anterior limb of the arch fracture is peripheral to the zygoma body.

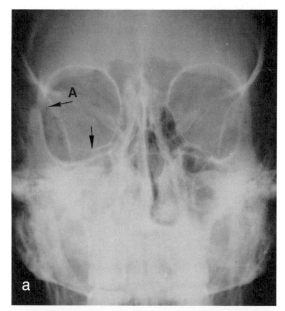

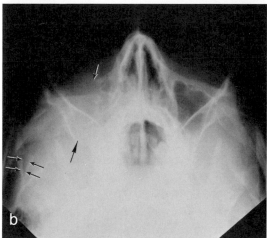

FIG. 3–15.   The ZMC (tripod) fracture. **a,** Caldwell view with zygomaticofrontal suture separation and lateral position of the zygoma fragment (A). Lateral orbit wall fracture (horizontal arrow). Orbital floor fracture (vertical arrow). **b,** Waters view with trans-maxillary fracture (arrows). Arch fractures (horizontal arrows).

terior portion of the fracture overlaps the zygoma body.

Outward displacement of the zygomatic arch fracture may occur, as seen in Figure 3–14, in which the anterior limb of the arch is lateral to the zygoma body. Information such as this may be very important in planning the positional restoration of this fracture.

Zygoma (ZMC, Tripod) Fracture

Many names are used for the fracture that detaches the zygoma body from its frontal, maxillary, sphenoidal, and temporal articulations. Although the zygoma (malar) bone is nearly quadrangular and has four major surfaces and four articulations, its radiographic appearance resembles a tripod. Zygoma fractures have been termed zygomaticomaxillary complex (ZMC), tripod, trimalar, malar eminence, and zygomaticofacial fractures (see Chapter 9).

The ZMC fracture is probably one of the most common facial injuries. It is usually the result of an altercation, but also often occurs as a result of falls and athletic and vehicular injuries. Nakamura and Gross reported an occurrence of 16.6% in their series.[5] This frequency was second only to nasal (28.8%) and mandible (28.4%) fractures.

Jacoby and Dolan described fragment analysis in connection with this injury.[6] The most consistent finding in ZMC fracture is separation of the zygomaticofrontal suture combined with a fracture through the zygomaticosphenoidal surface of the lateral orbital wall. The zygomatic arch is interrupted and an oblique fracture extends through the zygomatic attachment to the maxilla. Displacement of the resulting fragment may occur in any direction, depending on the direction of force producing the fracture.

The patient illustrated by Figure 3–15a has outward displacement of the orbital process of the zygoma at the zygomaticofacial suture on the Caldwell view. The lateral orbital wall fracture lies just lateral to the oblique orbital line. These changes suggest a ZMC fracture.

The Waters view in Figure 3–15b shows the transmaxillary and zygomatic arch components of the tripod fracture. Clockwise rotation of the zygoma fragment is present. A portion of the anterior orbital floor was separated and displaced along with the orbital margin. The zygomatic arch is angled outward and a posterior limb of the arch fracture nearly reaches the glenoid fossa. The zygoma fragment is displaced downward nearly to the coronoid process.

Companion CT views of this injury are demonstrated in Figure 3–16. The transmaxillary component is seen in Figure 3–16a. Subcutaneous and intrasinus air surround the fracture margins. The zygomatic arch fractures are defined in Figure–16b in which outward angulation of the arch is also present. Figure 3–16c demonstrates the separation between the orbital process of the zygoma and the lateral orbital wall.

Variations of ZMC fractures may occur. I have seen two medially displaced ZMC fractures in which an accompanying optic canal fracture endangered the optic nerve during reduction. Also, if the mouth is closed during injury, the zygoma may be displaced against the coronoid process and prevent opening. Similarly, injury with zygoma displacement when the mouth is open may prevent closure. Bilateral ZMC fractures may mimic the Le Fort II fracture.

Mixed Midfacial Fractures

Injuries of adjacent portions of the facial skeleton may occur as a result of a blow from a broad object. Nasal fractures may be associated with adjacent injury of the frontal process of the maxilla and orbital rim, as demonstrated by Figure 3–17. In this patient a large inferior medial orbital margin fragment has been displaced along with the frontal process of the maxilla and nasal arch on the right side. Compressive injury of the subadjacent nasolacrimal duct resulted.

The upper inner orbital margin in Figure 3–18 is interrupted along the lateral frontal and ethmoid sinus surfaces. An associated nasal arch fracture is present.

Extensive nasal comminution should suggest the presence of an injury to the entire nasal-frontal-ethmoid complex. A mosaic of frontal sinus surface fractures is present in Figure 3–19a along with marked comminution the nasal arch and lamina papyracea. A lateral view in Figure 3–19b shows posterior displacement of the frontal sinus surface and nasal bones into the ethmoidal complex interrupting the ethmoid roof. Although one might expect pneumocephalus with such an injury, it was not present at the time of this examination. Cerebrospinal fluid rhinorrhea did occur several weeks after injury, presumably due to clot retraction at the later date.

Complex Midfacial Fractures

The study of Nakamura and Gross revealed that nearly 20% of their cases involved multiple portions of the facial skeleton.[5]

Le Fort first investigated complex fractures in a study conducted at the turn of the century.[7] Using a variety of injuring objects, he found consistent planes of weakness of the facial skeleton. The basic forms of facial weakness found by Le Fort are still valid, although he could not predict the very violent injuries resulting from modern auto accidents.

The first plane of weakness is transmaxillary. When force is applied in the anteroposterior direction of the palatal plane, separation of the palate occurs along the midportion of the maxillary sinus walls and the pterygoid processes.

We prefer to begin the imagery evaluation of complex injury by identifying the pterygoid processes on the lateral view. Figure 3–20a is the lateral view of a Le Fort I injury in which the pterygomaxillary surface is interrupted. This change is common to all of the Le Fort injuries. The Waters view in Figure 3–20b shows counterclockwise rotation of the lower maxillary fragment and rather broad separation of a right lateral maxillary wall fracture. Comminution of the medial maxillary walls is present. The left lateral maxillary wall is fractured, but only a subtle overlap of bone signifies the location of the fracture. In this patient, the displacement resulted from force

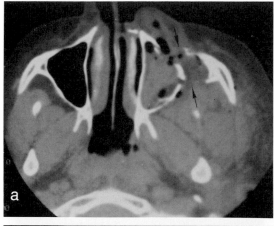

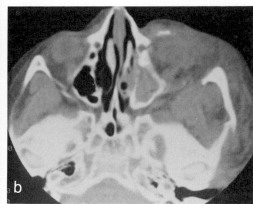

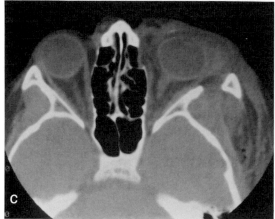

FIG. 3–16.   CT examination of the ZMC (tripod) fracture. **a,** Axial view through the transmaxillary component (arrows). **b,** Axial view of the zygomatic arch component. **c,** Transorbital axial view with separation of the lateral orbital wall.

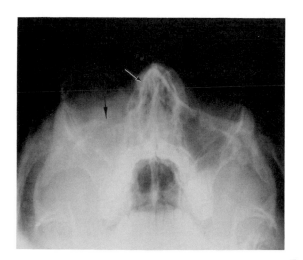

FIG. 3–17.   A Waters view with fracture of the inferomedial orbital margin, frontal process of the maxilla, and nasal arch on the right (arrows).

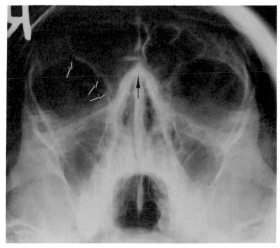

FIG. 3–18.   Waters view showing right upper inner orbital rim fractures (arrows) extending into the frontal and ethmoid sinuses. A nasal arch fracture is also present (midline arrow).

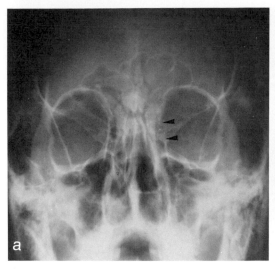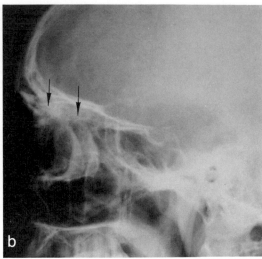

FIG. 3–19. Comminuted frontonasal ethmoid complex injury. **a,** Caldwell view with frontal sinus surface mosaic fracture. Nasal arch is nearly unrecognizable. Lamina papyracea fractures present (arrowheads). **b,** Lateral view with posterior displacement of the nasal and frontal bones into the ethmoid surface. Ethmoid roof comminuted (arrows).

applied in a right anterolateral direction. An anterior open bite position has resulted from the fracture. The zygomatic and orbital portions are intact.

The Le Fort II fracture is described as a central pyramidal fracture with interruption across the lateral maxillary-inferior orbital plane, across the nasoethmoid or nasofrontal plane, and down across the opposite inferior orbital-lateral maxillary border. The pterygoid plates are interrupted. A large central, roughly triangular fragment results. Comminution is usually present at the contract point.

Figure 3–21a is the Waters view of a patient with a Le Fort II fracture. Comminution is present over the nasal arch. An oblique inferior orbital-lateral maxillary interruption is present on both sides. Counterclockwise rotation of the central fragment is present. The zygomatic and lateral orbitral walls are intact.

The Caldwell view in Figure 3–21b shows the nasofrontal fracture to best advantage. Caudal displacement of the central fragment is present.

Gentry et al. introduced the "strut concept" to CT evaluation of complex fractures.[8,9] They describe the lateral orbital walls and nasofrontal bones as vertical struts. The zygomatic arches and inferior orbital rims are horizontal struts. The medial and lateral maxillary sinus walls are lower vertical struts that are bridged by the horizonal hard palate strut.

Analysis of the Le Fort II fracture lends itself well to the strut analysis, as seen in Figure 3–22. Figure 3-22a is a midmaxillary CT slice in which the anterior and lateral fracture components of a Le Fort II injury are evident. Both pterygoid plates are fractured. Figure 3–22b is in the plane of the inferior orbital rim and shows an oblique fracture through each side. Figure 3–22c is in an orbital plane and shows interruption of the nasal arch.

The Le Fort III fracture (weakness) plane spans the zygomatic arches, lateral orbital walls, and nasofrontal planes to result in craniofacial separation. The inferior orbital rim and maxillary lateral borders are intact. This form of injury is seldom seen. More commonly, the contact side is comminuted and a Le Fort III separation is present as a shearing fracture on the opposite side.

The injury in Figure 3–23 illustrates such a mixed complex injury. In Figure 3–23a, the Waters view shows a left ZMC fracture. A central nasofrontal comminuted fracture is also present, and on the right are the zygomaticofrontal suture and zygomatic arch fractures. The right inferior orbital rim and lateral maxillary wall are intact. Figure 3–23b is a

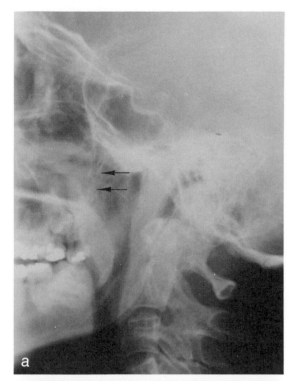

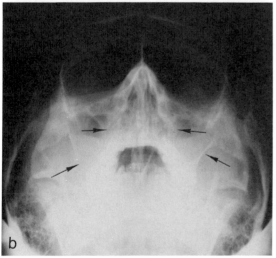

FIG. 3–20. Le Fort I fracture. **a,** Lateral view with pterygomaxillary interruption (arrows). **b,** Waters view with transmaxillary fracture (arrows) and anterior open bite.

Caldwell view detailing the extensive nasofrontal interruption.

Two large fragments are present. The larger follows a transmaxillary (Le Fort II) plane on the right, and traverses the nasofrontal area, right zygomaticofrontal suture, and right zygomatic arch. Clockwise rotation of the large fragment is present. The smaller fragment is a ZMC fragment that is displaced toward the left. Thus, this injury would best be described as a left Le Fort II–ZMC and right Le Fort III fracture. Such a designation would call attention to the disrupted left inferior orbital rim as an interruption requiring fixation, in addition to the need for zygomaticomaxillary suture wiring with suspension.

Figure 3–24 belongs in a category of facial fractures in which extreme comminution characterizes the contact area and in which the larger fragments may be hard to characterize.[3]

The Waters view in Figure 3–24a shows extreme left orbital and maxillary comminution associated with nasal arch comminution and deformity. The left ZMC is displaced nearly 1 cm from the normal position, and the left lateral maxillary wall is similarly displaced. Nasofrontal comminution is highlighted by the Caldwell view in Figure 3–24b. On the right the fracture extends across the canine plane of the maxillary alveolus. Clockwise rotation of the larger maxillary fragment is present. Such an injury almost surpasses description unless it is described in terms of each area of interruption.

Figure 3–25 is a CT examination of a "smash" injury with a contact point over the left maxillary sinus. The midmaxillary (transmaxillary) plane is illustrated by Figure 3–25a and shows the marked left maxillary comminution. Both pterygoid plates are fractured. The right coronoid process of the mandible is fractured and the left condyle is dislocated out of the glenoid fossa and divided in two.

The zygomatic arch plane is shown in Figure 3–25b. In this, the right zygomatic arch is fractured posteriorly near the intact glenoid fossa. The left zygomatic arch is separated from the comminuted zygoma body and glenoid border, and is laterally displaced. Note that the left glenoid fossa is "empty" (condyle dislocation is present above).

The orbital plane is shown in Figure 3–25c. In this view the right lateral orbital wall is interrupted, the nasal arch is deformed, and the entire left lamina papyracea is comminuted. The left lateral orbital wall is intact except along the anterior zygomatic edge.

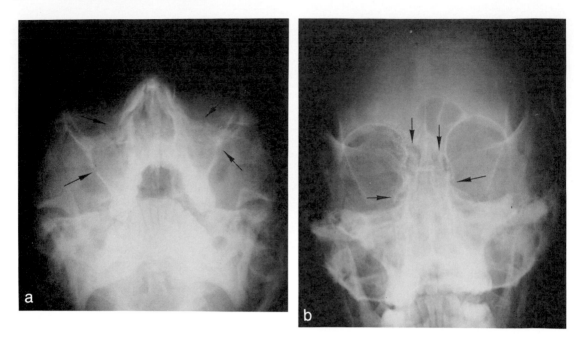

FIG. 3–21.   Le Fort II fracture **a,** Waters view with central (pyramidal) fracture (arrows). **b,** Caldwell view with nasofrontal fracture (arrows).

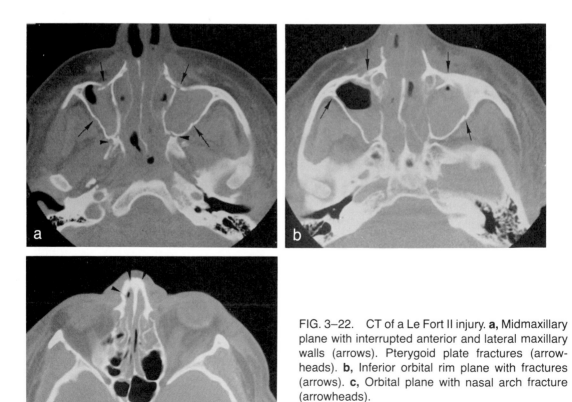

FIG. 3–22.   CT of a Le Fort II injury. **a,** Midmaxillary plane with interrupted anterior and lateral maxillary walls (arrows). Pterygoid plate fractures (arrowheads). **b,** Inferior orbital rim plane with fractures (arrows). **c,** Orbital plane with nasal arch fracture (arrowheads).

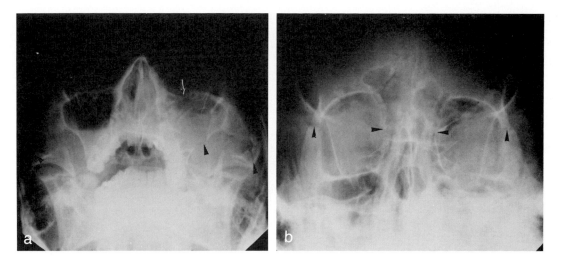

FIG. 3–23.   A mixed complex injury. **a,** Waters view with a left ZMC fragment and a large fragment resulting from a left transmaxillary, nasofrontal, and right zygomaticofrontal suture (lateral orbital) and zygomatic arch fractures (arrow and arrowheads). **b,** Detailed Caldwell view of the nasofrontal fracture. Vertical arrowheads indicate fractures at the frontozygomatic surface area; the horizontal arrowheads, nasal-orbital-ethmoidal fractures.

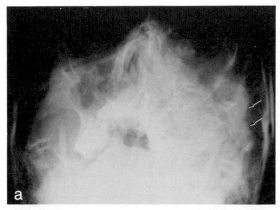

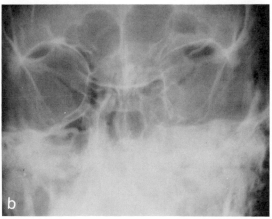

FIG. 3–24.   A left facial "smash" injury. **a,** Waters view with left orbital, nasal, and maxillary comminution. ZMC displaced medially (arrows). **b,** Detailed Caldwell view of the nasofrontal area.

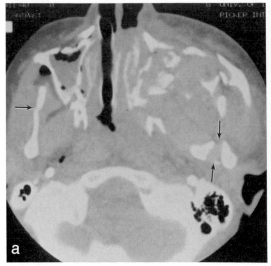
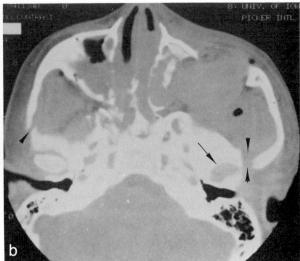
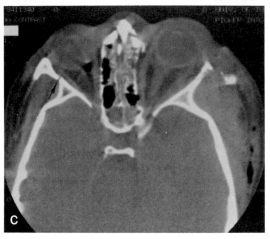

FIG. 3–25. CT examination of a "smash" fracture. **a,** Transmaxillary plane with marked left maxilla comminution. Right coronoid process fracture (horizontal arrow). Left condyle fracture dislocation (vertical arrows). Pterygoid fractures present. **b,** Zygomatic arch plane. Bilateral fractures of the zygomatic processes of the temporal bone (arrowheads). "Empty" glenoid fossa caused by condyle dislocation on the left (arrow). **c,** Transorbital plane with right lateral orbital wall fracture (arrow). Nasal arch interruption. Left lamina papyracea comminution. Sheared-off fragment from anterior zygoma on left.

In this case the CT examination was most important in representing the principal fragments and soft-tissue injury present.

Recognizing the principal fragments of a complex injury is germane to the concept of chain-link wiring and fixation of facial injuries. Plain-film examination gives the best information about perpendicular struts. CT provides the best information about details of the osseous interruption and may help define injuries only suggested by plain film examination.

RADIOGRAPHIC PATTERNS OF MANDIBULAR FRACTURES

The panoramic radiographic devices provide the means of defining the mandible on a single tomographic curved plane. Some injured patients are unconscious or unable to cooperate and therefore are examined using conventional radiographic methods. In most cases, physical diagnostic information uncovers the presence of a mandible fracture, so that radiographs only confirm the location and aid evaluation needed for proper fixation of the fracture.

The conventional Waters, lateral, and basal radiographs provide supplementary information about mandible injury and the temporomandibular joint (TM). Oblique lateral overhead views may give additional information about a mandibular injury near the angle. Tomography is helpful in assessing the (TM) and nearby areas.

Perhaps the most vulnerable portion of the otherwise intact mandible associated with midfacial fractures is the coronoid process. It may be fractured at the tip or sheared near the mandible attachment in association with zygoma fractures. Figure 3–26a is the Waters view of a patient with a comminuted ZMC and zygomatic arch fracture on the right. The right coronoid process is fractured near the tip and is rotated laterally at its base, compared with the unaffected side. The panoramic radiograph in Figure 3–26b shows the oblique fracture through the coronoid base.

Incidental associated fractures may also occur. A right inferior orbital rim fracture is present in Figure 3–27a. Notice, in addition, that the vertical ramus (condyle to mandible angle length) is shorter on the left than on the right. This difference should strongly suggest a fracture of the vertical ramus. The panoramic radiograph in Figure 3–27b reveals an "unfavorable" oblique fracture of the left mandible angle. This fracture is held in place against the adjacent second molar and hence has not been significantly displaced by the medial pterygoid muscle.

An oblique-lateral plain exam may help define a mandible angle fracture suspected from other views. Figure 3–28a is a lateral view in which a step-off of one mandible is suspected. An accompanying Caldwell view in Figure 3–28b shows an overlap density on the right side with vertical ramus elongation. The oblique-lateral mandible view best shows the mandible fracture and displacement, as seen in Figure 3–28c.

Displacement of a mandible angle fracture may produce elongation of the vertical ramus on plain views. The patient whose Waters view is shown in Figure 3–29a had a nasal tip fracture (not shown in this view). In addition, the right vertical ramus is elongated when compared to the left. The panoramic radiograph in Figure 3–29b shows displacement of the mandible angle fracture, which produces the elongation in the Waters view.

Thus, either shortening or lengthening of the vertical ramus image on plain films should suggest the presence of a fracture.

Horizontal ramus fractures, if bilateral, are produced by strong forces such as those associated with an auto accident. Posterior displacement of the central mandibular fragment may be marked and associated tongue displacement that may produce compressive change of the upper airway resulting in respiratory distress.

Such a condition is illustrated by Figure 3–30; the Waters view illustrated in Figure 3–30a shows bilateral oblique horizontal fractures with separation of a large symphyseal free fragment. Figure 3–30b is a lateral view of this fracture in which the central fragment has been displaced posteriorly and obliterates the valleculae as it nears the swollen posterior pharyngeal wall.[10]

Similar strong force is required to produce a vertical fracture in the symphysis area. This type of fracture should signal the possibility of a fracture involving the articular process or neck of the mandible. Separation of the mandibular central incisors is present in the Waters view of Figure 3–31a. This separation is continuous with a central fracture through the mandibular symphysis. Neither mandibular condyle can be seen in the glenoid fossa. A low-positioned panoramic radiograph in Figure 3–31b reveals the symphysis fracture, but does not allow visualization of the articular processes.

A higher-positioned panoramic view not only shows the malpositioned condyles but also illustrates overlap as evidenced by increased density between the condyles and subarticular portions of the mandible, as illustrated by Figure 3–31c.

Condyle displacement is best visualized in the basal projection. The medial condyle displacement in this patient, indeed, is best seen in the basal view of Figure 3–31d. In this examination, each condyle lies in a medial location and the glenoid fossa is empty.

High-energy force application to the mandible may also produce crushing injury of the articular condyle. If this type of injury is suspected, thin-section tomography is the best means of defining the fracture. Figures 3–32a and 3–32b are lateral polytomograms of the right and left temporomandibular joints of a patient who was injured in an auto accident and complained of TMJ pain but grossly had no mandible fracture on plain films. A perpendicular oblique fracture extends just below the articular condyle on the right side. A crushing subarticular fracture is present on the left. Both condyles are abnormal in position. Other views demonstrated fractures of the typmpanic bones on both sides.

Tympanic bone and tympanic membrane

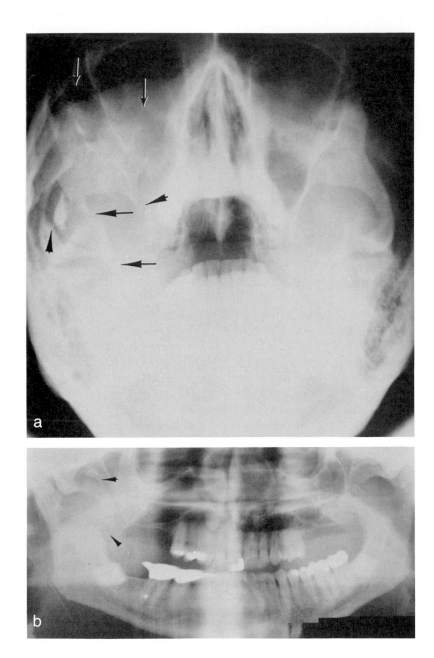

FIG. 3–26.   Right ZMC fracture with comminuted arch and coronoid process fracture. **a,** Waters view with two vertical arrows and two arrowheads indicating the ZMC and the arch fractures. The two horizontal arrows indicate fractures at the base and tip of the coronoid process. **b,** Panoramic radiograph with coronoid tip fracture (upper arrowhead) and coronoid base fracture (lower arrowhead).

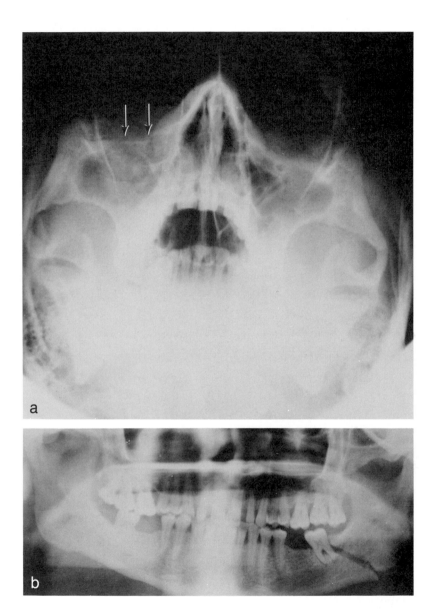

FIG. 3–27. Right inferior orbital rim fracture and left mandibular angle fracture. **a,** Waters view demonstrates a right inferior orbital rim fracture (arrows). The left vertical ramus is shorter than the right (dots). **b,** The panoramic radiograph shows an "unfavorable" mandible angle fracture held in place by an adjacent molar.

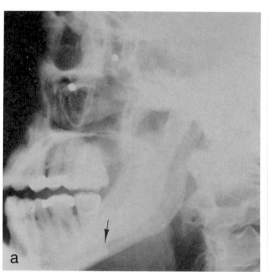

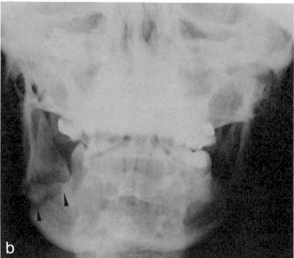

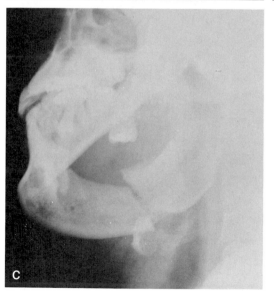

FIG. 3–28.   Right horizontal ramus mandible fracture. **a,** Lateral view with suspicious step-off (arrow). **b,** Caldwell view with double-density (overlap) on right side (arrowheads). **c,** Oblique-lateral view clearly defines the displaced fracture. (Metallic pellets are from a previous injury.)

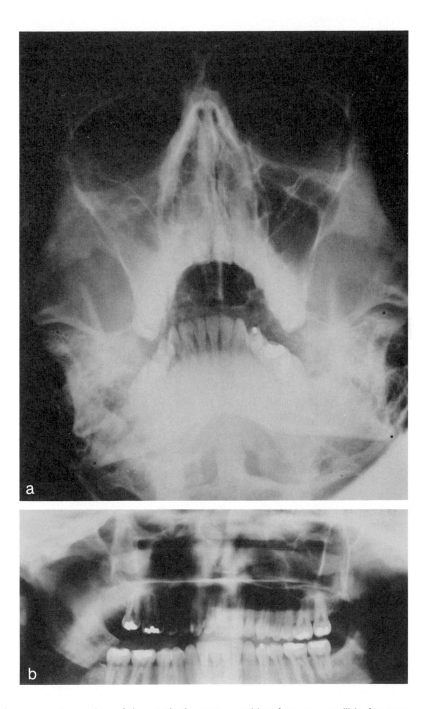

FIG. 3–29.   Apparent elongation of the vertical ramus resulting from a mandible fracture. **a,** Waters view with radiographic elongated right vertical ramus, compared to the left (dots). **b,** Panoramic radiograph showing an impacted right angle fracture that produced the vertical discrepancy.

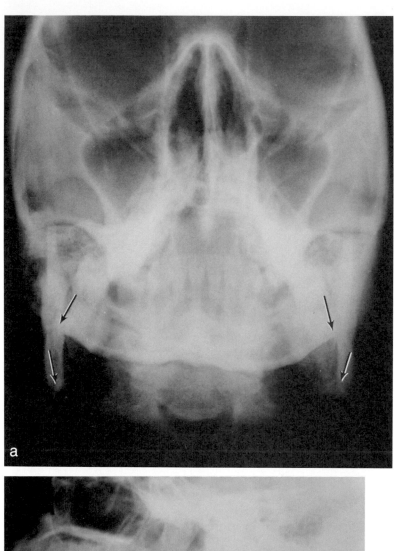

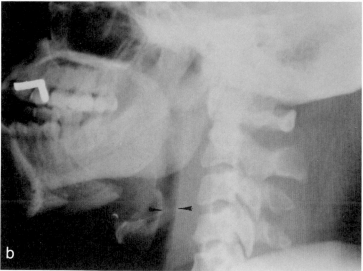

FIG. 3–30.   Bilateral horizontal ramus fracture with posterior displacement of tongue and soft tissues producing respiratory distress. **a,** Waters view with widely separated horizontal ramus fractures (arrows). **b,** Lateral view with posterior displacement of the symphysis fracture with narrow airway (arrowheads).

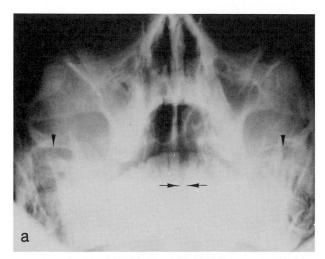

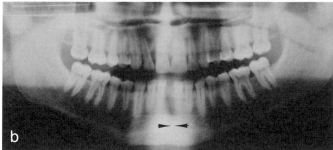

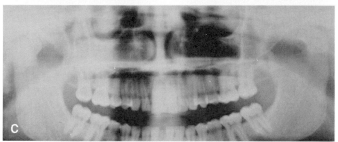

FIG. 3–31. Mandible symphysis fracture with bilateral condyle fractures and dislocation. **a,** Waters view with symphysis fracture (arrows). The glenoid fossa is empty (arrowheads). **b,** Low-positioned panoramic radiograph shows the symphysis fracture (arrowheads). **c,** High-positioned panoramic radiograph shows bilateral condyle fractures and increased density where the fractures overlap the subarticular portion. **d,** Basal projection with empty glenoid fossa (vertical arrowheads). The condyle fragments are displaced medially (horizontal arrowheads).

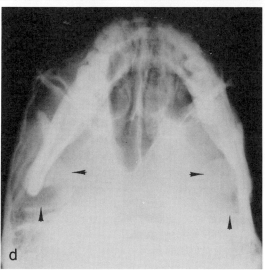

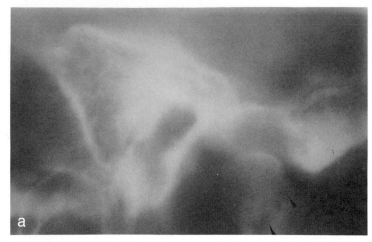

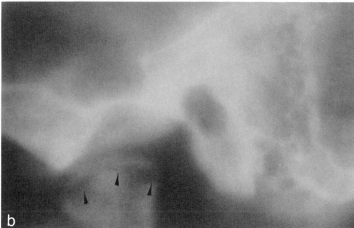

FIG. 3–32. Condyle fractures on thin-section tomography. **a,** Right TMJ with oblique condyle fracture (arrowheads). **b,** Left TMJ with crushing condyle injury (arrowheads).

injuries probably occur frequently in association with mandible fractures when the condyle is displaced posteriorly against the tympanic (posterior) surface of the glenoid fossa. Very strong force through the condyles against the glenoid fossa surface may result in an associated temporal bone fracture.

The patient depicted in Figure 3–33 had a severe mandible fracture in an auto accident. As seen in Figure 3–33a, a PA view of the mandible, the patient had a separated left parasymphyseal fracture and a comminuted right-angle fracture. Bilateral conductive hearing loss was present, as was tympanic membrane laceration. Figure 3–33b is a right lateral tomogram showing a tympanic bone fracture continuous with a fracture through the tegmen tympani of the temporal bone. Slight upward displacement of the tegmen is present.

Even greater separation of the tympanic

and temporal bone fractures is present in Figure 3–33c, which is a tomogram of the left side of this patient. Such an extensive fracture as this may even extend far enough medially to damage the tympanic course of the facial nerve, as occurred in this patient.

The tympanic bone is easy to reduce in these patients by expanding a Vienna nasal speculum of appropriate size in the external canal. The tympanic membrane tear may heal spontaneously or, if it fails to heal, may require tympanoplasty to prevent development of a cholesteatoma. Auditory ossicle dislocation may result in conductive hearing loss and require corrective ossiculoplasty. Injury to the facial nerve may require decompression of the neural canal or even surgical reattachment of the severed nerve or grafting to allow the patient to regain facial nerve function. Another complication of fractures through the tegmen tympani is development of a cerebrospinal

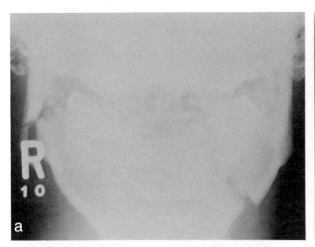

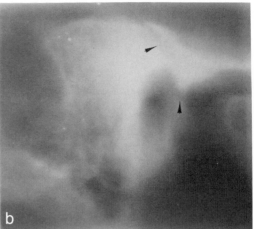

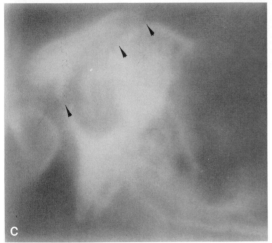

FIG. 3–33. Extensive mandible fractures with tympanic and temporal bone injuries. **a,** A posteroanterior mandible view with an oblique left parasymphyseal fracture and comminuted right-angle fracture. **b,** A thin-section tomogram of the right side with a slightly separated tympanic and tegmen tympani fracture (arrowheads). **c,** A thin-section tomogram of the left side with a similar, but more separated, fracture (arrowheads).

fluid leak if the overlying dura and arachnoid membranes are also torn during the injury. While these injuries and complications are uncommon, radiographic evaluation should lead one to suspect such damage and seek proper otologic care for the patient.

Very rarely the mandibular condyle may be displaced upward through the thin cephalic surface of the glenoid fossa into the temporal fossa of the skull. This injury may produce meningeal and brain injury or bleeding.

One other area of potential injury in association with mandible fractures is the soft tissues of the neck and the airway. As discussed, the large symphysis fragment may allow posterior settling of the tongue and upper airway to produce dyspnea or apnea. Similar respiratory difficulty may result from injury to the hyoid bone or larynx if the object striking the mandible is large enough to compress the neck as well. While the great vessels of the

neck are well cushioned by surrounding muscle to prevent direct injury, occasionally the displaced sharp mandible fracture edge or a sharp object striking the neck may injure the vessels.[11]

Mandibular or maxillary dental prosthetic appliances may be damaged and aspirated during facial or mandibular injury. Neck and chest radiographs may be helpful to identify these usually opaque foreign bodies.

The patient in Figure 3–34 was injured in an auto accident. He suffered a mandible fracture as well as a crushing larynx injury for which tracheostomy was performed. The PA mandible view shows a right mandibular angle fracture and the tracheostomy tube. In addition, the maxillary central and lateral incisors are absent but there is no clinical evidence of maxillary injury. In this view, a tooth and wire from the maxillary bridge are seen along the surface of the epiglottis. The

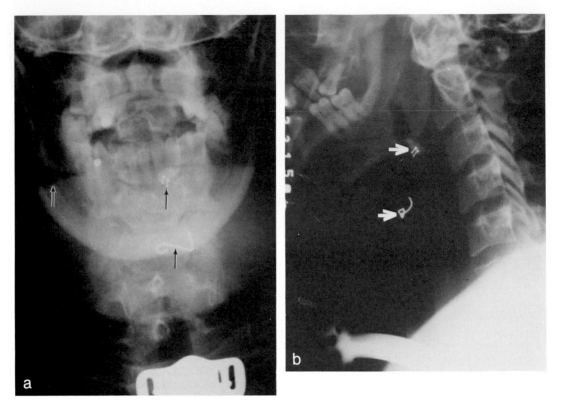

FIG. 3–34. Mandible fracture with aspiration of portions of a maxillary dental bridge. **a,** PA mandible and neck view with a right mandibular angle fracture (arrow) and aspirated dental appliances (central arrows). **b,** Lateral view of the same patient. Tooth and wire in hypopharynx (arrows).

lateral view in Figure 3–34b also shows the mandible fracture and the dental appliances in the hypopharynx. No other foreign bodies were present in a chest examination.

CERVICAL SPINE FRACTURES

Associated injuries are common among patients with facial fractures. Olson and his co-workers found associated injuries in 46.6% of their patients.[12] Schultz reviewed 1000 facial injuries and found 51% with associated injury.[13] Though no percentage for cervical spine fracture was included, he did refer to an earlier study in which 4% of 400 patients had an associated cervical spine fracture.[14]

We recently reviewed the last 10 years' literature on cervical spine fractures. There were 510 articles. Only 2 articles called attention to the association of facial and cervical spine fractures. From this material we conclude that the incidence of cervical spine injury with facial injury is uncommon.

Radiographic Views

Most patients with cervical spine injury are symptomatic. The diagnostic problem is greatest in the unconscious patient who is unable to describe the presence of pain.

If a cervical fracture is suspected, a complete examination including AP, lateral, and both oblique views of the cervical spine should be obtained. Tomography is used as a detail study of any cervical spine part that is suspicious on plain films. CT is helpful to display fractures hidden from view on plain examination and is of greatest use in evaluating the presence of fracture fragments lying within the cervical spinal canal.

Although customarily views are obtained on a 20-by 25-cm film, a 28-by 35-cm format is useful for including views of both the head and neck in one image, which allows evaluation of the skull, face, mandible, and neck in one examination and serves to provide more rapid filming. The large-format tabletop views are somewhat magnified, but present no difficulty to the experienced examiner.

Figure 3–35a illustrates a lateral examination obtained on the large-film format. Position and alignment of the cervical spine is well portrayed, and the joint spaces are of normal width. Each vertebral body is normal in size and not compressed. The odontoid process and atlas vertebra are likewise normal in appearance. Each articular process is in normal position. The neural arches and spinous processes are intact. Unfortunately, the scattered radiation used for the large-format view does not allow for evaluation of the prevertebral soft tissues, as does the standard format. Certain features should be evaluated in the lateral cervical spine examination: depiction of all 7 vertebrae; prevertebral soft-tissue thickness; position and alignment; joint space width; craniovertebral junction position; atlas; odontoid process; vertebral body height; articular process position; and neural arches and spinous process.

Figure 3–35b is a conventional AP view that includes C-3 through C-7 and the upper three thoracic vertebrae and ribs. Generally this view is useful for evaluating alignment, the pedicles, and spinous processes. The position of the outer articular process borders is evident. Unfortunately, the mandible overlies the upper cervical spine in this view. If the patient is able to cooperate, an AP open mouth view may be obtained. If the patient is unable to cooperate because of injury, tomograpic views of the upper cervical spine may be obtained if injury is suspected.

The oblique examination is illustrated by Figure 3–35c. This view shows only the left-sided features and would be accompanied by another view showing right-sided features. The oblique view is used to study the intervertebral canal size and shape, the homolateral pedicles, and the articular processes.

The cervical spine is divided into upper and lower parts. The upper part includes the occiput, the atlas, and the upper axis and the odontoid process. The lower cervical spine includes the lower half of the axis and the lower five cervical vertebrae.

Injuries of the upper cervical spine are infrequent but often produce cervical spinal cord injury. Lower cervical spine injuries are frequent but less commonly damage the spinal cord.

Instability of a cervical spine fracture refers to the potential for injury to the spinal cord. Stability of a given fracture depends not only on the integrity of bone structures, but also on ligamentous support. Therefore, although little bone abnormality may be present, the cervical spine may be very unstable because of ligamentous injury that may be difficult to detect on radiographs unless an unusual position or alignment is present.

Atlanto-occipital Junction

Craniovertebral junction dislocation results in wide separation between the occipital condyles and the atlas articular processes. As shown in Figure 3–36, separation between the basion (inferior tip of the clivus) and the dens (odontoid process) may occur.

Atlas

The principal atlas injury resulting from head injury is the so-called Jefferson fracture. This injury is created by application of a long axis force so that a vertical force acting between the occipital condyles and the axis superior articular facets results in lateral displacement of the atlas articular facets. This force produces a fracture through the anterior and posterior arches of the atlas and increases the size of this ring-shaped bone. As a result, the peripheral margin of the atlas is lateral to the outer margin of the axis superior facet, as seen in Figure 3–37a. While this injury can produce subtle changes in position on lateral views, tomograms ordinarily are necessary to visualize the anterior and posterior arch fractures, as in Figures 3–37b and 3–37c.

Typically this fracture is considered unstable, but usually no neurologic injury accompanies the Jefferson fracture.

The atlas posterior arch may also be fractured by an extension injury in which the arch is sheared off of the articular process attachments when the occiput is forced downward against the arch. This fracture is stable and looks like the posterior arch injury in the Jefferson fracture.

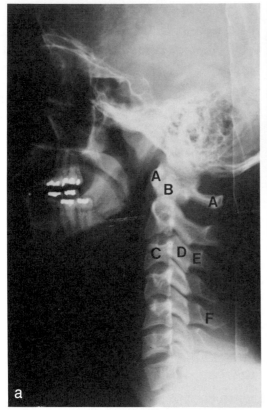

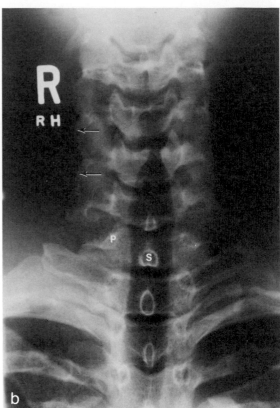

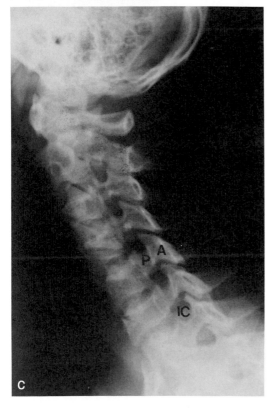

FIG. 3–35. Normal cervical spine examination. **a,** Lateral head and neck survey view. Atlas anterior and posterior arches (A). The dens (B). Vertebral body (C). Articular process (D). Neural arch (E). Spinous process (F). **b,** AP cervical spine view. Pedicles (P). Spinous process (S). Outer articular process border (arrowheads). **c,** A left oblique cervical spine view. Intervertebral canal (IC). Pedicle (P). Articular process (A).

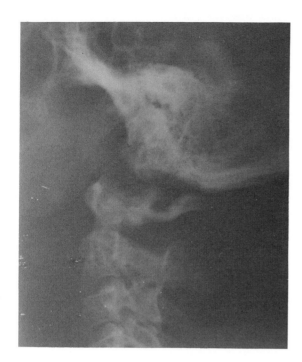

FIG. 3–36.   Atlanto-occipital dislocation.

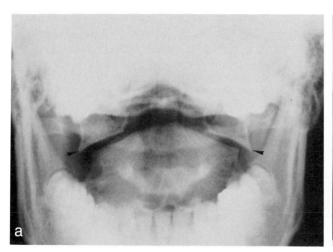

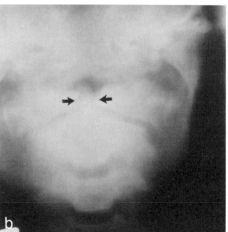

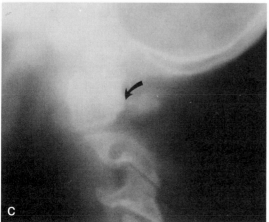

FIG. 3–37.   Jefferson fracture of the atlas. **a,** AP view with displaced atlas facets (arrowheads). **b,** AP tomogram through atlas anterior arch fracture. **c,** Lateral tomogram showing posterior arch fracture.

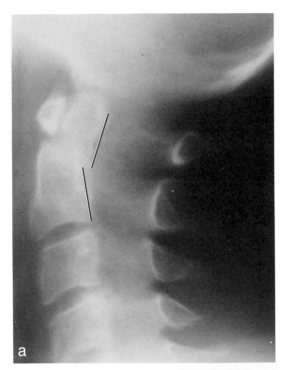

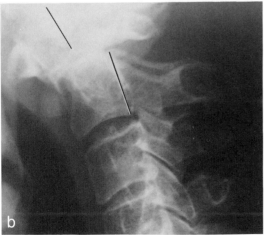

FIG. 3–38. Odontoid process fractures. **a,** Extension injury with posterior odontoid displacement (lines). **b,** Flexion injury with anterior odontoid displacement (lines).

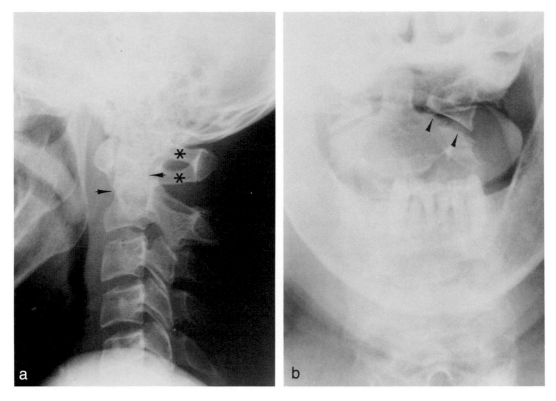

FIG. 3–39. Odontoid process fracture with axis superior facet fracture on the left. **a,** Lateral view with tipped atlas posterior arch (*). Odontoid fracture (arrowheads). **b,** AP open-mouth view with crushing fracture of the left superior axis facet (arrowheads).

Axis

The odontoid process projects upward from the axis vertebral body. It is held in close position to the anterior arch of the atlas by a strong cruciform ligament. Flexion and extension injury may shear the odontoid process from the axis. The cruciform ligament typically holds the odontoid in close proximity to the anterior atlas arch after a fracture and produces step-off along the posterior surface.

In Figure 3–35a one can easily identify the inferior axis vertebrae articular surface. From this the posterior axis vertebral body surface can be followed superiorly along the posterior odontoid surface to the tip of the process. The anterior odontoid surface can similarly be followed downward to the anterior axis vertebral body surface.

Posterior displacement of the odontoid occurs with an extension fracture of the odontoid, as seen in Figure 3–38a. Anterior odontoid displacement results from a flexion force,

as seen in Figure 3–38b. Both types of injury are unstable but do not often have associated neural injury.

Transverse positional change in the atlas may reflect axis injury. In Figure 3–39a the lateral view shows great separation of the posterior atlas arches while the axis neural arches are nearly superimposed. In addition there is a subtle odontoid process fracture just at its base.

This injury is the result of a lateral bending injury force. The open mouth odontoid view in Figure 3–39b fails to show the odontoid fracture but does demonstrate a fracture of the left axis superior facet that produced the tilted atlas position.

Rotatory dislocation of the atlas and axis may occur, with or without an axis superior facet injury. The lateral view in Figure 3–40a shows the atlas tilting similar to that in Figure 3–39. In addition, the atlas articular facet on one side extends in front of the odontoid, while that on the opposite side is posterior.

The AP view in Figure 3–40b shows a left superior axis facet fracture. The right lateral tomogram in Figure 3–40c shows posterior position of the atlas articular process in relation to the axis superior facet. On the left, as shown in Figure 3–40d, the atlas articular process is anterior and has been displaced downward, fracturing the front of the axis facet beneath it.

A fracture extending between the superior and inferior axis articular processes has been termed the interarticular fracture or traumatic spondylolisthesis (also known, incorrectly, as the hangman's fracture). In my case series there are 14 examples of this injury, 3 accompanying facial fractures and 1 associated with a mandible fracture. All but 1 of the fractures resulted from flexion injury and were easily reduced with the patient in an extension position. None in our series had an accompanying spinal cord injury.

Figure 3–41 demonstrates the interarticular axis fracture. Marked prevertebral swelling is present. The anterior vertebral body margins of C-2–C-3 are near one another, indicating an intact anterior longitudinal ligament. The posterior vertebral body margins are separated, indicating a tear of the posterior longitudinal ligament. The fracture extends between the superior and inferior axis articular processes. Separation of the atlas and axis posterior neural arches indicates a tear through the ligamentum flavum and atlantoaxial ligaments. The injury is unstable.

A variation of the interarticular fracture is demonstrated in Figure 3–42. The fracture in this patient is through the neural arch of the axis and into the inferior articular facets. Posterior longitudinal ligament laceration is indicated by the anterior displacement of the axis vertebral body. Moderate prevertebral soft-tissue swelling is present. This fracture type is unstable. The patient also had a frontal-ethmoid facial fracture.

Fractures through the axis vertebral body below the odontoid process may occur, as shown in Figure 3–43 in which anterior displacement of the upper axis vertebral body and odontoid process results from a flexion injury. Because a posterior ligamentous tear is also present through the atlantoaxial ligaments, this fracture is unstable.

Lower Cervical Fractures

Vertebral Body Fractures

Vertebral body compression fractures may best be identified by a difference between the anterior and posterior vertebral body height. This difference may occur with or without accompanying displacement of other structures.

The C4 compression fracture in Figure 3–44a has resulted in an anterior angulation in position at the C4-C5 levels. Slight prevertebral soft-tissue swelling is present. Posterior ligament injury is reflected by separation of the C4-C5 neural arches and spinous processes. Therefore, the fracture is unstable.

Multilevel compression fractures may occur and result in marked distortion in position, as demonstrated in Figure 3-44b. Marked prevertebral soft-tissue swelling is present. Instability is indicated by ligamentous injury, producing separation of the posterior elements at C5-C6.

Perhaps the most serious vertebral body fracture is the "bursting" fracture in which a vertebral body is so crushed by flexion that a traumatic disc extrusion occurs into the spinal neural canal. In Figure 3–45a an oblique fracture extends through the anteroinferior third of C6. This extension results in downward rotation of C6 against the superior articular surface of C7. This force shears off the anteroinferior vertebral fragment and allows posterior displacement of the larger vertebral fragment, producing reversed angulation of the posterior vertebral surfaces. In addition, the extreme force applied to the involved vertebral body results in a perpendicular fracture that divides the two halves of the vertebral body. This perpendicular fracture is best defined in AP tomograms, as illustrated by Figure 3–45b.

Vertebral Dislocation

Bilateral articular facet dislocation is usually easy to identify. Marked step-off of the vertebral bodies occurs, as seen in Figure 3–46 where a C5-C6 complete dislocation is present. The C5 inferior articular facets lie anterior to the C6 superior facets, and spinous process separation is present. The facet engagement

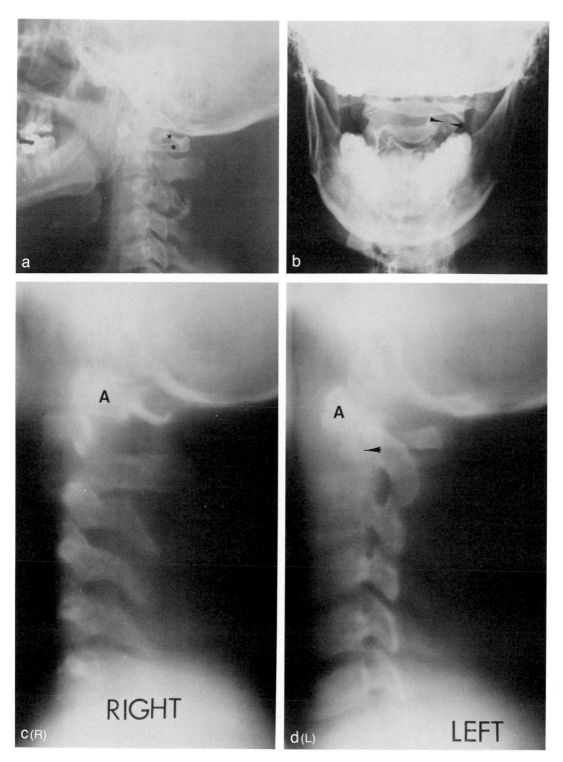

FIG. 3–40.   Rotatory atlas-axis dislocation with left superior axis facet fracture. **a,** Lateral view with rotated, tipped atlas, as seen by converging processes. **b,** AP open-mouth view with left superior axis facet fracture (arrowheads). **c,** Right lateral tomogram with posterior position of the atlas articular process (A). **d,** Left lateral tomogram with anterior position of the atlas articular process (A) and a fracture through the superior axis facet (arrowhead).

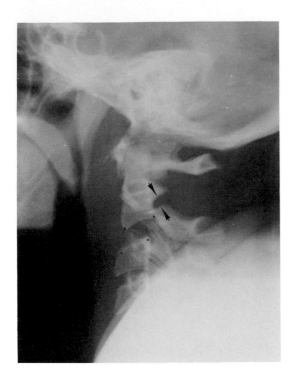

FIG. 3–41. Interarticular fracture of the axis. Vertebral body margins (dots). Fracture (arrowheads).

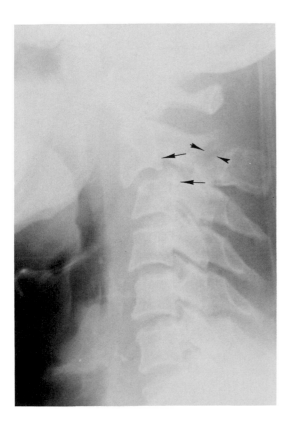

FIG. 3–42. Variation of the axis interarticular fracture in which the neural arch is fractured posteriorly (arrowheads) and posterior longitudinal ligament injury is reflected by the C2-C3 vertebral body step-off (arrows).

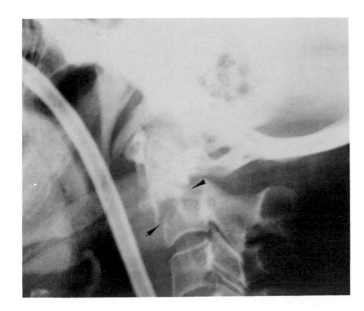

FIG. 3–43. Fracture through the axis vertebral body (arrowheads) with anterior displacement of the upper fragment.

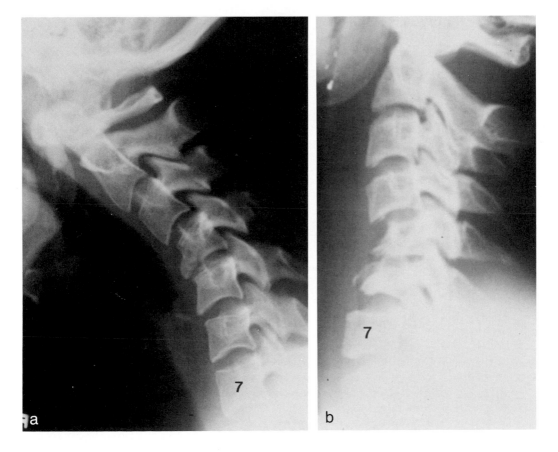

FIG. 3–44. Vertebral body compresson fractures. **a,** Single C4 compression fracture with angulation. **b,** Multiple compression fractures with angulation.

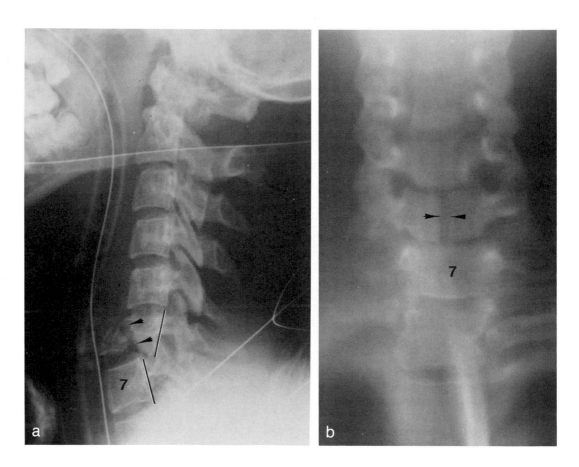

FIG. 3–45.   Vertebral body bursting fracture. **a,** Lateral view with an oblique anteroinferior fracture (arrowheads). Posterior angulation indicated along the posterior vertebral body surface (lines). **b,** AP tomogram to illustrate the perpendicular separation of the two vertebral body portions (arrowheads).

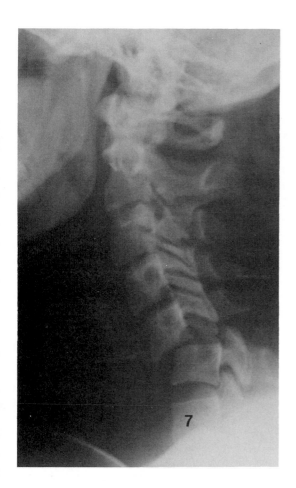

FIG. 3–46.   Bilateral C5-C6 dislocation with inter-lock. Note the C5 facets lie anterior to those of C6.

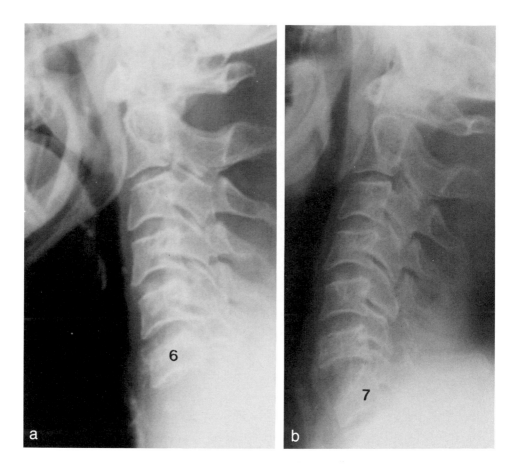

FIG. 3–47.   Fracture-dislocation of C7 hidden by large shoulders. **a,** Only the upper six vertebrae are well-defined. **b,** Postreduction view showing that C7 compression fracture also was responsible for the hidden vertebra.

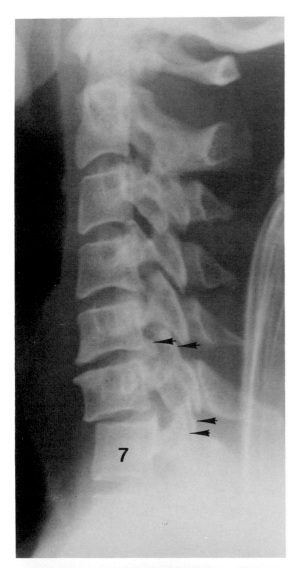

FIG. 3–48.   Unilateral C6-C7 facet dislocation. C7 facets superimposed (lower arrowheads). C6 facets rotated (upper arrowheads).

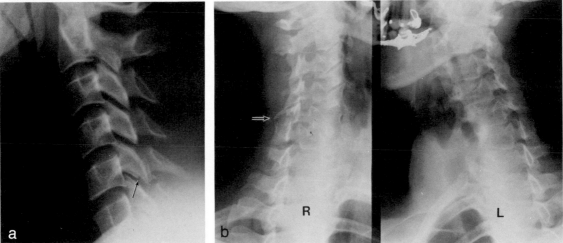

FIG. 3–49.   Unilateral articular process fracture. **a,** Essentially normal–appearing lateral view with questionable facet fracture on one side of C5 (arrow). **b,** Oblique views show an obliterated intervertebral canal at C5-C6 and a facet fracture of C5 (arrow) on the right side.

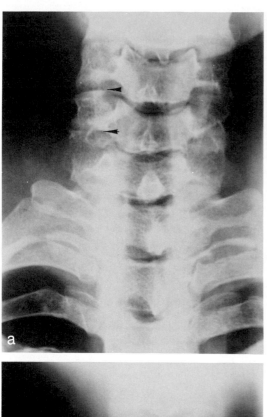

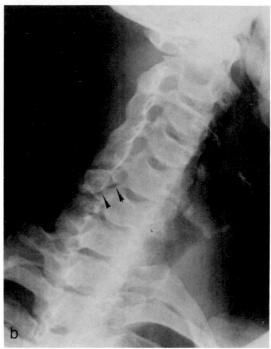

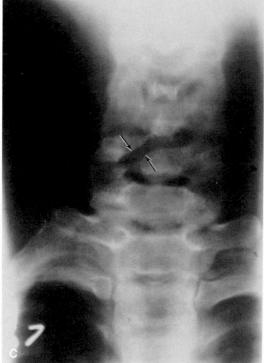

FIG. 3–50. Facet complex fracture. **a,** An AP view with rotation in position of the right C6 facet (arrowheads). **b,** An oblique view shows the pedicle fracture (arrowheads). **c,** An AP tomogram shows the oblique neural arch fracture (arrows).

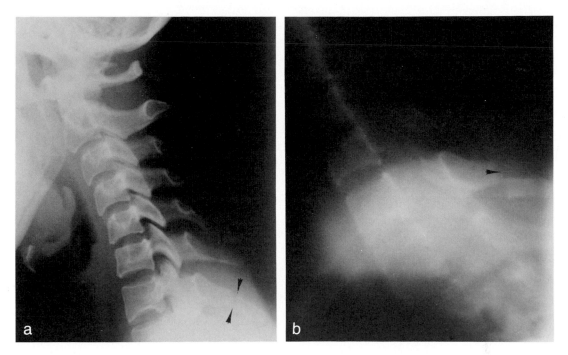

FIG. 3–51.   Spinous process fracture. **a,** Lateral view with angled C7 spinous process (arrowheads). **b,** Lateral tomogram reveals the fracture (arrowhead).

results in the so-called interlock position, which may be difficult to reduce. This type of dislocation often produces direct spinal cord injury or produces vertebral artery vascular injury with paralysis.

The lowest portion of the cervical spine may be difficult to visualize in a patient with a short neck or with large shoulders because soft tissues may obscure C7. The patient in Figure 3–47a can easily be evaluated through C6. If one notes the distance between the adjacent vertebral corners, it is seen that where one would expect to see the anterior upper corner of C7, no vertebra is evident. This lack should strongly suggest the presence of a dislocation and indicate the need for repositioning by pulling on the arms (if uninjured) to lower the shoulders or by doing a tomographic study. A repeat examination after reduction is shown in Figure 3–47b, which illustrates the presence of a compression fracture that was also present at C7.

Unilateral articular facet dislocation is the most difficult problem to analyze among the cervical injuries. The only clue to this injury is the presence of articular process separation adjacent to the level of normal facet position.

Also, a slight step-off is usually present with respect to the vertebral body position. The C6-C7 step-off is easily seen in Figure 3–48. While the C7 superior articular facets nearly overlap, there is separation of the C6 inferior facets as well as rotation of all facets above C6. Tomography may be helpful in demonstrating this abnormality.

Facet Fracture

Unilateral facet fracture may be difficult to identify because of overlap by a normal articular process. The radiograph of the patient in Figure 3–49 suggests a facet fracture of the C5. Oblique views as shown in Figure 3–49b demonstrate normal right facets. The left C5 facet has been crushed, nearly obliterating the intervertebral canal between C5 and C6.

Two of our patients with mandible fractures have had such articular process fractures. Usually the subadjacent nerve root is also damaged by this injury.

The entire articular process may be separated from the remaining vertebra by a fracture through the pedicle (anterior attachment) and the neural arch (posterior attachment).

This separation results in facet rotation so that the facet joint becomes evident in the AP view, as seen in Figure 3-50a. An oblique view, Figure 3-50b, shows the pedicle fracture. The neural arch component was evident only on an AP tomogram in Figure 3–50c. The facet complex fracture is unstable and usually also injures the adjacent cervical nerve root.

Spinous Process

Spinous process fractures occur in the lower cervical spine as a result of direct trauma or the fatigue fracture known as the clay shoveler's fracture. In Figure 3–51a angulation of the C7 spinous process suggested a fracture that was confirmed in a lateral tomogram shown in Figure 3–51b. These fractures result in neither instability nor neural injury.

REFERENCES

1. Littleton, J.T.: Tomography: Physical Principles and Clinical Applications. Baltimore, Williams and Wilkins Co., 1976.
2. Lee, S.H., and Rao, C.V.G.: Cranial Computed Tomography. New York, McGraw-Hill, 1983.
3. Dolan, K.D., Jacoby, C.G., and Smoker, W.R.K.: The Radiology of Facial Fractures. Radiography 4:576–663, 1984.
4. King, E.F., and Samuel, E.: Fractures of the orbit. Trans Ophthalmol Soc U.K. 64:134–153, 1944.
5. Nakamura, T., and Gross, C.W.: Facial fractures. Arch Otolaryngol 97:288–290, 1973.
6. Jacoby, C.G., and Dolan, K.D.: Fragment analysis in maxillofacial injuries: the tripod fracture. J Trauma 20:292–296.
7. Tilson, H.B., McFee, A.S., and Soudah, H.P.: The maxillofacial works of Rene Le Fort. Houston, The University of Texas, 1972.
8. Gentry, L.R., Manor, W.F., Turski, P.A., and Strother, C.M.: High-resolution CT analysis of facial struts in trauma: 1. Normal anatomy. Am J Roentgen 140:523–532, 1983.
9. Gentry, L.R., Manor, W.F., Turski, P.A., and Strother, C.M.: High-resolution CT analysis of facial struts in trauma: 2. Osseous and soft issue complications. AJR 140:533–541, 1983.
10. Seshul, M.B., Sinn, D.P., and Gerlock, A.J.: The Andy Gump fracture of the mandible: a cause of respiratory obstruction or distress. J Trauma 18:611–612, 1978.
11. Goldwater, M.D., Lorson, E.L., Tucker, D.F., and Dolan, K.D.: Internal carotid artery thrombosis associated with mandibular fractures. J Oral Surg 36:543–545, 1978.
12. Olson, R.A., Fonseca, R.J., Zietler, D.L. and Osbon, D.B.: Fractures of the mandible, a review of 580 cases. J Oral Maxillofac Surg 40:23–28, 1982.
13. Schultz, R.C.: 1000 major facial injuries. Rev Surg 27:394–410, 1970.
14. Schultz, R.C.: 400 major facial injuries. J Plastic Reconst Surg 40:415–425, 1967.

Part 2
Computed Tomography
Guy A. Catone

Victims of high-velocity, high-impact traumatic events affecting a broad area of the facial skeleton who have also sustained multisystem injuries are usually not immediate candidates for conventional planigraphic or pluridirectional tomographic radiology of the maxillofacial complex [1,2] (Fig. 3–52). The combination of high speed of impact and a large surface area of contact between the injuring surface (e.g., dashboard, windshield) and the maxillofacial complex produces extensive fragmentation at the site of impact [3]. Such multitrauma patients with possible injuries to the brain, spinal cord, thorax, abdomen, and skeleton cannot be readily or safely positioned for the standard radiographic techniques that may be easily accomplished on a patient with isolated maxillofacial trauma in whom no other body systems are involved. Also, it is dangerous to elicit movement from or to position the multi-trauma patient for

conventional images before the patient's global injuries have been fully elucidated. This danger is apparent when any view is ordered that results in hyperextension of the cervical cord. [4]

A RATIONALE FOR THE USE OF CT IN COMPLEX MAXILLOFACIAL INJURIES

Although preliminary radiographs of the skull in the AP and lateral projections, often taken in an emergency situation, yield incomplete information for diagnosis of and planning the reconstruction of complex facial injuries, [2] such preliminary radiographs may be useful to the radiologist in gaining an overview of the injuries in order to plan an appropriate imaging protocol. [4] Initial conventional radiographs revealing skull, maxillofacial, or cervical trauma can be followed by CT. Reformatted images can be used for more complete information. Pluridirectional tomography (PT) can be used as a primary or adjunctive imaging modality in patients with isolated complex maxillofacial disruptions, or selectively in patients with coexisting multisystem involvement when complications associated with positioning or movement have been ruled out.

Most major trauma centers have found that a CT series of the skull reveals much information concerning the patient with head injuries [1,5-16] and allows a reduction in routine skull radiography and such specialized invasive diagnostic modalities as pneumoencephalography and arteriography. [17-19] CT has also led to a reduction in unnecessary ophthalmologic [20-22] and neurosurgical [17-19] intervention.

Patients arriving at the hospital who are suspected of having craniocerebral injuries are usually prepared for a CT scan of the intracranial contents soon after initial resusci-

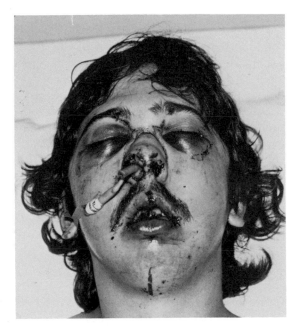

FIG. 3–52. Typical multitrauma patient with multiple systemic injuries that coexist with facial skeletal trauma. Patient is a 25-year-old male involved in a high-velocity motor vehicle accident.

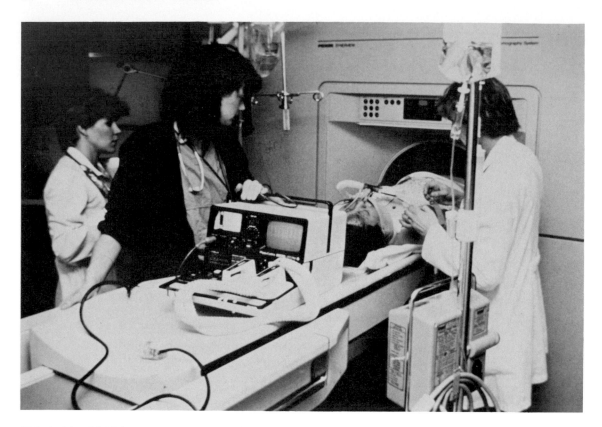

FIG. 3–53.   Multiple systems trauma patient with suspected maxillofacial injuries undergoing CT scanning of the maxillofacial skeleton as well as of other injuries.

tation and stabilization of vital functions. The majority of patients who are stable enough for a head CT scan can undergo a maxillofacial/cervical imaging session, which takes from 5 to 10 min longer to perform[1] (Fig. 3–53). The patient is monitored continuously during the imaging session and, if physiologic compromise occurs, the session can be concluded and the patient returned to the trauma unit or the operating room, depending on the presumed underlying cause.[1,16] Most trauma centers report that rarely are such scanning sessions aborted because of deterioration of the patients' vital functions.

CT technology and techniques greatly assist surgeons during the early period of patient management, when initial resuscitation has stabilized the patient and the priorities for care are being determined by providing the best possible images of bony and soft-tissue disruptions.[4] Even before newer high-resolution scanning, several authors cited the capability of CT to demonstrate complex max-

illofacial skeletal fractures.[11,23–28] Although some of these authors reported that the early CT images did not display fine-bone detail as well as PT,[25–27] faster scanning times and higher-resolution CT now allows exquisite detail of such gracile structures as the ethmoid labyrinth [4,29] (Fig. 3–54). As in the care of all injured patients, a thorough systematic clinical examination is the sine qua non for developing a plan for overall reconstruction of complex maxillofacial injuries based on craniofacial surgical principles.[30,31]

EVOLUTION OF COMPUTED TOMOGRAPHY

The application of CT technology has revolutionized the care of the multitraumatized facial patient to such an extent that the modality no longer merely confirms the clinical impression, as was the role of conventional radiography, but rather discovers many sub-

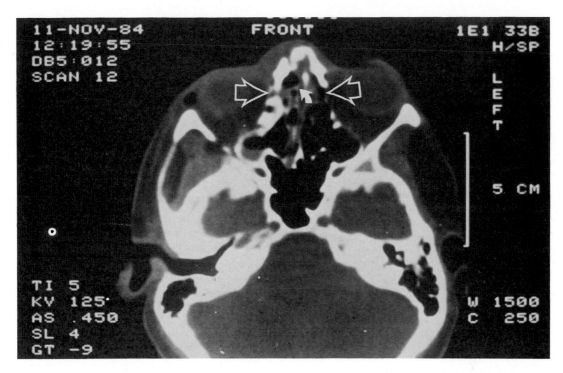

FIG. 3–54. Transaxial CT clearly displaying ethmoid labyrinth (open white arrows) and area of air-fluid retention (closed white arrow).

tle and potentially dangerous disruptions not detected on clinical examination. It then directs the surgeon regarding the proper craniofacial approach and allows him to assess the reconstructive effort in the postoperative phase to determine if future surgery is required.

HISTORICAL PERSPECTIVE

It is useful to examine the development of CT in relation to other imaging modalities and to analyze its impact on diagnosis in the maxillofacial region vis-à-vis conventional imaging technologies.

Subsequent to the seminal observations in 1895 by Roentgen involving high-energy radiation (x rays) and the later demonstration of its valuable medical applications, the limitations of such an imaging modality in producing two-dimensional radiographs of three-dimensional objects became clear.[32] The weakness in the technology lay in the superimposition of structures, which could not be differentiated if they had similar densities.

The development of laminagraphy and,

more recently of pluridirectional (hypocycloidal) tomography were attempts to improve the dimensional aspects of planigraphic technology by bringing into focus specific sections of the body. Tomography provides excellent spatial resolution without a similar enhancement of contrast resolution for the spectrum of densities of soft-tissue structures.[33] The blurring of detail in tissue planes not in the focal plane of the tomogram remains a significant drawback when attempting to visualize multiple comminuted bony fragments (Fig. 3–55). In such instances the blurring summates and obscures the detail of the bony fragments within the focal plane. Despite such limitations, PT remains a significant technological achievement and has many applications in maxillofacial trauma.

As Ames and others mentioned, in 1917 Radon demonstrated mathematically that a three-dimensional object could be reconstructed by assembling an infinite set of projections of the object using algorithmic calculations.[11] According to Rowe and others, in 1961 Oldendorf designed a method for monitoring the density of a point in a plane sur-

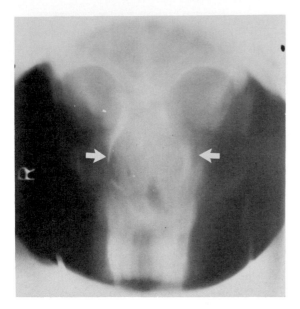

FIG. 3–55.   Polytomogram of the midface of a middle-aged women involved in a multiple vehicle collision. Extensive comminution of the midface is present. The blurring of detail-caused by the "summation" effect of the many bone fragments created by the process of image generation is evident (white arrows).

rounded by a higher density object, e.g., brain versus cranium.[19] These principles of Radon and Oldendorf appear to have been incorporated by Hounsfield, who observed that making conventional recordings on photographic film of the shadow of an object to be studied was not the most efficient method of using all the information provided by the passage of radiation through the object.[34] Hounsfield felt that the majority of useful information was lost in the depiction of a solid object in a two-dimensional image that superimposed all internal structures, which produces a summation image of the object rather than clearly focusing any given plane of tissue within tissue of varying densities.

PRINCIPLES OF CT SCANNING

Hounsfield designed CT so that the direction of the narrowly collimated x ray beam enters the object to be imaged through its edge, dividing the anatomy into specific slices within which the radiation is confined. As the radiation is transmitted through each tissue slice, all that is defined is the detail of the anatomy of the tissue within the slice, at the exclusion of contiguous anatomy. In a concentrically located gantry, the x ray source is housed and is arrayed about the object. Several hundred radiation crystal detectors of sodium iodide or bismuth germanate that in early CT scanners moved with the x ray sources but now remain stationary are positioned exactly opposite the collimated beams and determine the attentuation of the photons of radiation caused by their passage through the object (the maxillofacial skeleton) being evaluated. The detectors are linked to photomultiplier tubes that convert the energy of radiation into electrical signals. Thousands of readings, each specific for a given point in space between the radiation source and detector, are obtained per slice of tissue irradiated. These readings are processed by an appropriate computer program that applies a series of simultaneous algorithmic equations, transforming the solutions into absorption coefficients. Thus, the signal can be measured by a quantitative numeric value of the attenuated radiation (absorption coefficient) as well as by qualitative image of the object under scrutiny. No superimposition is evident because each image coincides with a cross section through the area examined (Fig. 3–56).

The x ray beam can be collimated to the desired slice thickness from 1.5 to 12 mm and can be moved from Hounsfield's original device, which rotated through an arc of 180° in several minutes in 1°-increments, to a full 360° in 5 to 10 min or, in "fast-scanning," in 1 sec. The original "water bag" that cradled the patient's head and was designed to decrease the dramatic change in contrast from calvarium to air has now been eliminated, allowing for greater penetration into the gantry, whose aperture has greatly enlarged over the years. Patients with major trauma lie supine (or prone for direct coronal views in patients with isolated facial injuries) on a "trolley" that can be controlled remotely, enabling the patient to be moved after each set of contiguous projections. The injured patient can thus be programmed to be moved superiorly until the craniocerebral, maxillofacial, and cervical areas are completely studied. Current gantrys

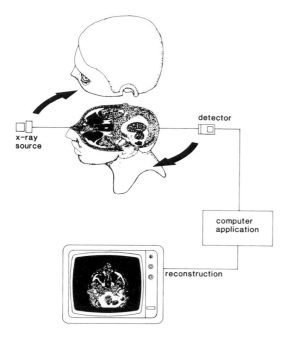

FIG. 3–56.   Diagram showing the basic principle of CT in creating "slices" of the maxillofacial region. (Redrawn after Fujii, N., and Yamashiro, M.: Computed tomography for the diagnosis of facial fractures. J Oral Surg 39:735, 1981.)

can permit slices to be taken at various angles (60 to 90°) incident to the patient. Scans are made usually parallel to the orbitomeatal line (OM line).

The scanning area or display on the CRT is divided into specific data squares, each having its unique X-Y coodinates. A matrix is a compilation of coordinates (squares displayed on the CRT). Absorption coefficients are unique for the individual points in the matrix. These points or pixels (picture elements) form the image and vary in size and number in relation to the matrix area size. Early CT scanners had matricies of 80^2. Current CT technology generates images in the form of a 256^2 to 512^2 matrix with pixel sizes of 0.75 × 0.75 mm to 1.5 × 1.5 mm (X-Y coordinates). A finer reconstructive matrix with smaller pixel size allows a greater number of pixels/unit scan area, thus permitting a marked improvement in spatial and contrast resolution. The size of the pixel as well as slice thickness is critical in the resulting spatial resolution of a given CT system. Each pixel depicts the value of the absorption coefficient of the related vol-

ume of tissue in the slice. Volume element, or voxel, which is used in the development of three-dimensional imaging technologies, combines pixel and slice thickness.

The resultant image produced by CT is a summation of multiple pixels representing attenuation values (absorption coefficients) and assigned various shades of gray based on such radiation attentuation. The quantitative values assigned to the pixels are based on the assignation of Hounsfield units (HU) to various tissues. Cortical bone is assigned a value of + 1000 HU, water is 0 HU, and air is − 1000 HU. These values are given varying hues of gray corresponding to the amount of x ray attentuation of a known standard.

The center of the gray scale is called the window level setting; the width of the gray scale is called the window setting. A high centering of the gray scale (high level setting) with a wide window setting is optimal for imaging the maxillofacial skeleton. A lower centering of the gray scale with narrow window settings results in sensitive soft-tissue differentiation and detail, as is required for imaging the orbital viscera or cerebral tissues.

Early generation CT scanners lost details because of patients' movement artifacts. Currently, even in the severely injured, somewhat uncooperative patient, decreased scanning times have solved this problem,[35] resulting in the ability to study areas previously having motion artifact, i.e., lung, mediastinum, and larynx. Narrower collimation, narrow width, and more precise detector alignment has allowed an improvement in spatial relation. Software enhancements now permit image generation, modification, reconstruction, reformatting, magnification, and analysis in a variety of techniques that have resulted in great improvements in diagnostic capabilities of CT. On appropriate scanners, CT images can be converted to three-dimensional representations using special three-dimensional software. This technology is especially useful in planning future reconstruction after initial maxillofacial injuries have been repaired.

There is a linear correlation between the statistical validity of attenuation coefficients assigned to each pixel or voxel and the photon fluence (dosage) of radiation that is used to visualize spatially the tissue region of interest. A higher photon fluence for a given region of tissue will improve the statistical validity of the attenuation coefficients (CT number or HU calculated for that region of tissue). It has been found that images from a high-photon fluence system will have less statistical "noise" and result in "smoother" CT representations. Factors that decrease photon fluence for a given voxel produce noisier, less accurate images, with a lowered x ray dose to the patient, narrower slice thickness, and reduced size of pixels (increasing the number of components in the matrix). A trade-off exists between high-quality spatial resolution, which requires smaller pixels and narrow slice thickness, and superior contrast resolution, which is largely dependent upon photon fluence, or radiation dosage.

Many alterations can be performed on the processed CT data before generating a hard-copy image. Algorithms or computer recalculations can diminish artifacts caused by abnormally high subject contrast, such as the interfaces of bone, brain, and air at the base of the skull, or can enhance areas of low subject contrast, such as gray matter/white matter distinction in the brain.

Normal anatomic structures such as bone, calcification, blood, brain, muscle, and fat lie in only a small segment of the attenuation spectrum, as does air. To view a specific tissue, it is necessary to select only that window width of the spectrum, controlled by the CRT. A wide window width, for instance 200 to 400 HU, will produce a flat, long-contrast scale between its upper limit (white) and lower limit (black). A narrow window width, such as 50 HU, will produce a short, high-contrast scale between its upper and lower limits. To visualize a specific anatomic structure, the center of the window is set on the value that is known to be the normal attentuation value for that tissue. This value is referred to as the window level. Manipulation of the window width and level is a simple electronic function of the CRT and can significantly affect the diagnostic quality of a scan.

Conventional planigraphic radiographs provide a screening tool that gives orientation and direction to subsequent CT imaging. Current generation CT scanners are capable of providing a preliminary digital image (Fig. 3–57) available in the frontal, lateral, or oblique projection to actively select CT slices of specific characteristics and gantry angulation in axial or coronal planes programmed in relation to the OM line, thus providing maximum data with the least amount of time or radiation exposure. The radiographic tube and detector is locked in a single position rather than rotating during exposure. Therefore, the radiologist can preview the overall anatomy and select or focus on a critical anatomic area for reduced slice-thickness examination. This selection is especially important for demonstrating significant bone displacement intracranially or intraorbitally, or for defining bone encroachments on the optic nerve, canal, etc. Moreover, the improved lateral preview feature is essential for assessing the cervical spine.

The selection of the slice plane, either axial or coronal, depends on the information sought and the safety of positioning the patient. Multiple-trauma patients are usually in a neutral supine position for axial cranial and maxillofacial and cervical CT slices. It is important to routinely scan and view cranial slices first because of possible associated intracranial injury. If the complex maxillofacial injury is isolated, the coronal view can be obtained using the supine head-hanging position or the prone neck-extended or "elevated-chin" position. Standard head holders are not employed in trauma patients to avoid accidental flexion injury of the cervical spine.

The CT cuts can be angled within the plane of interest to avoid artifacts, e.g., dental restorations, orthopedic devices, and foreign bodies. Imaging slices above and below foreign bodies such as bullets can aid in visualization without the production of radial artifacts (Fig. 3–58). Slices are contiguous and not overlapping and vary in thickness depending on the anatomic area or the resolution required (10 mm, intracranial; 5 mm, maxillofacial and orbital; 5 mm, cervical/laryngeal region)(Fig. 3–59). Selective use of the 1.5-mm slice thickness can provide high-resolution images.

The usefulness of CT for maxillofacial trauma screening can be enhanced by narrow density windows to separate structures of

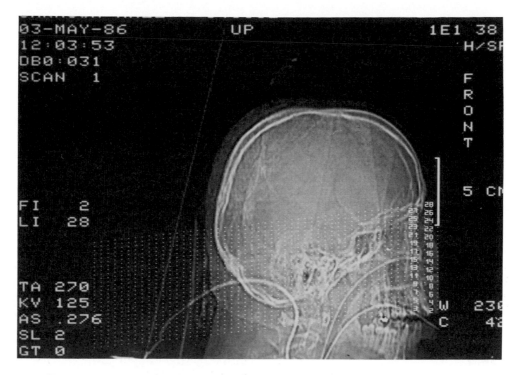

FIG. 3–57.   Preliminary digital image used to design the protocol for the maxillofacial skeletal scanning session.

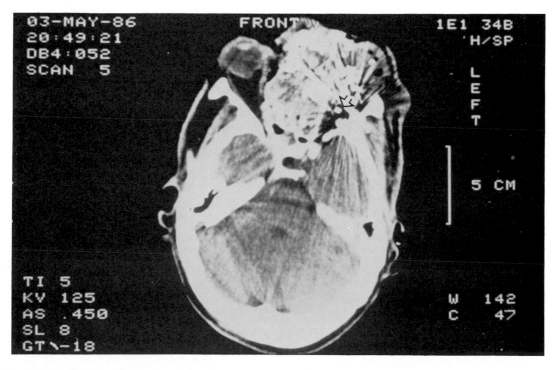

FIG. 3–58.   CT scan showing radial artifacts produced by high-density objects. In this case, the artifact is a bullet fragment in a self-inflicted wound that entered the nasofrontal region and left orbit (arrow).

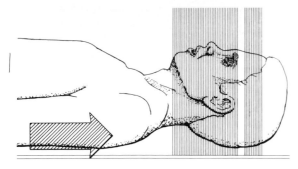

FIG. 3–59.   Diagram of multiple trauma patient supine on trolley; 10-mm intracranial slices, 5-mm maxillofacial slices, and 5-mm cervical slices are indicated. Arrow shows direction of trolley movement (cephalad-caudad). Vertical lines indicate anatomic "slices" made by array of radiographic sources. (Redrawn from Kassel, E.E., Noyek, A.M., and Cooper, P.W.: CT in facial trauma. J Otolaryngol *12*:2–15, 1983.)

similar density. Also, a three-dimensional tomographic effect can be achieved by using both axial and direct coronal CT (CCT). Another enhancing device is image reversal on CT scan to display dense structures such as bone or black details against a gray background. This maneuver can sometimes enhance fracture detail. Facial structures are relatively inhomogeneous and in part made up of gracile bony structures adjacent to air spaces or soft-tissue. Large changes in tissue density create great variations in attenuation of transmitted x rays and allow relatively easy contrast resolution. By expanding the gray scale window and increasing the (facial) level center in the positive gray scale, the spatial and contrast bone resolution is improved, allowing evaluation of facial bone detail without significant loss of soft-tissue differentiation. The radiologist can perform direct distance measurements using cursor placement, which is very useful in foreign body localization.

High-resolution imaging has been made a major advance in CT technology by providing further enhancements in reconstructive algorithms. One can manipulate gathered computed data with either bone or soft-tissue algorithms. The soft-tissue algorithms will best display the differences in density attenuation within the soft tissues. Previously, any tissue density greater than 1000 HU (bone) was pre-

sented as a single shade of white, thus showing minimal density or intrinsic bone detail; this limitation has been resolved by extending the capabilities of data accumulation and reconstruction to 4000 HU, the so-called extended bone window. Use of the extended bone numbers allows expansion of the Hounsfield unit scale up to 4000 HU, hence opening up the relatively limited gray scale of bone imaging. This expansion has practical application in the definition of fine bone detail in the ethmoid labyrinth, cribriform plate area, roof of the sphenoid sinus, and temporal bone.

High-resolution scanners also allow reconstruction of raw data (available computed information) about an area of interest, that is, to present an enlarged image without significant loss in resolution. This manipulation of data, whether for magnification or selection of bone or soft-tissue algorithms, must be performed at the time of scanning. The data are available for only a limited time, the exact limitation depending on the specific CT manufacturer. High-resolution magnification has been beneficial in better displaying of finer tissue detail in bone or soft-tissue modes. Image manipulation for the magnified image is performed solely from accumulated data with no further irradiation of the patient. Thinner slices from 1 to 5 mm are available and provide better detail and less volume averaging. Scanning experimental facial trauma has shown that high-resolution bone algorithms, the magnified mode, and thin slices provide fine detail.[36]

Reformatting CT images in other planes may be important. In the patient whose neck cannot be manipulated and in whom coronal and sagittal information is important, adequate storage of data using 5-mm axial slices through the maxillofacial region will permit adequate coronal reconstruction. Improved reformatted images have resulted from improved algorithms as well as from the use of thinner contiguous axial slices. Reformations are available in coronal, sagittal, oblique, or paraxial axes. Some reformations are almost instantaneous. Image quality is slightly decreased, but useful information can be obtained in those planes that cannot be directly scanned. These benefits can be offset by increased scan time, which may be contraindicated in acute trauma. Biplanar reformatting is important in defining bone disruptions of the orbital walls. Taping of CT data is essential in complex maxillofacial trauma imaging; if the imaging input is not taped or used at the time of examination, the high-resolution information may be lost.

In patients requiring urgent neurosurgical intervention, a CT screening examination can be performed with 10-mm axial brain slices and 5-mm axial facial slices, all within 2 min as a rapid scan. There is no need to delay the operation while images are recorded; these can be prepared over the next 10 to 15 min and brought to the operating room while surgical preparations are underway. In rapid scanning, in contrast to dynamic scanning, the desired multiple slice levels are preselected and scanned with minimum delay between scans. In this manner, the field of interest (accumulation of data) is covered as quickly as possible, with image reconstruction delayed slightly because of scanning priority. This technique is valuable in cases in which the least amount of motion between slice levels is desired or in patients who may be able to cooperate for only a limited period of time.

Dynamic scanning became possible after scan times became very brief. Rapid sequential CT scans are obtained with minimum interscan delay. This study is performed at a single slice level (selected) and is used in conjunction with a CT time-coordinated rapid bolus injection of a contrast medium. Information is usually presented by evaluating a series of images taken fractions of a second apart, or graphically by maniplating the data regarding the arrival and transit of the contrast medium through the predetermined area of interest, as in evaluation of CSF leaks.

High-resolution CT scanning using the magnified mode and a bone algorithm is the best method for demonstrating maxillofacial fractures. The extent of maxillofacial injuries can be demonstrated without underestimation. It is possible to rapidly scan those multiple-trauma patients who will require immediate surgical care and store the data to be retrieved and viewed later. Patients who do not require urgent surgical management can

be scanned and the images reviewed as treatment proceeds. Scanning the critically injured, relatively unstable patient in a "retrospective" manner and the stable, multiple-injured patient in a "prospective" manner, according to Kassel et al.,[2] is the most time-efficient way to provide images of the maxillofacial skeleton. In either modality, the bone algorithm must be used. A soft-tissue algorithm may be preferred when examining the orbits. Intracranial structures are not studied in the high-resolution modes; in patients with isolated complex facial injuries, direct CCT studies are usually performed as part of the initial study. Axial and coronal studies may be performed in the high-resolution mode with more ideal monitoring of the field of scanning. Whether to perform direct CCT is decided after axial scans have been viewed.

RADIATION DOSAGE IN CT SCANNING

Radiation dose to the lens (eye) measured by thermoluminescent dosimeters on Rando phantoms during coronal CT (General Electric EMI-5000) is 10 to 12 rads, supine; 1 rad, prone. The dose was calculated using a 6-mm collimator with a series of 5 sections at 5-mm intervals.[37] Koga et al. reported a gonadal dose of 0.3 mrad with a complete scan at 120 Kvp and 25 mA.[38] Moriuchi et al. pointed out that the gonadal dose can be reduced to 0 mrad if a lead protector is worn.[39] North and Rice noted that the major advantage of CT over planigraphic films is the lower radiation dose.[27] The peak skin doses for CT ranged from 0.4 to 4.7 rads for a typical series. Even contiguous scans over several levels will increase the total surface dose only modestly. In contrast, multiple tomographic cuts with a pluridirectional unit will deliver a cumulative dose at a level approaching 6 rads/slice on the skin surface proximal to the x ray source. Noyek et al. noted that the radiation risk factor may approximate 2 rads/CT slice.[4] Maue-Dickson et al. reported that a single 1.5-mm section at a 320-mA setting with a 3-sec pulse width delivers about 4 rads (0.04 Gy) at the entrance site on the face.[26] A PT series at 4-mm x rays in two projections necessitates up to 15 cuts in each of the two planes, measuring about 30 rads.

Although improved spatial resolution has resulted in increased surface dosage, the absorbed radiation exposure of CT has been reduced to at least 50% of that received from conventional polytomography. Rowe et al., Kassel et al., Finkle, and Carter demonstrated that CT in 24 sections had an average radiation dose of 5.6 rads.[19,35,40,41] The average dose for linear tomography in the supine (reverse Waters) position for 9 sections is 3.4 rads. In the prone (Waters) position the average dose is only 0.08 rads for 9 sections. It has been noted that radiation-induced cataracts are a dose and time-related phenomenon. A single dose of 200 rads or multiple exposures of 400 to 500 rads can cause this ophthalmologic problem.

COMPUTED TOMOGRAPHY COMPARED TO PLURIDIRECTIONAL TOMOGRAPHY

One of the major advantages of CT over PT is the avoidance of the problems inherent in conventional head and neck radiography, that is, its lack of availability, the limited capabilities of the system, multiple exposures of the patient to relatively high doses of radiation, inadequate visualization of the affected area, and difficulties in positioning the patient because of his compromised physical status.[27] Early generation CT applications to maxillofacial trauma were judged inferior to PT.[42–45] The different characteristics of CT and conventional PT pictures are a feature of the different principles of image generation inherent in both techniques. In laminagraphy exposures, the radiographic tube and film undergo linear movement in opposite directions with respect to a plane in the object, blurring all other planes. Polycycloidal tomography permits more sectioning in the coronal and lateral planes by multidirectional movements of the film and tube around a fixed spatial point within a given plane. Thus, inherent in PT as opposed to CT image production is the fact that, while objects outside the plane of interest are blurred, when multiple fracture fragments are present their blurred images summate and are superimposed on the actual focal plane, thus decreasing detail. PT offers optimal spatial resolution but does not significantly improve contrast resolution within the soft-tissue range (Table 3–1).

Certain features of CT imaging are important in the diagnosis of maxillofacial problems. With CT, three-dimensional structures can be seen without distortion and superimposition of overlying bony or soft-tissue structures; also, the tangential law of conventional tomography is not valid; and CT enables cross-sectional anatomic studies together with determination of tissue attenuation differences. An important difference between CT and PT is that although PT used to have the relative advantage of a higher resolving power than CT (though current generation scanners have rivaled this quality), this advantage is partly nullified by blurring or superimposition (inherent in PT technology). The main disadvantage of PT is that it is unable to differentiate various tissue densities. With PT, bony rims are frequently obscured by the adjacent blurred soft tissues; with CT scans, however, the bone and soft-tissue interface will be clearly visible. Claussen et al. showed that CT clarified the diagnostic problems of localizing fracture fragments in brain and facial skeleton; identifying intracranial or intraorbital trauma with or without hemorrhage; imaging associated inflammatory complications of the brain; and imaging posttraumatic cyst or residual parenchymal defects.[8,25,42]

Grove noted that in the evaluation of orbital trauma, although bone injuries are usually seen adequately with the conventional PT, determining the extent of complex fractures and the relationship of fractures to soft tissues using radiographs alone may be difficult.[46] Moreover, radiographs are of little value in the detailed study of soft tissues and low-density foreign bodies. PT frequently does not provide sufficient data to establish a diagnosis or to localize an abnormality in patients with orbital injuries. In his evaluation of isolated orbital injuries, Grove demonstrated muscle entrapment (inferior rectus) (Fig. 3–60).[46] CT also defined many bone fragments and defects not seen well on radi-

Table 3–1. Comparison of Conventional Radiography and Tomography with CT

Conventional Radiography	Tomography	CT
Uses central projection		Uses collimated
Distortion occurs		Orthograde (minimal distortion)
Provides morphologic image information		Provides morphologic-quantitative information (local distribution of absorption coefficients)
	Images body section	Images body section
	Superimposition from overlying tissue structures (blurring detail) occurs	No superimposition occurs
	Tangential law (of tomography) applies	Independent of projection effects
	Thin layers (4 mm is feasible) obtained	Current CT—less than 1-mm thickness

(Modified from Claussen, C., and Singer, R.: Progress in the diagnosis of craniofacial injuries and tumors by computed tomography. J Maxillofac Surg 7:210–217, 1979.)

ographs. Grove used CT image reversal to enhance fracture fragment delineation with even more clarity than conventional CT.

Using CT, Rowe et al. studied 27 maxillofacial trauma patients, 18 of whom had PT for comparison.[19] All fracture lines, bony fragments, and associated facial skeletal disruptions were clearly demonstrated by CT in the entire group of patients, allowing diagnosis and classification of injury. It was noted that, overall, CT provided data not seen by PT in 15 of 18 cases in which both CT and PT studies were taken. The authors also indicated that PT was superior to CT when finite intrinsic bone detail was required. Noyek et al.[4] noted that this observation would appear to be invalid if extended bone window, high-resolution CT were used. They further concluded that CT now offers superior diagnostic imaging in all areas of consideration.

CT imaging provides superior bone detail compared to PT performed in the same plane;

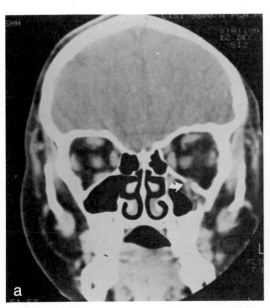 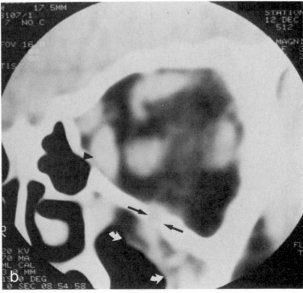

FIG. 3–60 **a,** Direct coronal displaying fracture of the inferior orbital wall with inferior rectus entrapment (arrow). Compare with intact right orbital floor. **b,** Direct coronal CT in magnified mode revealing herniation of muscle (opaque mass) between medial and lateral fractured floor segments (black arrows) and edema and hemorrhage of sinus membrane (white arrows). Medial wall appears intact with normal-appearing medial rectus muscle (arrowhead).

only sagittal CT reformats remain inferior to lateral PT, though the information gleaned from CT may be more than adequate in most imaging settings. Complex fractures with fragmentation are more readily found with CT than PT because of the superior contrast resolution of CT. CT is superior to PT in delineating more complex Le Fort fractures, especially when zygomaticomaxillary complex fractures are superimposed. Also, orbital roof fractures are better visualized with CT than PT. Transaxial CT is better suited than PT to identify intracranial injuries and is equally able to determine the presence or absence of anterior or posterior frontal sinus fractures (Fig. 3–61). PT in two projections helps to identify potential nasofrontal duct injuries that may not be appreciated on axial CT. Potential optic nerve damage is more clearly seen by axial CT than by biplanar tomography.

The axial CT can easily define clinically obscure temporal bone fractures and associated epidural hematomas that are not seen on PT of the facial skeleton. Traumatically induced

encephalocele as may occur in the frontal, sphenoid, or ethmoid sinuses or in the orbital or nasal cavity can be delineated with CT but not PT (Fig. 3–62). CT absorption values can be calculated and can differentiate CSF from brain parenchyma.

Direct coronal CT (CCT) is at least equal to PT in assessing the complicated orbital floor, rim, and anterior wall of the maxillary sinus fractures (Fig.3–63) If entrapment of the inferior rectus is suspected, if the globe is displaced into the maxillary antrum, or if damage to the optic nerve is suspected, coronal CT images the injury more clearly. Orbital roof fracture is better displayed on CT than PT. The latter may require imaging in both coronal and axial planes because fracture lines running parallel to the plane of section may be impossible to identify unless greatly displaced. The degree of rotation and displacement of zygomaticomaxillary complex fractures is more easily judged on coronal CT. In uncomplicated Le Fort II fractures, coronal PT is equal to axial CT. More complex Le Fort III

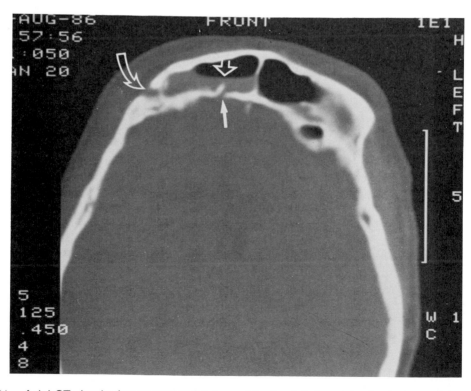

FIG. 3–61.   Axial CT clearly demonstrating fracture of the frontal sinus lateral anterior wall (open curved arrow), fracture of posterior wall (closed straight arrow), and air-fluid level (open straight arrow).

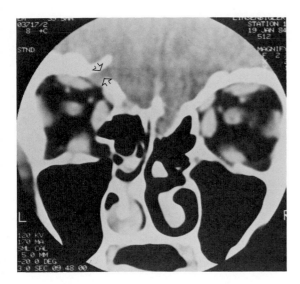

FIG. 3–62. Traumatically induced encephalocele. Brain is herniating (between arrows) through rupture in the supermedial orbital wall.

fractures in the presence of other facial fractures are more completely defined with CT.

Additional situations favoring the use of axial CT over coronal PT in maxillofacial trauma include pneumocephalus, questionable temporal bone fractures, massive soft-tissue loss, orbital emphysema suggesting medial wall blow-out fractures, conditions requiring definition of the extent of NOE fragmentation, and cervical injuries including laryngeal, tracheal, and bony trauma (Fig. 3–64). Axial CT identifies fractures of the anterior and posterior frontal sinus walls, which is essential for proper clinical management. In correlating the findings at surgery with preoperative images, it is apparent that lateral PT may complement CT in evaluating the extent of sagittal displacement of fragments. Biplanar PT may be superior to axial CT alone in defining fragmentation and direct injury to the nasolacrimal duct. Basilar skull fractures associated with facial fractures can be missed by PT but may be directly visualized by CT or may be manifest as a focal pneumocephalus (Fig. 3–65). The detail of PT may be required for precise localization of complex basilar skull fractures once they are recognized.

Zilkha reported the results of planigraphic, conventional tomography, and CT in 30 patients with maxillofacial trauma.[47] Planigraphic and conventional tomography were not useful in identifying several fractures of the medial and inferior orbital walls and the cribriform plate. Significantly, neither imaging method was helpful in specific patients in whom an orbital hematoma was present. Zilkha noted that in the presence of fractures of the orbital floor or medial wall, the visualization of muscle entrapment is problematic. The presence of edema and/or hemorrhage involving the periorbita and mucous membrane of the maxillary and/or ethmoid sinuses can be interpreted incorrectly as a picture of "pseudoprolapse" of orbital contents. Hemorrhagic or edematous paranasal sinuses will obscure the bony orbital wall fragment displacement within them on conventional planigraphic and tomographic radiographs.

Zilkha demonstrated in his series that CT was superior to conventional tomography overall in the radiologic evaluation of patients with maxillofacial trauma. CT demonstrated blow-out fractures of the orbital floor and medial wall so that the fracture sites, extent of displaced bone fragments, and status of the extraocular muscles could be visualized accurately. Fracture fragments were seen routinely despite clouding of a paranasal sinus. Entrapped muscles appeared to be elongated and their long axes appeared to be perpendicular to the fractured orbital wall. (Fig. 3–66)

In a study by Hammerschlag et al., experimental "pure" blow-out fractures were produced in eight cadavers and compared using conventional planigraphic, tomographic, and CT modalities.[48] CT slices 2 mm thick were taken in the direct oblique plane, parallel to the long axis of the inferior rectus muscle, and also in the direct coronal plane. The majority of fractures were detected by direct coronal CT with lateral tomograms and sagittal CT images. In all cases, the specimens revealed larger fractures on dissection than were visualized radiographically. CT correlated well in the presence of depressed bony fragments with or without soft-tissue prolapse (Fig. 3–67).

While there is a modicum of controversy relating to the inferior spatial resolution of CT compared to PT, Hammerschlag et al. thought this weakness was more than compensated for by CT's improved contrast resolution,

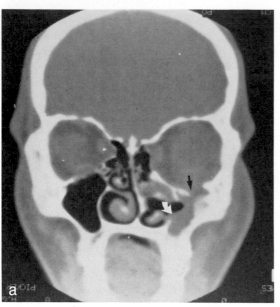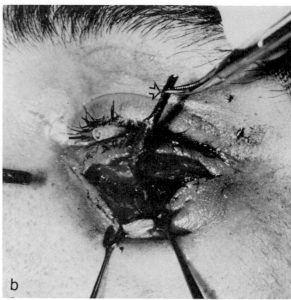

FIG. 3–63.   **a,** Direct CT of orbits showing fractures of the right orbital floor (black arrow) and cloudiness and debris in the right maxillary antrum (white arrow). **b,** Clinical photograph at surgery showing foreign bodies (tree bark) being removed from right maxillary sinus via blepharoplasty incision (open arrow). Plastic cylindric object between eyelids (enclosed arrow) is part of ocular "contact lens" used to protect the globe during surgery.

which allowed identification of soft-tissue densities of the roof of the maxillary sinus, representing prolapsed periorbital fat, extraocular muscle, hematoma, or an unrelated antral retention cyst.

Hammerschlag and co-workers questioned the biomechanics of blow-out fractures as promulgated by numerous authors and noted that true extraocular muscle entrapment was rare. They noted that the altered ocular motility observed in orbital trauma may be related to direct muscular or neural injury. They also suggested that the posterior inferior orbital fat pad may play a significant role in explaining the symptoms experienced by the patient and the signs observed by the clinician in such injuries. This fat pad is situated between the periorbita and the muscle mass of the inferior rectus and inferior oblique. Apparently, fibrous bands connect the muscular fascia to the periorbita. More evidence suggests that the ocular hypomotility in orbital trauma is related to increased tension on these fibrous bands resulting from orbital edema, hemorrhage, or actual entrapment of the fat pad itself, rather than tethering of the extraocular muscles (inferior rectus/oblique).

Further, the authors felt that coronal images taken through the inferior rectus muscle and orbital floor do not provide an adequate evaluation of the inferior rectus muscle and any defects of the orbital floor. In their study, they found extraocular muscle "kinks" that were not well defined in serial coronal slices. To evaluate orbital blow-out fractures adequately, the authors suggested the use of reformatted oblique sagittal sections that would scan along the plane of the long axis of the inferior rectus muscle. They also proposed study of the orbit in the axial plane, parallel to the orbital floor, imaging from the floor to the roof and thus defining the presence of medial wall fragmentation. They conceded that while more resolution is lost with reformation, the detail was adequate to make a diagnosis.

As with Zilkha,[49,50] Hammerschlag found that both PT and CT underestimate size and complexity, especially of nondepressed fragmented bony segments; however, visualization of depressed fragments was reasonably accurate with both radiographic techniques.[48] He further concluded, as had other authors,

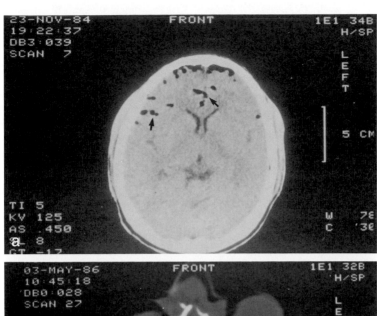

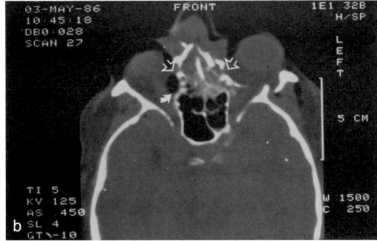

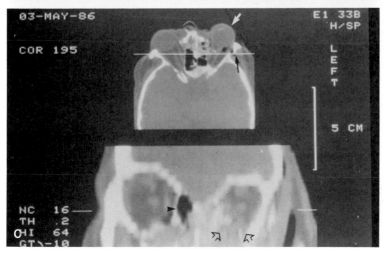

FIG. 3–64

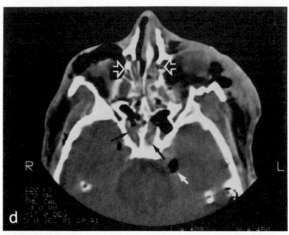

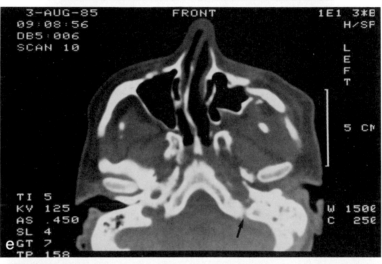

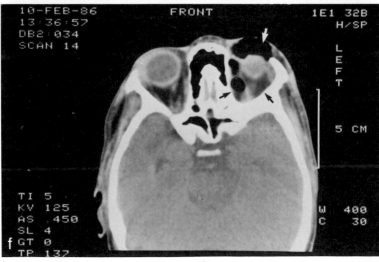

FIG. 3–64. See legend on page 101.

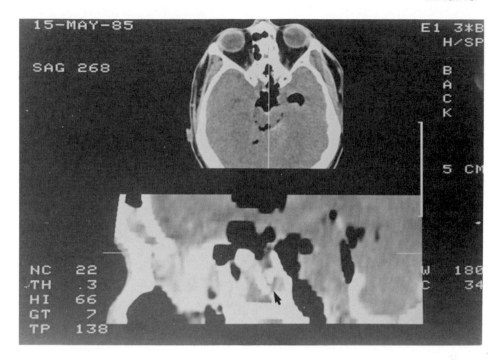

FIG. 3–65.   CT demonstrating pneumocephalus in the transaxial and reformatted sagittal planes. Upper figure displays cursor plane. At least one area of bony rupture is present (arrow).

that CT was an improvement over PT, especially in imaging herniation of orbital viscera (Fig. 3–68).

Brandt-Zawadski et al. evaluated 24 patients with various maxillofacial conditions, 14 of which patients had facial trauma.[29] The authors noted that the relatively inferior spatial resolution of CT compared to PT had limited CT's use in maxillofacial trauma. However, they noted that the advances in CT technology permitting ultrathin-slice imaging improved spatial resolution. Moreover, new software allowed greater flexibility in data manipulation, thus allowing image reformat-

ting in various related planes and regions of interest in density analysis. High-resolution CT with reformations allowed thorough evaluation of facial trauma and was superior to thin-section PT in several cases. These authors noted that in 5 patients studied using both CT and PT, CT provided as much or more data than the conventional tomograms. CT also defined a greater number of maxillofacial skeletal fractures and a specific fracture (temporal bone) not visualized by PT. A significant advantage of the superior contrast resolution of CT over PT is its ability to rapidly evaluate damage to vital structures including

FIG. 3–64.   **a,** Transaxial CT displaying pneumocephalus in an anterobasilar skull fracture (arrows). **b,** Transaxial CT revealing collapse of nasoethmoid region (open arrows) and right pneumo-orbita (closed arrow). **c,** Coronal reformat in region of cursor line (black arrow). Lower figure shows destruction of left orbital floor (open arrows) and nasoethmoidal air (arrowhead). Incidental finding on upper axial CT is proptosis of left ocular globe (white arrow). **d,** Transaxial CT displaying fragmentation, cloudiness in the region of the nasoethmoid labyrinth (open white arrows), and hemorrhage into sphenoid sinus (black arrows). Focal pneumocephalus is characteristic for basilar skull fracture (closed white arrow). **e,** Transaxial CT with basilar skull fracture (arrow) with coexisting maxillofacial fractures. **f,** Massive orbital emphysema (black arrows) involving posterior medial orbital cavity. Emphysema of anterior orbital cavity and eyelids is also present (white arrow).

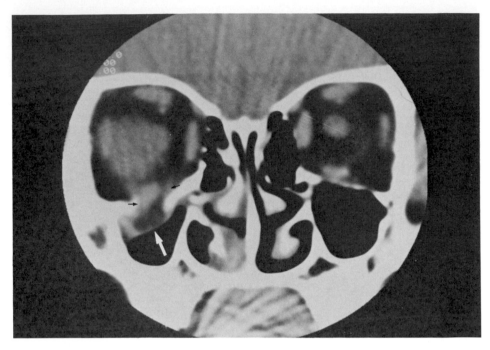

FIG. 3–66.   Coronal CT clearly displaying fractured orbital floor despite partial cloudiness of right maxillary sinus (white arrow). Muscle mass of inferior oblique/rectus is seen interposed between fragments (black arrows). Compare orbital contents to opposite noninjured side. Note detail of extraocular muscles and inferior rectus muscle resting on intact orbital floor.

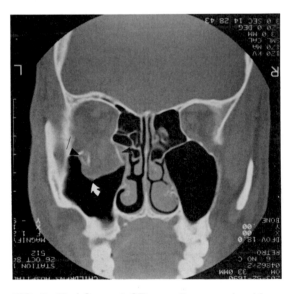

FIG. 3–67.   Coronal CT revealing massive blow-out fracture of left orbital floor (white arrow) with medial (black arrow) and lateral (arrowhead) bone fragments of orbital floor with herniation of orbital fat and muscle.

the globe and optic nerve or to detect associated brain trauma. The disadvantage of PT used alone becomes critical in view of the delayed complications of undetected injury resulting in diplopia, mucocele, cosmetic deformity (enophthalmos, bony defects), and life-threatening meningitis.

The use of polytomography alone does not facilitate mental reconstruction of a three-dimensional image. In contrast to CT, the positioning of the patient for PT may affect the interpretation of architectural derangements, because rotation may stimulate structural displacement. As alluded to earlier, in the presence of maxillofacial skeletal comminution the generation of the polytomogram can result in blurring or "ghost" artifacts over the focal plane of tissue to be examined, which may cause the surgeon to misinterpret the underlying fractures. CT, on the other hand, by the manner in which it generates images, does not produce such artifacts even in the presence of severe comminution. CT, with its superior contrast resolution compared to PT can allow direct viewing of soft-tissue anatomy.

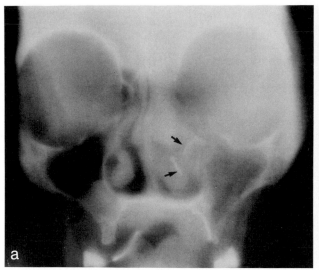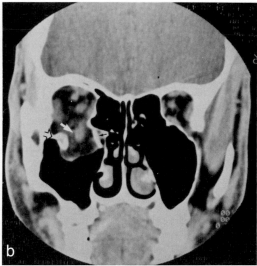

FIG. 3–68.   **a**, Polytomogram of left orbit revealing comminution of the orbital floor medially into the maxillary sinus and nasal cavity. Note bony fragments in nasal cavity (arrows). Compare fractured side with opposite side. **b**, Coronal CT for comparison with Figure 3–68a (different patient). Note bulk of inferior rectus dropping through rupture of orbital floor (white arrow). Also note "bending" of fractured lateral floor segment and "trapdoor" medial to the medial fracture segment (open black arrow and closed black arrow, respectively).

Orbital visceral injuries or displacements involving the globe, extraocular muscles, and optic nerve can be more readily visualized by CT as opposed to conventional radiographs. There is some consensus that CT is more able than PT to differentiate pseudoprolapse of orbital tissues from muscle entrapment by demonstrating the muscle lying free within the orbit. Massive facial trauma often raises suspicions regarding the intregrity of the globe and optic nerve, which may be injured by displaced bone fragments. CT can readily detect the presence and exact location of these bony fragments as they relate to the orbital viscera, as opposed to PT, which may reveal the bony fragments but fail to display the soft-tissue trauma. Intraocular disruptions such as hemorrhage, lenticular subluxaton, and extraocular damage (e.g., subdural hematoma of the optic nerve sheath) are detected by CT and not revealed by conventional radiographic techniques.

CT is critical in missile injuries, blast effect, industrial accidents, or motor vehicle accidents in which foreign bodies may be present within the maxillofacial complex. The high-density resolution of CT may display nonopaque foreign bodies not detected on con-

ventional films. While PT in the coronal and lateral projections is an acceptable modality to display facial fractures, CT reveals in addition the ocular muscles, globe, intraorbital hemorrhage, encephalocele, pneumo-orbita, and displacement of the optic nerve and canal[51] (Fig. 3–69). In Brandt-Zawadski's study, one third of patients with maxillofacial trauma had associated intracranial findings that were identified by CT.

Subtle maxillofacial trauma involving the orbital floor and the walls of the maxilla and ethmoid bones are readily defined by CT, especially thin-slice CT involving 1.5-mm cuts. Reformatting in planes perpendicular to the bone of interest is essential in diagnosis. Problems arise in CT scanning of maxillofacial fractures when the scan is parallel to thin, undisplaced fracture lines, which may not be seen even with reformation from the axial to other planes. Combative patients can create motion artifact that decreases spatial resolution and is aggraved with reformation. This situation has been improved by faster scanning times (5 to 10 sec for high-resolution images). Loss of contrast resolution of soft-tissues can occur because of the need for short tube-cooling intervals during rapid sequence

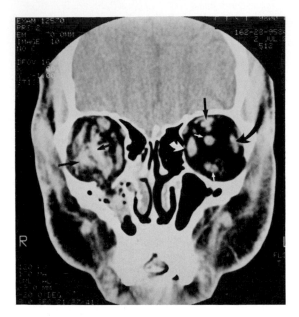

FIG. 3–69. Coronal CT displaying massive right retro-orbital hemorrhage (opacification between black arrows). Left orbit displays normal structures: optic nerve (small central white arrow), medial and lateral rectus muscles (curved white and black arrows, respectively), inferior rectus and inferior oblique muscles (vertical white arrow), and superior oblique muscle (vertical solid black arrow).

scanning without loss of bone detail resolution.

Daffner and co-workers agree with other authors in recognizing the dual role of CT in assessing soft tissue as well as bony disruptions.[52] In their series of 32 patients examined by CT (13 of whom were also given PT), they determined CT to be as effective as PT in identifying all fractures. Daffner also recommended the use of CT as a follow-up tool in re-evaluating patients with severe facial trauma. In at least 50% of these cases, CT demonstrated skeletal or soft-tissue abnormalities that proved to be critical in the management of the patient.

Kassel and Cooper are consistent with others in their observation that PT is adequate to identify fractures in most patients but that CT should be selected when comminution is extensive and the bone fragments themselves interfere with fine detail.[1] They note that newer CT studies display superior spatial resolution and bone detail compared to current PT studies. They differ with earlier authors in suggesting that properly programmed high-resolution CT images using the magnified mode and bone algorithm offer the ultimate method for demonstrating facial fractures.

Fractures involving the nasoethmoid complex are readily visualized on CT, despite the presence of opacification of the ethmoidal air cells (Fig. 3–70). Conventional films do not demonstrate well the fine ethmoid septae, and fracture lines are obscured by sinus opacification. It is not unusual to have clinical evidence of a nasoethmoid fracture with no confirmation on conventional radiographs. PT and plain films may not detect "blow-in" fractures of the medial wall of the orbit or differentiate this type of fracture from the more common blow-out fracture. Kassel and Cooper do indicate that the anatomic configuration of linear fractures of the vault extending to the frontal sinus is best displayed by conventional films. Plain films, however, are relatively unsuccessful in demonstrating fractures of the posterior wall of the frontal bone and basilar skull fractures.

Central nervous system injuries may coexist with maxillofacial trauma. Compared with PT, CT provides high-resolution, thin-slice information on the status of dural lacerations, pneumocephalus, and CSF leaks. CT is ten times more sensitive than PT in density resolution. Intracranial infections can be the sequel of impact such as from intracerebral bony fragments or foreign bodies or late developments relating to inadequate sinus drainage or undetected or chronic CSF leakage (Fig. 3–71). PT may be useful in patients with complex fractures who require coronal studies but for whom positioning (hyperextension) for direct coronal CT is contraindicated. CT may be less useful in patients with facial orthopedic devices or who have extensive dental restorations.

CT is the superior method in demonstrating comminuted bone fragments. PT studies of fractures with marked comminution show increased shadows and reduced detail in the actual focal plane because of superimposed multiple bone fragments. The components of more complex fractures that are associated with larger bone fragments or that cross anatomic sites, so that fragments exist in two or

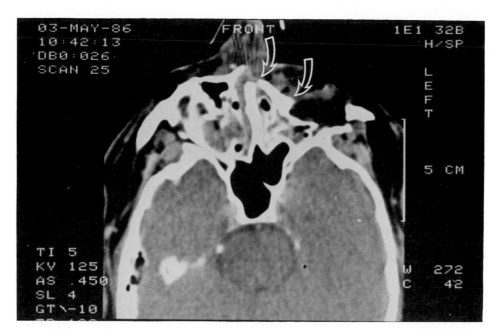

FIG. 3–70. High-contrast transaxial CT displaying multiple fragments of nasoethmoid complex, with telescoping of segments (arrows), despite presence of hemorrhage and edema.

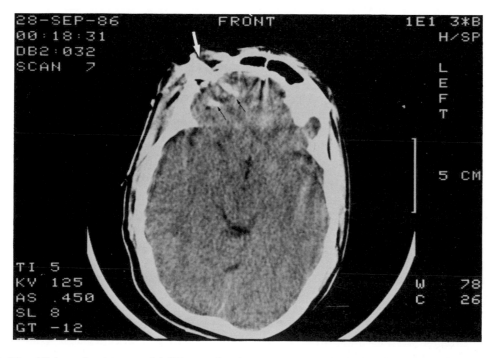

FIG. 3–71. High-contrast transaxial CT revealing frontal fracture (white arrow) and the presence of bone fragments within the brain (black arrows). This patient was a 14-year-old boy whose fall from a bicycle resulted in multiple frontotemporal skull fractures, CSF leak, loss of the right supraorbital ridge, and rupture of the right globe.

more anatomic regions, may be seen better by CT. Opacification of an associated paranasal sinus does not obscure detail on CT, and displaced bone fragments that may be visualized on conventional tomography or plain films will be easily noted. CT displays the common anterior ethmoidal clouding or emphysema of the orbit not seen on conventional films. Conventional radiography may visualize only the soft-tissue opacification of the ethmoid sinus and may not differentiate the opacification from the more common blow-out fracture.

Cooper et al. agree that CT is faster and has displayed more accuracy than PT in patients with maxillofacial trauma.[31] They indicate that high-resolution CT provides bone detail equal to or better than PT with the additional advantage of better contrast resolution. The anatomic disruptions noted on surgical exploration correlate more precisely with the images obtained with high-resolution CT than with conventional planigraphic or tomographic imaging.

Even before the advent of high-resolution CT, the axial view was valuable in demonstrating fractures of the orbital roof that were not displayed with conventional methods. Manfredi et al. described five patients with clinical evidence of indirect injury to the optic nerve in whom the optic canal fracture, together with associated orbital roof fractures, were better appreciated by CT than by PT, and in whom complex midfacial fractures were seen better with CT as well.[21] When PT is used as a primary imaging modality to obtain high-quality, high-data images, taking multiple views (AP, lateral), is often necessary to allow a three-dimensional interpretation. This increased exposure may greatly increase the total radiation dose to the patient, compared to CT.

Gentry et al. produced experimental maxillofacial injuries in cadavers and studied these fractures with thin-section CT.[36] CT proved to be as effective as PT in the detection and classification of these injuries, and its other advantages, such as ability to view soft tissues, eclipsed PT. The authors made a significant contribution to the radiologic classification of maxillofacial trauma by a unique method of evaluating such injuries—by viewing the maxillofacial complex structurally as a series of triplanar (horizontal, sagittal, and coronal) bony struts.

Finkle et al. commented on the deficiencies of clinical and radiographic studies in maxillofacial trauma, which led to preoperative speculation rather than definitive planning.[40] They compared clinical examination, linear tomography, and CT, using image reformation and CT axials with 5-mm slices and 2-mm overlap and direct CCT scans angled 60° to 90° from the axial plane. The statistical accuracy of various imaging methods and clinical impressions was ascertained by comparing preoperative findings with findings present at surgery. When the Le Fort classification was used, linear tomography was found to be more accurate than CT, although earlier studies found CT to be more accurate than linear tomograpy in evaluating clearly delineated Le Fort fractures compared with comminuted fractures and facial injuries. In determining orbital fractures, CT was found to be more precise than other methods; CT scan displayed orbital fractures 65.1% more accurately than clinical examination did.

Injuries involving comminution of structures such as the ethmoid, sphenoid, and maxillary sinus were revealed better by CT than by other procedures. All three investigative methods (clinical examination, linear tomography, and CT) were diagnostic for frontal sinus fractures, but in light of the classification of frontal sinus fractures that would dictate invasive or noninvasive care, CT with complementary PT, according to most authors, is clearly superior to strictly clinical examination. While Le Fort's classification remains useful in the clinical diagnosis of maxillofacial injuries, it may be nonessential for CT scanning because of the greater detail provided by CT imaging; on CT scans, "true" Le Fort fractures were rarely visualized. The authors were in agreement with Gentry et al. in observing that CT displayed comminuted midfacial fractures that were not seen before.[36] On the basis of information gleaned from CT reformation from the axial to the coronal, sagittal, and parasagittal planes, Finkle et al. believed CT was the most accurate method to use in the diagnosis of maxillofacial injuries.[40]

Kreipke et al. studied 31 maxillofacial trauma patients using several imaging methods—that is, planigraphic, coronal and lateral PT, and axial CT and direct coronal CT.[53] They found that CT was superior to PT in demonstrating fractured surfaces quantitatively. When one projection alone was used from each study, PT was better than CT in displaying and classifying fractures. This latter observation must be considered with reference to the complexity of the actual injury. Consistent with other investigators, Kreipke et al. found that each method was less than satisfactory when the plane of section was parallel or oblique to the focal plane of the region being examined. Biplanar imaging including the coronal view resulted in the greatest accuracy by either CT or PT modalities. The authors felt that PT offered better spatial resolution, while CT was superior in its contrast resolution. This better contrast was especially true when viewing with CT small fractures in which the partial volume effect of bone decreased detail. This problem was apparently overcome by the superior spatial resolution of PT. Kreipke et al. found that the enhanced contrast resolution of CT in relation to PT permitted differentiation between the ethmoidal wall and hemorrhage. They noted that the lamina papyracea was almot not visualized on PT.[53]

As opposed to other authors, they found PT more effective than CT in demonstrating orbital blow-out fractures, which they attributed to the superior ability of PT to display small orbital floor fractures. Kreipke et al. recommended that the coronal plane be used in visualizing maxillofacial injuries and that PT was superior in this position. The limitations of PT in the multitrauma patient have been discussed. Indeed, using different slice thickness and technique, Brandt-Zawadski showed that reformatted coronal images from axial CT sections were superior to PT.[29] Despite Kreipke and co-workers' negative commentary relating to CT, they recommended that a 2- projection (coronal and transaxial) CT, if it can be obtained, is the superior method to display fractures with the exception of those of the inferior orbital rim and floor. CT can compare well with PT in orbital bony trauma if appropriate reformatting can

be done. The usefulness of CT in clear contradistinction to PT in demonstrating orbital viscera has been mentioned.

Jend-Rossman and Jend reinforce the concepts that routine AP radiographs do not provide data detailed enough for primary reconstruction of midfacial trauma and that CT offers a superior diagnostic imaging method.[54] This conclusion was based on 120 CT studies of midfacial fractures of various kinds. The authors used high-resolution, thin-slice techniques and concluded that the axial scan was sufficiently diagnostic. They cited some difficulty with uniplanar studies of Le Fort I and II fractures and used a biplanar technique when these were suspected. They also used semicoronal scans by gantry angulation in those multi-trauma patients who could not tolerate cervical hyperextension or in patients who were intubated. Jend-Rossman and Jend concluded that CT was clearly superior to any other diagnostic method in visualizing the frontal portions of the skull base. Statistically, the anterior cranial base or dorsal wall of the frontal sinuses appeared to be more accurately revealed by CT. With some exceptions, these authors are consistent with others in citing the clear advantage of CT over conventional radiographs in diagnosing fractures of all orbital walls.

Frame and Wake presented 6 years of experience with CT in oral and maxillofacial surgery and traumatology.[55] The authors justified their use of CT by noting the complexity of the three-dimensional structure of the midface, in which the bones are situated in various planes separated by adjacent soft tissues and air spaces. Frame and Wake advocated the use of CT in midfacial fractures and airway assessment in trauma patients. They also suggested monitoring long-term healing of midfacial fractures and bone grafts with CT instead of conventional radiography because CT is able to display the lateral and posterior aspects of the maxilla and the pterygoid areas.

Carter and Karmody were early users of CT technology to visualize complex facial fractures.[23] Carter noted that the full extent of maxillofacial fractures is not displayed on planigraphic and conventional tomography.[41] She advocated the use of thin-section, high-resolution CT in axial and coronal planes and felt that CT had essentially replaced conventional tomography in the assessment of maxillofacial and cervical injuries. Consistent with the literature, Carter stressed the value of CT in concomitant evaluation of the cranial vault in the presence of maxillofacial trauma. The oral and maxillofacial surgeon must be alerted to the presence of underlying intracranial pathology such as subdural or epidural hematoma, intracranial blood, cerebral damage, evidence of increased intracranial pressure, and pneumocephalus, none of which are evident on conventional radiographs.

Rowe et al. and Carter and Bankoff compared PT with CT in patients with maxillofacial injuries and determined that CT yielded additional useful data in nearly every case, mainly regarding the damage to soft tissues and displacement.[19,56] Carter, like Zilkha,[42] noted the ability of CT to demonstrate associated hematoma and entrapped extraocular muscles not displayed by PT. The ability of CT to clearly denote complex fractures in three dimensions with displacement of small and larger fragments was noted using axial and coronal CT (Fig. 3–72).

Signficant findings involving fractures of the cervical spine and associated soft-tissue injury internal or external to the spinal canal is clearly demonstrated by CT (Fig. 3–73). In-vasion of the spinal canal by bone fragments, seen especially in crush fractures of the vertebrae, are displayed accurately using CT, and compression of the cord can be displayed by injecting a contrast agent into the subarachnoid space. Rotary subluxation of C1 or C2, which was noted by Carter to be similar to Grisel's syndrome arising from trauma,[41] can be demonstrated by CT.

Direct laryngeal trauma can be assessed early using CT to display the extent of injury to the cartilaginous elements as well as adjacent soft tissues.[57] CT in the axial plane is valuable in patients with supraglottic edema that prevents direct laryngoscopy. CT demonstrates the extent of hematoma and edema of the paralaryngeal and pre-epiglottic space and their effect on the airway. CT, unlike PT, demonstrates the true cross-sectional dimensions of the airway.

On the basis of the comparison of CT with polytomography, Carter has made the following recommendations.[41]

1. To identify the maximum number of fractures, obtain two projections (axial and coronal for CT, coronal and lateral for PT).
2. If both CT and PT are available, CT is the better technique except for injuries to the inferior rim or floor.

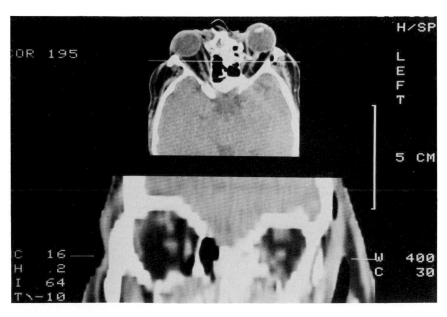

FIG. 3–72. Axial and coronal CT views of midfacial structures demonstrating capability of CT to display information in three dimensions.

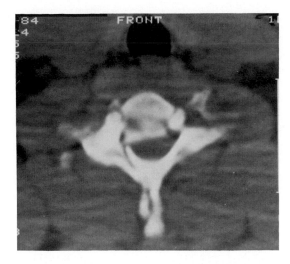

FIG. 3–73. CT can readily reveal fractures and soft-tissue injuries of the cervical spine.

3. In investigating bony injury to the orbital inferior rim or floor, PT is the better procedure; however, the ability of CT to demonstrate the intraorbital contents makes it a better choice if specific information about these structures is desired.
4. Coronal imaging is important in enumerating fractures. If only axial CT can be done and reformatting is not helpful, coronal PT should be obtained as well.

OBSERVATIONS OF MAXILLOFACIAL INJURIES WITH CT SCANNING

The first CT images of the head were taken in the transaxial plane, and it is this view that yields much information regarding maxillofacial trauma as well as the presence of intracranial trauma. Complex maxillofacial trauma as in "crush" injuries occupying a large bilateral facial area are rarely "pure," consistent with the Le Fort classification. Such trauma produces extensive fragmentation and soft-tissue injury and is elegantly visualized by high-resolution CT in the axial plane.

Axial CT can display invasion of the inter- and intraorbital regions and cranial vault by these complex injuries. Pneumocephalus is easily detected on axial CT (high-contrast brain window) and can originate from such sites as the posterior wall of the frontal sinus, ethmoid labyrinth, cribriform plates, and sphenoid sinus. Comminuted bony fragments cause rents in the dura and permit the entrance of air into the intracranial side of the dural wall (Fig. 3–74). If the arachnoid is lacerated, air enters the subarachnoid space and may produce a spontaneous ventriculogram. Localization of bone fragments in axial and coronal displays with extended bone window and 1.5-mm slice thickness in areas of concern is mandatory.

FRONTAL SINUSES

High-velocity, high-impact motor vehicular trauma may produce injuries located in the frontal sinuses and the floor of the anterior cranial fossa. A high index of suspicion should exist for these kinds of injuries because the frontal bone will fracture only from high-gravity force or at many pounds of pressure per square inch. The clinician may assume that deeper structures such as the dura, brain, or base of the skull or optic nerve are involved. In the past, frontal sinus fractures were assessed by lateral and AP tomography. While these methods may be used successfully, CT has virtually replaced polytomography for imaging this kind of injury, especially when there is much comminution involving the frontal bone, the anterior and posterior table, and the nasoethmoid complex with herniation of brain tissue into the sinus or orbits. Midfacial fractures involving the Le Fort II or III types of central facial smash with NOE components seem to have a higher incidence of intracranial complications.

Using CT, the anterior and posterior walls of the frontal sinuses can be visualized well and air-fluid levels seen easily. Kassel and Cooper noted a typical hinge-type pattern of fracture with displacement of the lateral frontal fragment through the lateral aspect of the frontal sinus[1] (Fig. 3–75). This type of fracture is often associated with a fracture extending along the floor of the anterior cranial fossa. Superior maxillofacial injuries in any event should suggest to the maxillofacial surgeon the presence of intracranial disorder. Frontal sinus fractures may be classified as anterior, posterior, or both.[58] Fractures involving the anterior and posterior walls, as noted with Le Fort I, II, III, facial smash, and NOE fractures,

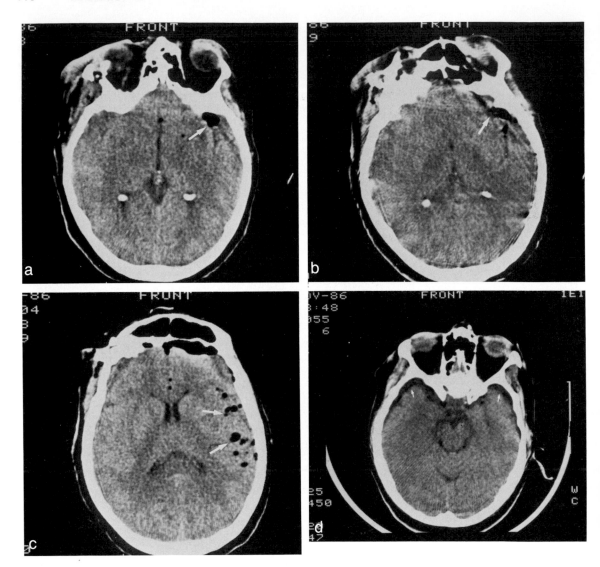

FIG. 3–74. **a, b,** and **c**. Extension of air into brain (arrows). **d**, Transaxial CT demonstrating hygroma (white arrows) of frontal lobes with coexisting maxillofacial fractures.

have a greater incidence of intracranial complications.

Performing exploratory surgery on all depressed fractures of the anterior wall may not be necessary for assessing the status of the posterior wall or for assessing the presence of hematoma or CSF within the frontal sinus (Fig. 3–61). I have used CT to determine whether an exploration of a fracture of the posterior table involving exenteration of the sinus and posterior wall with ablation or cranialization of the sinus is warranted. In my experience in dealing with maxillofacial trauma in the Allegheny General Hospital's Trauma Center, the CT scan has replaced the conventional radiograph and polytomogram in determining whether to perform exploratory surgery in depressed fractures of the anterior wall.

In NOE injuries at the root of the nose in which the nasofrontal region is depressed into or impacted along the base of the skull or medial lamina of the orbital walls, it is important to evaluate the patient for nasofrontal duct injury; if there is significant hemorrhage into the sphenoid or ethmoid sinus along with lesser wing fractures, the optic nerve should be evaluated clinically and using a CT scan. Obviously, if clinical conditions such as an amaurotic pupil or Marcus Gunn pupillary

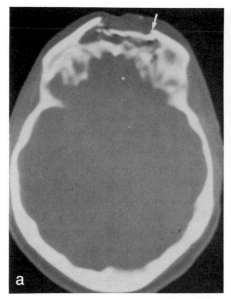
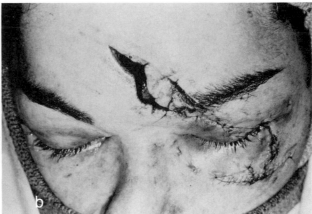

FIG. 3–75.   **a,** Transaxial CT displaying characteristic hinge-type pattern of fracture of the lateral frontal segment of the frontal sinus (arrow) The patient is a 30-year-old woman involved in a motor vehicle accident. **b,** Clinical photograph of the bony injuries displayed in Figure 3–78a.

phenomenon exist, immediate orbital decompression may be indicated. Fractures with a NOE component with the nasal root impacted into or onto the base of the anterior cranial fossa should alert the surgeon to the possibility of nasofrontal injury. Fractures in the nasofrontal complex or those associated with Le Fort II or III fractures are invariably comminuted. CT emphasizes this comminution while alerting the surgeon to check for medial canthal injury or lacrimal canal system drainage problems.

The entire supraorbital region and floor of the anterior cranial fossa can be investigated for fractures. Bone fragments and/or foreign bodies can be detected lying within the brain or orbital cavity (globe). The ethmoid labyrinth can be studied for comminution or implosion of the medial orbital walls (lamina papyracea) with accompanying herniation of the orbital viscera into the ethmoid space. Disruption of the medial and lateral canthal ligaments can be ascertained, and the presence of brain tissue within the ethmoid labyrinth or intraorbital region can be detected. Some 20 to 40% of inferior orbital floor fractures involve a similar injury to the ethmoid surface. This percentage may be higher in major trauma centers.[3]

In my center, fractures involving the more superior aspect of the midface or frontal sinuses are associated with an increased incidence of intracranial complications, compared to those fractures involving the lower midface. Linear fractures involving the vault extending into the frontal sinus are best imaged by conventional polytomography.

SPHENOID SINUSES

Sphenoid sinus fractures are rare and may be misdiagnosed. True fractures of the sphenoid sinus are usually associated with basilar skull fractures. Sphenoid sinuses are frequently opacified or contain an air-fluid level. An opacification by fluid collection in the sphenoid sinuses usually does not represent the result of a basilar skull fracture or a cerebrospinal fluid leak; it most likely represents contusion and swelling of the sphenoid sinus mucous membrane. Skull base fractures are easily visualized on 5-mm resolution slices. These fractures are very difficult to image using conventional polytomography.

NASOETHMOID INJURIES

Fractures in the nasoethmoid complex from high-speed accidents are usually grossly comminuted. CT visualizes the comminution pattern and promotes the reconstruction of this area by identifying individual fragmentation. Nasoethmoid fractures tend to be impacted in an anteroposterior direction with telescoping of the lamina papyracea and ethmoid air cells. Nasoethmoid injuries invariably involve one or both orbital walls, floors, or orbital viscera. They are often associated with frontobasilar skull fractures. In many instances, nasoethmoid components are part of the classification of Le Fort midfacial injuries, usually of the Le Fort II and III type.

Imaging with CT can determine possible medial canthal ligamentous injury, global displacement, or nasolacrimal ductal obstruction or tear. Injury to the nasofrontal duct in its course from the frontal sinus into the nasal cavity can also be imaged using CT. Such fractures of the nasoethmoid complex are readily assessed by CT whether or not there is opacification of the ethmoid air cells. Conventional films or polytomography do not demonstrate well the fine ethmoid septa because fracture lines are obscured easily by sinus opacification. Similarly, conventional studies including tomography may not detect blow-in fractures of the medial wall of the orbit or differentiate this type of fracture from the more common blow-out fracture. Commonly, medial and inferior blow-out fractures are associated in major complex facial trauma. Both anterior and posterior ethmoid air cells may be involved, although the majority are anterior. The nasoethmoid injury can be classified and surgery can be planned immediately using primary open reduction and direct fixation, including, when indicated, bone grafting procedures or closed reduction and fixation methods.

ORBITAL INJURIES

Numerous imaging methods have been used specifically to visualize the orbits. Planigraphic and tomographic radiographs are standard preliminary or definitive techniques in most instances. Fine-bone detail and soft-tissue densities may be difficult to define even with hypocycloidal tomography. Hence, distinguishing soft-tissue densities appearing within the associated sinuses as representing

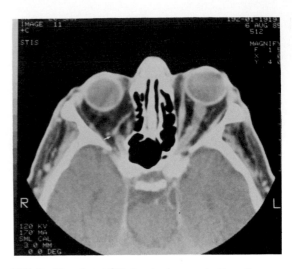

FIG. 3–76.   Axial CT clearly demonstrating discontinuity of optic nerve on right side (arrow).

hematoma, mucosal edema, or, indeed, prolapsed orbital viscera with or without muscle entrapment is difficult.

To attempt to differentiate such soft-tissue densities, the techniques of xeroradiography, positive contrast orbitography, and CT have been used. Of all conventional radiographic techniques and these latter modalities, CT has emerged as the primary imaging technology for orbital trauma, because orbital injuries possess all the elements to maximize the imaging strengths of CT.[29,46,47,51,52,59] The high fat content of the periorbital and intraorbital region lends itself to superb imaging because of the high-contrast resolution of CT. With high-spatial resolution, the four orbital walls and rims can be exquisitely displayed and fragment size and displacement accurately assessed using axial and reformatted coronal and sagittal views.

On axial CT, the bony structures making up the orbital apex and the optic canal are clearly seen, and suspected indirect optic nerve injury is given appropriate weight in the differential diagnosis (Fig. 3–76). High-contrast CT with narrower window and lower level can superbly assess the orbital viscera including the ocular globe, intraocular contents, extraocular muscles, ligaments (lateral, medial, check, suspensory), and optic nerve and its dural coverings. It can display herniation of orbital viscera into the ethmoid or maxillary sinuses or encroachment of brain tissue (encephalocele) into the orbits. Orbital emphysema, proptosis, global displacement or rupture ("flat tire" effect), lenticular subluxation, retrobulbar hematoma (orbital apex syndrome), and subdural hematoma of the optic nerve sheath are readily seen (Fig. 3–77). Disruptions of the extraocular muscles (entrapment in all planes) can be visualized and located precisely for subsequent surgical release.

The conventional radiographic signs of blow-out fractures of the orbit that are associated with complex midfacial trauma can be summarized as including fragmentation or comminution of the orbital floor, depression of fragments into the antrum, or prolapse of the orbital soft tissues in the maxillary sinus. These same radiographic signs apply to CT diagnosis. The orbital contents hence must be visualized at a narrower window and lower level to properly assess the orbital viscera consisting of the globe, optic nerve, and extraocular muscles. In addition, using varying technical maneuvers, one can determine the presence of brain tissue versus orbital fat within the orbit in its posterior reaches. One can view orbital wall fragmentation on axial CT especially when viewing medial and lat-

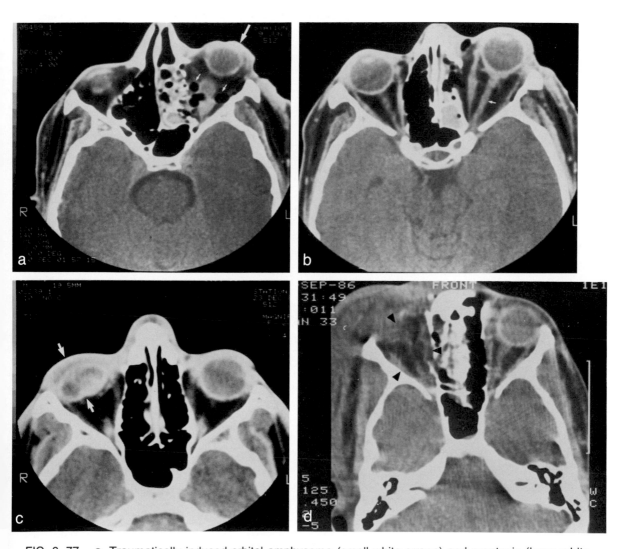

FIG. 3–77.   **a,** Traumatically induced orbital emphysema (small white arrows) and proptosis (large white arrow). **b,** Extensive proptosis with stretching of optic nerve (arrow). **c,** Traumatic rupture of right ocular globe; note typical "flat-tire" effect (arrows). Compare with opposite normal left globe. **d,** CT displaying massive avulsion of ocular globe and orbital viscera (between black triangles).

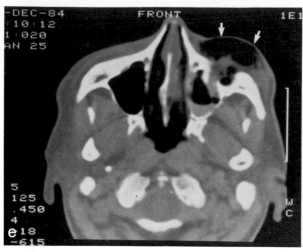
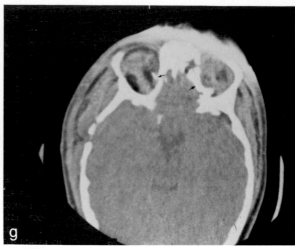

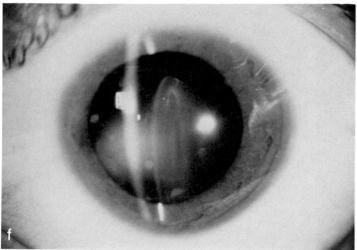

FIG. 3-77. (Continued).   **e**, Massive eyelid emphysema (arrows). **f**, Clinical photograph of traumatically induced lens dislocation. This injury is readily imaged by axial CT and must be detected because of the potential for the development of traumatic glaucoma. (Courtesy of Dr. J. Kennerdale, Dept. of Ophthalmology, Allegheny General Hospital.) **g**, Axial CT demonstrating intraorbital bony fragments (arrows).

eral wall disruption. The anterior reaches of the orbit, including the infraorbital rim, can also be assessed. When scanning parallel to the orbital floor, adequately assessing the floor of the orbit is difficult because it is parallel to the scanning beam. However, multiple spicules and fragmentation of the comminuted orbital floor can be found within the maxillary antrum. When coronal reformatted images are then observed in the magnified mode, these multiple fragments can be more accurately assessed.

Currently, isolated orbital injuries are studied in the axial and coronal planes. Direct coronal CT may be contraindicated in the mul-

titrauma patient; however, current software for coronal reformation provides an excellent method for visualizing the soft-tissue and bony components. The axial scan reveals much information, as noted above, because the plane of the scan is parallel to the roof and floor; in the presence of relatively nondisplaced but clinically significant fractures of these walls, this scan could be unproductive. The soft tissues of the orbital floor (posterior fat pad) cannot be visualized well in this plane. This problem is partially offset by high-resolution, thin-slice techniques and appropriate changes in gantry angulation.

The importance of axial scanning in suspected orbital trauma associated with maxillofacial trauma relates directly to ocular, optic nerve, and extraocular muscle injury. Direct trauma to the globe can result in chemosis, subconjunctival hemorrhage, hyphema, vitreous hemorrhage, lenticular subluxation with or without secondary glaucoma, retinal artery or vein occlusion, orbital apex syndrome, retinal edema, or detachment and rupture of the globe with herniation of the vitreous. CT can demonstrate many such intra- or extraocular complications that require immediate ophthalmologic attention. Axial CT can also demonstrate such orbital problems complicating maxillofacial injuries as pneumo-orbita, emphysema and edema of the eyelids, orbital encephalocele, and intra- or extraocular foreign bodies. Because changes in the anterior-posterior position of the globe are clearly defined, enophthalmos associated with increased orbital volume, loss of periorbital fat or fibrosis, or contusion of muscle posterior to the globe is accurately displayed.

The coronal reconstruction will define this problem more clearly and direct primary care more intelligently. When coronal reformatted images are then observed in the magnified mode, these multiple fragments can be more accurately assessed. The decision to approach the orbital floor with a primary bone grafting reconstructive procedure at the first operation is thus justified. This decision is extremely important when dealing with a multiply traumatized patient who may have a flail chest and for whom it must be determined whether a rib or iliac crest graft must be placed within the orbital floor to support the globe. Of course, direct CCT in orbital floor fractures is extraordinarily sensitive in the detection of complete destruction of the orbital floor and is the method of choice in the isolated maxillofacial injury without cervical cord injuries or other injuries that would preclude the use of direct CT scanning. Appropriate soft tissue scanning easily identifies the extraocular muscles and thus helps determine whether entrapment exists medially, laterally, and inferiorly. Foreign bodies or bone fragments involving the globe or extraocular muscles can also be detected. CT can clarify pseudoprolapse by displaying muscle lying "free"

within the orbit—a limitation in conventional tomography.

Opacification of the associated nasal sinus does not obscure detail on CT, and displaced bone fragments that may not be visualized on conventional tomography or plain films will be easily noted. Associated fractures of the inferior orbital rim or the relationship of the infraorbital canal to the fracture site may be assessed. The loss of vision without direct trauma to the globe may be due to indirect trauma to the optic nerves or the optic chiasm, interruption of the intracranial visual pathways, or cortical blindness. Bone fragments may be displaced toward the optic nerve or globe, injuring or displacing these structures. The globe may be displaced in an anteroposterior direction medially, laterally, or inferiorly. Even with massive injuries involving the facial structures, the globe is usually displaced inferiorly toward the ipsilateral maxillary antrum. Enophthalmos may be masked by edema or hematoma and does not present as an early finding unless an extensive blowout occurs, manifested by marked increase in fat herniation and immediate enophthalmos. Otherwise, an enophthalmos usually presents as a delayed progressive complication secondary to orbital fibrosis and progressive fat atrophy.

Some controversy concerning this mechanism has arisen in more-recent three-dimensional studies involving the orbital volume (see below). Emery and von Noorden noted that enophthalmos may be masked and does not present as an early finding unless an initial impact has caused massive loss of support for the globe with immediate fat herniation.[60] They observed delayed enophthalmos in 14% of patients with orbital floor fractures. CT may be useful to assess extraocular edema and intraorbital hematoma and to predict which cases of orbital fractures may be more likely to develop enophthalmos. Many percentages have been given for the coexistence of an ethmoid surface or medial wall fracture and an orbital floor blow-out. This figure is much higher in centers that have a higher percentage of major complex facial trauma. Demonstrating such fractures with conventional radiography may be difficult. CT is superb at displaying anterior ethmoidal clouding where involvement is more common or in demonstrating emphysema of the orbit that was not detected on conventional films. CT also demonstrates blow-in fractures of the orbit. Conventional radiography may visualize only the soft-tissue opacification of the ethmoid sinus and not delineate the more comon blow-out fracture.

An important consideration is the possibility that blindness can result after seemingly insignificant impacts such as a simple moderate blow to the brow region. A close correlation of clinical and CT findings can elucidate the prognosis for visual morbidity. Numerous traumatic mechanisms may result in visual loss. Direct injury to the globe with intraocular disruption is clearly the most straightforward. However, indirect trauma to the optic nerve, chiasm, visual pathways, and visual cortex, as mentioned above, often coexist with complex maxillofacial trauma. While it would seem logical to impune as the primary cause of visual loss, either hematoma involving the nerve or fragmentation of the adjacent facial skeleton resulting in compression or laceration of the optic nerve, other less obvious mechanisms seem to explain visual loss.

It is becoming increasingly apparent that most injuries of the optic nerve are canalicular and involve hemorrhage into the nerve sheath or contusion of the nerve with edma and subsequent compression. The unifying morbid etiologic element is a neural ischemia that rapidly results in blindness. CT scanning involving severe maxillofacial trauma should include serious attention to the optic canal or, by inference, the body of the sphenoid and lesser wing of that bone. A close anatomic relationship exists between the optic canal, lesser and greater wings of the sphenoid bone, sphenoid and ethmoid sinuses, and orbital plane of the frontal bone. Injuries to these bones, especially the lesser wing and the body of the sphenoid bone, may cause injury indirectly to the optic nerve itself. In penetrating injuries to the midface, localized force and injury are usually involved. Penetrating injury more frequently results in injury to the deeper structures of the maxillofacial region. Gunshot wounds appear to combine the features of blunt and penetrating injuries. CT combined with angiographic studies has an important role in the investigation of these injuries, which may cause vascular fistula, traumatic aneurysm, or dural tear.

Axial CT can readily demonstrate fractures involving the optic canal and thus raise suspicion of indirect neural trauma. The clinician should also be highly suspicious of optic nerve injury when hemorrhage into the sphenoid and ethmoid sinuses is viewed on CT, as these bones, constituting the walls of these sinuses, share in the bony boundaries of the optic canal (Fig. 3–78). The optic nerve is covered by dura, arachnoid, and pia and is thus a direct extension of the brain. These layers are fused to the nerve and to the periosteum of the sphenoid bone in the optic canal. Maxillofacial trauma with concomitant orbital involvement can result in canalicular fracture with a shearing force directed upon the meningeal layers of the optic nerve and, through their common fusion to the nerve, exert a torquing force on the nerve. CT can often display subdural hematomas involving the intraorbital portion of the optic nerve sheath, which can also result in blindness.

The importance of axial CT scanning of the orbits prior to reconstructive maxillofacial trauma surgery cannot be overemphasized. The literature reports cases of blindness occurring postoperatively after manipulation of midfacial fractures.[61,62] In Gordon and McCrae's report, the blindness was attributed to a subdural hematoma of the optic nerve sheath that occurred during fracture reduction. In Miller's report, permanent loss of vision occurred gradually over several days postreduction but was observed before operative repair of the facial injuries. An argument can be raised for delaying maxillofacial fracture repair involving suspicious ocular trauma lest the operative intervention be blamed for the visual loss that would have occurred inevitably.

In any maxillofacial injury in which there is orbital encroachment, especially with traumatic impacts involving the orbital roof, suspicious orbital visceral damage, or loss of visual acuity, a preoperative biplanar CT (axial and reformatted coronal) is recommended. An ophthalmologic consultation should be

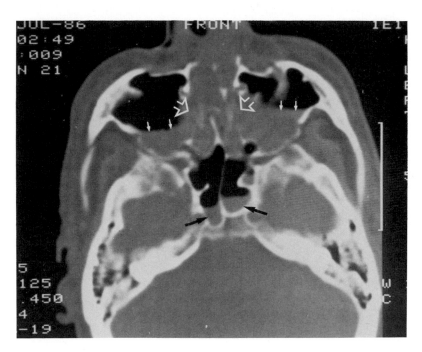

FIG. 3–78.   Axial CT demonstrating hemorrhage into maxillary sinus (closed white arrows), ethmoid sinuses (open white arrows), and sphenoid sinuses (black arrows). A significant potential for optic nerve injury has been found with this injury.

sought. The funduscopic examination may appear entirely normal in patients with neural injury and blindness; optic disc pallor may occur 2 to 6 weeks after neural injury. In the immediate post-trauma period, an absolute afferent pupillary defect (amaurotic pupil) or a relative afferent pupillary defect (Marcus Gunn pupil) should lead to vigorous investigation involving thin-slice, high-resolution CT in the region of the optic canal with magnification. These results can lead the ophthalmologist to select decompression orbitotomy in those cases with minimal canal disruption.

The orbits can be investigated by direct coronal CT in which the supine hanging-head or elevated chin position (if safe) can be used or by coronal reconstructed axial scans. In either technique, the scan is comparable to the plain Caldwell view. These views allow investigation of tangential cross sections of all orbital walls and orbital viscera, including all extraocular muscles (Fig. 3–79). Direct coronal high-resolution CT scanning produces superior images compared to reformations, especially when scans are nearly perpendicular to the OM line. Coronal scans are significantly useful in detecting extraocular muscle

involvement especially in the inferior rectus and inferior oblique muscles. Subtle orbital floor fractures are best seen on image reformation in a plane defined by the inferior rectus muscle, perpendicular to its course. A trapped muscle may appear elongated with its long axis perpendicular to the fractured wall. CT can display contrast between muscle and contiguous orbital fat. Current scanning technology involves delineation of bone fragments whether they are adjacent to air (sinus) or soft tissue. Hence, it is possible to detect multiple bone fragments in a sinus with air-fluid contents.

As in optic nerve injuries, the clinical examination must be closely correlated with the imaging protocol. Entrapment of the inferior rectus and oblique muscles will cause restriction in upward gaze because of the "tethering" effect and restriction in downward gaze because of the compromised mechanical advantage. In clinically significant fractures of the orbital floor, diplopia will occur in functionally important fields of gaze. The affected globe will appear lower or more posterior than the unaffected globe (enophthalmos) (Fig. 3–80). The decision to surgically explore

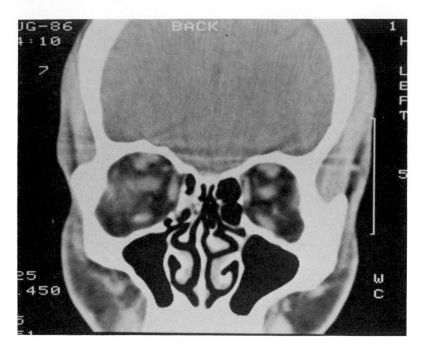

FIG. 3–79. Coronal CT demonstrating cross sections of orbital walls, viscera, and extraocular muscles.

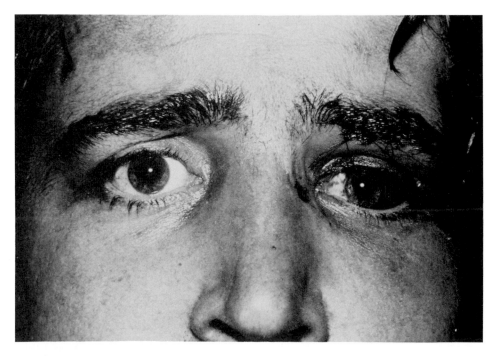

FIG. 3–80. Enophthalmos associated with extensive loss of orbital floor.

the orbital floor, therefore, will derive not only from CT images but from careful clinical examination and judgment. In complex maxillofacial injuries in which loss of tissue has occurred or in which the orbital floor or other orbital wall is missing, CT, especially biplanar or triplanar (axial, direct coronal, or coronal/sagittal reformatted CT), will generate a three-dimensional image of the area of injury so that the principles of craniofacial surgery can be applied (e.g., calvarial, rib, and iliac crest grafting). CT may also display blow-in fractures of the orbits.[63]

With injuries to the upper facial third, determining early the extent of damage is important because such injuries can be complicated by dural tears with pneumocephalus, CSF leak or meningitis, brain abscesses, laceration of brain tissue, foreign body or bone fragments imbedded in the cerebral tissues, or secondary abnormalities in sinus drainage related to the maxillofacial injury. Such complications are best studied using various modes of CT scanning. Thinner slices, 1.5 mm, combined with intravenous enhancement may be used to properly assess CSF leaks. Intravenous enhancements may also be used to assess possible brain abscesses.

ZYGOMATICOMAXILLARY COMPLEX (ZMC) FRACTURES

Isolated ZMC fractures are readily visualized by conventional radiography. In the multitrauma patient in whom routine films are limited, CT may be used to demonstrate the ZMC fracture as a component or components of more complex maxillofacial injuries. The actual fracture elements of ZMC fractures are viewed by very specific scanning planes—maxillary zygoma separation by axial or coronal scans, temporal element by axial scans, frontozygomatic by coronal scans, and bodily displacement of zygoma/coronoid by axial scans.[1] CT is good for displacements of the ZMC in the horizontal axis. Both coronal and axial scans may be required to fully visualize actual displacement of the zygomatic body. The separation of the zygoma from the maxilla may be seen in either transaxial or coronal planes; the temporal component is best visualized in the transaxial plane whereas the zygomaticofrontal component is best demonstrated in the coronal plane. One can visualize impingement of the zygoma on the coronoid process, which explains clinical signs and symptoms. Zygomatic arch fractures are well visualized in the transaxial plane and may be assessed as involving single or comminuted fragments. The step defect at the infraorbital rim can be seen in the transaxial and coronal planes. The infraorbital rim fracture is noted to extend medially from the lateral wall of the maxillary antrum along the zygomaticomaxillary suture through the zygomatic process of the maxillary sinus to involve the inferior orbital rim or to extend just lateral to the infraorbital canal. Such fractures are imaged either conventionally or with CT. The more lateral involvement of the infraorbital rim is different from the majority of inferior wall blow-out fractures, which tend to be centered medially to the infraorbital wall. As noted with midfacial fractures, CT appears to be the most accurate method to measure zygomatic displacements, especially in the horizontal axis.

Classifications of ZMC fractures have been based on the conventional Waters projection alone. Classifying ZMC injuries using CT scanning enables the clinician to establish three-dimensional patterns of displacement of the malar complex.[65] CT is useful in classifying ZMC fractures even though the useful classifications are based on the analysis of the displaced fragment from three directions using three different radiographs. Conventional imaging of the fractured ZMC is complicated by the difficulty of positioning the multiply injured patient properly for each of the three radiographs. In addition, radiographic interpretation may be influenced considerably by variations in the radiographic technique, making evaluating fine fracture patterns difficult.

CT has made it possible to place patients easily in a standardized position to obtain axial images without worrying about excess movement or any disturbance from edema of the face. Thus, CT can evaluate anterior and posterior displacement of the bone fragments in malar complex fractures with a series of axial images. Clear images of the complex inner body structures and surrounding soft tissues, as well as the fracture patterns of the malar complex on the Z axis, can be observed. Characteristic changes can be seen in the antrum in every type of malar complex fracture, especially the lateral walls of the fractured antrum. This imaging may provide some insight in resolving the problem of why some malar fractures are unstable and tend to relapse after reduction without complete fixation.[65] Such relapse may occur because of the inability of thin comminuted walls of the antrum to resist the tension applied by surrounding soft tissues in this type of malar fracture when the fracture was fixated only in the frontal area. If one compares CT with the conventional radiographic classification system proposed by Knight and North,[64] most malar fractures with bodily displacement visible on conventional radiographs also have an anteroposterior shift that is observable on CT; a case having severe medial lateral displacement is inclined also to have severe posteroanterior displacement. By combining the conventional and CT classification systems, it is possible to establish a complete three-dimensional or anatomic pattern of displacement for each malar complex fracture and plan treatment more effectively or accurately.[65]

The lateral orbital walls, including the zygomatic arches and zygomaticomaxillary suture areas, are well viewed with CT (Fig. 3–81). Fractures involving disruption of the nasal septum, cribriform plate, and walls of the sphenoid sinus can be visualized well in the axial plane. Visualizing the floor of the sphenoid sinus in problematic, and sagittal reformatted CT or lateral PT is an important adjunct in diagnosis. In the multitrauma patient, using reformatted coronal CT scans is usually more appropriate. In this plane, the entire midfacial skeleton can be viewed. The basilar skull region, paranasal sinus, and orbital cavities are well defined. The four walls of the orbit can be delineated and reconstruction planned. A grid placed over the scan film can be used to assess telecanthus and ocular hypertelorism. Vertical and horizontal displacements of the zygoma can be evaluated. The volume of avulsed hard and soft tissue can be judged to plan for craniofacial repair, especially when three-dimensional imaging

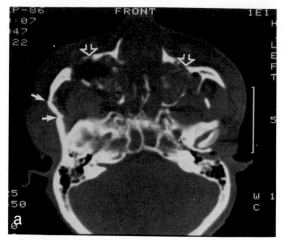

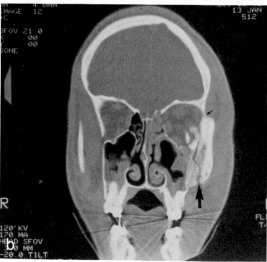

FIG. 3–81.   **a,** Axial CT demonstrating fractures of the right zygomatic arch (closed arrows) and fractures of the orbital rims (open arrows). **b,** Coronal CT revealing fractured, displaced left bone of zygoma (large black arrow) and separation of frontozygomatic suture (small black arrow).

modalities are employed. The majority of CT scanner gantries do not allow direct sagittal scans. While sagittal reformations are improving, they remain inferior to the skeletal images of PT. Most authors feel that sagittal reformats of the orbital floor are the best view using this method.

MIDFACIAL INJURIES

As mentioned, most complex maxillofacial injuries do not readily correspond to the classic Le Fort categorization. In high-velocity accidents, it is more common especially to have combinations of the classic Le Fort I, II, and III classifications than to have strictly delineated Le Fort fractures. It is also more common to have comminution of the midfacial skeleton than to have strictly defined boundries as classified by Le Fort.

There is a direct relationship between the severity of the impact and the displacement and comminution of the facial structures. Axial CT readily demonstrates fractures of the maxilla that are commonly associated with complex midfacial injuries. Axial CT is useful in imaging fractures of the posterior maxilla, alveolus, and pterygoid plates and thus defines the posterior extension of the Le Fort and midfacial fracture group. The anterior walls of the maxilla, infraorbital rims, lateral maxillary walls, and contents of the maxillary antra are clearly seen (Fig. 3–82). The CT will display anterior, medial, or lateral walls without the hyperextension of the neck, usually required for conventional studies. Anterior wall fractures may be directly visualized and related to the position of the infraorbital canal. Maxillary sinus contusion, air-fluid levels, or opacification or fragmentation within is accompanied by a fracture of the sinus wall in the majority of instances.

Maxillary fractures of the Le Fort variety are usually bilateral and associated with some degree of adherence to the Le Fort description, although asymmetry may be present. Usually, the nasal bones and septum are involved, as are the pterygoid processes of the sphenoid bone. One can readily assess with CT the Z axis displacement of the midface. All the various sutural components, including zygomaticomaxillary and midpalatal, can be ascertained using transaxial CT as well as reformatted CT or redirected CCT.

In recent years, it has become evident that CT scanning is superior to polytomography in delineating more complex Le Fort II fractures, especially when ZMC fractures are superimposed. The facial structures are relatively inhomogeneous and partially consist of thin bone surrounded by air or soft tissue. Large changes in tissue density create great variations in attenuation of transmitted x rays and allow relatively easy contrast resolution. By expanding the gray scale window and in-creasing the facial level center in the positive gray scale, the spatial and contrast bone resolution is improved, allowing evaluation of facial bone detail without significant loss of bone tissue differentiation.

In uncomplicated Le Fort II fractures, coronal polytomography is equal to axial CT; in more complex Le Fort III and central facial crush injuries in the presence of significant facial fractures and comminutions, however, CT is the modality of choice.

MANDIBULAR FRACTURES

Mandibular fractures are usually best seen with either conventional radiographs or polytomograms, especially when the temporomandibular joints are to be assessed. Anterior, posterior, and lateral polycycloidal tomography are usually diagnostic. However, when patients have multiple injuries and assessment of the overall maxillofacial injuries is required early in the initial post-trauma phase, CT does offer some advantages when the patient cannot be moved. CT has been reported as being successful when diagnosing mandibular fractures,[66] and certainly the position or fragmentation of condyloid processes and coronoid processes can be assessed in the transaxial and coronal planes (Fig. 3–83). The sagittal reformatting of the temporomandibular joint can assess rupture of the glenoid fossa of the temporal bone with dislocation of the condyloid process into the middle cranial fossa.

CERVICAL SPINE

If axial sections are taken more inferiorly, the entire cervical spine can be completely imaged. A lateral preview film is taken initially to give an overview and to allow selection of areas of particular concern. The axial plane CT study generates data about the bony cervical spine and its subjacent cord content. As mentioned, an airway obstruction caused by laryngeal edema or fracture can be simultaneously assessed. In summary, scanning in the axial plane generates significant information and is exceptionally useful in determining anteroposterior dimensional changes

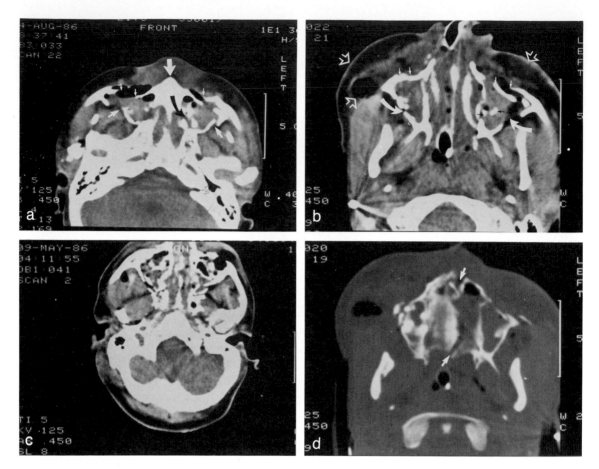

FIG. 3–82. **a,** CT in axial plane demonstrating severe midfacial disruptions. Fracture of the anterior maxillary walls (three small white arrows) and posterior maxillary walls (bilateral white arrows); "blow-in" fracture from medial maxillary sinus wall (black arrow). Midfacial skeleton appears to be impacted posteriorly (large white arrow). **b,** Extensive midfacial injury revealed by CT. Note anterior maxillary wall fractures (four white arrows), bone fragments in maxillary sinus (black arrows), posterior maxillary wall fractures (curved arrows), massive emphysema present throughout soft tissues (open white arrows). Note vertical mandibular rami. **c,** Severe comminution of midfacial skeleton. Multiple bone fragments within maxillary sinus and posterior wall of maxillary sinus fractures with generalized hemorrhage throughout. **d,** CT of maxilla revealing sagittal palatal fracture (arrows).

in the maxillofacial skeleton and cervical regions (Fig. 3–84).

COMBINATION INJURIES

Conventional planigraphic radiology and PT are standard imaging modalities for isolated maxillofacial skeletal fractures. In combinations of injuries, the clinical examination, while no less important, can be severely limited or encumbered by gross edema or hematoma, so that imaging may yield the only meaningful preliminary data. Unfortunately, even when possible, conventional radiography rarely reveals the extent of the damage, and the bony fragmentation found on surgical exploration may be much more extensive.[42] Multiple maxillofacial and associated injuries will demand a more deliberate diagnostic system using the quality of images produced by a current generation CT scanner. Increasingly, sophisticated, clinically directed, image-manipulated CT is playing a major role in these injuries. Unenhanced axial CT can generate excellent diagnostic data, safely and rapidly with minimal stress to the multitrauma patient. The brain can be studied by 10-mm slices, the maxillofacial skeleton by

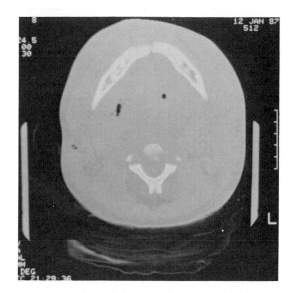

FIG. 3–83. Axial CT demonstrating fracture of the mandibular symphysis. CT is useful in diagnosing mandibular fractures in those patients who cannot be positioned for conventional radiography of the mandible. CT is also useful in localizing displaced condyloid processes of the mandible.

5–mm slices or thinner slices if required, and the cervical region by 5-mm slices in one imaging session. Direct coronal and direct sagittal images are ordinarily not permitted by the extent of systemic injuries or suspected cervical trauma. Direct sagittal images are usually not allowed also because of technical problems in gantry size, mobility or configuration. Scanning can be performed in a variety of window levels and width and size

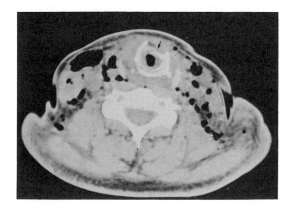

FIG. 3–84. Axial CT demonstrating fracture of the larynx (arrow) with massive air emphysema in the neck (multiple black areas of varying sizes and shapes).

thicknesses, with or without image reversal. Following rapid scanning techniques, reformations can be generated within the coronal plane or sagittal plane or at various angles to Reid's base line with or without the magnified mode. Axial CT will allow imaging of such late morbidity as brain abscess or chronic CSF leak. Indolent CSF leaks are best evaluated by preview-controlled CT after intrathecal introduction of metrizamide.

A disadvantage of coronal CT is that it is uncomfortable or impossible in some patients because of other injuries, especially if the gantry cannot be tilted, and it is contraindicated in patients with spinal cord injuries. Artifacts are another problem. Metal artifacts, which are caused by high-density objects such as dental restorations or bullets, commonly appear as radial streaks in coronal views and may obscure fracture fragments.

It is possible to sedate patients and to give anesthesia to patients when exquisite fine detail is absolutely essential. Intubated combative patients are commonly managed with paralyzing drugs, and children may be sedated to gain more precise images.

My experience at the Trauma Center at Allegheny General Hospital in Pittsburgh is consistent with that of most authors, who report that the majority of complex maxillofacial injuries associated with significant comminution of the facial skeleton are caused by blunt high-impact force distributed over a large surface area of the face. The majority of these injuries are caused by motor vehicular trauma, with industrial accidents and recreational accidents making up smaller percentages. Although maxillofacial injuries can be classified in a variety of ways using numerous groupings, the oral and maxillofacial surgeon has difficulty placing blunt high-velocity, high-impact trauma with resultant bony comminution into meaningful categories such as the classic Le Fort grouping. The Le Fort classification maintains its utility but must be modified somewhat in describing the combinations encountered in the multitrauma victim. Kassel and Cooper noted in their series that midfacial fractures were, by far, the most common injury.[1] These fractures were of the pure Le Fort variety with different combinations of Le Fort I, II, and III on the left and

Table 3–2.   Groups of Midfacral Skeletal, Neurologic, Orbital, and Laryngeal Injuries

Group I:	Complex "smash" fractures
Group II:	Multiple and/or bilateral fracture (Le Fort group)
Group III:	Craniocerebral trauma
Group IV:	Cervical spine (with or without spinal cord injury)
Group V:	Orbital trauma (with or without globe, optic nerve)
Group VI:	Laryngeal trauma
Group VII:	Complications (early, e.g., dural tear with pneumocephalus; late, e.g., CSF leak)

(Modified from Noyek, A.M., et al.: Sophisticated CT in complex maxillofacial trauma. Laryngoscope (Suppl) 19:1–17, 1982.)

right sides of the facial skeleton. True Le Fort I, II, and III with distinct or single fracture planes were rarely caused by motor vehicle accidents. More commonly, the fracture planes represent a series of comminuted fractures through the facial skeleton. A direct relationship exists between the severity of the force and the displacement and comminution of the facial fracture.[22]

Multiple maxillofacial and associated injuries can be defined more appropriately by creating generic and specific groupings and combining them to explain or describe the extent or nature of the damage (Table 3–2).

To be "complex," a maxillofacial injury would encompass either Group I or Group II, in addition to any of the remaining groups, soft-tissue injuries, or complications. Using sophisticated CT, the number and location of fracture lines provide data for definitive surgical repair and suggest approaches for surgical exploration. It also allows visualization of the extent and direction of dislocation of fracture fragments. This knowledge enhances the surgeon's craniofacial technique relating to the sequence in which multiple fragments are "chain-linked" together by transosseous wiring or rigidly fixed using bone plates. Other important major maxillofacial anatomic disruptions such as avulsed tissue, optic nerve injury, or displacement or rupture of the globe can be detected, and the necessity for primary reconstruction, as seen with bone grafting and remote, free vascularized soft/bony tissue transfers can be assessed.

CEREBROSPINAL FLUID (CSF) LEAKS

Although contrast enhancement techniques are not usually employed in the acute situation, they may be used to visualize vascular problems. Contrast studies are used in maxillofacial trauma to localize late active CSF leaks. The contrast medium, metrizamide, a nonionic, water-soluble contrast agent, is usually introduced by a lumbar puncture but also may be given by puncture at the lateral C1 or C2 or suboccipital spaces with the contrast agent positioned intracranially at the suspected locus of the leak. Cooper and Kassel used 190 to 220 mg/ml, and up to 10 ml of the high concentration has been given without any serious side effects.[67] The imaging protocol consists of careful preview-controlled axial and coronal studies. Cotton pledgets are placed in each nostril. Axial and coronal studies are useful in detecting CSF leakage related to the posterior wall of the frontal sinus; the coronal display is important in leaks in the region of the ethmoid labyrinth, the cribriform plates, and the roof of the sphenoid sinus. Slice thickness may be reduced to 1.5 mm and the extended bone window with high resolution should be used. In stable noncervical trauma, patients may be scanned in the prone position for direct coronal CT.

In slow leaks or in patients not actively leaking at the time of examination, Valsalva's maneuver with the patient in a more provocative position is attempted to elicit leaks. Scanning may be delayed for 3 hrs after the initial scan in a patient with an opaque sinus; measurement of CT absorption numbers may show an increase in the delayed scan, indicating that the contrast agent is leaking into the sinus. There may be an increase in Hounsfield units for example from 40–50 HU to 75–87 HU.

Traumatic CSF leaks usually start within 48 hrs after trauma and usually cease spontaneously within 1 week in 40% of cases. Most of the remaining cases usually stop within 6 months. Significantly, in untreated cases, the incidence of meningitis may be as high as 50%.[68] Surgical intervention without prior accurate localization may fail to demonstrate the defect in the dura or bone because the defect may be minute and the leak may arise from the anterior, middle, or posterior cranial fossa. The CSF leak may occur on the opposite side from the dripping nostril and more than one fistula may occur. Plain films, tomography, and radionuclide investigations are not as useful as CT. CT in addition to contrast studies offers the ability to identify both the size of a fracture and the leaking contrast agent. Resolution is better in several planes. CT used with contrast media is superior to radionuclide cisternography in a case of CSF fistula that leaks slowly or in which the leak has resolved.

As surgeons advance their technique, especially that of early primary repair, the need to have the maximum information available preoperatively is further increased. The concept that radiographic studies serve merely to confirm or document the clinical diagnosis of facial fractures is no longer valid given changing technology. Higher resolution density and fine spatial CT images are striving to keep pace with newer methods of craniofacial surgery. It has become increasingly apparent that CT can provide the surgeon with an appropriate blueprint for primary reconstruction and prevent surprises at the operating room table.[69] Kassel et al. feel that the radiologic study no longer grossly underestimates the complexity of the facial bony fragments, but rather presents an image from which the surgeon can base treatment plan and expectations before, or instead of, operative exploration.[2]

THREE-DIMENSIONAL IMAGING OF MAXILLOFACIAL TRAUMA

Oral and maxillofacial surgeons have long known that successful treatment of maxillofacial injuries, congenital and developmental facial anomalies, and traumatically induced facial deformity is best addressed by accurate approximation of the displaced or deformed underlying maxillofacial skeleton, and not only reapproximation or reconstruction of the overlying soft tissue. The specialty of oral and maxillofacial surgery was instrumental in the development of orthognathic surgery, the principles of which have been employed to redress the functional and aesthetic problems of congenital or developmental origin as well as the problems of deformity arising from trauma. As orthognathic surgery became increasingly sophisticated, its fundamental technologies were used to reconstruct the midfacial skeleton after Le Fort II and Le Fort III injuries and in ZMC osteotomies used to treat malunited midfacial fractures as well as dentofacial deformities.

Craniofacial surgery evolved parallel to these developments and was used mainly to address severe congenital facial deformities. The principles of orthognathic and craniofacial surgery can be used to treat nearly all of the acute and residual deformities arising from traumatic injuries. While oral and maxillofacial surgeons had been successful using numerous anthropometric analyses, direct facial measurements, manual and computed cephalometric analyses, and plaster casts of the dental arches and face, the possibilities existed to image the facial skeleton and its soft tissues in three dimensions, to fabricate models from these images using computer programs, and then to plan surgical bony and soft-tissue reconstructions with the best possible data base. It was further within the realm of technology to simulate proposed reconstructive surgical procedures using the three-dimensional graphic manipulations provided by programs similar to the Computer Assisted Design and Drafting (CADD), the software employed by the aircraft industry in the design of high-performance aircraft.

Most patients with complex maxillofacial injuries have asymmetric deformities that could be better managed with the aid of three-dimensional imaging to accurately plan surgical reconstruction. Conventional planigraphic (cephalometric) radiographs, pluridirectional tomography, CT studies, and magnetic resonance imaging (MRI), while very useful, are not as definitive as three-dimensional CT reconstructions. The mental reconstruction by the oral and maxillofacial surgeon of two-dimensional images into three-dimensional models invites error, especially when evaluating a patient with a complex major acute or post-traumatic defect. An additional disadvantage of this method is the inability to store or render two-dimensional mental images into hard copy to be shared with members of the maxillofacial team. The pressures of time, memory, and imagination make this form of preoperative planning unreliable.

Even with biplanar (axial-coronal) or triplanar (axial-coronal-sagittal) images produced by CT, the surgeon must still imagine a three-dimensional conceptualization. Imaging in three dimensions is a major departure from conventional modalities, especially in situations of complex asymmetric or avulsive defects of the maxillofacial skeleton. With high-quality three-dimensional representations the surgeon can plan operations on the maxillofacial skeleton with precision, predicting most major defects relative to size, shape, and volume and thus directing the surgery more definitively.

Serial-slice image data has been used to fabricate three-dimensional displays by a number of investigators and clinicians.[70–86] The early work in this field was somewhat cumbersome when using three-dimensional edge detection or encoding and display resulting from a three-dimensional model from the original CT scan data.[79] Vannier and co-workers developed newer methods involving high-resolution CT scans of the maxillofacial region that could reconstruct three-dimensional bone and soft-tissue contours from imaging data. To obtain appropriate three-dimensional reproductions of the maxillofacial region, continuous, equally spaced, nonoverlapping, high-resolution CT scan slices with narrow collimation were generated by modern CT scanners. Hemmy et al. used 1.5-mm abutting slices for a total of 45 sections of the facial structures.[76] Scanning methods by Marsh and Vannier, included scanning the maxillofacial complex anterior to the external acoustic meatus;[74,75] Hemmy et al. began from the alveolar ridge of the maxilla and proceeded in a cephalad direction for an axial distance of 6.75 cm.[76] This distance has been appropriate to display the cranial base, orbits, and midface, which are the areas of most importance in maxillofacial surgery.

After using appropriate CT scanning and a method developed by Vannier and co-workers,[87,88] three dimensional constructs can be produced. The method reported by Vannier

consisted of the application of three-dimensional programs to scans on over 300 patients with congenital and acquired craniofacial abnormalities. Most of the studies consisted of 30 to 100 nonoverlapping sections obtained at 2-mm intervals with 2-mm collimation. Smaller slices (1.5 mm) and various reconstruction matrices have been used (256^2 to 512^2). In the majority of instances only the front half of the patient's skull was included in the original transaxial CT images. The original CT scans were then archived on floppy disks or magnetic tape to a computer system that stores the images alternatively; the data can be transferred to the CT scan viewing console (Siemens Evaluscope B or RC). Vannier et al. copied the data on a 28-megabyte cartridge unit (Model RK07), integrated in the viewing console.[87,88] Hardware used in three-dimensional reconstruction includes a magnetic tape unit, a hard disc drive, a graphic display device, and a terminal with interacting devices (mouse, trackball, joystick, or light pen); a camera is used for photographing the images (Fig. 3–85).[83]

Three-dimensional images are constructed by a three dimensional array of adjacent voxels. The actual dimensions of a voxel are dependent on the scanner and the thickness of the slice generated. Most scanners produce matrices with pixels each 0.8 × 0.8 mm in size. If the scanner is programmed to generate 1.5-mm slices, then each voxel is 0.8 × 0.8 × 1.5 mm in size. The voxel is "recognized" in the computer by a number indicating the computed tomographic density. Thus, as an object is scanned, it is translated into a three-dimensional representation of CT density numbers, each one indicative of a voxel. To produce images with shape and depth, the density number of each voxel is encoded as a shade of gray. This program thus distinguishes soft tissue and bone.

Using a process called subregioning, one can select the area of interest from a given CT slice by direct manipulation of the image on the CRT screen. The pixels included in the region of interest will be used to form the three-dimensional reconstructions. By a technique referred to as interpolation, new interpolated slices are created based on the densities of the original slices. To produce a

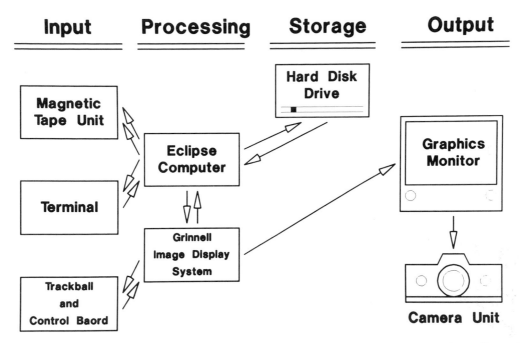

FIG. 3–85.   Diagrammatic representation of flow of information required to generate a three-dimensional image. (Redrawn from Jackson, I.T., and Bite, V.: Three-dimensional computed tomographic scanning and major surgical reconstruction of the head and neck. Mayo Clin Proc 61:546–555, 1986.)

three-dimensional image, it is necessary to form interpolated voxels of 0.8 mm³, which presupposes a CT slice thickness of 0.8 mm. In a technique called thresholding developed by Marsh and Vannier, a density on the gray scale is selected[75]; a value of 1 is assigned to a voxel possessing a density greater than that number and a value of 0 is assigned to a voxel with a lesser value. The value for bone density is used for a threshold approximately +110 CT units. A three-dimensional computer program reviews the columns and rows of voxels in each slice; the distance from a reference plane to the first voxel whose CT density exceeds the threshold is recorded. This process is repeated by the program for each CT slice, thus developing a surface contour (for example, for the maxillofacial skeleton) and storing the data as hues of gray. In cases in which images of bony anatomy are seen, the picture that emerges is shaded with light and dark areas; not necessarily for artistic perspective or enhancement of volume effect, but to indicate actual distances from the reference plane, brighter voxels are closer and darker voxels are farther away from this plane. The three-dimensional images can thus be built up

slice by slice and viewed on the graphic display device.

After viewing, the three-dimensional images can be stored temporarily on a hard disc or permanently on a floppy disc or magnetic tape. The region of interest can be rotated at various angular increments around the X, Y, or Z axes. These images can be displayed on the viewing console singly from selected angles of incidence or as a rotating cinemode motion picture. Permanent copies can be generated by the use of 35-mm photographic film or standard radiographic sheets. These can then be used for preoperative planning and in the operating room. Solid models can be fabricated from the three-dimensional imaging data by a computer numerically controlled (CNC) milling machine to produce exact replicas of bony structures directly from the CT scan data. These models (acrylic) can be gas-sterilized and used in the operating room (Fig. 3–86).

Vannier and co-workers produced programs written in Fortran and Assembler languages that could operate on a minicomputer incorporated in the CT viewing console.[88] The programs could operate without modification

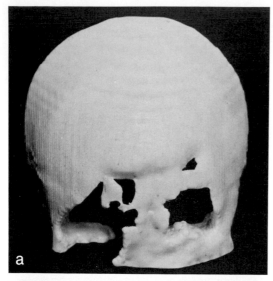

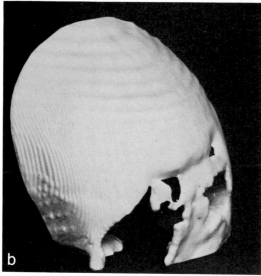

FIG. 3–86.   **a,** Frontal view of an acrylic model produced by a CNC milling machine of a 14-year-old boy after a bicycle accident resulting in avulsion of the right supraorbital area and defects in the frontal bone. This computer-generated model can be gas-sterilized and used to design operative procedure to reconstruct lost frontal bone in the right supraorbital ridge. **b,** Lateral view of the model in Figure 3–86a. Note that one can examine the inner table also, which is reproduced with accuracy.

on such CT scanners as the Siemens Somatome 2 and Somatome DR3. The original transaxial high-resolution CT scan slices are used as input for these programs and three-dimensional surface reconstructions are produced. In a study by Vannier et al., more than

50 views were produced including soft-tissue and bony surfaces in the frontal, rear, lateral, oblique, top and bottom projections.[74] It was apparent that any view from any angle of incidence could be obtained, but the authors felt that only those views that had clinical significance would be routinely produced.

Three-dimensional surface contour or reconstructions can be displayed and manipulated in the same fashion as images produced by a CT scan. The spectrum of gray colors in these reconstructions can be measured as actual distances or depths. The representations produced by three-dimensional programs appear as black and while photographs of the skull with the soft tissues removed (Fig. 3–87). One can also obtain oblique projections of the three-dimensional displays, which is useful in evaluating the orbits and the maxilla, by rotating the original scan by a selected angle from 0 to 90° before contour extraction. Other contour extractions can be performed so that at the soft-tissue area interface, approximately -200 CT units produce three-dimensional soft-tissue reconstructions of the face.

Vannier and co-workers, using technology very similar to the computer processes used in advanced military aircraft design, developed a sophisticated computer-aided design system for the planning and evaluation of craniofacial surgical procedures.[73,79] In one particular case in Vannier's studies, a patient with asymmetric hypertelorism was evaluated using the encoding of fewer than 2500 coordinates with 40 CT scans as input. The inferolateral displacement of the left orbit in Vannier's article was seen in the frontal views. A left frontal bone cleft was clearly demonstrated. Vannier and co-workers note that the major advantages of the CADD system approach to craniofacial surgical planning and evaluating include interactive display, quantitation of linear, surface, and volumetric measurement, and ability to move image components independently. Soft-tissue and bony surface contours may be superimposed and displayed simultaneously to assess their relationship to the overall facial structure. The authors also demonstrate in the example of the asymmetric hypertelorism that translocation of the orbit can be executed

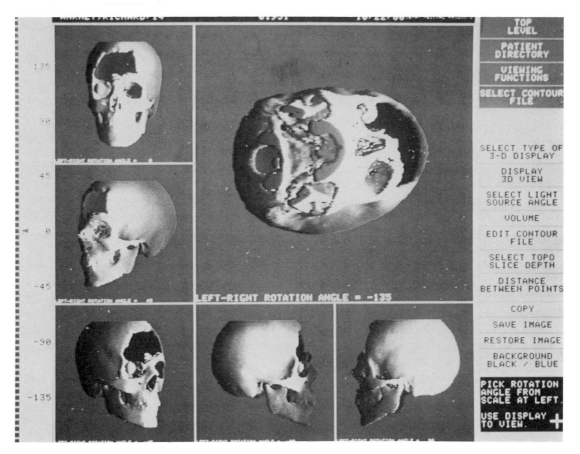

FIG. 3–87. Extensive frontobasilar and avulsive injury of the right supraorbital region in the patient in Figure 3–86 reproduced by use of a three-dimensional CT program. The appearance is that of a black and white photograph of the skull with the soft tissues removed.

more precisely by use of computer-simulated surgery.

Vannier, Conroy, Marsh, and Knapp described the methods of applying three-dimensional computed imaging to physical anthropology.[89] In their article they descibed how this method has been used successfully to view and surgically manage over 700 patients with craniofacial deformities, facial trauma, neoplastic disease of the head and neck, and intracranial soft-tissue abnormalities. The life-size, geometrically accurate three-dimensional models have also been produced from the CT scan data using advanced Computer Assisted Design and Drafting and Computer Assisted Manufacturing (CADD-CAM) techniques.

By convention, the X direction is assigned to be horizontal in the mediolateral orientation. The Y direction refers to anteroposterior,

and the Z direction to the superior-inferior. Thus, the X–Y plane corresponds to the plane of section. The Z axis is perpendicular to the plane of section and corresponds to the direction of table motion in CT scanning.

In the three-dimensional representations produced by Vannier and co-workers in numerous articles, the depth information is encoded in gray scale (the lighter the gray scale, the closer the surface is to the observer). As Vannier and co-workers described, this depth can then be electronically "dissected" on the computer screen in any plane desired and the following data can be generated with submillimeter accuracy and instantaneously on extracranial or intracranial surfaces.[89] Because of the digital nature of three-dimensional imaging, one can remove specific areas or make selected regions transparent to permit viewing of deeper, normally occult anatomic structures. As an example, the calvaria and brain tissue may be removed to show the intracranial base of the skull, or the mandible could be removed to show the hard palate and base of the skull in living subjects.

Woolson et al. produced three-dimensional images, similar to Vannier's, of a patient with a congenital dislocation of the left hip.[84] The images demonstrated the various three-dimensional image options provided by the Cemax 100 computer system (Contour Medical Systems, Inc., Mountain View, Ca.) from the CT scan data of this patient. The coutour data from which the three-dimensional images were reconstructed on the CRT may be interfaced with a CNC milling machine to produce solid models of these three-dimensional representations of bony anatomy. The CNC 3 axis milling device produces from machineable wax blocks two negative molds of the three-dimensional image, each parted through the coronal plane and containing half the data points of the three-dimensional image. These models are assembled and liquid plastic material is poured into them to produce a solid plastic model of bone. Although Woolson produced models of the femoral head, exquisite models of the mandible or maxilla can be produced as well.

Woolson notes in his discussion that translating a mental idea into a three-dimensional analysis of the object is a difficult task in most cases, especially when complex anatomic areas such as the hip or shoulder joint are considered. The superimposition of bony anatomy in planigraphic films can hinder the visualization of many pathologic conditions that affect the articular surfaces of joints such as, in maxillofacial surgery, the temporomandibular joint. As mentioned, the image of an entire bone can be deleted using an editing program to allow independent viewing of an adjacent bone or joint surface, which is helpful in diagnosing certain intra-articular pathologic conditions. Woolson also indicates that the production of accurate bone models from preoperative CT scans will provide a means of better surgical planning (of osteotomies or complex total joint replacement) and a more precise method of manufacturing customized prostheses for problem cases. Mirror imaging, which involves scanning the normal con-

tralateral side or making a model of the normal bone, can produce a normal bone model and hence optimize the correction of any deformity.

The obvious future applications of three-dimensional technology to orthopedic surgery and maxillofacial surgery in general are unlimited. The ultimate goal will be the production of a computed surgical simulation system whereby surgery is performed before operation on three-dimensional bone images on a CRT by cutting manipulating, and reconstructing these images. Three-dimensional biomechanical finite element studies applied to the reconstructive bone images could then help to predict the outcome of the proposed surgery. Because this computer system can be adapted to accept all forms of digitized scanning data, MRI scans can also be used for the reconstruction of three-dimensional bone images and solid models.

Marsh et al. demonstrated their experience with CT augmented by three-dimensional surface reconstruction methods and CADD-CAM technology by using 313 CT studies in the management of 216 patients having a variety of congenital and acquired head and neck disorders.[81] Three-dimensional reconstructions were implemented as a series of computer programs that ran on the unmodified CT scanners. The images viewed were very similar in Vannier's studies, either viewed on the CRT screen of a scanner console or printed as hard copy on radiographic or photographic film for the surgeon's evaluation. Whereas the hard copy can be made life-size to facilitate measurements, all three-dimensional surface images contain a vernier scale representing 5 cm. This calibration allows quantitative evaluation of elective skeletal movements in the immediate postoperative period to correlate the achieved result with that anticipated, and in the long term to evaluate the consequences of relapse and future growth.

Hemmy and Tessier studied dried skulls from patients with Crouzon's disease and orbital neurofibromatosis.[80] These skulls were studied using three-dimensional reconstruction of CT data. They compared images with one another and with actual skulls and concluded that the use of dry skulls is helpful in pointing out errors of inclusion or exclusion. Thinner sections permit more accurate representation. Because the reconstructive data do not appear to be significantly enhanced by using overlapping sections, radiation can be reduced by using abutting sections. To compare the reconstructive CT scans with photographs, Hemmy and Tessier used axial scans at 1.5-mm intervals (abutting scans) at a section thickness of 1.5 mm using a GE CT/ 8800 scanner with a 320 × 320 matrix, 9.6 sec scan, pulse of 2 msec at 250 mA and 120 kvp. The threshold selected for bone was set at 150 on the scanner. The conclusions were based on the facts that one can make visual comparisons of the reconstructed data and that errors of inclusion or exclusion are easily noted by comparison with the photographs.

Gillespie and Isherwood reported several illustrative cases using three-dimensional anatomic images from CT scans.[85] These included at least one patient with a traumatic injury to the left zygoma. In that case, the fracture line was seen in the left maxilla and lateral wall of the left orbit with a comminuted left antral fracture and zygomaticofrontal suture separation. Soft-tissue edema was also apparent. These authors described their experience of using three-dimensional images generated by the program for three-dimensional image generation entitled "3-D 83." The GE CT/8800 scanner was used.

Conventional CT slices were used as input to the 3-D 83 program. For optimal maxillofacial anatomic detail, contiguous 1.5-mm sections (120 kvp and 400 mA, 576 views) were obtained through 5-mm sections. After processing these CT images using the 3-D 83 program, these authors felt, like other workers in this field, that the anatomic surface of those surfaces immediately adjacent to areas or volumes of markedly different CT attenuation are best adapted for reconstruction by the 3-D 83 program. The regions of interest could be isolated and viewed in a variety of orientations that are not possible using other technologies. Precise measurements could be made between various coordinates. A craniocaudal view, for example, permits measurement of intervertebral rotation.

Total CT scanning time for a facial examination was about 45 to 60 min. Computation

time for three-dimensional images could vary from under one hour to several hours, depending on the inclusion of various axes of rotation, the number of frames per rotation, and the size of the volume to be reconstructed. The computer, of course, could be programmed to perform reconstructions overnight or during periods of nonuse, making use of what otherwise might be downtime.

Koltai and Wood reported the use of CT scanning for the evaluation and surgical planning of maxillofacial injuries.[90] They noted the difficulties inherent in conventional radiography and polytomography and, indeed, CT scanning alone. They recognized that CT imaging had become the favorite technique for the evaluation of maxillofacial fractures, especially because it permits highly accurate internal imaging in axial cross section. Koltai and Wood used a computer system called Insight Phoenix Data Systems, which uses the conventional CT scan as a substrate to create three-dimensional reconstructions. The authors used this computer system for at least a year in the evaluation and surgical planning of facial fractures in many patients with complex maxillofacial injuries.

They obtained their data from an acutely injured but otherwise stable patient who had associated complex maxillofacial trauma. The unenhanced axial CT scans were obtained in a dynamic mode using a bone algorithm in 1.5-mm contiguous slices. Slices 35 through 55 were limited to the area of injury. All scans were accomplished using a GE CT/8800 scanner, after which the data was directly transferred to magnetic tape and then placed into the memory of the insight computer, which produced three-dimensional reconstructions. The displayed images were viewed on a high-resolution monitor and manipulated in real time, either by rotating or planar sectioning. Koltai and Wood presented photographs that were obtained directly from the computer monitor. Koltai and Wood described, among other fractures, a severe midfacial injury that included a nasofrontal-ethmoid fracture with a right Le Fort II and Le Fort III injury. Preoperatively, the CT scans were processed for three-dimensional representations. The patient had bilateral orbital exploration and graft suspension of the left orbital floor. The patient was then placed in intermaxillary fixation and had open repair of the right Le Fort II and Le Fort III fracture with maxillary suspension. Finally, the patient had frontal sinus obliteration and open repair of a complex nasoethmoid fracture. Other impressive injuries described in Koltai and Wood'a article were managed by open and closed reductions. In these cases, the CT scans were processed for three-dimensional imaging prior to surgery to direct the surgical repair.

DeMarino et al. presented five examples of complex maxillofacial trauma demonstrated by conventional plain films followed by two-dimensional and three-dimensional CT.[91] The CT in three dimensions vividly demonstrated spatial relationships not easily conceptualized by conventional modalities. Patients selected for this study included those exhibiting extensive maxillofacial injuries. Each patient was initially evaluated with conventional im-

aging modalities including plain radiographic examination, tomography and conventional axial two-dimensional CT scans. The authors thought that the nature and complexity of the maxillofacial injuries justified that the value of the three-dimensional CT imaging technology be assessed first and then compared with conventional CT scans. The transfer of CT data to the computer console for generation of three-dimensional reconstructions was similar to previous studies with the addition of the rotation by 10- to 30°-increments around X, Y, and Z axes. The authors concluded after reviewing several severely fractured cases that the three-dimensional imaging technology had many potential applications for maxillofacial traumatology and preoperative evaluations of craniofacial anomalies, neoplastic diseases of the head and neck, and cervical spine injuries. The authors noted that another application would be in the study of CSF leak.

Another case presented by DeMarino and

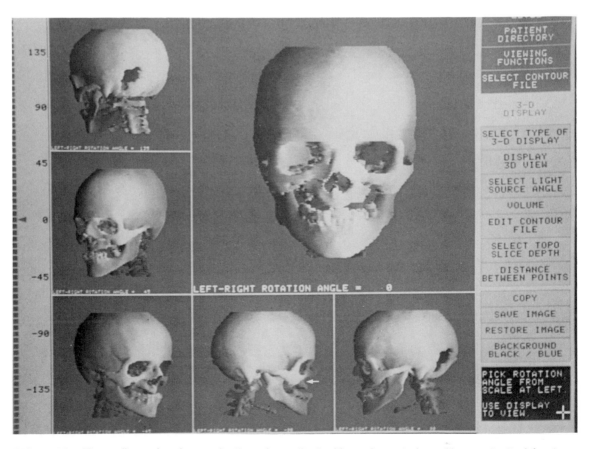

FIG. 3–88. Three-dimensional reproduction of a patient with an impacted maxillary malunited fracture. The Le Fort I fracture was not treated because the patient was not expected to survive the severe closed head injuries.

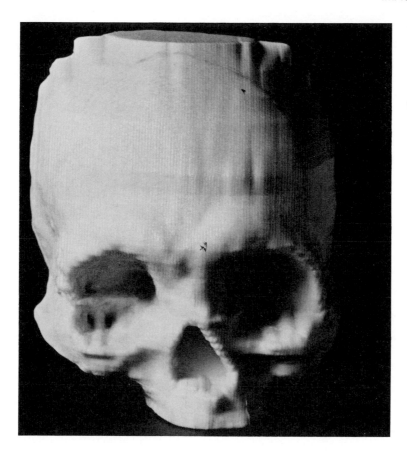

FIG. 3–89.   Lucite model fabricated by a three-dimensional computer milling program (Cemax Corporation, Mountain View, California) revealing in great detail the midface and orbits in a 39-year-old man involved in a motor vehicle accident that resulted in retropositioning displacement of the midface. The model was used for planning the reconstructive skeletal surgery of the midface.

associates described a 31-year-old man involved in a motor vehicle accident. Conventional radiography showed a fracture of the left skull base and fluid in the maxillary and frontal sinuses. Two-dimensional CT scans showed a subdural hematoma of the right frontotemporal region and multiple fractures fo the left orbit, maxilla, and frontal bone. The three-dimensional CT scan, imaged from an orientation that allowed a thorough assessment of the fracture planes, showed a fracture of the left roof of the orbit extending into the lesser wing of the sphenoid. As the case presentation suggested, many of the spatial relationships not easily appreciated on conventional radiographs or conventional two-dimensional CTs are easily conceptualized with the three-dimensional technique. Thus, not only the extent of the fractures but a suggestion of the mechanism of the injury can be

readily assessed (Fig. 3–88). The authors found it useful to evaluate the three-dimensional scans prior to seriously assessing the multiple two-dimensional sections in order to focus on specific areas of clinical and surgical concern. The authors were surprised to find significant limitations in their ability to interpret two-dimensional images without a full understanding of the spatial relationship so well depicted on the three-dimensional images.

While exquisite three-dimensional images can be generated from ever more sophisticated three-dimensional programs, for the pragmatic surgeon the most useful property of the new technology is its ability to measure with precision.[83] During the initial scanning process, the spatial relationships of soft tissue and bone are permanently recorded. By appropriate surface life-size display, distance, area, and volume can be measured. To measure distance between two points, the number of voxels between the points are counted in the X, Y, and Z directions. The Pythagorean theorem is then used to calculate the distance between the points. To measure area in a three-dimensional image, the number of pixels are counted in the area of interest and this number is multipled by the area of one pixel (0.0064 cm²). The authors note the use of area calculation in the evaluation of the orbital aperture. For computer volume measurements of the three-dimensional image, the voxels in each slice are counted and these numbers totaled. This total is then multiplied by the volume of one pixel (0.00096 cm³). Using this program, total orbital bony volume, total orbital soft-tissue volume, bone graft volume, orbital fat volume, orbital neuromuscular tissue volume, and globe volume have been determined.[83]

A region-growing technique is used for measuring various intraorbital tissues. In this technique, the cursor is positioned in an area of the desired radiodensity range, and the voxels are counted within that range. The volume is determined as outlined. The use of this program has demonstrated that the cause of post-traumatic enophthalmos is an increase in volume of the bony orbit and not a decrease in the soft-tissue (viscera) volume.[92] With the conflicting concepts in the literature on the management of orbital trauma, this investigation has led to a novel insight as to the proper managment of orbital trauma. Because it is well accepted that the management of delayed, untreated traumatic enophthalmos is problematic, restoration of normal orbital volume should be a priority. Surgical approaches would involve reduction of fracture segments, reconstruction of lateral and, if necessary, medial orbital walls, and occasional reconstruction of the orbital floor with immediate primary bone grafting. The authors advocate osteotomy and possible bone grafting behind the globe to reduce orbital volume and to move the globe anteriorly in long-standing traumatic enophthalmos based on an enlarged intraorbital volume.

Imaging technology has radically altered the manner in which the surgeon will approach the diagnosis and management of maxillofacial trauma and resulting acquired deformities (Fig. 3–89). While three-dimensional imaging has changed from being an investigative instrument to being used widely in craniofacial pathologies, CT in multiple planes currently is most practical. Every-increasing enhancements of three-dimensional software programs will make three-dimensional imaging and model construction less expensive, less time-consuming, and equal in resolution to other methods and, therefore, more practical to use on a routine basis for severe maxillofacial injuries.

REFERENCES

1. Kassel, E.E., and Cooper, P.W.: Radiologic studies of facial trauma associated with a regional trauma centre. J Can Assoc Radiol 34:178–188, 1983.
2. Kassel, E.E., Noyek, A.M., and Cooper, P.W.: CT in facial trauma. J Otolaryngol 12:2–15, 1983.
3. Dolan, K.D., and Jacoby, C.G.: Facial fractures. Semin Roentgenol 13:37–51, 1978.
4. Noyek, A.M., et al.: Sophisticated CT in complex maxillofacial trauma. Laryngoscope (suppl.) 92:1–17, 1982.
5. Ambrose, J.: Computerized axial tomography. J Radiol 46:401, 1973.
6. Ambrose, J.: Computerized transverse axial scanning (tomography): Part 2. Clinical application. Br J Radiol 46:1023–1047, 1973.
7. Ambrose, J.: Computerized x-ray scanning of the brain. J Neurosurg 40:679, 1974.
8. Claussen, C., and Lohkamp, F.: CT in traumatic lesions between cerebral and facial skull. Int. Symp. and Course on Computed Tomography; Miami Beach, 3–8 April 1977; Comput Assist Tomogr 1:361, 1977.
9. Saul, T.G., and Ducker, T.B.: The role of computed tomography in acute head injury. Comput Tomog (4):296–308, 1980.
10. Ghoshhajra, K.: CT in trauma of the base of the skull and its complications. Comput Tomog 4(4):271–276, 1980.
11. Ames, J.R., Johnson, R.P., and Stevens, E.A.: Computerized tomography in oral and maxillofacial surgery. J Oral Surg 38:145–149, 1980.
12. Diaconis, J.N., and Rao, K.C.: CT in head trauma: A review. CT 4:261–270, 1980.
13. Espagno, J., et al.: The usefulness and prognostic value of CT scanning in craniocerebral trauma. J Neuroradiol 7:121–132, 1980.
14. Kaiser, M.C., et al.: CT for trauma to the base of the skull and spine in children. Neuroradiology 22:27, 1981.
15. Frame, J.W., and Wake, M.J.C.: Computerized axial tomography in the assessment of mandibular keratocysts. Br Dent J 153:93–96, 1982.

16. Reference deleted.
17. Zimmerman, R.A., et al.: Cranial computed tomography in diagnosis and management of acute head trauma. Am J Roentgenol 131:27–34, 1978.
18. Danziger, A., and Price, H.: The evaluation of head trauma by computed tomography. J Trauma 19:1–5, 1979.
19. Rowe, L.D., Miller, E., and Brandt-Zawadzki, M.: Computed tomography in maxillofacial trauma. Laryngoscope 91:745–757, 1981.
20. Alper, M.G.: Computed tomography in planning and evaluating orbital surgery. Ophthalmology 87:418–431, 1980.
21. Manfredi, S.J., et al.: Computerized tomographic scan findings in facial fractures associated with blindness. Plas Reconstr Surg 68:479–490, 1981.
22. Spierer, A., et al.: Diagnosis and localization of intraocular foreign bodies by computed tomography. Ophthalmic Surg 16:571–575, 1985.
23. Carter, B.I., and Karmody, C.S.: Computed tomography of the face and neck. Semin Roentgenol 13:257–266, 1976.
24. Forssell, A., and Liliequist, B.: Computed tomography of the paranasal sinuses. Adv Otorhinolaryngol 24:42–50, 1978.
25. Claussen, C., and Singer, R.: Progress in the diagnosis of craniofacial injuries and tumors by computed tomography. J Maxillofac Surg 7:210–217, 1979.
26. Maue-Dickson, W., Trefler, M., and Dickson, D.R.: Comparison of dosimetry and image quality in computed and conventional tomography. Radiology 131:509–514, 1979.
27. North, A.F., and Rice, J.: Computed tomography in oral and maxillofacial surgery. J Oral Surg 39:199–207, 1981.
28. Fujii, N., and Yamashiro, M.: Computed tomography for the diagnosis of facial fractures. J Oral Surg. 39:735–741, 1981.
29. Brandt-Zawadzki, M.N., Minagi, H., Federle, M.P., and Rowe, L.D.: High-resolution CT with reformation in maxillofacial pathology. Am J Radiol 138:477–483, 1978, also Am J Neuroradiol 3:31–37, 1982.
30. Gruss, J.: The use of craniofacial surgical techniques in the management of major cranio-maxillo-facial trauma. Proceedings of the International Symposium of Maxillo-Facial Trauma. Wayne State University, Detroit, Michigan, Nov. 13–15, 1981.
31. Cooper, P.W., Kassel, E.E., and Gruss, J.S.: High resolution CT scanning of facial trauma. Am J Neuroradiol 4:495–498, 1983.
32. Oldendorf, W.H.: The quest for an image of brain: A brief historical and technical review of brain imaging techniques. Neurology 28:517–533, 1978.
33. Massiot, J.: History of tomography in medicine. Mundi 19:106–115, 1974.
34. Hounsfield, G.N.: Computerized transverse axial scanning (tomography). Description of system. Br J Radiol 46:1016–1022, 1973.
35. Kassel, E.E., Noyek, A.M., and Cooper, P.W.: High resolution computerized tomography in otorhinolaryngology. J Otolaryngol 11:297–306, 1982.
36. Gentry, L.R., Manor, W.F., Turski, P.A., and Strother, C.M.: High resolution computed tomographic analysis of facial struts in Trauma: 1: Normal anatomy. Am J Radiol 140:523–532, 1983.
37. Grove, A.S.: Orbital trauma evaluation by computed tomography. Comput Tomog 3:267–278, 1979.
38. Koga S., et al.: Radiation dosage of computerized tomography—with special reference to CT-H250. Rinsho Hoshasen 21:1073–1076, 1976.
39. Moriuchi, I., et al.: X-ray exposure dose for the gonadal gland by the examination of computerized tomography and its protection—EMI-1,000 scanner. Rinsho Hoshasen 23:797–800, 1978.
40. Finkle, D.R., et al.: Comparison of the diagnostic methods used in maxillofacial trauma. Plast Reconstr Surg 75:32–38, 1984.
41. Carter, B.L.: Computed tomography of the head and neck. In Contemporary Issues in Computed Tomography. Edited by B.L. Carter. New York, Churchill Livingstone, 1985.
42. Claussen, C.D., Lohkamp, F.W., and Krastel, A.: Computed tomography of trauma involving the brain and facial skull (craniofacial injuries). J Comput Assist Tomogr 1:472–481, 1977.
43. Hesselink, J.R., et al.: Computed tomography of the paranasal sinuses and face. Part I. Normal anatomy. J Comput Assist Tomogr 2(5):559–567, 1978.
44. Hesselink, J.R., et al.: Computed tomograph of the paranasal sinuses and faces. Part II. Pathological anatomy. J Comput Assist Tomogr 2:568–576, 1978.
45. Schindler, E., and Reck, R.: Value and limits of computer-assisted tomography. Head Neck Surg 2:287–292, 1980.
46. Grove, A.S.: Orbital trauma and computed tomography. Ophthalmology 87:403–411, 1980.
47. Zilkha, A.: Computed tomography in facial trauma. Radiology 144:545–548, 1982.
48. Hammerschlag, S.B., et al.: Blow-out fractures of the orbit. Radiology 143:487–492, 1982.
49. Zilkha, A.: Computed tomography of blow-out fracture of the medial orbital wall. Am J Neuroradiol 2:427–429, 1981.
50. Zilkha, A.: Computed tomography of blow-out fractures of the medial orbital wall. Am J Roentgenol 137:963, 1981.
51. Frame, J.W., and Wake, M.J.C.: The value of computerized tomography in oral surgery. Oral Surg 52:357–363, 1981.
52. Daffner, R.H., Gehweiller, J.A., Osborne, D.R., and Roberts, L., Jr.: Computed tomography in the evaluation of severe facial trauma. Comput Radiol 7:91–102, 1983.
53. Kreipke, D., et al.: Computed tomography and thin-section tomography in facial trauma. Am J Radiol 142:1041–1045, 1984.
54. Jend-Rossman, I., and Jend, H.-H.: Systematic approach to diagnosis of midfacial fractures in CT, oral and maxillofacial surgery: Proceedings from the 8th International Conference on Oral and Maxillofacial Surgery. E. Hjorting-Hansen, ed., Quintessence, 1985.
55. Frame, J.W., and Wake, M.J.C.: Six years experience of computerized tomography in oral surgery. Oral and Maxillofacial Surgery: Proceedings from the 8th International Conference on Oral and Maxillofacial Surgery. E. Hjorting-Hansen (ed.). Chicago, Quintessence Publishing Co., Inc., 1985, p.34.
56. Carter, B.I., and Bankoff, M.S.: Facial trauma: Computed versus conventional tomography. In Sectional Imaging Methods: A Comparison. Edited by J.T. Littleton and M. Durizch. Baltimore, University Park Press, 1983, p.319.
57. Mancuso, A.A., and Hanefee, W.N.: Computed tomography of the injured larynx. Radiology 133:139–144, 1979.
58. Pollack, K., and Payne, E.: Fractures of the frontal sinus. Otolaryngol Clin North Am 9:517–522, 1976.
59. Ord, R.A., et al.: Computerized tomography and B-scan ultra-sonography in the diagnosis of fractures of the medial orbital wall. Plast Reconstr Surg 67:281–288, 1981.
60. Emery, J.M., and von Noorden, G.K.: Traumatic pseudoprolapse of orbital tissues into the maxillary

antrum: A diagnostic pitfall. Trans Am Acad Ophthalmol Otolaryngol 79:893–896, 1975.

61. Gordon, S., and McCrae, H.: Monocular blindness as a complication of the treatment of a malar fracture. Plast Reconstr Surg 6:228, 1950.
62. Miller, G.R.: Blindness developing a few days after a midfacial fracture. Plast Reconstr Surg 42:384, 1968.
63. Lightman, I., Reckson, C.: Blow-in fracture of the orbit. Ann Plast Surg 3:572–575, 1979.
64. Knight, J.S., and North, J.F.: The classification of malar fractures: An analysis of displacements as a guide to treatment. Br J Plast Surg 13:325, 1961.
65. Fujii, N., and Yamashiro, M.: Classification of malar complex fractures using computed tomography. J Oral Maxillofac Surg 41:562–567, 1983.
66. Tyndall, D.A., Matteson, S.R., and Gregg, J.M.: Computed tomography in diagnosis and treatment of mandibular fractures. Oral Surg 56:567–570, 1983.
67. Cooper, P.W., and Kassel, E.E.: Computed tomography and cerebrospinal fluid leak. J Otolaryngol 11:319–326, 1982.
68. Ommaya, A.K.: Spinal fluid fistulae. Clin Neurosurg 27:363–392, 1976.
69. Gehrke, G., Schwenzer, N., and Thron, A.: Possibilities and problems of CT diagnosis in maxillofacial traumatology. Oral and Maxillofacial Surgery: Proceedings of the 8th International Conference on Oral and Maxillofacial Surgery. E Hjorting-Hansen (ed.). Quintessence, 1985.
70. Herman, G.T., and Liv, H.K.: Three-dimensional display of human organs from computed tomograms. Comp Graphics and Image Proc 7:130, 1978.
71. Dwyer, S.J. III, et al.: Medical processing in diagnostic radiology. Institute of Electronics and Electrical Engineers Transactions on Nuclear Science 27:1047, 1980.
72. Artzy, E., Frieder, G., and Herman, G.T.: The theory, design, implementation and evaluation of a three dimensional surface detection algorithm. Comp Graphics and Image Proc 15:1, 1981.
73. Vannier, M.W., Marsh, J.L., and Warren, J.O.: Three-dimensional computed analysis of craniofacial surgical planning. Proc Radiol Soc N Am. Chicago, 1982.
74. Marsh, J.L., and Vannier, M.W.: Surface imaging from CT scans. Surgery 94:159, 1983.
75. Marsh, J.L., and Vannier, M.W.: The "third" dimension in craniofacial surgery. Plast Reconstr Surg 71:759, 1983.
76. Hemmy, D.C., David, D.J., and Herman, G.T.: Three dimensional reconstruction of craniofacial deformity using computed tomography. Neurosurgery 13:534, 1983.
77. Latamore, G.B.: Creating 3-D models for medical research. Comput Graphics World 7:31–38, 1983.

78. Totty, W.G., and Vannier, M.W.: Complex musculoskeletal anatomy: Analysis using three dimensional surface reconstruction. Radiology 150:173–177, 1983.
79. Vannier, M.W., Marsh, J.L., and Warren, J.O.: Three-dimensional CT reconstruction images for craniofacial surgical planning and evaluation. Radiology 150:179, 1984.
80. Hemmy, D.C., and Tessier, P.L.: CT of dry skulls with craniofacial deformities: Accuracy of three-dimensional reconstruction. Radiology 157:113–116, 1985.
81. Marsh, J.L., et al.: Computerized imaging for soft tissue and osseous reconstruction in the head and neck. Clin Plast Surg 12(2):279–291, 1985.
82. Altman, N.R., Altman, D.H., Wolfe, S.A., and Morrison, G.: Three-dimensional CT reformation in children. Am J Radiol 146:1261–1267, 1986.
83. Jackson, I.T., and Bite, V.: Three-dimensional computed tomographic scanning and major surgical reconstruction of the head and neck. Mayo Clin Proc 61:546–555, 1986.
84. Woolson, S.T., Dev, P., Fellingham, L.L., and Vassiliadis, A.: Three-dimensional imaging of bone from computerized tomography. Clin Orthop 202:239–248, 1986.
85. Gillespie, J.E., and Isherwood, I.: (Short communications) Three- dimensional anatomical images from computed tomographic scans. Br J Radiol 59:289–292, 1986.
86. Cutting, C., et al.: Three-dimensional computer-assisted design of craniofacial surgical procedures: Optimization and interaction with cephalometric and CT-based models. Plast Reconstr Surg 77:877, 1986.
87. Vannier, M.W., Marsh, J.L., Warren, J.O., and Barkier, J.: Three- dimensional computer aided design of craniofacial surgical procedures. Diagn Imaging 5:36–43, 1983.
88. Vannier, M.W., Marsh, J.L., Warren, J.O., and Barkier, J.: Three dimensional CAD for craniofacial surgery. Electronic Imaging 2:48–54, 1983.
89. Vannier, M.W., Conroy, G.C., Marsh, J.L., and Knapp, R.H.: Three-dimensional cranial surface reconstructions using high-resolution computed tomography. Am J Phys Anthropol 67:299–311, 1985.
90. Koltai, P.J., and Wood, G.W.: Three dimensional CT reconstruction for the evaluation and surgical planning of facial fractures. Otolaryngol Head Neck Surg 95:10–15, 1986.
91. De Marino, D.P., et al.: Three-dimensional computed tomography in maxillofacial trauma. Arch Otolaryngol Head Neck Surg 112:146, 1986.
92. Bite, V., Jackson, I.T., Forbes, G.S., and Gehring, D.G.: Orbital volume measurements in enophthalmos using three-dimensional CT imaging. Plast Reconstr Surg 75:502–507, 1985.

4

SOFT-TISSUE INJURIES

CHARLES C. ALLING III

The extent of soft-tissue injury to the facial area varies depending on the forces involved, the agent doing damage, and the circumstances and location of injury. Soft-tissue injuries of the maxillofacial region vary from minor injuries to the most complex types of wounds, including avulsion of portions of both soft tissues and underlying bony structures (Fig. 4–1).

Timing is extremely important in the management of soft-tissue wounds of the face. Early debridement and primary closure of facial wounds make it possible for patients to regain acceptable function at a much earlier time, minimize loss of function, and prevent facial disfigurement. Maxillofacial trauma incurred during war is accompanied by a high incidence of soft-tissue injury; in the Vietnam War, for example, approximately 95% of the maxillofacial injuries sustained in combat involved a soft-tissue injury, and more than 50% of those involved only soft tissues.[1]

Patients often exhibit considerable concern about an injury involving the facial region, and every effort must be directed toward restoring normal function and aesthetics as rapidly as possible. However, although early definitive care of maxillofacial soft-tissue injuries is important, it never takes precedence over the general care of the patient. Patients with maxillofacial injuries may also have multiple body injuries consisting of wounds of the head, chest, abdomen, and

extremities. Priority must always be given to life-saving and emergency procedures: the establishment and maintenance of a patent airway, arrest of hemorrhage, recognition and treatment of shock, treatment of associated head injuries, and treatment of severe trauma to the extremities, thorax, and abdomen (see Chapter 2).

Although the soft tissues of the face are extremely vascular, uncontrolled hemorrhage secondary to injury is rare. During the initial examination, clamping of obvious bleeding vessels and application of occlusive pressure dressings may be necessary to control bleeding. The pressure dressings also provide temporary immobilization of the hard and soft tissues. Because most facial injuries are contaminated, early antibiotic coverage and antitetanus therapy are indicated to supplement careful surgical debridement. The use of analgesics and narcotics should be avoided until the possibility of concomitant cerebral injury has been eliminated.

In most cases, meticulous attention should be paid to the basic principles of adequate but conservative debridement, hemostasis, gentle handing of tissues, closure in layers to minimize loss of function, and an orderly and logical approach to the various elements of the injury. The surgical team must be alert to the fact that many soft-tissue injuries may be life-threatening as a result of factors ranging from occult injuries of the great vessels of the

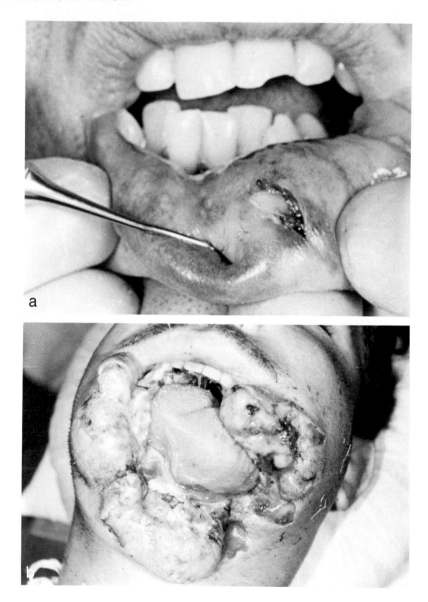

FIG. 4–1. Soft-tissue minor and major injuries. **a,** Soft-tissue injury to the lip with retention of a foreign body. (Courtesy of Dr. Edward Stiesmeyer.) **b,** Avulsive wound to the mandible and inferior lip incurred by a high-speed bullet. (Courtesy of Dr. James Chipps.)

neck to airway challenges, shock, and systemic infections. In patients with underlying facial fractures, consideration must be given to obtaining impressions for splints or direct reduction and fixation of fractures *prior* to primary definitive management of the overlying soft-tissue injuries.

CLASSIFCATION OF SOFT-TISSUE INJURIES

Each facial wound is evaluated prior to initiation of repair to determine the nature and

extent of the injury (Fig. 4–2). Many injuries will affect both sensory and motor nerve function, particularly the facial and trigeminal nerves. When one or more of the major peripheral branches of the facial nerve are involved, it should be repaired at the time of initial surgery. Microsurgical repair is preferable, but circumstances and total patient care generally require that macroscopic techniques be used. For repair of injuries to the parotid gland and duct, macroscopic techniques, perhaps aided with magnifying glasses, will suffice. Extensive soft-tissue in-

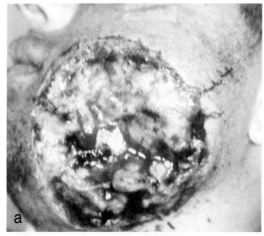

FIG. 4–2. Examples of soft-tissue injuries. **a,** Avulson. Full-thickness loss of buccal soft tissue. (Courtesy of Dr. James Chipps.) **b L** and **R,** Contusion. The bruising is indicative of an underlying mandibular fracture. **c,** Laceration. **L,** Intraoral laceration without bony injury, very similar to an incision that may be made for anterior mandibular surgery. **R,** Normal repair 2 weeks following injury. **d,** Laceration. **L,** Before repair of an extraoral laceration without underlying bony injury. **R,** After repair.

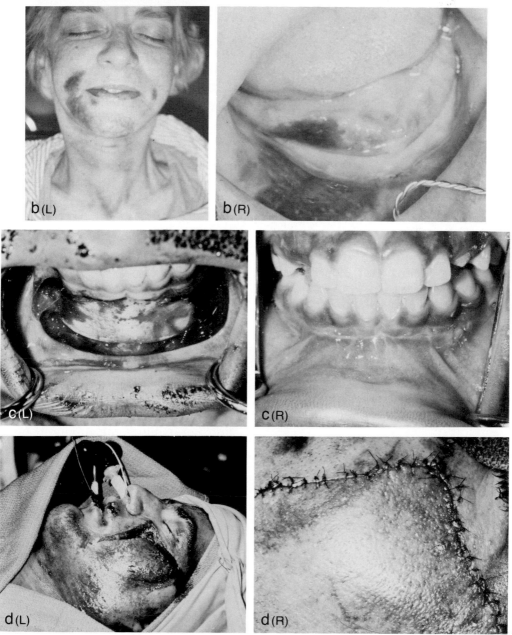

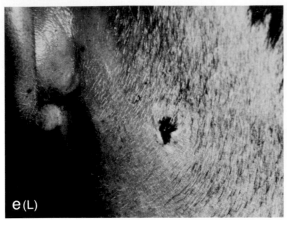
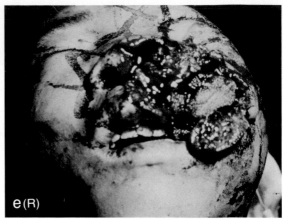

FIG. 4–2 (continued).   **e,** Missile wounds. **L,** Perforated missile wound of entrance by a high-velocity bullet. **R,** The avulsive exit wound.

juries of the face with underlying bony injuries should be repaired in conjunction with the overall treatment plan for reduction and fixation of facial skeletal fractures.

ABRASIONS

These wounds vary from superficial, consisting of a scraping of the skin that leaves a raw, bleeding surface, to a deforming shredding. Abrasions are usually painful because of exposed nerve endings. Treatment consists of thorough mechanical scrubbing with one of the surgical detergents, followed by the application of an antiseptic solution. An eschar forms, protecting the wound and permitting re-epithelialization. Occasionally, infection occurs and the coagulum must be removed.

AVULSIONS

An avulsive exit wound may be produced by a bullet tumbling in the body and by fragments of teeth, artificial dentures, and bones shattered by a bullet. An avulsive entrance wound may be produced by a high-velocity bullet or by irregular objects. Occasionally, scalping avulsions will result from the glancing, tangential passage of a missile.

CONTUSIONS

Contusions are subcutaneous hemorrhages produced either by trauma from a blunt object

that does not break the overlying mucosa or skin, or by hemorrhage from underlying injuries such as a fracture. Contusions generally do not require treatment since the hemorrhage is usually self-limiting.

LACERATIONS

Lacerations result from tearing of the soft tissue by a sharp object. They may be simple and superficial or complex, involving underlying vessels, nerves, and salivary glands or their ducts. Their margins may be smooth or irregular, depending on the wounding instrument. Lacerations are the most common type of soft-tissue injuries seen in vehicular accidents.

PUNCTURE WOUNDS

Puncture wounds are produced by sharp objects such as knives. Unless complicated by bleeding, many facial tissue puncture wounds can be closed with excision of the edges of the wound. In some cases, healing occurs with little deformity if the wound is left open and allowed to repair by granulation.

BURNS

Burns often involve the soft tissues of the face and are usually associated with burns of other parts of the body. (Management of burns will be discussed later in the chapter.)

MISSILE WOUNDS

Missile wounds are caused by missiles moving at a wide range of velocities. Missiles may be high-to-low-velocity bullets and fragments from grenades, rockets, mines, and booby traps. Missile wounds are incurred in civilian settings and, of course, in all types of warfare, from terrorist activities to conventional war.

Missile wounds may be divided into four types: penetrating, perforating, avulsive, and blast injuries. Penetrating wounds are caused by a low-velocity missile that is retained within the tissues. There is a wound of entrance but no wound of exit. The size of the wound depends on the shape and size of the missile.

Perforating wounds are caused by a missile that passes through the tissue, leaving a wound of entrance and a wound of exit. High-velocity missiles cause small entrance wounds and large, avulsed exit wounds. Since the energy imparted by a missile depends more on its velocity than on its mass, the high-velocity missile will cause significant tissue destruction along its course as well as at the point of exit. Fragmentation of teeth and bone, from missile damage produces secondary missiles that may cause extensive trauma. Low-velocity missiles may pass through tissue with a wound of exit about the same size as the wound of entrance, causing less external soft-tissue destruction.

Avulsive wounds are usually related to high-velocity missiles in which portions of soft and often hard tissues are completely removed from the patient.

In blast injuries, dirt or other foreign body particles penetrate the tissues, producing a general shredding of the tissues and creating difficulty in cleaning the deeply penetrating particles. Adequate debridement and soft-tissue closure may be impossible, and scrubbing or irrigation may fail to remove all of the particles. Tattooing is almost inevitable and extensive infection frequently occurs. When the eyes are exposed to the blast, the sight is usually lost. Gross contamination is common

with fragments of plastic, metal, debris, and clothing often carried deep into the wounds. There may be associated burns of all degrees.

COMBINED SOFT-TISSUE AND BONE INJURIES

In combined soft-tissue and multiple bone fractures, the rule of treatment planning should be to treat from the inside out for the soft-tissue injuries and, in general, from the bottom up for the skeletal injuries (see Chapter 13). The repositioning of bone fragments often may be performed through the external wounds, thereby forming a foundation for assembling the soft tissues. Oral soft-tissue wounds usually should be repaired concurrently with the application of intermaxillary fixation or insertion of splints. Extensive soft-tissue injuries of the face with underlying bony injuries should not be repaired definitively until at least the initial reduction and fixation of the facial fractures is accomplished or until intraoral impressions, if indicated, are obtained. If definitive reduction of fractures cannot be accomplished early, temporary suturing of lacerations should be performed, and final repair of the soft tissue performed after reduction and fixation of the fractures.

GENERAL CONSIDERATIONS

Although the general principles of soft-tissue management apply to all facial wounds, techniques vary with the location and type of wound. There may be considerable damage to the surrounding tissues with disturbance of the normal anatomic and physiologic defense mechanisms against bacterial invasion. Thorough but very conservative debridement, hemostasis, careful tissue handling, and meticulous restoration of tissues in layers to a position as normal as possible will produce the best results, as has been attested repeatedly in the past 100 years. (See Chapter 1.)

Wounds respond best when treated within a few hours following injury. Primary closure should be accomplished within the first 24 hrs. If more time is necessary before definitive soft-tissue repair for the reduction and stabilization of fractures, the wounded tissue should be kept moistened for 2 to 3 days, depending on the amount of contamination and the extent of the wound.

Recovery from soft-tissue injuries depends on the capacity of the body to repair or restore the injured tissues. The role of the surgeon is to design and perform procedures that assist the natural reparative process.

INCISED, CLEAN WOUNDS

Wounds heal by a continuous and progressive series of events initiated immediately after injury. The tissues first react to the injury with a proliferation of connective and epithelial tissue. Collagen acts as a binding material, influencing the contraction of the wound and providing tensile strength.

When soft tissues are opened by either a surgical incision or trauma, inflammatory edema always occurs around the area to some degree, leukocytes digest devitalized tissue, and macrophages invade the clot, ingesting the remnants of fibrin and red cells. Two types of new tissue are formed by cellular proliferation: connective tissue cells, which restore the continuity of the deeper structures by the processes of fibroplasia, and epithelial cells, which restore the surface of the wound. New vessels are produced from angioplasts arising from connective tissue cells and from the budding of the endothelium of pre-existing blood vessels. Capillaries from proliferating blood vessels advance into the wound from the periphery.

Sandison and Howes and their associates in the 1920s divided the healing of the incised wound into three phases: the lag phase, lasting from the time of wounding until day 5 or 6; the fibroplasia phase, lasting from day 6 to 14; and the maturation phase, lasting from day 14 until the wound is fully repaired.[23] A rapid increase in wound strength occurs during the period of fibroplasia and reaches a maximum around the fourteenth to sixteenth postoperative day.

WOUNDS WITH LOSS OF TISSUE

As might be expected, wounds with a loss of tissue heal more slowly than simple incised wounds. The surface appears red and finely granulated within a few days after the loss of tissue. Granulation tissue, young fibrous connective tissue with abundant blood vessels, forms in the defect, but healing will not be completed until there is a cover of a continuous layer of new mucous membrane or epithelium. Because more fibrous connective tissue is produced in wounds with a loss of tissue than in simple incised wounds, scar contracture on the former type of wound is greater.

INFECTED WOUNDS

Infection and suppuration retard wound healing. Infection, as an acute or chronic inflammatory process, will develop when organisms find a suitable medium for growth. The process may be localized, spreading, regional, or generalized, depending on the type and virulence of the infective organism, the receptiveness of the wound, the contiguous anatomy and physiology, and the general condition of the patient.

PRINCIPLES OF MANAGEMENT

DEBRIDEMENT

Although all of the steps of wound repair are important, debridement is probably the most critical because it must be done by human beings, except for the natural exfoliation of certain foreign or devitalized particles.

Debridement consists of the removal of all foreign matter and devitalized tissue including small detached fragments of bone; it may be very time consuming and may require a general anesthesia. Mechanical cleansing is performed first by scrubbing the wound and the surrounding area with a surgical soap. A stiff scrub brush is used for the scrubbing, although some particles will require removal by a sharp instrument such as a curette or a scalpel blade. Copious amounts of saline irrigation are used during the debridement to help remove debris and foreign bodies. (D_5W may be used for irrigation because the solution will provide local hemostasis to abraided tissues.) A water-jet lavage instrument is especially helpful in the wet debridement of a blast-type wound with many small penetrating wounds.[4] Palpation of the wound will detect particles of foreign matter that might not be noted by inspection. If pigmented foreign bodies are allowed to remain in the wound, a tattoo may result, producing a severe cosmetic problem (Fig. 4–3). Polymyxin B sulfate ointment may be sponged into the wound during the debridement to remove residual debris such as grease and tar that cannot be removed by regular procedures. Final flushing of the wound with hydrogen peroxide will remove residual blood clots. This technique was used on injuries in the Vietnam War with considerable success.[5]

Fragments of bone that remain attached to soft tissue should be considered viable tissue and left in the wound to aid in repair of the bony injury. Many of these fragments will remain viable and will repair when they are maintained in a fixed position.

Metallic missile fragments that are easily located should be removed. Small fragments often are well tolerated, however, and their removal may cause unnecessary destruction of tissue and be a waste of time. Metal fragments that are situated adjacent to major vessels should be removed because they may cause erosion of the vessel wall. If the fragment is some distance from the wound of entrance, it may be removed during a subsequent operation.

After the removal of all foreign matter, conservative removal of devitalized tissue is indicated. The tissues of the face have an excellent blood supply and resist locally induced infection very well. Excessive excisional debridement is never indicated, and usually only the obviously nonviable tissue should be removed. Skin margins that are macerated or are very irregular are excised approximately 2 to 3 mm to allow for a cutaneous edge that is even and perpendicular to the underlying subcutaneous tissues.

HEMOSTASIS

Hemostasis is a primary consideration in wound repair to prevent secondary hemor-

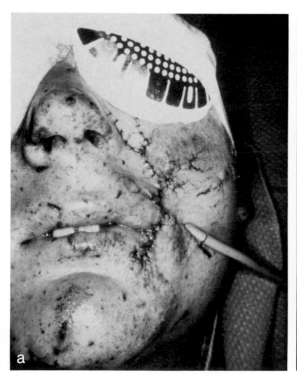 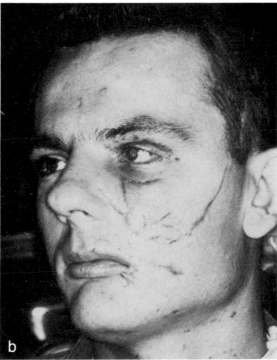

FIG. 4–3. Traumatic tattoo. **a,** Abrasions and lacerations produced by a blast injury. **b,** Because of time constraints resulting from masses of patients, complete debridement was not possible, and the patient bears traumatic tattoos.

rhage with subsequent hematoma formation that may be followed by infection and wound breakdown. Because cleansing and debridement of the wound may cause a resumption of bleeding, control by clamping and ligating may be necessary during initial cleansing. Hence, preparation for adequate blood replacement should be made prior to the operation.

Control of bleeding arterial vessesls can be accomplished by ligating larger vessels with silk sutures, and smaller vessels with absorbable sutures or electro-coagulation. Extreme care should be exercised when using electrocautery to avoid burning the skin edges and nerves. In situations in which the bleeding vessel is deep within the wound, clips are utilized. The surgeon should be prepared for urgent situations that require ligation of a major vessel below the injured site, such as the external carotid artery or one of its branches (Fig. 4–4).

Management of hemorrhage arising from veins may be problematic, because there is no effective valve system for drainage from cranial areas. Thus, a laceration of the posterior facial vein or the lingual vein may permit a rapid and fatal hemorrhage if one is not able to control the hemorrhage at the point of injury. Ligation above the injured site may not be a surgical option. Unilateral and even bilateral ligation of the external carotid arteries will not be effective. The usual approaches are to use warm pressure packs, induced hypotension to control blood pressure, identification of the injured site, and direct care of the injured vessel.

Profuse hemorrhage from the nose and posterior pharynx may accompany facial trauma and may require combined anterior and posterior nasal packing. (See Chapters 2, 11, and 13.)

Induced hypotension with circulatory control is an effective method of controlling hemorrhage during an operation. Because under normal conditions the blood pressure is maintained by a balance between the volume of circulating blood and the capacity of the vascular bed, induced hypotension is based on the disruption of one of these mechanisms— either the volume of the circulating blood is reduced or the capacity of the vascular bed is increased. The resultant hypotension may be hypovolemic or normovolemic. Normovolemic hypotension with reduction of the systolic blood pressure to approximately 60 mm Hg at heart level is usually preferred.

UNDERMINING

In wounds with avulsion of tissue, undermining by dissection in the subcutaneous layers, usually with scissors and hemostats, and sometimes between the muscular layers is necessary to permit mobilization of soft tissues for the primary closure of large defects without excessive tension on the soft tissues. Successful cosmetic repair of most soft-tissue injuries largely depends on avoiding tension in closing the cutaneous surface. In the facial region, especially the cheek and neck, an extensive amount of undermining may be used because of the relative mobility of the soft tissues.

Undermining should be accomplished superficial to the restored muscle layers and below the subcutaneous layer, primarily using blunt dissection. In avulsive-type wounds, it may be necessary to arbitrarily establish the layers with sharp dissection to permit the necessary undermining.

PRIMARY CLOSURE

Soft-tissue wounds of the face should be repaired in a manner that will restore the fa-

---

FIG. 4–4. Arterial anatomy of the facial tissues. **a L,** Lateral view of an angiogram of the external facial artery and its distribution. **R,** Frontal view of angiogram. **b L,** Lateral view of an angiogram of the internal maxillary artery and its distribution. **R,** Frontal view of angiogram. **c,** Lateral view of an angiogram of the lingual artery. **d,** Incision line for dissection to and ligation of the external carotid artery for hemorrhage control

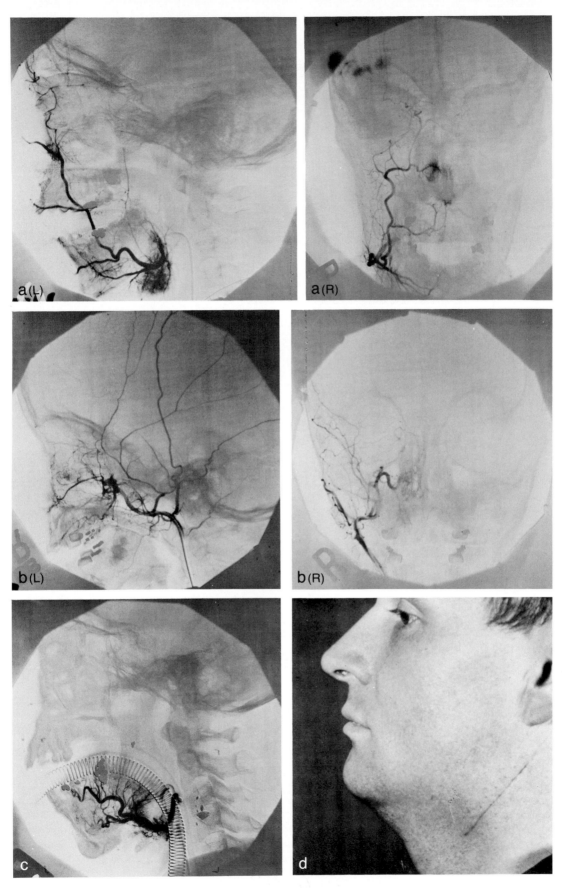

(Legend on Facing Page)

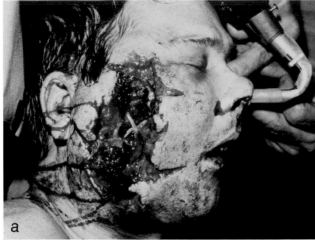

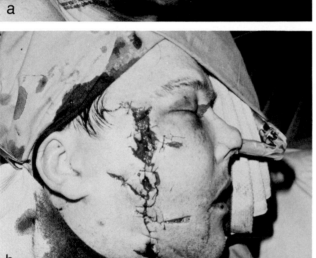

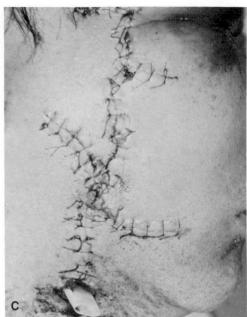

FIG. 4–5. Wound closure. **a,** Complex lacerating injury of the facial tissues. **b,** Treated by primary closure utilizing, for orientation, key sutures on the cutaneous surface, followed by closure in layers. **c,** Note drain in the submandibular space. (Courtesy of Dr. James Chipps.)

cial structure to a position as near normal as possible (Fig. 4–5). Although facial soft-tissue wounds often demonstrate gross disorientation of the soft tissues, most may be closed primarily, that is, by directly suturing across the wound.[6] The principles of tissue management must be followed and closure accomplished meticulously, with accurate repositioning of the various layers of tissue to eliminate all dead spaces.

The repair should begin with careful re-positioning of detached periosteum over exposed bone at the fracture sites. To permit more accurate positioning of the tissues, it is often helpful to place a few temporary skin sutures at key points at the corner of the mouth, the vermillion border of the lip, or the distinctive curves or points of the laceration prior to closing the deep layers (Fig. 4–5). If the deepest portion of the wound involves the oral cavity, the mucosa should be closed first with a watertight closure that prevents

FIG. 4–6. Various suturing techniques. **a,** Running horizontal sutures provide a watertight approximation of mucosal tissues. **b,** Running continuous loop sutures are useful for rapid closure of long lacerations and incisions. **c,** Horizontal sutures interspersed with interrupted sutures provide a broad approximation of the cutaneous and subcutaneous tissues with a slight eversion of the superficial margin. **d,** Modified horizontal mattress suture to level unequal margins. **e,** Running subcuticular suture is placed in the base of the dermis.

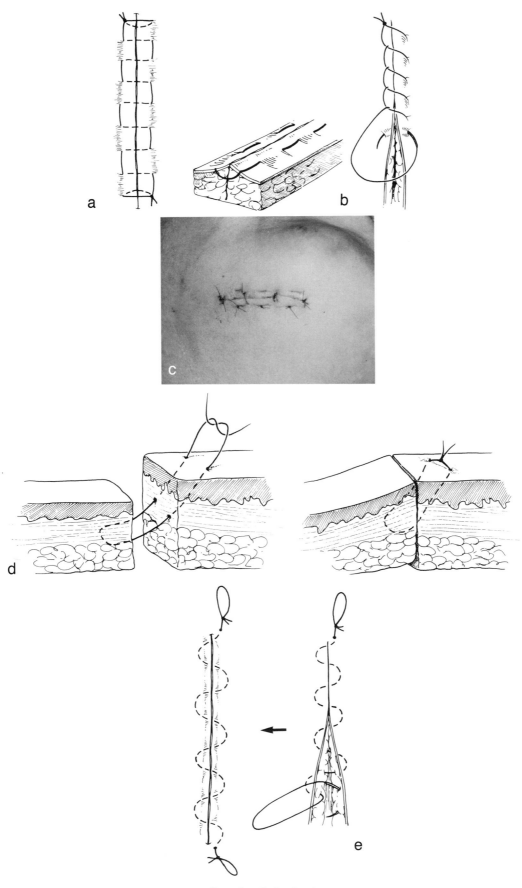

a

b

c

d

e

(Legend on Facing Page)

oral fluids from further contaminating the
wound. Sutures of polyglycolic acid or silk
are preferred because they remain in place,
are well tolerated, and may be removed with
minimal difficulty. Plain and even chromic
catgut sutures often loosen before the incision
lines and laceration have repaired sufficiently
to be secure. A running horizontal mattress
suturing technique provides the best watertight closure when closing the mucosa. After
closing the mucosa, the suture line and adjacent tissues may be dried and painted lib-
erally with tincture of benzoin or sprayed
with cyanoacrylate to further ensure a watertight closure (Fig. 4–6).

After closure of the mucosa, the periosteum, muscle, fascia, and subcutaneous tissues are closed in layers. Absorbable sutures
of 3–0 plain gut or polyglycolic acid sutures
should be used because chromic gut sutures
may cause considerable tissue irritation and
may lead to wound breakdown.[7] In wounds
with considerable avulsion of tissue, which
results in tension when the muscle layer is
approximated, a 32-gauge wire suture may be
used. Sutures of 4–0 plain gut or polyglycolic
acid should be placed in an inverted manner
in the subcutaneous tissues to approximate
the skin edges evenly.

The skin edges may be approximated by
placing a continuous subcuticular suture in
the dermis using a 5–0 nylon suture or polyethylene in the base of the dermis, alternating
from side to side with the ends brought to
the surface to permit removal. If the wound
is longer than 5 or 6 cm, the continuous subcuticular sutures may be brought to the surface at regular intervals to facilitate removal.

Skin sutures using 6–0 nylon, polyethylene, or silk are placed without tension on the
skin edges to produce a slightly everted edge.
They may be placed in an interrupted manner
approximately 2 mm from the wound edge
and approximately 2 to 3 mm apart. A continuous lock suture may be used in relatively
long wounds to reduce the overall operating
time. In areas of considerable tissue stress,
placing periodic vertical mattress sutures may
be necessary to accomplish the desired eversion and to help support the deeper tissues.
Horizontal mattress tissues will provide ever-

sion of the skin margins but with less support
of the deeper tissues.

DELAYED PRIMARY CLOSURE

Because soft-tissue injuries of the face are
usually contaminated, on some occasions primary closure is not indicated (Fig. 4–7). Delayed primary closure consists of debriding
the wound, then dressing it open with moist
fine mesh or antiseptic gauze until all infection has been controlled, at which time the
wound is closed in layers. This closure is undertaken in 3 to 5 days, prior to mature epi-
thelialization of the wound edges. Delayed
primary closure may be used either when the
wound is managed first more than 48 hrs after
the time of injury, or when there is a heavy
press of patients, as in conventional warfare.

SECONDARY CLOSURE

It may not always be possible to treat injuries within the indicated period for primary
closure or delayed primary closure, particularly when many casualties are present, as in
warfare. These wounds may become infected
and sloughing, so that primary closure is not
indicated. In these instances, it is necessary
to treat the wound by periodically removing
all devitalized and infected tissues, establishing adequate drainage applying moist dressings, and administering indicated antibiotic
therapy while continuing careful daily observation. In approximately 5 days, the wounds
may begin to close or can be closed as previously described. When more than 5 days
have elapsed between injury and treatment,
the wound edges will begin to epithelialize
and secondary closure is necessary.

The wounds are isolated from the oral cavity with watertight closures, as discussed
above; the wound margins are excised and
the skin undermined to permit closure of the
tissues in a layered manner without undue
tension on the skin. Secondary closure may
produce satisfactory results if the wound has
been kept moist and debridement of necrotic
tissue has been performed daily.

DRAINS

Superficial lacerations of the face usually do
not require drainage. In general, wounds

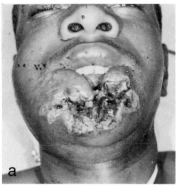 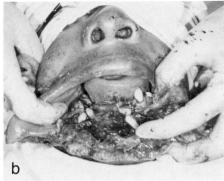 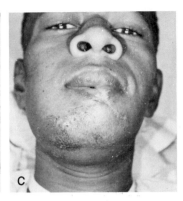

FIG. 4–7. Delayed primary closure. **a,** Soft- and hard-tissue complex of injuries kept moist for several days. **b,** Closure performed as with primary repair. Nonvital bone fragments and teeth that could not be salvaged are debrided. Bone is covered with soft tissue; closure is performed by layers, ending with the cutaneous surface. **c,** Final appearance prior to reconstructive and definitive surgery. (Courtesy of Dr. James Chipps.)

above the mandible can be closed primarily without drainage. Whether to drain depends on the type of wound involved, and each case should be decided individually. Many soft-tissue injuries resulting from missiles will require placement of drains in cavitation areas to minimize hematoma formation. Wounds involving only the cheeks, lips, or upper face usually may be closed in a manner that eliminates all dead spaces, not requiring drainage.

Wounds of the floor of the mouth, base of the tongue, retromandibular area, infratemporal fossa, and neck will often involve dead spaces and require the placement of drains. In wounds involving the mandible with loss of bony structure and involvement of the oral cavity, the placement of a drain is important. The soft-tissue defect in the oral cavity must be sutured with a watertight technique and the periosteum closed into and over the space that had been occupied by the mandible, and a drain should be placed superficial to this area. If the drain is placed too deeply the tissues may break down, with formation of an oral cutaneous fistula. In wounds with extensive dead space, an indwelling catheter attached through a suctioning device, such as a Hemovac, with continuous or intermittent suction may be used instead of a drain to assist in minimizing hematoma formation.

Wounds involving the submandibular regions are always drained (Fig. 4–5). The drain is inserted between sutures or through a stab incision adjacent to the sutured wound. The drain is sutured to the skin edge to prevent its loss within the wound. One or more sutures may be placed, but not tied, adjacent to the drain so that, when the drain is removed, the sutures are available to close the drain site. Drains are removed when the wound no longer produces purulent exudate, usually in 2 to 5 days.

DRESSING AND NURSING CARE

A protective dressing should be applied to sutured wounds of the face. The dressings range from adhesive strips applied across the incision line for simple lacerations to compressive dressings for the more complex injuries.

Following repair of a complex soft-tissue wound, a properly placed compressive-type dressing is invaluable in preventing postoperative edema, reducing tension on the suture lines, and immobilizing the healing wound. Compression enhances circulation in the area by preventing edema and supporting venous flow.

An excellent dressing regimen for complex or extensive soft-tissue injuries of the facial area consists of polymyxin B sulfate ointment on gauze placed over the suture lines, followed by a 4 × 8-inch cotton gauze and sponge and padded with fluffs to provide a bulky dressing. The dressing is then secured by wrapping the face and head with a *very slightly* stretched elastic-type dressing. The elastic dressing should not be applied tightly as this may cause venous stasis, wound repair complications, and discomfort. The eyes may be included within the dressing by applying a sterile eye pad and a shield to eliminate undue pressure on the eye. The compressive dressing should be left in place for at least 24 hrs and up to 72 hrs in the case of complex and extensive wounds, unless it is necessary to remove drains earlier. After the bulky dressing is removed, a smaller dressing is placed to absorb drainage and to support the laceration lines.

Postoperative wound care is extremely important and is initiated after dressing removal. It includes cleansing the lacerations every other day with sterile cotton applicators saturated in hydrogen peroxide diluted one half with water, followed by applying an ointment to the suture lines to minimize crusting and scab formation. Bacitracin or polymyxin B sulfate ointment are satisfactory in most cases, although nitrofurazone ointment is beneficial in wounds that continue to weep tissue fluids as it tends to dry the wound and promote early healing. Complex soft-tissue injuries should be cleansed and ointment reapplied two to four times daily depending on the condition of the individual wound.

If superficial wound breakdown occurs secondary to infection or to closure of skin with too much tension, wounds may be irrigated and dressed with sponges soaked with 1% acetic acid solution. This treatment aids in the debridement of nonviable tissues and keeps the wound clinically clean. These wounds may be closed secondarily or allowed to granulate with skin grafting planned at a later time, depending on the extent of the wound breakdown.

For simple lacerations, alternate skin sutures are removed 3 days postoperatively and the remaining sutures in 5 days. Complex wounds respond better if all sutures are left in place for 7 days; earlier removal increases the incidence of wound dehiscence. The use of nylon and polyethylene sutures permits retention of sutures for this length of time without evidence of tissue reaction.

Intraoral soft-tissue injuries are managed according to the same principles as the extraoral. Simple lacerations are repaired with black silk, polyglycolic acid, or, for surface closures, chromic gut sutures. The incision line is gently cleansed every other day with an antiseptic solution or diluted peroxide and the sutures are removed 5 to 10 days following the injury. For either complex or deep lacerations, soft-tissue intraoral injury is closed by layers using polyglycolic or gut sutures to approximate the muscle masses. If a dehiscence with exposure of the underlying bone occurs, irrigation with peroxide diluted one half with water should be provided at least four times/day (Fig. 4–8). This irrigation procedure may be an act of protracted and dedicated nursing care and has often been the difference between losing and saving a section of the facial skeleton.

TECHNIQUES OF MANAGEMENT

SOFT-TISSUE DEFECTS

In some instances, the size, depth, and position of extensive tissue destruction and avulsion prevents primary repair without undue tension on the tissues. If left untreated, the wound may granulate and eventually heal. If necessary, secondary repair with replacement of tissue can be accomplished at a later time.

Attempted primary closure of a large facial defect may cause derangement and distortion of adjacent structures and tensions that will produce tissue death and dehiscence. Injuries with major defects of the lip, eyelid, nose, and cheek are treated by suturing skin to mucous membrane around the margins of the defect. This suturing closes the raw areas, preserves the vitality of the surrounding tissues, maintains the defect, and avoids the distortion of the adjacent structures (Fig. 4–9). When this procdure is used, it is essential that moist dressings be placed over the wound until the wound has granulated satisfactorily. An alternative method, used during the Vietnam War, involved placing room-temperature curing silicone prostheses in maxillofacial wounds and suturing them to the tissue. The prostheses were maintained until appropriate

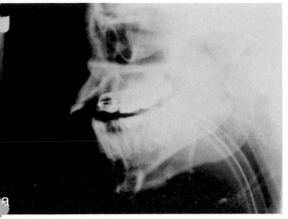 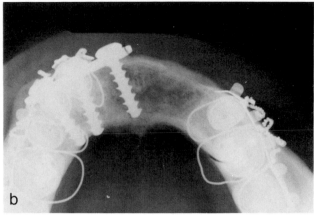

FIG. 4–8.   Anterior mandibular comminuted fracture. **a** and **b,** Soft-tissue dehiscence following the intraoral open reduction jeopardized repair of the fracture. Irrigation 4 to 6 times/day for 4 months by a dedicated nurse saved the anterior mandible.

tissue replacement could be performed. Later reconstructive procedures may have required repair of the defect by local or distant flaps, depending on the extent of the defect.[8]

INTRAORAL INJURIES

Injuries in the oral cavity may vary in severity from lacerations of the oral mucosa and lips to avulsive wounds of the palate, alveolar process, and floor of the mouth. With extensive injuries involving communication between the oral cavity and cutaneous surfaces, a watertight mucosal closure is imperative.

Prior to soft-tissue closure, all fractured teeth that cannot be salvaged or used for immobilization should be removed to reduce the incidence of infection and wound breakdown with fracture nonunion (see Chapter 4-12). Teeth should be retained if their removal would necessitate the sacrifice of large segments of alveolar bone. Wounds in the floor of the mouth often involve fractures of the mandible with exposed bone and laceration of the tissues of the floor of the mouth and tongue. Hemorrhage, edema, and potential airway obstruction are significant problems in these cases (see Chapter 7).

Because the tongue fills nearly the entire oral cavity when the mouth is closed, injury to it is common. Because of the profuse blood supply to the tongue, injuries to the apex or dorsum heal rapidly after debridement and closure by layers (Fig. 4–10). However, wounds to the base of the tongue may result in serious hemorrhage, with threats to the airway.

All hemorrhages, at least in theory, may be controlled by pressure. However, continuous pressure to a hemorrhage arising from severed vessels in the base of the tongue is not practical. Nevertheless, because the hemorrhage may challenge the airway or produce shock, and hence be life-threatening, it must be controlled as directly and as promptly as possible. Intubation, tracheostomy, and general anesthesia may be necessary. If the hemorrhage is arterial in orgin, ligation of the lingual artery or the external cartoid artery may be performed, while it may reduce but not completely control the hemorrhage, the reduction of the volume of the flow may allow the laceration of the artery to be identified and repaired.

Because the venous system of the head and neck lacks valves, venous laceration, such as in the ranine or lingual veins, may be a potential threat to life as a result of airway obstruction or hypovolemic shock. A laceration of one of the major veins of the tongue is nearly equivalent to a laceration of one of the jugular veins. As with the major arterial lacerations, the patient should be placed under general anesthesia with the indicated systemic supports. Through the use of pressure gauzes and suctioning, the laceration must be

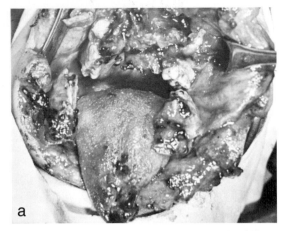

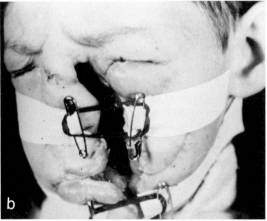

FIG. 4–9.   Avulsive soft-tissue losses. **a** and **b,** Extensive loss of soft tissue was initially treated by suturing cutaneous tissues to mucous membrane. (Courtesy of Dr. James Hayward.)

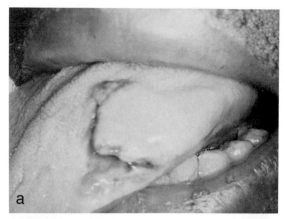

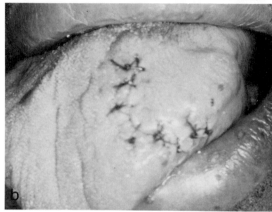

FIG. 4–10.   Tongue laceration. **a** and **b,** Lacerated tongue was closed in layers using chromic gut suturing material.

identified and controlled directly because the jugular veins are not accessible for ligation, and ligating all of the arterial vessels leading to the circle of Willis is not reasonable.

Teeth and bone fragments that may have been driven into the tongue may be difficult to locate but if left in place may predispose to infection. Great care should be taken to identify and remove these fragments. If the ventral surface of the tongue and floor of the mouth are injured, the tongue should be closed in layers and the soft tissue in the floor of the mouth used to cover the exposed bone of the mandible.

If the symphysis area of the mandible is avulsed, placing a bone plate pin or wire between the segments of bone may permit an-

terior support for suturing the musculature and closing the mucosa.

In avulsive injuries of the palate, the remaining palatal mucosa is mobilized and sutured to the buccal mucosa or the alveolar mucosa. If tissue to cover a palatal defect is sufficient, an acrylic splint fabricated to cover the defect may permit as much granulation of mucosa as possible. Definitive repair should be planned at a later date and may consist of many procedures (Fig. 4–11).

The importance of proper nursing care for intraoral repair cannot be overemphasized. Breakdown of the oral mucosa may result in an oral cutaneous fistula or loss of sections of the facial skeleton. Success depends on the correct placement of proper suture material and dedicated nursing care to provide a clean environment within the oral cavity.

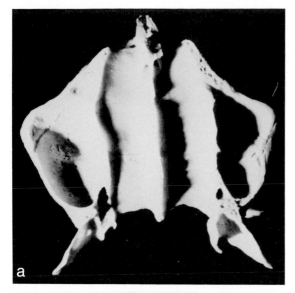

FIG. 4–11. Oroantral openings and fistulas. **a,** Anatomic specimen demonstrating the maxillary sinal cavities. **b, c,** and **d,** Orosinal opening secondary to facial skeletal trauma. **b L** and **R,** Surgical treatment consisted of removing the mucosal lining tissue in the opening, and **c L** and **R,** Raising the medial full-thickness mucoperiosteal flap to the palatal midline and the lateral flap from the subperiosteal layer superiorly to just inferior to the infraorbital foramen. **d L** and **R,** The periosteal layers, bilaterally, are incised parallel to the defect to permit movement of the flap over the osseous defect. The margins are everted and immobilized with the aid of rubber tubing. (Courtesy of Dr. Jack Caldwell.)

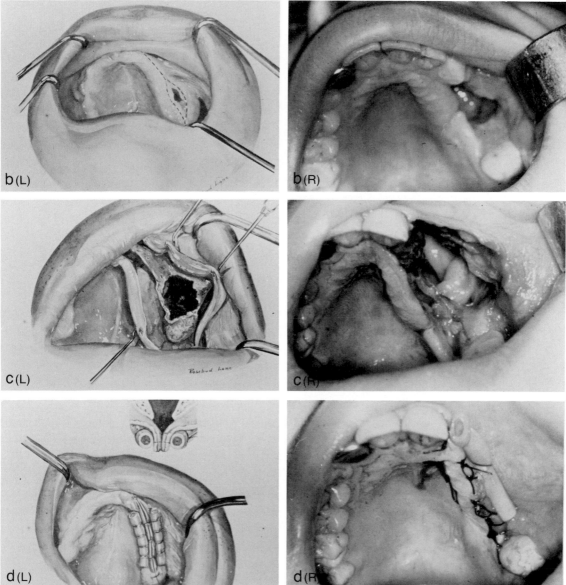

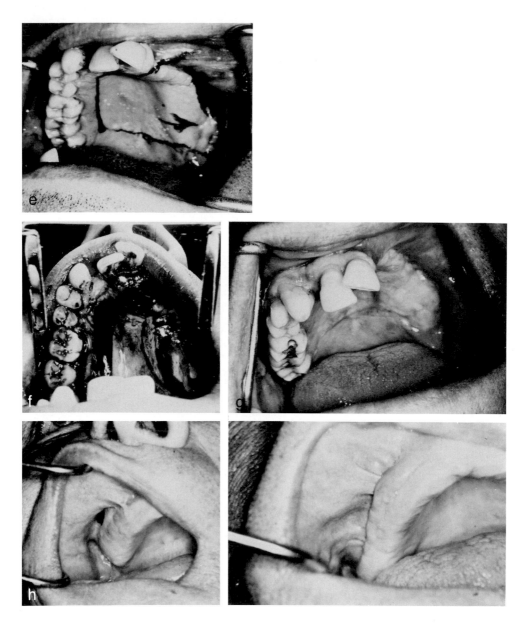

FIG. 4–11 (continued).   **e, f,** and **g,** Closure by a reverse sliding flap of an oral-sinal-nasal fistula incurred as part of a complex of facial injuries. In this technique, ample soft-tissue attachment, anterior and posterior to the defect, is necessary to assure the viability of the repositioned flap. The margins of the defect are incised and closed. This procedure may be performed in two stages by first raising the flap and replacing it in its original bed to stimulate blood supply, and then performing the retraction maneuver. **h** and **i,** An orosinal opening lateral to the maxilla may be difficult to close because of the pull of facial muscles. A subperiosteal flap, extending to the infraorbital foramen on the lateral side, is carried across the alveolar ridge and tucked under a medial flap that is raised over the entire width and height of the alveolar ridge. The periosteum is scored horizontally on both flaps to add relaxation and stability.

INJURIES TO SALIVARY GLANDS AND DUCTS

Facial injuries frequently involve the major salivary glands and the ducts associated with those glands. When wounds of the submandibular areas result in considerable destruction of the submandible gland, as often occurs, the remaining portions of the submandible gland should be removed at the time of debridement and the duct ligated as it passes toward the oral cavity.

Wounds of the cheek often involve the parotid gland and may require removal of portions of the gland; however, attempts should be made to preserve as much of this gland as possible and to close the overlying fascia parotideomasseteria. Wounds in the region of Stensen's duct should be examined to ascertain possible injury to the duct. A line extending from the inferior border of the external acoustic meatus to a point midway between the ala nasi and the upper border of the lip approximates the level of the duct. The severed ends of the duct often can be identified by inserting a probe from the oral orifice of the duct and by identifying salivary secretions from the glandular or proximal ends of the duct. Anastomosis of a sectioned Stensen's duct may be performed through the overlying lacerations by suturing the duct around a polyethylene catheter. Operating glasses that magnify two to four times are useful but not mandatory in this operation.

If no attempt at repair of the duct was made at the time of injury, the same operation may be performed as soon as the laceration and nonfunction of the duct is evident (Fig. 4–12).

In a missile wound, a portion of the duct may be destroyed or avulsed, precluding primary repair and making identification of the duct impossible. These cases should be managed by primary closure of the wound with a drain extending into the oral cavity from the region of the proximal end of the duct. The drain should be left in place for a minimum of 14 days, if it is effective in evacuating saliva from the area. If the drainage is inadequate, a sialocele will develop in the cheek after the pressure dressing has been removed. This can be managed by placing a catheter of small diameter, such as an oxygen catheter,

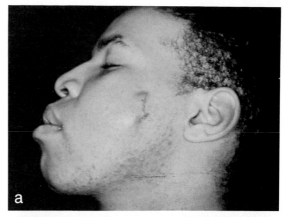

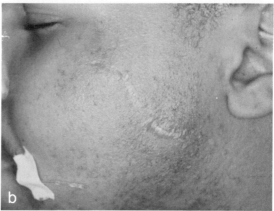

FIG. 4–12. Parotid duct lacerations. **a,** Serous parotid fluid collected in the buccal tissues 4 weeks following a laceration. **b,** The area was opened, the duct was reconstituted around a polyethylene tube (which can be seen exiting from the mouth with salivary fluid in it), and the laceration was revised.

through the mucosa to extend into the area of the sialocele. The catheter should remain in position for an additional 10 to 14 days to permit the track to become epithelialized and to create a new duct into the oral cavity.

Another method that has been successful in restoring the drainage capability of the parotid gland consists of raising a 5-mm-wide, 20-mm-long flap of mucosa with its base at the orifice of the duct. A blunt dissection is performed near the duct, extending back to the sialocele area. The passage of the flap to the sialocele is accomplished with double-armed suture material placed into the tip of the flap; the suture needles are passed up the dissected path into the sialocele and then exit through the overlying cutaneous tissues. The sutures are tied and left in place for only 3 or

4 days. Bulky pressure dressings are kept in place to immobilize the cheek and the reversed flap of mucosal tissue for 7 to 10 days. If this procedure is successful, the mucosal surface extending into the sialocele will produce a fistulous tract that will function as a duct.

External wounds that involve the parotid gland frequently weep saliva for several days, but almost without exception the drainage will cease spontaneously in 10 to 14 days without formation of a fistula. When parotid saliva is draining from a wound, it may be helpful to maintain a pressure dressing over the area. If these procedures fail, ligation of the proximal end of the duct usually causes atrophy of the parotid gland.

INJURIES TO THE FACIAL NERVE

Wounds of the face frequently involve branches of the facial nerve; accurate assessment of the injury prior to surgery can be helpful in determining the branches involved and distinguishing peripheral from central involvement of the nerve. Many patients experience spontaneous return of nerve function within the first 4 to 5 months after injury without surgical intervention. Facial muscle stimulation should be performed regularly on these patients until clinical evidence of return of nerve function is observed.

When facial nerve injuries are located peripherally, attempts should be made to identify the branches using a nerve stimulator. Although larger branches may be anastomosed with 6–0 nylon or silk sutures, small branches should be repaired with 9–0 nylon sutures using an operating microscope.

Unfortunately, missile wounds frequently cause extensive tissue destruction or avulsion of tissues, making primary repair of nerves impossible at the time of initial injury. When portions of the nerve are avulsed and cannot be repaired primarily, the severed ends should be tagged with silk sutures or silver clips to allow for identification of the nerve at the time of subsequent nerve grafting.

BURNS OF THE FACE

Burns of the face are often encountered in conjunction with burns of other areas of the body and are usually treated as part of the general therapy for burns. In civilians, burns occur most frequently in industrial accidents, whereas those associated with war injuries are seen in conjunction with blast injuries (Fig. 4–13). Three types of burns are distinguished: first-degree burns, which are red, similar to the erythema of a sunburn; second-degree burns, which are reddish white with many blisters; and third-degree burns, in which all the layers of the skin are involved, extending into the underlying fascia.

Burns of the face present special problems depending on the severity of the burn. An early evaluation must be made to rule out involvement of the respiratory tract, which is often observed in patients injured by high heat in a closed space. These patients exhibit coughing, bronchial spasm, striata, redness of the posterior pharynx, and singed nasal hairs. Increased expiratory effort may indicate upper airway edema requiring tracheal intubation.

Initially, facial burns are cleansed gently with room-temperature saline and facial hair is shaved to decrease the risk of folliculitis. After cleansing, the degree of injury may be assessed.

Local therapy of first-degree burns is the application of an antibiotic ointment such as bacitracin to the involved area; second- and third-degree burns are managed by applying mafenide ointment, taking care to protect the eyes. The object is to promote rapid drying of the wound and the production of a crust of scabs as a defense against infection. Third-degree burns may be treated by applying silver sulfadiazine and fine mesh gauze, changing the dressing daily after cleansing and debridement. The cleansing includes special consideration for the removal of exudates from the nares and the external ear canal. Because soft tissue and cartilage of the nose are easily destroyed by infection, any crust inside the nose should be removed to facilitate breathing and to prevent damage. The use of a stent to prevent contraction of the mouth during healing should be considered. Following debridement of the eschar from third-degree burns, either a xenograft, usually pig skin, is placed followed in 48 hours by a split-thickness autogenous skin graft, or an autog-

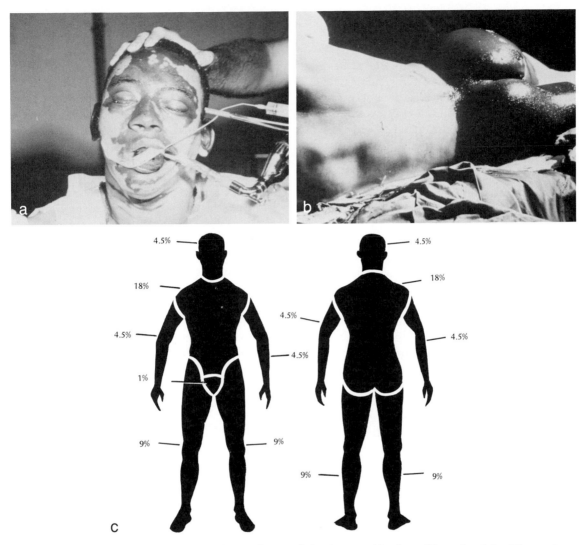

FIG. 4–13.   Burns. **a** and **b,** Second-degree burns of the face and body. **c,** The rule of 9s. The various proportions are based on third-degree burns. For second-degree burns, the values are halved.

enous skin graft is placed directly without the xenograft. Xenografts prepare wounds for autogenous grafts by decreasing bacterial growth and stimulating microcirculation.

Chemical burns to the oral and pharyngeal tissues caused by industrial accidents or the willful ingestion of caustic materials are treated initially with the appropriate antidote. Intermediate care should be directed toward reducing the effects of scar contractures; for example, a burn of the rima oris may be treated by placement of a splint, borne by the teeth, which is designed to be a base against

which repair can take place. Typically, the splint is worn continuously for 6 to 12 weeks. The long-term effects depend, of course, on the depth of the burn. The equivalent of a first- or second-degree burn will have negligible residual functional or untoward cosmetic effects. Third-degree type burns will produce contractures that may be quite severe. Foreshortening and deviation of the soft palate may be corrected by push-back palatoplasty procedures. Loss of vestibular depths and scars of the tongue and floor of the mouth may be corrected by grafting procedures similar to those used for preprosthodontic surgery.

The most common electrical burn to the oral and maxillofacial tissues is to the rima oris, usually the commissure, in children who place an active electrical wire in their mouths. The earliest care should be only wet debridement, not surgical debridement, and general systemic support of analgesics and psychotropic agents, as indicated. Tissue damage ranges form an erythema, to blistering, to total tissue destruction that may include the full thickness of the lip. The physical characteristics of the injuries, including the length of contact, determines the initial apparent injury and the intermediate and long-range tissue injury. A 3- or 4-week period of recovery for the surrounding tissues is necessary before surgical repair can be undertaken in case of actual tissue loss; the surrounding tissues lose their ability to repair following the passage of a destructive electrical current. The wound is cleansed four times/day with applicators carrying diluted peroxide; a stent, placed on the maxillary teeth and equipped with flanges to support the wounded tissues, is helpful to reduce early scar contracture. After a period of about 4 weeks, corrective surgery may be planned and performed (Fig. 4–14). Patients who have had no loss to minimal tissue loss should be treated by a maxillary dentition-supported stent that has flanges to support the commissures and reduce the possibility of scar contracture; these individuals, having the equivalent of first- and second-degree burns, usually require no corrective surgery.[11,12]

WOUNDS OF THE NECK

Missile wounds of the neck are frequently associated with oral and maxillofacial injuries. Usually, treatment of these injuries by the oral and maxillofacial surgeon occurs only during warfare; other surgeons manage these injuries in civilians.

All missile wounds of the neck are potentially extremely serious. Insignificant penetrating wounds may involve one of the major vessels of the neck and result in profuse secondary hemorrhage. The penetration of a small fragment can cause a tear in the carotid artery or jugular vein, which may tamponade within the carotid sheath. Diagnosis of carotid artery and, especially, jugular vein involvement is often not possible on preoperative evaluation; many patients may continue to demonstrate a normal pulse without neurologic deficits. Although little or no hemorrhage may be present on initial examination, sudden and heavy hemorrhage may be encountered during debridement, and immediate repair or control the involved vessels must be performed.

Injuries to the trachea and larynx are life-threatening and require tracheostomy. Tears in the trachea should be repaired after the tracheostomy has been performed. Insertion of an internal stent of acrylic or room-temperature vulcanizing silicone is effective in cases with comminution or shattering of the laryngeal structures.

Injuries of the pharynx or esophagus are explored and closed primarily in a double layer whenever possible. A nasogastric tube is placed to provide a means of feeding for 10 to 14 days. At times, holes in the pharynx or esophagus may be so small that they cannot be identified at surgery to permit primary closure. These patients should be managed by placement of a nasogastric tube for drainage of the neck wound.

Most wounds of the pharynx, esophagus, larynx, and trachea cause a degree of emphysema within the tissues of the neck, usually detected by clinical palpation or radiographic examination of the neck. If emphysema is present, the neck should be explored to locate the site of injury and perform the necessary repair. The wound should be drained for approximately 48 to 72 hours.

Only those missile wounds of the neck that do not involve vital structures should be treated conservatively. Conservative management includes excision of the skin margins, debridement by thorough irrigation, and primary closure of the wound with a drain. Any wound that may involve vital structures should be surgically explored for repair of the injury.

LIPS

Lips are extremely vulnerable to injury. Lacerations frequently occur because of impinge-

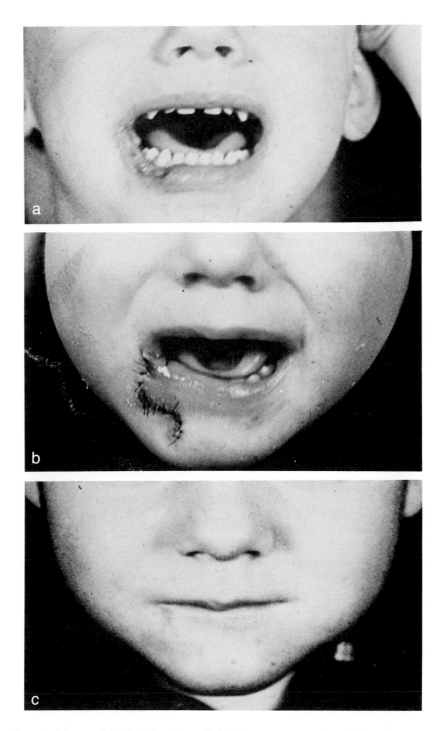

FIG. 4–14.   Electrical burn of the inferior lip. **a,** Full-thickness destruction of the inferior lip from contact with an electrical cord. **b,** Following a period of several weeks, the lip was reconstructed. **c,** Final appearance of the patient months following the injury. (Courtesy of Dr. James Hayward.)

ment of the lips between the anterior teeth and some external object. A laceration should be cleaned thoroughly, inspected and palpated, and even examined radiographically to insure that a segment of a tooth or other foreign body has not been retained in the tissues of the lip. The mucocutaneous border is aligned first with a key suture to assure accurate closure and prevent a conspicuous defect. Repair in layers then begins with the mucous membrane using polyglycolic acid or silk sutures placed to ensure a watertight closure. The muscle layers are approximated with absorbable sutures. Extensive avulsion of portions of the lip may require placement of transposition flaps, which usually requires a secondary reconstructive operation. The subcutaneous and cutaneous tissues are closed in layers.

EYELIDS

As with treatment of wounds of the neck, the repair of injuries to the eyelids, nose, and ears may not be the primary responsibility of the oral and maxillofacial surgeon. However, under many civilian and military circumstances an oral and maxillofacial surgeon does handle injuries of these structures.

Injuries to the eyelids are usually associated with more serious lacerations of the face and often include damage to the globe. The eyes are inspected to rule out bleeding into the chambers and corneal damage. The size, quality, and reactivity of the pupils are recorded to assess possible intracranial injury. Basic principles of wound management should be followed with thorough cleansing and removal of any foreign bodies prior to suturing (Fig. 4–15). Debridement is kept to a minimum, with all fragments of tissue being salvaged. Suturing begins in the inferior aspect of the lid sulcus and continues to the conjunctiva-skin junction at the rim using a running suture of fine nylon. A temporary suture placed at the ciliary margin may aid in approximating the wound. The edges of the outer surface of the tarsal plate are secured with 6–0 catgut sutures. The skin can then be closed with fine nylon interrupted sutures.[13]

Lacerations of the medial aspect of the lower lid may involve the lacrimal apparatus.

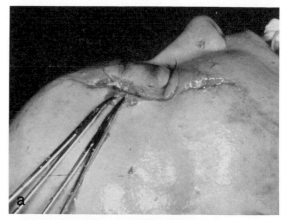
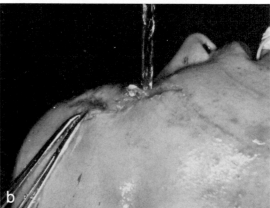
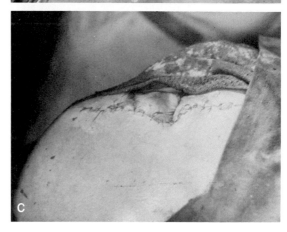

FIG. 4–15. Laceration of the lateral orbital soft tissues. **a,** The patient, an automobile driver not wearing a seat belt, received a laceration in the orbital area that missed the eye. The laceration was produced by the entry of fragments of glass and paint from the shattered rear-view mirror deep into the orbital area. **b,** The injury was debrided by inspection and palpation; 3000 ml of normal saline was also used in the debridement process. **c,** The closure was routine, the recovery was uneventful, and the injury produced no disability.

In wounds involving this area, the duct is explored before the skin is sutured. If the duct is severed, the medial end of the severed canaliculus may be difficult to find. After it is located, the severed canaliculus should be threaded over a small polyethylene tubing or suture material, which should be anchored into position for 14 days. The adjacent tissues are approximated with fine absorbable sutures.

In extensive lacerations, it may be necessary to provide postoperative splinting by placing a temporary mattress suture to join the opposing lid edges. A bland ophthalmic ointment should be placed between the lids, followed by the application of a dressing in the form of eye pads to provide general support. Wounds involving fracture of the nasal bones should be evaluated for possible severance of the medial canthal ligament. This should be repaired prior to superficial suturing.[14]

NOSE

Trauma to the nose may involve both fractures of the nasal skeleton and soft-tissue injury (Chapter 11). Soft-tissue repair consists of restoring the nasal mucosa with reapproximation and minimal suturing of the nasal cartilage in the perichondrial layer. The skin can then be approximated with a running interdermal suture in addition to a few skin sutures. Lubricated intranasal packing should be used to mold the nasal mucosa.

EARS

Soft-tissue trauma to the face often involves laceration or partial avulsion of the ears (Fig. 4–16). Complete traumatic loss is unusual; the lobule, a portion of the concha, and the external auditory canal are usually preserved even in cases of severe injury. The ear has an excellent blood supply and can be adequately nourished by a small remaining pedicle. In all ear wounds, the cartilage should be covered with cutaneous tissue, which may require a pedicle flap from the postauricular area. Severely damaged cartilage may be trimmed, reapproximated, and covered by adjacent cutaneous tissues. A direct blow or excessive

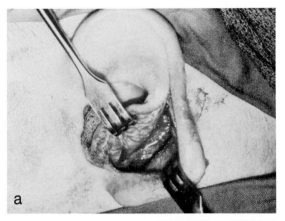

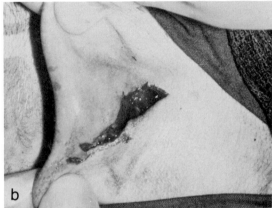

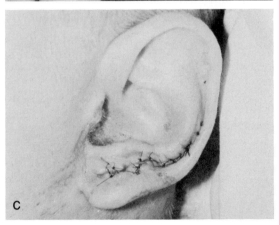

FIG. 4–16.   Laceration of the external ear. **a** and **b,** Laceration extended from the scapha and superior lobule of the external ear through to the posterior ear. **c,** The attachments of the heads of the posterior auricular muscle were identified and reapproximated, and the laceration was closed in layers. Repair was routine and uneventful.

traction on the ear can cause hemorrhage that collects between the perichondrium and cartilage, and the clot may become fibrosed, causing a thickening that, in turn, obliterates the convolutions of the ear. When this oto-hematoma matures it is known as a "cauli-flower ear." Early treatment is incision for drainage of the blood and serum with application of a molded pressure dressing to prevent recurrence of the hematoma.

GENERAL CARE OF THE PATIENT

ANTIBACTERIAL THERAPY

All soft-tissue wounds sustained in maxillofacial trauma, including gunshot wounds, bites, oral cutaneous lacerations, and blunt soft-tissue trauma, should be considered contaminated wounds. Antibiotic coverage is essential to prevent infection and wound breakdown.[15,16] In severely traumatized patients without allergies, penicillin may be administered in dosages of 1 million to 6 million units IV every 4 hours depending on the severity of the injury. War wounds have demonstrated a rather high incidence of gram-negative infections, the predominant organisms being Pseudomonas, Proteus, and Klebsiella. Appropriate antibiotics can be determined by the use of culture and sensitivity testing.[17,18]

Protection against infection by Clostridium tetani organisms also should be provided. Penicillin may be as protective against tetanus as ordinary doses of tetanus antitoxin, if started at the time of injury. Penicillin controls the growth of Clostridium tetani but cannot protect against the toxin already produced.

ANESTHESIA

Many operations involving the face are performed satisfactorily using local and regional anesthesia. If the patient is adequately sedated and confident there are many advantages to the use of local anesthetic techniques. Bleeding is minimized, and the patient returns to bed fully conscious, requiring minimal postoperative medication after the effects of the local anesthetic have disappeared. However, predicting the reaction of patients to treatment under local anesthesia may be difficult.

Extensive wounds of the face with underlying bony injuries are best treated under general anesthesia to allow for adequate cleansing, debridement, and meticulous repair. When the patient's condition and the situation permit, reducing and securing fixation of the underlying facial fractures prior to the closing of soft-tissue wounds is preferable. This precludes the necessity of manipulating the facial wounds to reduce and fix facial fractures during the healing phase, which may result in wound breakdown. Controlled hypotension may be used to minimize hemorrhage.

REFERENCES

1. Lilly, G.E., and Tinder, L.E.: Maxillofacial injuries: Survey of 8,746 cases. Milit Med 135:483, 1970.
2. Sandison, J.C.: Observations on the growth of blood vessels as seen in the transparent chamber introduced into rabbit's ear. Am J Anat 41-475, 1928.
3. Howes, E.L., Sooy, J.W., and Harvey, S.C.: The healing of wounds as determined by their tensile strength, JAMA 92:42, 1929.
4. Bhaskar, S.N., Cutright, D.E., Hunsuck, E.E., and Gross, A.: Pulsating water jet devices in debridement of combat wounds. Milit Med 136:264, 1971.
5. Osbon, D.B.: Early treatment of soft tissue injuries of the face. J Oral Surg 27:480-487, 1969.
6. Tinder, L.E.: Maxillofacial injuries sustained in the vietnam conflict. Milit Med 134:668, 1969.
7. Lilly, G.E., Cutcher, J.L., and Jones J.C.: Reaction of oral tissues to suture materials, Part IV. Oral Surg 33:152, 1972.
8. Salem, J.E., et al.: In vivo fabrication of temporary prosthesis for maxillofacial avulsion wounds: A clinical trial in vietnam. J Trauma 12:501, 1972.
9. Ducker, T.B., Kemp, L.G., and Hayes, G.J.: Neuron metabolism and peripheral nerve surgery. J Neurosurg 30:270, 1969.
10. Morgan, L.R., and Cramer, L.M.: Treatment of facial paralysis produced by combat wounds. Plast Reconst Surg 53:647, 1974.
11. Ryan, J.E.: Prosthetic treatment for electrical burns of the oral cavity. J Prosthet Dent 42:434, 1979.
12. Graubard, S.A., Gold, L., and Henkel, G.: Modified retention splint for an electrical burn in a 1 year old child. Oral Surg 54:385, 1982.
13. Callahan, A.: Surgery of the Eye: Injuries. Springfield, Il., Charles C Thomas, Publisher, 1950.
14. Curtin, J.W.: Basic plastic surgical principles in repair of facial lacerations. IMJ 129:657, 1966.

15. Goldberg, M.H.: Antibiotics and oral cutaneous lacerations. J Oral Surg 23:117, 1965.
16. Zallen, R.D., and Black, S.L.: Antibiotic therapy in oral and maxillofacial surgery. J Oral Surg 34:349, 1976.
17. Osbon, D.B.: Intermediate and reconstructive care of maxillofacial missile wounds. J Oral Surg 31:429, 1973.
18. Joy, E.D.: Early care of maxillofacial missile wounds. J Oral Surg 31:425, 1973.

5

MAXILLOFACIAL FRACTURE FIXATION PROSTHESES, METHODS, AND DEVICES

HUGH P. BRINDLEY

Treatment of traumatic injuries in the maxillofacial area involves restoring normal function, maintaining normal occlusion, and preventing facial deformities. To achieve these objectives, maxillofacial surgeons must reduce, fixate, and retain in position anatomically aligned bone fragments long enough to allow for bony union.

Bony fragments can be immobilized by indirect means, direct means, or a combination thereof. Indirect fixation devices are attached to structures other than bone and usually incorporate intermaxillary fixation to assist in controlling bony fragments. Direct fixation devices are attached directly to bone and frequently require no intermaxillary fixation to provide for bony segment immobilization. Generally, a combination of fixation methods is necessary to provide adequate immobilization.

The wide variety of indirect, direct, and combination technique devices provide the surgeon with many alternative approaches to patient management. Although routine fractures usually require the use of only a few

techniques, the resourceful surgeon is proficient using many techniques. The less frequently used techniques can be valuable alternatives in managing complex problems that defy solution by usual methods.

Fixation methods are a means to an end. The objectives of treatment and the clinical presentation of the patient must always be paramount in choosing methods of treatment to avoid the pitfall of altering the patient to fit the method.

The purpose of this chapter is to review maxillofacial fracture fixation methods, devices, and the prostheses that are currently utilized in definitive treatment.

NONINVASIVE TREATMENT MODALITIES

Sometimes in the treatment of patients with maxillofacial injuries, the best treatment is nontreatment. No functional or cosmetic gain is achieved by using reduction, retention, or fixation on nondisplaced zygomatic arch fractures, zygomaticomaxillary complex (ZMC) fractures, and isolated antral wall fractures. Also, in some edentulous patients who are poor medical risks, minimally displaced or nondisplaced fractures of the maxilla and mandible can be treated by removing the prosthesis and prescribing a liquid diet. In such cases, the removal of functional stress minimizes the movement of fracture segments and allows healing to occur, although at times slowly. Noninvasive treatment can also be used in the treatment of intracapsular fractures of the mandible; a soft or liquid diet involving only passive movement of the mandible is desirable to reduce the chances of ankylosis of the mandible to the glenoid fossa or zygomatic arch; fixation, if used at all, may be only temporary during the first few days of edema to reduce the pain. In these examples, noninvasive treatment methods may be the most desirable means of management.

DIRECT BONDING

Direct bonding of teeth is used with alveolar segment fractures and with subluxed or avulsed teeth.[1] Direct bonding is advantageous because it requires minimal material to fixate the teeth, making for better oral hygiene. The disadvantage is that its lack of strength and the likelihood of the materials fracturing because of poor anchorage from many loosened teeth with no intervening support limits its long-term use. Direct bonding in conjunction with reinforcing wire improves the strength of the fixation device and enhances long-span stability involving many replanted avulsed teeth.

INDIRECT FRACTURE FIXATION TECHNIQUES

The oldest form of fixation methods are the indirect fixation techniques — those that yield immobilization of fractured bony segments by attaching to prostheses, devices, and teeth, rather than to the fractured bone. Indirect fixation involves the use of both intraoral and extraoral techniques.

PHYSICAL PROPERTIES OF WIRE MANAGEMENT

Because many fixation techniques require the use of wire, it is important to consider some of its physical properties. In the early years of maxillofacial surgery, gold, copper, and silver wire were used for fracture fixation.[2,3] More recently soft alloy wire was used, though it now has limited application. Currently, stainless steel wire in widths of 0.016 to 0.020 inches is used predominately. Its ductility and flexibility make it very strong, and it is also relatively corrosion resistant and biocompatibile. Prestretching wire has been proposed to eliminate or reduce the need for retightening. However, the reduced ductility of prestretched wire increases the work hardening with twisting and increases the likelihood of wire breakage.[4] Still another problem with stainless steel wire is the effect of repeated autoclaving. In many operating rooms, stainless steel wire is left on a wooden spool and repeatedly autoclaved with surgical instruments. The combined effects of the surface corrosion and repeated heating makes wire break easily when tightened. Air-cooling stainless steel instead of rapidly cooling it in water also slowly reduces the ductility of the wire with repeated autoclavings.[5] The most desirable method to prepare and store wire is to package limited amounts of precut wire lengths, autoclave them at most twice, and discard unused portions of wire. Another alternative is to autoclave with the instruments only the amount of wire that possibly may be used and discard any unused portions following completion of the procedure. While this may seem wasteful, having to replace broken wiring used in surgical procedures is wasteful and also frustrating.

Because the treatment of fractures may involve different teams of surgeons, it is customary, for consistency in placing and removing wire, to twist the wire in a clockwise direction (Fig. 5–1). When tightening a wire, constant outward pull should be maintained to prevent the wire from twisting upon itself, which creates work hardening and increases the likelihood of breakage. Also, using outward pull facilitates adapting the wires snugly to the teeth. Circumferential dental wires

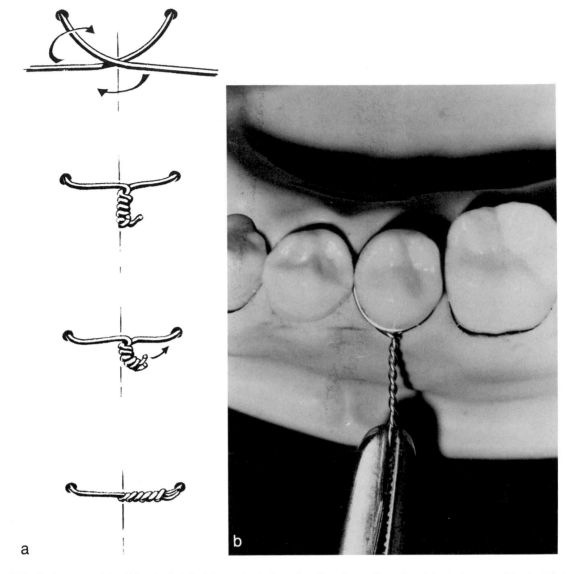

FIG. 5–1. **a** and **b,** Wire is twisted in a clockwise direction for uniformity of technique and to facilitate removal.

should be placed subgingivally whenever possible to avoid plaque accumulation on tooth surfaces.

DENTITION WIRING TECHNIQUES

Intermaxillary fixation is basic for immobilizing and fixating maxillofacial fractures, and numerous sound, time-proven dentition wiring techniques are available for providing methods to permit attachment of fixation (Fig. 5–2). Various wiring techniques are indicated for immobilization of the mandible with fractures within the dental arch; for im-

mobilization of the mandible with nondisplaced vertically and horizontally favorable fractures posterior to the dental arch; for emergency treatment of fractures of the symphysis; for displaced fractures requiring temporary reduction of fragments; for certain types alveolar fractures; in conjunction with circumferential wiring, open reductions, skeletal pins, bone plates, or craniofacial suspension methods of treatment; and for the prevention of fractures prior to mandibular surgery in the event that a large central lesion might contribute to a pathologic fracture.

The deciding factor in the choice of intra-

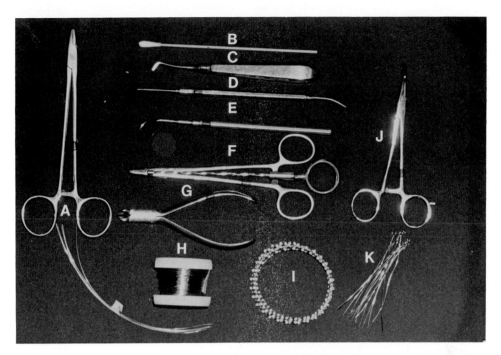

FIG. 5–2.   The equipment for wiring procedures includes small nose wire twister (A); cotton applicator or lead solder (not shown) for continuous loop wiring (B); band pusher for adapting wire to tooth surfaces and splints (C); gauze packer to hold wires below the gingival margins (D); dental mirror for visualization and retraction (E); modified wire twister for rapid uniform twisting of wire (F); wire ligature scissors (G); roll of stainless steel wire in appropriate sizes (H); roll or segmental sections of stainless steel arch-bar material (I); hemostats for placement of elastic bands (J); preformed eyelet loop wires (K).

dental wiring techniques is generally the presence or absence of teeth. When the number, size, or distribution of teeth precludes the use of wire, other techniques must be considered. Intradental wires usually are not relied on as the sole means of immobilization in complex mandibular or multiple facial fracture.

DIRECT INTERMAXILLARY TECHNIQUE (GILMER)

One of the oldest techniques, and a revolution when first developed, the direct intermaxillary technique depends on having a minimum of four teeth in each segment.[6] A stainless steel wire of 0.018 inches is cut into segments approximately 16 to 18 cm long. Both ends of the wires are then passed from the lingual surface through the interproximal spaces on each side of the tooth to be utilized for fixation. The wire on the lingual surface of the tooth is held down with a blunt instrument at the cervical portion of the tooth, while the two free ends are grasped with large curved hemostatic forceps, large needle hold-

ers, or wire twisting forceps, and the wire is twisted around the tooth. A sufficient number of opposing teeth in each arch are wired. The mandible is immobilized and fixed to the maxilla by twisting the individual wires to those of the opposing arch (Fig. 5–3). For each unit it is advisable to select two approximating maxillary and two approximating mandibular teeth that also occlude. A more stable fixation may be obtained by crisscrossing the upper and lower wires.

The disadvantage of the Gilmer method is that in order for the mouth to open after wiring, the wires have to be cut and then replaced. Also, one or more wires may break before they are tightened sufficiently, in which case the mouth has to be opened and the treatment repeated. However, this technique is fast, simple, and effective in treating simple fractures occurring in jaws having an adequate number of teeth.

Eyelet Technique (Oliver, Eby, Ivy)

This eyelet loop wiring technique has the advantages of versatility and ease of appli-

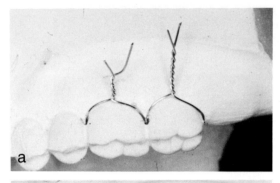

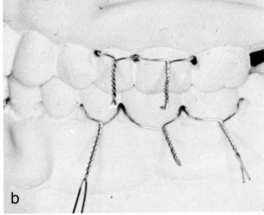

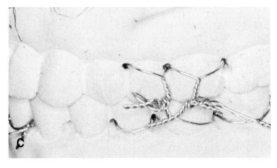

FIG. 5–3.   Gilmer direct wiring. **a** and **b,** Individual teeth are ligated and wires twisted. **c,** Opposing twists are united for intermaxillary fixation.

cation (Fig. 5–4). It was first described by Joseph D. Eby in 1921 following information from Robert T. Oliver, and it was popularized by Robert H. Ivy, then a Lt. Colonel in the U.S. Army[7,8] In this method, 27-mm length of wire is twisted around an instrument to establish a small loop. Both ends of the wire are then passed through the interproximal space from the buccal side. One end of the wire is then passed from the lingual side to the buccal side around the anterior tooth, and the other end is passed around the posterior

tooth. An end of the wire is then passed either through, or medial to, the eyelet, and the two ends are twisted to form a button. This procedure produces a loop and a button to be used for supporting intermaxillary fixation wires, elastic loops, or ligatures. The eyelet should project from the maxillary dental arch above the horizontal plane and in the mandibular dental arch below the horizontal plane to prevent the ends from impinging on each other. After a sufficient number of eyelets are established, the teeth are brought into occlusion and ligatures or elastic bands are passed between the upper and lower eyelets and loops. If the free end of the wire passes medially to the loop of the eyelet, the wire around the teeth will become increasingly tight.

The eyelet technique is indicated for immobilization procedures when maximum oral hygiene is desirable; in simple fractures of the mandibular ramus or condyle in which fracture lines are vertically and horizontally favorable; in greenstick fractures of children; and in partially edentulous mouths.

The disadvantage of this technique is its limited use in grossly displaced fractures of the tooth-bearing areas because of a lack of arch rigidity. Also, the limited number of points of fixation available increases the load of fixation to a few teeth. If an eyelet wire breaks, replacement may be necessary and may require removal of all intermaxillary stabilization and fixation.

Continuous Loop Wiring Technique (Stout)

A series of eyelets on a single strand of wire is produced as follows. A piece of lead solder or the wooden handle of a cotton applicator wooden stick swab is placed against the teeth to aid in the forming of wire loops.[9] A wire is then placed around the last molar with both ends projecting to the buccal side, the posterior end as a horizontal buccal wire and the anterior end as an active passing wire to form loops. The posterior end is placed horizontally along the buccal surfaces of the teeth, and the longer anterior end is inserted over the buccal wire and the lead or wooden former to pass through the same interproximal space from which it emerged. The wire is

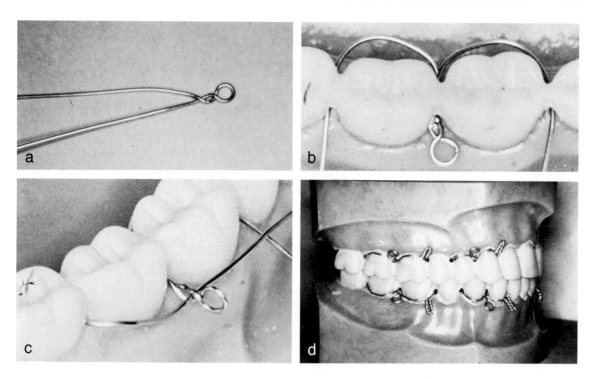

FIG. 5–4. Eyelet loop wires. **a,** Eyelets are formed around a cotton applicator wooden stick. **b,** The eyelet wire ends are inserted from the buccal to the lingual side and then laterally through adjacent embrasures. **c,** The posterior wire is passed medially to the twist that formed the eyelet. **d,** The wire ends and eyelet loop are tightened.

drawn taut around the former, finishing the first loop. The active wire then goes around the lingual surface to the next embrasure emerging below the former. The wire is then passed over the former and back again through the same interproximal space. In this fashion a complete quadrant can be fitted with wire loops. The lead or wooden former is removed when the section is completed. Each loop is twisted two or three times to form a small anchor leg and then turned upward on the upper arch and downward on the lower arch. The final tie of the quadrant, usually mesial to the cuspid, is made by uniting the buccal wire with the free end of the last loop. As each loop is tightened, including the final tie, a blunt instrument is used to make snug the lingual turns of the wire below the height of contour of the teeth (Fig. 5–5).

Continuous loop wiring provides a large number of loops for attachments and can be used as an alternative to arch bars and splints in certain situations. The Stout multiple loop wires can function as a splint on partially

avulsed teeth and can be adapted to individual arches. Moderately displaced mandibular fractures can be reduced with elastic traction properly placed between the multiple loops.

The disadvantages of Stout's loop wiring include the extensive manipulative technique, the restrictions imposed by unusual or abnormal dental anatomy (mixed dentition, peg-shaped teeth, or extensive dental or periodontal disease), and the need to replace the entire section if a wire breaks.

A modification in placement of continuous loop wiring has been described by Rowe and Killey, who gave credit for the technique to Professor Hugo Obwegeser of Switzerland. The fracture wire is contoured outside of the mouth to produce loops conforming to the lingual anatomy of the dental arch to be wired, and the posterior end of the wire is bent forward to lie parallel to the buccal surfaces of the teeth. The lingual loops are attached to lengths of heavy floss. The loops are turned to produce vertical alignments. The short end of the contoured wire is in-

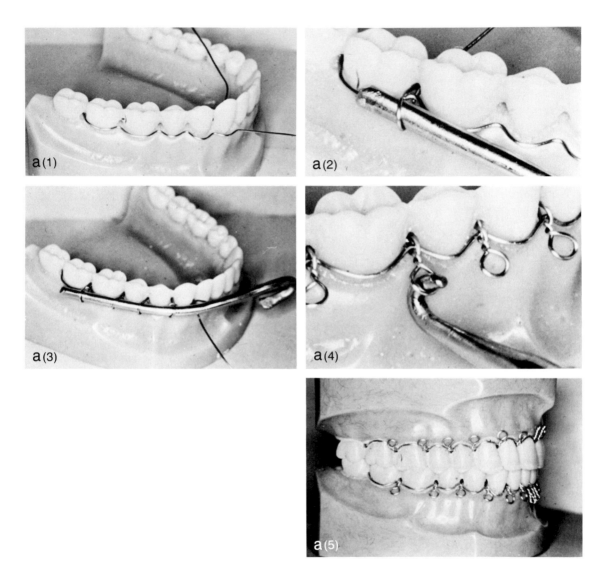

FIG. 5–5. Continuous loop wiring techniques and placement of elastic traction in edentulous areas. Continuous loop wiring is illustrated as it is used in the classic Stout technique. Variations include using a cotton applicator wooden stick instead of the less commonly used lead roll; forming loops during the passage of the wire without using either wooden sticks or solder; and using a wire with preformed loops that are drawn through the embrasures with a ligature or floss attached to each loop. **a. 1,** The horizontal strand is held anteriorly; the working end is passed between the most posterior teeth in the arch and emerges apically to the horizontal wire. **2,** The working end is then passed around the solder and back through the embrasure. **3,** The procedure continues, ending on a sound, strong tooth. **4** and **5,** The eyelets are formed from the loops and may be tilted apically to receive elastic traction or occlusally to receive intermaxillary wire or suture fixation.

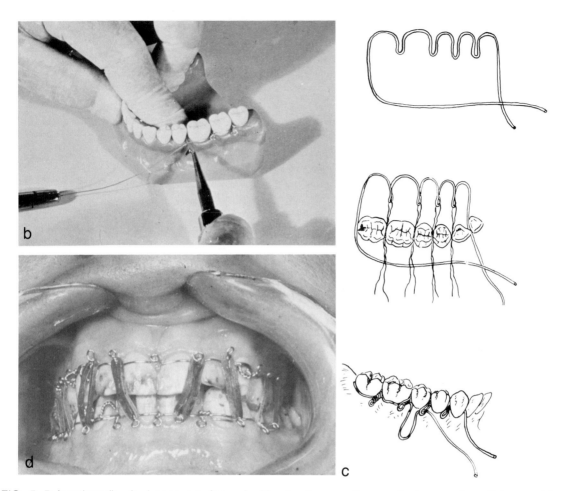

FIG. 5–5 (continued). **b,** Loops are formed without using a cotton applicator wooden stick or solder. (Courtesy of Dr. Leon D. Fiedler.) **c,** Precontoured wire loops may be passed between the teeth. **d,** Continuous loop wiring with elastic traction.

serted through the interproximal space anterior to the most anterior tooth to be wired, and the long end is inserted between the two most posterior teeth; simultaneous traction with the floss ligatures placed through the intervening interproximal spaces seats the wire loops.

The loops are separated and the long end of the wire inserted through the loops and joined to the short anterior wire to form the end twist.

Stout's wiring applied to patients with edentulous spaces requires the formation of a wire bridge across edentulous space (Fig. 5–5e). Elastic bands may be applied to the space, or a technique employing dental floss may be used leaving the elastic around the bridging wire and locking the elastic on itself.

Single- and Double-Wire Splinting Technique (Essig)

A fracture wire is placed from the labial surface through the embrasures of sound teeth three or four teeth away from the fracture site and placed against the inner surface of the teeth across the fracture.[10] The wire is then passed through one embrasure closer to the fracture than the desired splint length and is adapted to the labial surface across the fracture. The ends of the wire are loosely twisted on the labial surface, forming the labiolingual loop. Another wire is passed on the opposite side of the fracture from the labial through the posterior adjacent embrasure to the previously passed labiolingual loop. It is adapted to the inner surface of the teeth across the

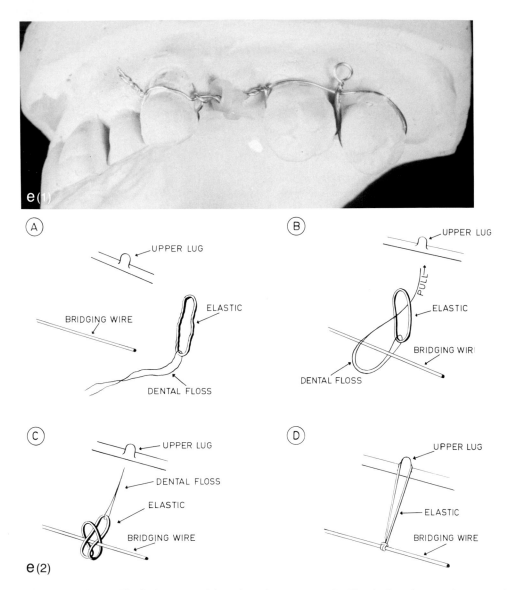

FIG. 5–5 (continued). **e,** Technique used in edentulous areas. **1,** Elastic bands may be placed on a horizontal bridge of twisted wire. **2,** Technique to place elastics on a horizontal bridge of twisted wire or an arch bar.

fracture and passed through the adjacent embrasure toward the fracture from the twisted wire embrasure. The wire is then adapted to the labial surface of the teeth across the fracture and the ends of the wire are loosely tightened. Secondary wires are then placed above and below the double labiolingual wires below the contact and twisted on the labial surface. The secondary wires are tightened in series separately until the inner wire is firmly adapted to the inner tooth surface. The main arch wires on either side of the fracture are

then tightened and the wire ends cut and twisted into the interproximal space along with the secondary wires (Fig. 5–6).

Another modification of this technique is to apply a single inner-outer wire to the two or three teeth on either side of the fracture or loosened teeth. This wire is closely adapted to the lingual and labial surfaces with finger pressure. The wire is then loosely twisted on the distal labial aspect of the splint, with care being taken not to pull the inner wire away from the lingual or palatal surfaces of the

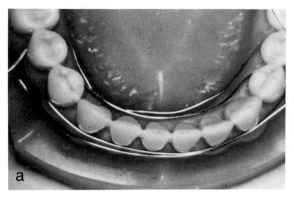
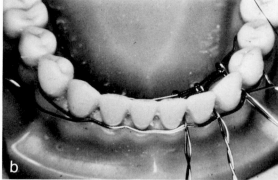
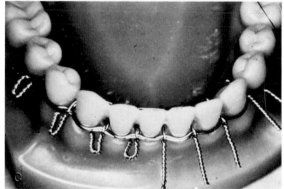

FIG. 5–6. Double-and single-wire Essig technique. **a, b,** and **c,** Placement of Essig's double wires to provide lugs.

teeth. Secondary interproximal wires are then passed above and below the interproximal contacts to engage the inner and outer wires when they are twisted on the labial side. This process should begin at the embrasure furthest from the twisted end of the inner-outer wire and continue toward the twisted end of the wire while tension is being applied to the inner-outer wire. If the inner-outer wire is tightened too much initially, the inner wire will not adapt to the inner surface of the teeth at this point, requiring loosening of the primary wire. Secondary wires are tightened in this fashion until secure and then cut and tucked on the labial side beneath the contact point. The inner-outer wire is then tightened, cut, and tucked on the labial aspect.

The Essig technique, which was originally devised to reduce and fix fractures of the mandible without immobilizing the jaws, is a very efficient method of wiring. The framework is usually ligated to the six anterior teeth and is particularly advantageous when teeth are avulsed in conjunction with minimally displaced symphysis fractures. Depending on the shape of the teeth, Essig wires can be difficult to apply, and teeth must have firm

interproximal contact if this method is to be used effectively. Orthodontic movement of teeth can be avoided by using secondary wires above and below the contact if occlusion permits. Still another way to avoid movement of teeth, and also to improve hygiene and the strength of the double-wire splint, is to apply self-curing acrylic to the splint.

Twisted Labial Wire Technique (Risdon)

Wires are placed around the posterior teeth on each side of the dental arch. The wires are twisted with the twist touching the mesio-buccal aspects of the teeth.[11] The two ends of the wire are twisted together to form a common arch bar. Each tooth is then separately wired to the buccal twisted wire and the cut ends looped and used as fixation lugs (Fig. 5–7). In a closed-bite case, the Risdon method of horizontal wiring can be used in lieu of an arch bar. This method can also be used to temporarily immobilize symphysis fractures and to stabilize oblique fractures within the arch. Strong traction may be exerted to disimpact fractures because Risdon wires can be

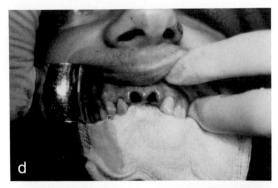

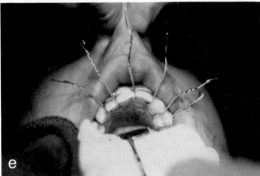

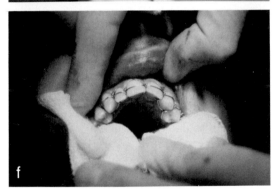

FIG. 5–6 (continued). **d, e,** and **f,** Placement of single wire variation to replant avulsed teeth.

used on isolated teeth and on a number of teeth not in contact with each other.

A variation of this technique can be used for intermaxillary wire fixation. Prior to forming a common arch wire, a 13-gauge needle is cut into 2-mm segments, and three to four of these metal tubes are threaded onto the wire before being twisted in the midline. After the common arch wire is ligated to the individual teeth, individual intermaxillary wire can be threaded through the attached metal tubes to rigidly fix the jaw into occlusion. The disadvantage of Risdon wiring is the need for teeth in adjacent fragments, the need for additional loops for adequate intermaxillary fixation, and because of lack of rigidity, the inability to immobilize fragments if the fracture is comminuted.

Wire Button Technique (Kazanjian)

The wire button technique is suitable for immobilization by elastic traction or wire fixation.[12] It can be used for temporary or permanent fixation in simple fractures without displacement. A wire is placed around each of two adjacent teeth and the ends of the wires twisted together. The twists are then twisted together. Approximately, 1 inch of wire is left after cutting the ends, and this is twisted into a button. Four such buttons can be made in each arch, and the jaws immobilized by elastics or wires fixed to each pair of opposing buttons (Fig. 5–8).

A modification of this technique can be used when only isolated single teeth in a segment or arch are available for fixation purposes. A 15-cm segment of wire is looped to form a clove hitch in the center. Both free ends of the wire are grasped with wire twisters and a noose is placed over the crown of the tooth. By applying traction to both ends of the wire noose, the surgeon places the wires beneath the gingiva, using a gauze packer or other appropriate instrument. The wire is then twisted on the labial aspect, leaving approximately 1 inch of twisted wire after cutting. This is coiled in a clockwise direction as it is forced against the tooth, leaving a gnarl or a rosette of wire to which fixation elastics or wires can be attached.

ARCH BARS

Arch bars are intraoral labial appliances with various types of attachment devices that are adapted and secured to a patient's dentition for the purpose of stabilizing and/or providing fixation for fractures of the facial area. These appliances vary according to the types of materials from which they are made, their rigidity or malleability, and whether they are prefabricated or custom-made.

Commercial prefabricated arch bars vary in the design of attachment lugs and the rigidity of the horizontal bar. Named after the original

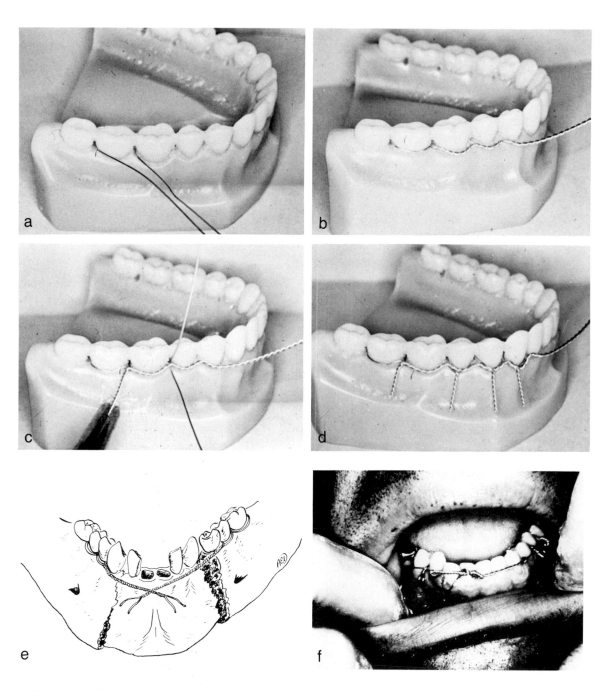

FIG. 5–7.   Risdon wiring technique. **a, b, c,** and **d,** Steps in providing lugs using Risdon wiring technique. **e** and **f,** Placement of Risdon wiring to stabilize bilateral parasymphyseal fractures.

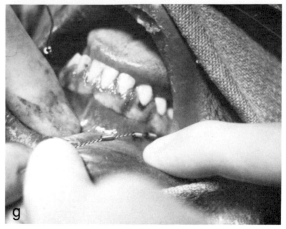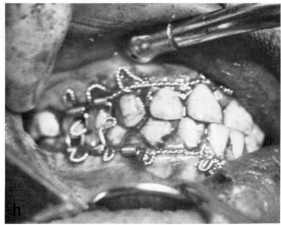

FIG. 5–7 (continued).   **g** and **h,** Placing metallic tubes on Risdon wiring. The tubes will support intermaxillary wires.

designers, the Winter, Jelenko, and Erich bars have differently designed lugs for attachments. The Winter arch bar is not as hygienic as either the Jelenko or Erich bars because of its longer vertical attachments, which tend to trap food; also, the high position of the lugs allows for more torque to be applied to the fractures by a higher fulcrum advantage of intermaxillary fixation elastics or wires (Fig. 5–9). The Jelenko bar is much heavier than other prefabricated arch bars and should be preadapted to a cast and, if necessary, corrected to the normal anatomy before being applied to the arch. This adjustment minimizes orthodontic displacement of teeth, while the additional rigidity of the bar gives greater stability to a fracture. Erich arch bars are malleable and easily manipulated and can be contoured to the dentition intraorally during application, although preadapting is desirable if casts are available.

The material from which the commercial arch bars are made varies. Winter splints are made of aluminum alloy, which resists corrosion relatively well but deforms easily. The heavy Jelenko bar is made of an alloy that corrodes and tarnishes easily. Erich arch bars in strips or rolls are made of stainless steel and have excellent corrosion resistance. Erich arch bars are the most commonly used form of arch bar splint today because of their ease of adaptability, corrosion resistance, and economy. The custom-made cast arch bar splints are used in fixation appliances and are

extremely useful when long-term use is anticipated. They can be designed to minimize gingival irritation and impingement. They also allow the least movement of teeth and can be very useful in preventing pathologic fracture during the removal of central mandibular lesions, as well as in providing postoperative support.

Though widely used, arch bars do have disadvantages that can lead to problems if cautions are not observed. Prefabricated arch bars, if not well adapted, cause movement of teeth. They cannot be used in some severe closed-bite cases, and they may cause impaction, malalignment, or distraction of bony fragments if reduction is not accurate prior to fixation. Oral hygiene may be difficult to maintain and lugs may impinge painfully on the gingival papillae. Arch bars used in the treatment of fractures should therefore be individually tailored appliances that are contoured for specific fractures. When an open reduction is done, the arch bar may need to be cut across at the fracture area to allow adequate alignment apposition. The bar can be rejoined with self-curing acrylic or a stainless steel wire (Fig. 5–10).

Use of arch bars is indicated for immobilization of simple and comminuted fractures within the dental arch; for immobilization of fractures occurring posterior to the dentition, the vertical rami, and the condylar neck or condyle of the mandible; for nondisplaced fractures of the maxilla; for alveolar fractures;

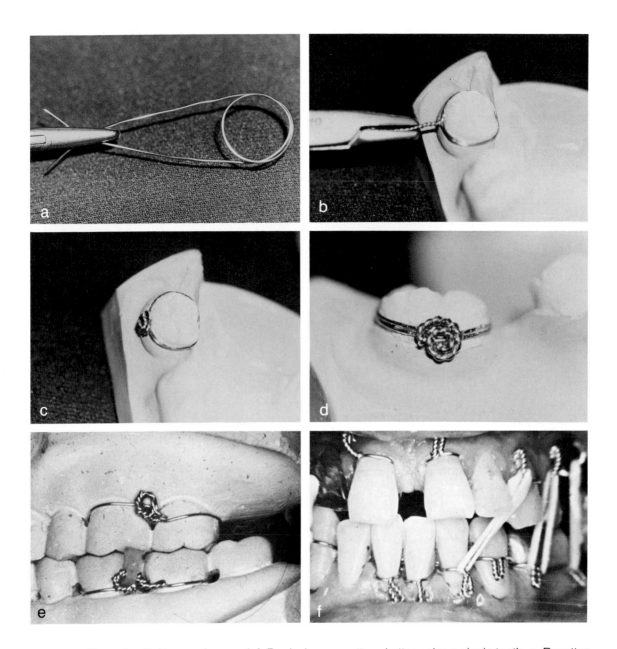

FIG. 5–8.   Kazanjian Buttons. **a, b, c,** and **d,** Producing a rosette or button using a single tooth. e, Rosettes or buttons formed on adjacent teeth in the maxilla. **f,** Application of elastic traction to loops of wire, instead of rosettes. The elastic traction will draw and guide the fracture segments to a desired position; intermaxillary stabilzation using wires combined with open reduction using either plates or compression wiring is then performed.

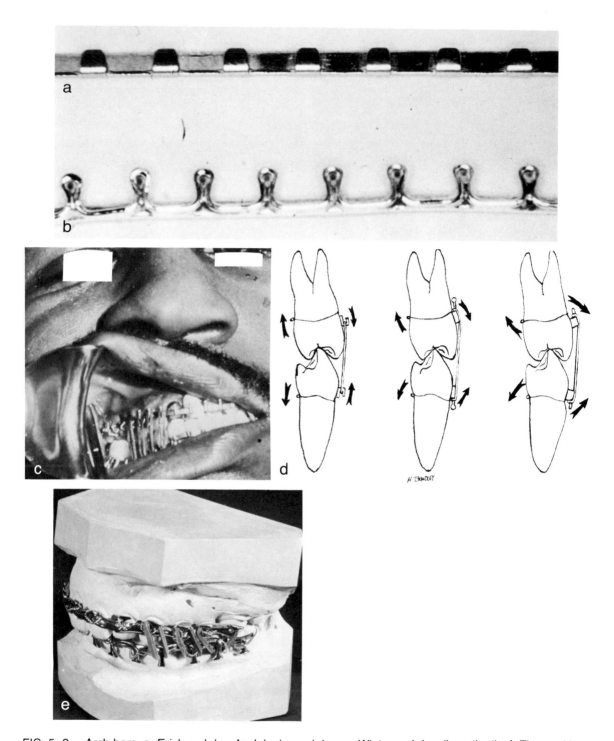

FIG. 5–9.   Arch bars. **a,** Erich arch bar. **b,** Jelenko arch bar. **c,** Winter arch bar (in patient). **d,** The position in which the lugs on the Winter and Jelenko arch bars are placed may cause more torque to be applied to the teeth than is applied with Erich-type arch bar. These forces become more apparent the more anterior the fracture, the more comminution present, and the heavier the elastic traction used. **e,** Cast metallic arch bar with T lugs.

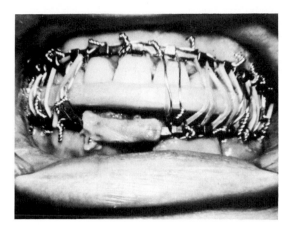

FIG. 5–10. Arch bar rejoined with wiring and self-curing acrylic after an intraoral open reduction of a mandibular fracture.

for splinting avulsed teeth; and in conjunction with other types of fixation devices.

Arch bars cannot be relied on as a sole means of immobilization in grossly displaced fractures. Obviously, they cannot be used in edentulous patients or in patients with extensive fixed prostheses. Because of their ability to trap food debris at the gingival margin of dentition, arch bars are not indicated in the presence of oral infection or in fractures associated with hypertrophied gingival tissue. Arch bars should not be used in closed-bite cases if the overbite impingement of the upper teeth on the lower bar prevents repair of the fracture in centric relation (Fig. 5–11). Arch bars have limited use in a mixed dentition as they are difficult to retain against the teeth.

To ligate the arch bar to the teeth, the sur-

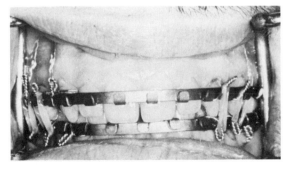

FIG. 5–11. Arch bar impingement on teeth. Impingement of a fracture arch bar on teeth may prevent the establishment of normal occlusal relations and an accurate reduction of a fracture.

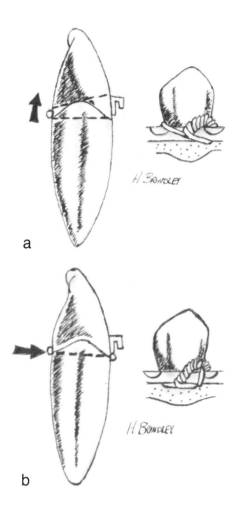

FIG. 5–12. As described in the text, teeth with a small cingulum may require a modified ligature to ensure secure retention of an arch bar. **a,** Usual method of ligating an arch bar to a tooth. **b,** Modification of ligating an arch bar to a tooth with a small cingulum.

geon inserts a wire from the medial side of the dental arch around the cervical margins of the teeth to the buccal side and twists the free ends over and under the bars (Fig. 5–12). With teeth with small cingulums this method will occasionally allow the bar to ride occlusally under the stress of intermaxillary traction or fixation. To direct the force of the bar apically and resist the pull of intermaxillary forces and to ligate teeth with small cingulums, both ends of the wire are placed on the gingival side of the bar and the anterior end is twisted around the bar in the form of a clovehitch. When the wire is tightened, it adapts the bar to the gingival margin of the tooth. It is important to correctly place interdental wire above and below the bar to facilitate adaptation to the teeth and minimize movement of the teeth.

At the terminal tooth on each end of the bar, the posterior end wire should be placed on the gingival side of the bar and the anterior wire should be placed on the occlusal side of the bar (Fig. 5–13). This placement allows the clockwise torque created by twisting the wire to seat the wire beneath the bar. This maneuver also allows the arch bar to be positioned in a more apical direction, which is important in the molar region because of the short vertical height of the crowns. It is also important to place the wire end nearest an edentulous space on the occlusal side of the bar to avoid tilting the teeth toward the edentulous space. The larger the caliber of wire used to apply arch bars, the more influence the torquing effect has in moving teeth.

An arch bar can be used as an anchor for weight traction on severely impacted fractures of the maxilla. A wire is fastened to a previously secured maxillary arch bar, tied to a rope, and placed over pullies on a Balkan frame. By adding 1 to 3 lbs of lead shot, the surgeon may disimpact the maxilla prior to immobilization fixation (Fig. 5–14).

It is apparent that an arch bar used in the treatment of fractures can provide a large number of loops for elastic traction, and the rigidity of the appliance can allow equal distribution of stress throughout the arch. The common errors of arch bar application are improper adaptation of the bar, incorrect ligation of teeth, ligation of an insufficient number of teeth, and inefficient tightening of the wires. Regardless of these limitations, however, prefabricated or custom-made bars are easy to apply and are an effective basic procedure in the treatment of maxillofacial fractures.

ORTHODONTIC APPLIANCES

Application to teeth of orthodontic bands may be difficult in a fracture patient because of the inability to open the mouth widely, the presence of pain and bleeding, and the difficulties controlling secretions. Orthodontic appliances, especially bonded brackets, do have application for stabilizing segmental alveolar process fractures and subluxed or avulsed teeth when there is ample access and control of the patient. The applications of

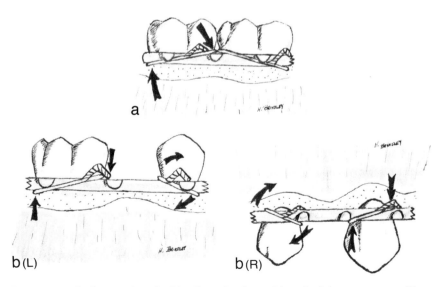

FIG. 5–13. Placement of wires on terminal teeth and adjacent to edentulous areas. **a,** Placement of arch bar ligature wire on a terminal tooth in the mandibular arch. **b L** and **R,** Placement of arch bar ligature wires on teeth adjacent to edentulous spaces.

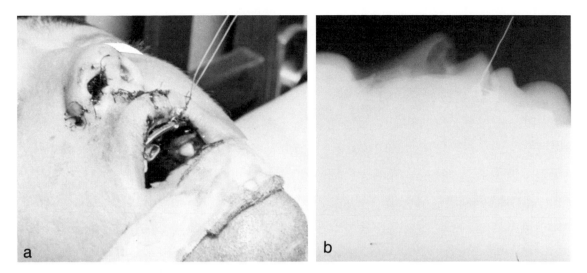

FIG. 5–14. Disimpaction of a midfacial fracture. **a,** Bedside, and **b,** Radiographic views of disimpaction of a midfacial fracture, with weights transmitting forward forces to the maxillary arch bar.

bands, orthodontic arch wires, and bonded brackets require instrumentation not usually available in emergency rooms. In cases in which intermaxillary fixation wiring is required, one may find that bonded brackets will shear away and not be as reliable as arch bars and fracture wiring techniques. The limited use of orthodontic appliances is due principally to the time required to place them in emergency room settings.

INTERMAXILLARY FIXATION (IMF)

From the earliest written accounts, methods of stabilizing maxillofacial fractures have involved immobilization by fixating the mandible to the maxilla. This method used head bandages until the advent of the Bean and Gunning splints during the American Civil War and the continuing contributions of Oliver, Eby, Ivy, and Stout to intermaxillary wiring during the first decade of the twentieth century.[3,4,8,13,14,15] Intermaxillary fixation, which includes the use of supporting arch bars, wire loops, and splints, is the most reliable and the most versatile management principle for maxillofacial fracture control.

Because aspiration remains a possibility, safety is always the primary concern with IMF. Patients and family members should be counseled regarding the location of fixation wires and elastics and the way to remove

them in case of emergency. The family and patient should be instructed to remain calm if vomiting occurs, as it usually can be managed by forcing liquid out through the nose and/or mouth. The use of antiemetic agents such as promethazine or trimethobenzamide suppositories may be beneficial in extreme cases in which patients remain nauseated for prolonged periods of time, such as may occur with viral or influenza infections. The patient should carry appropriate instruments at all times to allow removal of IMF. If the IMF uses wire fixation, small wire cutters should be used; if the IMF uses elastics, scissors should be used. Rip-cord devices can be utilized with elastic IMF when a single wire loop is passed loosely around or through the elastics on a side of the mouth and a twisted end lightly placed anteriorly. The patient is instructed to pull the rip-cord on each side to remove fixation (Fig. 5–15).

Elastic Intermaxillary Traction and Fixation

Elastics have many uses in fracture management (Fig. 5–16). In the initial phases of fracture repair, heavy elastic traction can be used to reduce impacted midfacial or maxillary fractures, thus simplifying definitive repair procedures; using traction is especially beneficial when significant delay in definitive reduction and fixation procedures is neces-

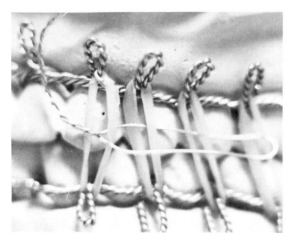

FIG. 5–15. Rip-cord device. An application of a wire to facilitate rapid removal of intermaxillary fixation elastics.

sary. Elastics can also be used to apply segmental traction to reduce a separation of a fracture line. Elastics are used most commonly to correct discrepancies in occlusal relations.

Elastic traction is also useful in rehabilitation and physical therapy and is especially beneficial in training muscles to compensate for the absence of a normal temporomandibular joint in displaced and dislocated subcondylar fractures of the mandible. Elastics are placed obliquely in single-looped cross-arch fashion to form a parallelogram when viewed from the front. In this way, opening the mouth against the pull of the elastics will keep the mandible in the midline and direct teeth into proper occlusion when the mouth is closed. The number of elastics used and the degree of oblique pull is determined for each case and gradually reduced as the patient's musculature adapts. Using this approach, patients can be trained to open relatively normally and occlude without prematurities or malocclusion.

The diameter of the elastic loops used most commonly is 3/16 inches. The amount of traction obtained varies with the width or strength of the elastics used. 5½-oz or medium wall-thickness elastics are the most commonly used for routine fixation purposes. Elastics may be improvised by cutting narrow sections from rubber tubing. Repeated autoclaving, ozone exposure, and excessive age

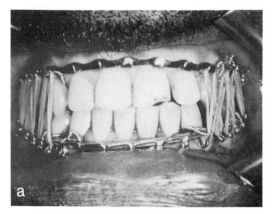

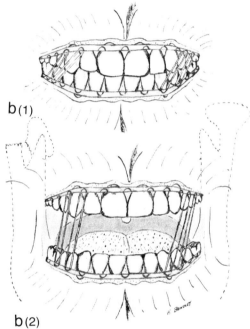

FIG. 5–16. Disimpaction and alignment of fractured segments. **a,** Double-looped elastics are applied to disimpact and align a minor fracture for simplified reduction procedures. Elastics will also reduce minor discrepancies in occlusal relations resulting from fracture alignments. **b** (**1** and **2**), Single-looped cross-arch elastics are placed in a parallelogram fashion to provide counter traction with opening movements to compensate for a dislocated subcondylar fracture.

causes elastics to break easily. The intraoral environment results in elastics' losing their strength in several days, necessitating periodic replacement if consistent traction is desired.

Application of elastics to fracture appliances varies with each situation. In general, where tight fixation is desired, elastics should be double stretched by looping one end of the elastic over an attachment and stretching both strands around an attachment in the opposing arch, and hooking the loop of the elastic over an attachment in the original arch. The pattern created may be vertical, cruciate, or V-shaped, depending on individual preference, the directional need for traction movement, and availability of attachments. Elastics can also be attached to orthodontic arch wires without vertical fixation attachments by looping elastics with the aid of a suture over the wire and attaching the elastic through the opposite arch with either a wire suture or hooking over existing attachments (Fig. 5–5e).

Oral hygiene with elastic IMF is more of a problem than with wire IMF. Elastics should not be crisscrossed if they are to be used for long-term fixation to avoid food trapping and ineffective brushing of the outer tooth surfaces. Brushing a large amount of elastics placed in all directions will frequently dislodge or break them. Patients should be cautioned to brush with vertical strokes to avoid displacement and breakage and also to be cautious of dislodged bands, which may then be swallowed or inhaled. Where brushing is difficult or impossible, pulsating water syringe devices are helpful to remove food debris from between teeth and appliances; however, these devices should be used only after all intraoral incisions are repaired to avoid dissection by the streams of pressurized solutions. Topical acidulated fluorophosphate rinses are beneficial for preventing decalcification around appliances and on the occlusal surfaces of teeth.

Wire Intermaxillary Fixation

Wire IMF can be applied or substituted for initially placed elastic IMF. Because plaque does not adhere to wires as readily as to elastics, wire IMF is more hygienic and permits vigorous brushing with less possibility of dislodging. After the fracture and occlusal discrepancies have been reduced by elastic IMF, continuous pull on the arch appliances may be uncomfortable and is not necessary. Substitution of wires for elastics allows retention

of fixation without continuous traction on appliances and supporting teeth.

Wire fixation does have disadvantages compared to elastic IMF. If orthodontic appliances with bonded brackets instead of bands are used, the shearing force applied by wire IMF may dislodge brackets. Wire fixation will loosen after the initial application because of elongation of the wire and will have to be retightened from time to time, usually weekly, to prevent movement of the mandible. With involuntary movements of the mandible such as coughing, sneezing, or yawning, wire IMF is more likely than elastic IMF to dislodge fracture appliances.

Application of wire IMF to arch appliances usually uses at least three or four maxillary and mandibular attachments. The horizontal portion of the loop wire should be placed against the arch appliance to avoid pressure against the attached gingiva. Usually not more than two or three rectangular, square, or triangular loops of wire per side are required to provide adequate IMF.

Additional IMF Devices

Wessberg and Epker developed the use of screw pins attached intraorally at the malar buttress and external oblique ridge of the mandible to provide for IMF and vertical support for downgraft procedures of the maxilla.[16] These screw pins can also be applied for fixation in Le Fort I and II midfacial fractures. The pins have threaded points on each end that can be screwed into their respective support bone, and the height can be adjusted (Fig. 5–17).

Suspension wires and devices occasionally can be used for IMF without other devices. In children with subcondylar fractures in whom brief fixation is desired, a single anterior nasal spine wire and midline anterior circummandibular wire can be attached by intermediate wires for quick intermaxillary fixation.

DalPoint described the use for IMF of two S-shaped hooks placed bilaterally in the nasal pyriform aperture superiorly and inferiorly around the inferior border of the mandible; the hooks were joined by intermediate wires[17] (Fig. 5–18). The appliance requires open sur-

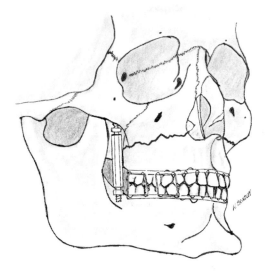

FIG. 5–17. Vertical bipolar screw pins provide intermaxillary fixation as well as vertical support for Le Fort I or II fractures. (From Wessberg, G.A., and Epker, B.N.: Intraoral skeletal fixation appliance.) Oral Maxillofac Surg 40:827, 1982.)

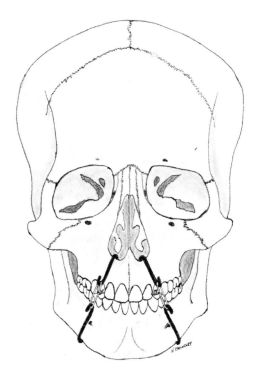

FIG. 5–18. Bilaterally placed S hooks provide intermaxillary fixation. (From DalPont, G.: A new method of intermaxillary bone fixation. In Oral Surgery. Edited by E. Husted and E. Hjørting-Hansen, Trans. 2nd Congress of the International Association of Oral Surgeons. Copenhagen, Munksgaard, 1900 p.3250.)

gical procedures for both placement and removal.

Regardless of the method or apparatus used for IMF, educating the patient is advised to ensure better acceptance. An information booklet describing wire fixation, precautions, hygiene, and diet can be effective in minimizing problems associated with IMF.

INTRAORAL SPLINTS

Intraoral splints and prosthetic devices answer the challenge of specific requirements in the treatment of maxillofacial fractures. A maxillofacial treatment prosthesis can be a custom-made appliance fabricated on casts of the patient's dentition, or a device modified from the patient's partial or complete denture. Fracture splints may be made of either cast metal or acrylic resin. The purpose of intraoral splints in the treatment of maxillofacial fractures is to maintain and reduce fragments, immobilize the segment, and afford a means of fixation during rehabilitation.

A prerequisite for the use of splints in the treatment of mandibular or maxillary fractures is the ability to obtain a satisfactory impression. For this reason, closure of facial lacerations involving the commissures of the lips prior to intraoral examination may be contraindicated. Facial lacerations may be closed primarily within 12 to 24 hours in selected cases if the general condition of the patient is stabilized. The surgeon responsible for the definitive reduction of the maxillofacial skeletal fractures will usually operate transorally or through open lacerations (Fig. 5–19). If arch bar or fracture wire placement or impressions can be taken prior to closure of facial fractures, the laboratory phases of splint construction can be done during the initial healing. Frequently, however, repaired lip lacerations are inadvertently reopened while the surgeon is operating directly on the fracture site, taking impressions, placing a fracture fixation prosthesis or device, or applying arch bars through a recently repaired oral orifice.

Intraoral fracture splints can be used in lieu of arch bars or intradental wiring in the treatment of any fracture requiring immobilization of the mandible. Their use is usually restricted, however, to certain situations that

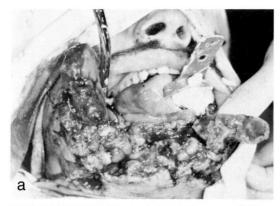

FIG. 5–19. Impressions of bony segments prior to soft-tissue closure. **a,** Impressions for splints are made prior to soft-tissue closure of a facial fracture. **b,** Casts of a patient with a left mandibular fracture articulated against a cast of the intact maxilla. **c,** The mandibular sectional casts are secured with plaster and prepared for processing a splint.

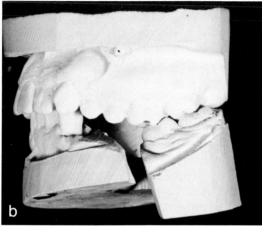

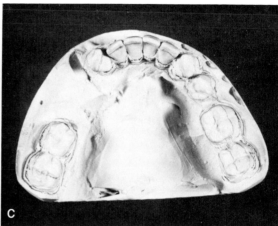

cannot be adequately managed by simpler techniques, such as in edentulous patients; when prolonged immobilization is required; when stabilization of fragments is required but intermaxillary fixation is not necessary; in management of fractures in children presenting a mixed dentition; in periodontally involved dentition that requires equal distribution of stress and maximum tolerance of tissue and teeth; when repositioning and reducing widely distracted fracture fragments; and when treating comminuted alveolar fractures in which bone fragments must be stabilized to an intact arch.

Intraoral splints are adjuncts to the treatment of complex fractures and are often used to aid other methods of immobilization. Acrylic resin splints are easily fabricated, do not interfere with occlusion, and require less time for construction than metallic splints. The disadvantage of acrylic splints must be considered, however, when choosing an intraoral prosthesis for a selected patient. These splints are more bulky and may not give as

rigid fixation to distracted bone segments as metallic splints.

There are few contraindications for the use of intraoral splints in the treatment of jaw fractures. Intraoral splints should not be used if simple wiring or arch bar techniques will suffice, if time is a prime consideration, or if their bulk would interfere with occlusion or re-establishment of centric relation.

Gunning Splints

Dr. Thomas D. Gunning, a dentist from New York, and Dr. James B. Bean, a dentist in the Confederate States of America, developed the use of intraoral splints during and after the Civil War.[14,15] One of the several types of the original Gunning and Bean splints was a one-piece upper and lower bite block inserted into the mouth and fixed with a head bandage. In later years, the gutta-percha and the vulcanite materials in splints were replaced by acrylic, and the splints, rather than being solid blocks, became two-piece up-

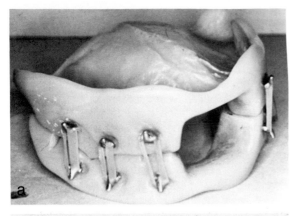

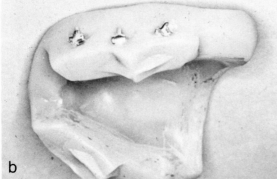

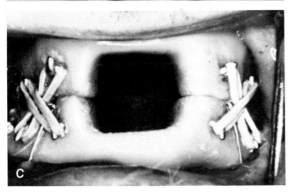

FIG. 5–20. **a, b,** and **c,** Gunning's splints with a localizing key on the occlusal rims. The mandibular splint is secured with circummandibular wires, the maxillary splint with circumzygomatic wires.

per and lower bite blocks (Fig. 5–20). The present concept involves two blocks with lugs processed into the acrylic, and the splint inserted in the same manner as prescribed for dentures. Usually a "key" is processed into the blocks to establish and ensure the correct relation of the lower and upper portions. An intermediate wafer may be necessary when during the preoperative preparations only estimates of centric relation are possible.

Variations of the general category of Gunning splints include nonoccluding splints for certain edentulous and partially edentulous mandibular fractures (Fig. 5–21). Nonoccluding splints are made similar to a denture base or plate without bite rims or other provisions for function or intermaxillary fixation. The splints are secured to the mandible using any of a variety of methods, and the patient is given a diet of liquids and soft foods requring application of little or no stress to the mandible. The splint provides adequate stability to allow bony union. Nonoccluding splints may be helpful in patients with comminuted or multiple fractures, in whom surgery is risky and intermaxillary fixation is not desirable. The splints may be indicated in children with mixed dentition.

Dentures as Splints

If available, the dentures of an edentulous patient with facial fractures should be used to provide fixation of the fractures because the dentures replicate the centric relation of the ridge prior to injury; frequently the dentures are broken and need to be repaired first. The patient's dentures can be modified by adding sections of arch bar embedded in the buccal surface of the acrylic flange (Fig. 5–22). Another fixation method is to drill interproximal holes and adapt continuous loops or eyelet loops to the dentures. This method is especially helpful when laboratory facilities are not available or when time does not permit other modifications to the dentures. T lugs of Alling are metallic studs that form a T-shaped external attachment for fixation of elastic traction or stainless steel IMF wires to the dentures or splints. The studs are embedded in the buccal and labial acrylic. T lugs permit traction in any direction, and, because the lateral surfaces are smooth, they are not irritating to the buccal soft tissues (Fig. 5–23). They may be made from heavy-gauge soldered stainless steel wire in cast metal Ts or from paper clips bent into a looped T shape. Removing several anterior teeth from the lower denture is desirable to allow an improved airway, an exit point for vomitus, and intake of nutrition. It is prudent before surgery to drill through the interproximal areas of the pos-

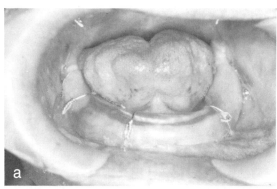

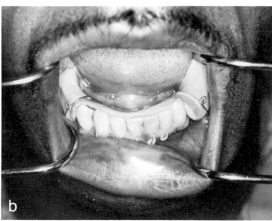

FIG. 5–21. Nonoccluding splints. **a,** Nonoccluding processed acrylic splint to stabilize a nondisplaced body of the mandible fracture. **b,** Nonoccluding vinyl splint to stabilize a nondisplaced body of the mandible fracture.

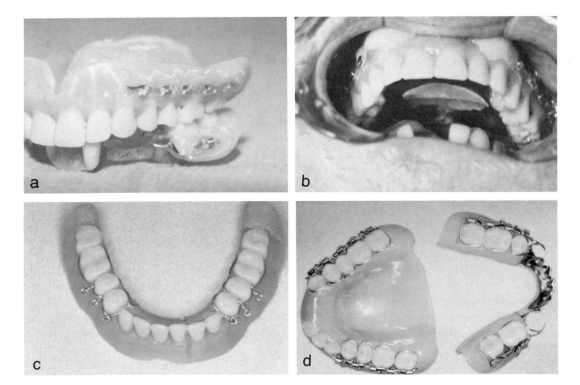

FIG. 5–22. Placement of lugs on splints. **a,** Placing acrylic embedded arch bars on a maxillary denture. **b,** Securing a maxillary denture with transalveolar Kirschner wires and acrylic used to cover ends of the wires. **c,** Denture modified with continuous loop wires. **d,** Dentures modified with arch bars.

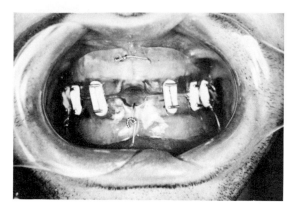

FIG. 5–23.   T lugs provide points of attachment for traction or fixation in any direction. Also, being flat on the lateral aspect, they are less irritating to the adjacent soft tissues.

terior denture teeth or denture flange to allow for the passage of circummandibular or transalveolar wires.

Retention of Gunning Splints and Fracture Prostheses

The upper splint can be fastened to the maxilla with alveolar wires or pinned with two or more Kirschner wires, 1.5 to 1.8 mm in diameter. The upper splint is pinned to the maxilla by drilling the pins through holes in the buccal flange of the prosthesis and through the maxilla at the level of the canine eminence with the pins engaging the palatal acrylic. Upward pressure on the palate of the denture is necessary to seat the denture firmly in the maxilla and to prevent the pins from displacing the denture. Care must be taken to avoid the maxillary sinus and nasal fossa; the tip of the pin is allowed to just penetrate the palatal acrylic of the denture. After the pins are affixed to the maxilla through the prosthesis, the ends are cut next to the acrylic with a steel disc or heavy pin cutters and the rough projections of the pins are covered with quick-cure acrylic on both the palatal and the buccal aspects. The same basic approach can be used with a transalveolar wire, which is brought from the palatal perforation through an interproximal hole between the cuspid and first bicuspid teeth with the ends of the wire twisted on the outer labial flange (Fig. 5–24).

Palatal screws may be used to secure an upper denture or splint to bone. Because they

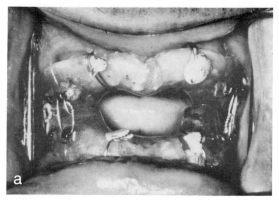

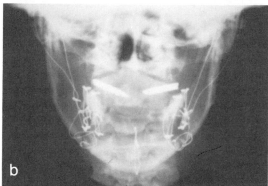

FIG. 5–24.   Stabilization of dentures and splints. **a,** Maxillary splint stabilized with transalveolar wires; mandibular splint stabilized with circumferential wires. Self-curing acrylic has been placed over the twisted ends of the wires. **b,** Bilateral complex comminuted fractures stabilized with direct transosseous fixation and a mandible partial denture and maxillary full denture. The mandibular denture was retained by circumferential wiring, the maxillary by transalveolar pins, and the entire complex of upper and lower splints by circumzygomatic wiring.

may not provide retention adequate to resist opening forces during intermaxillary fixation, palatal screws are often used in combination with other retention devices or in situations not requiring intermaxillary fixation.

Adjacent skeletal fixation is also helpful to retain an upper splint prosthesis. Jugal buttress ridge wires can be attached to the buccal flange of the upper denture or to attachments such as arch bars, eyelet wiring, continuous loop wiring, or T lugs. In the same manner, anterior nasal spine wires are helpful in stabilizing dentures anteriorly. Other skeletal fixation such as circumzygomatic, frontal suspension, piriform rim, or orbital rim wires can be used to retain an upper prosthesis. (The method of placement of these skeletal wires will be discussed later in this chapter and elsewhere.)

A lower splint or the patient's lower denture may be retained by circummandibular wires passed around the mandible and fixed over the prosthesis or through previously drilled holes in the denture. A wire attached to a curved needle may be passed through a stab incision to the inferior border of the mandible and passed lingually into the floor of the mouth (Fig. 5–25). The incision is made in a cutaneous area that has been sterilized. A wire is drawn into the mouth and the needle discarded. A second needle with the other end of the wire attached is then passed through the same incision and lateral to the mandible. The buccal wire is thus passed into the mouth through the buccal or labial vestibule. The two intraoral free ends of the wire are then tied over the denture or the lower half of the Gunning-type splint. An alternative method is to pierce the skin below the inferior border of the mandible with a large-bore central vascular line plastic cannula with stylet and pass it superiorly through the floor of the mouth medial to the mandible. The stylet is withdrawn, the hub of the plastic cannula is cut off, and a stainless steel wire is threaded through the lumen of the needle from outside to inside. The cannula and the end of the wire are withdrawn intraorally. A second cannula with a stylet is then inserted through the skin at the previous entrance site and passed into the mouth lateral to the mandible. The stylet is removed, the plastic cannula hub is cut off, and the free end of the wire is threaded through the lumen of the lateral cannula into the mouth. The cannula is withdrawn intraorally. A slight sawing motion on the ends of the wire is desirable to eliminate soft-tissue entrapment and dimpling of the skin. Skin counter-traction is usually required to totally remove skin dimpling. The wire is then tied around the splint, forming a loop at the inferior border of the mandible.

Another retention technique available for the lower denture or Gunning splint is transalveolar pins. These are used by passing a Kirschner wire through the buccal flange of the lower prosthesis, through the alveolar bone, and through the medial flange of the prosthesis bilaterally in the midbody area posterior or anterior to the mental foramen. Self-curing acrylic is applied to the cut and sharp ends of the pins adjacent to the denture to prevent soft-tissue injury. If alveolar bone height is inadequate or the flange of the prosthesis is too short, a threaded Steinmann's pin can be passed through only the outer flange of the denture into the body of the mandible. The cut end of the pin is covered with self-curing acrylic.

Lingual and Palatal Splints

The lingual splint is frequently used in the treatment of symphysis fractures to prevent inward tilting of the alveolar ridge and to counteract the tendency of the inferior border to become distracted (Fig. 5–26). Similarly, a palatal splint can be used to stabilize palatal or alveolar segment fractures of the maxilla (Fig. 5–27).

Metallic or acrylic splints may be applied to the lingual aspect of the mandibular arch or palatal vault and ligated to the teeth through drill holes in the splint. The holes are placed opposite the interproximal spaces and low enough on the splint to allow the wire ligature to be secured apically to the coronal contours of the teeth. If the holes are placed above the contact points, the splint will not be stable. Holes placed adjacent to the interproximal areas should be oval to accommodate the passage of wires, to permit the wires to nestle beneath the height of contour of the supporting teeth, and to permit the wires to pass easily (Fig. 5–28). Even if a laboratory technician fabricates the splint, the doctor should drill the interproximal holes, as an error in hole design and placement may be costly in terms of time and frustration.

The retaining wires may be formed into rosettes or lugs on the buccal aspect and be used for anchorage of IMF to an opposing splint, to loops of wire, or to an arch bar. It is possible to wire the splint to the teeth using eyelet or continuous loop wiring techniques, and thus to produce loops for traction or fixation to the opposite arch. When using a lingual or palatal splint in conjunction with arch bars, a

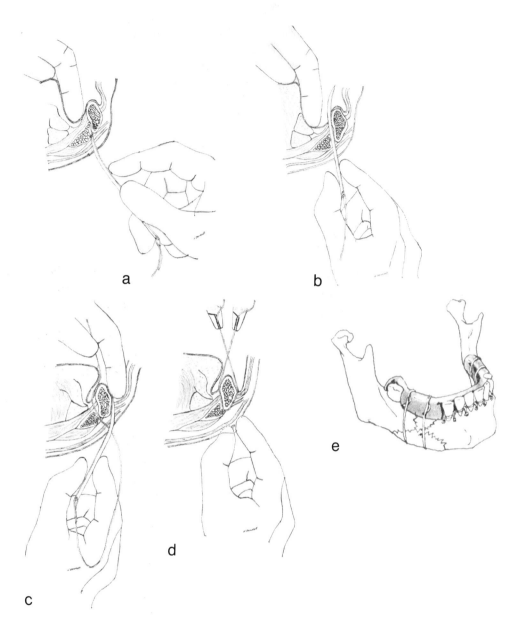

FIG. 5–25.   Circumferential wiring of the mandible. Illustrated is a technique for placing circummandibular wires using an autopsy needle. Similar techniques are used with cannulas and other passing instruments. **a,** The oral cavity is prepared by drying and swabbing with an antiseptic solution, and the cutaneous tissues are prepared with a standard surgical scrub. The tip of the needle is carried to the inferior border of the mandible. **b,** The needle is advanced on the medial side of the mandible to enter the oral cavity. The intraoral finger presses the sublingual and submandibular glands medially and provides taut mucosa for the upward penetration of the needle. The needle should enter the oral cavity at the junction of the mucosa and the mucoperiosteum. **c,** The first needle is discarded after carrying one end of the wire into the oral cavity. A second needle carries the other end of the wire through the same cutaneous entry point to enter the oral cavity at the junction of the free mucosa and mucoperiosteum of the lateral body of the mandible. Care is taken to avoid making a loop in the wire as it is brought around the base of the mandible. **d,** Simultaneous skin counter-traction helps to release entrapped soft tissue, eliminating dimpling of the overlying skin. **e,** The wire is secured around the intraoral device.

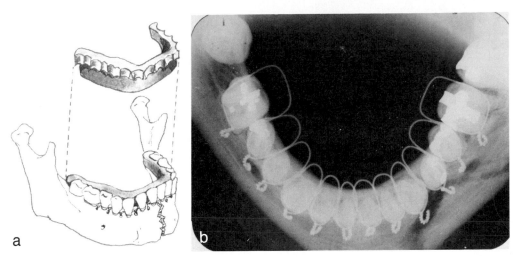

FIG. 5–26. **a,** Lingual splint supports fractures of the body of the mandible. **b,** The splint prevents medial collapse of the fractured segments.

smaller-diameter wire should be used to anchor the splint because of limited interproximal space and leave ample room in the embrasure for the arch bar wiring. Lingual acrylic splints may be reinforced with heavy-gauge wire or a bar embedded in the acrylic for additional stability (Fig. 5–29).

The palatal maxillary splint can be used as an expansion device. If the palate is splayed outward and reduction toward the midline is desired, a palatal expander is reversed and processed into a split half of an acrylic splint, which is wired to adjacent teeth (Fig. 5–30). The split palate can be reduced in a matter of hours by turning the cogs with a ratchet to decrease the fully expanded axle. The same type of appliance can be used to overcome scar contractures following avulsive injury by re-expanding the arch.

Winged Sectional Splints

The winged sectional splint was devised by Colonel Roy Stout and was the forerunner of the lingual splint (Fig. 5–31). A piece of wrought wire holds the buccal and lingual wings of the splint together posterior to the last tooth on each side of the arch. The buccal wings are widely sectioned through an anterior button; this permits the lingual and buccal sections to be drawn into undercuts when a wire is passed around the button and tightened.

Cast Splints

Using cast-metal splints in the treatment of jaw fractures is a most stable means of immobilizing fractured segments. Metal splints are made of German silver, gold, and chrome-cobalt alloys, depending on the availability of materials, the experience of the laboratory, and the demands of the case. Cast-metal splints usually are retained in position by either cement or wires. The metallic splints are especially indicated when more rigid stabilization is required, especially over a long period of time, than can be obtained by an acrylic splint, and when bone loss is extensive and prevention of arch collapse is desired.

The various types of cast-metal splints are used for the treatment of specific conditions. A fundamental concept in the use of cast splints is their ability to secure an accurate impression. Complicated fractures usually require making many impressions of the broken parts (Fig. 5–19), and assembling the finished models in the laboratory with the splint constructed in sections. Such splints are locked together in the mouth with metal plates, screws, or similar locking devices (Fig. 5–32). The following types of splints illustrate their purposes in specific cases.

Lingual Cast Splints

A lingual cast splint is designed to cover the lingual surface of the teeth (Fig. 5–33).

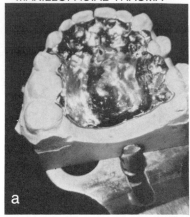

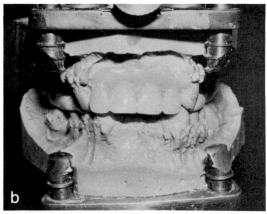

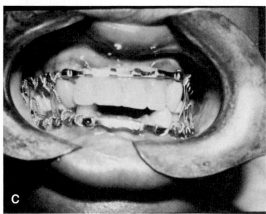

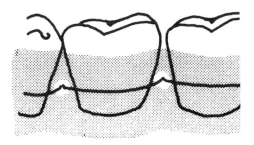

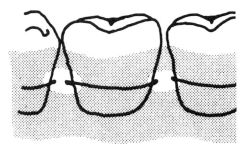

FIG. 5–28.   Horizontal oval holes permit firm attachment of wires to the teeth and provide additional space for passage and retention of wires.

FIG. 5–27.   **a,** Palatal splints, like nearly all splints, are built on reconstructions of a maxillary cast that was cut along the lines of fracture. Teeth may be added to palatal splints for aesthetic purposes, as shown in **b,** The laboratory phase, and **c,** Following placement in the oral cavity.

This type of splint is particularly efficient in treating midline fractures of the mandible. It is wired into position after the fracture is reduced manually, and the twisted wire ends are used to support the intermaxillary elastics or wires. Used in this manner, the splint pre-

vents buccal-lingual torsion and midline collapse. Wire holes must be placed in the splint carefully, because holding wires must be inserted from the lingual aspect, beneath the greater curvature of the tooth and through the interproximal spaces. Pins should be placed in the wax model prior to casting to facilitate preparation of the oval holes. Drilling holes through a metal splint, particularly

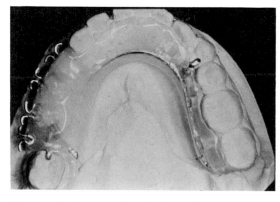

FIG. 5–29.   Accessories for lingual splint: reinforcing bar, T lugs, and occlusal rests.

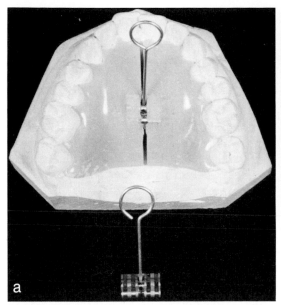

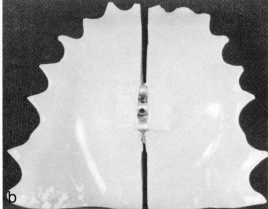

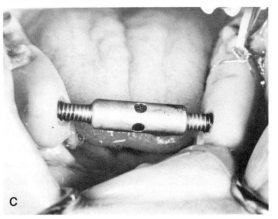

FIG. 5–30. Expanding and contracting splints. **a,** Split palatal splint on a cast, with ratchet in place to turn the cogs to expand or contract the splint. **b,** Splints before oval holes are placed to secure the device to teeth. **c,** Expansion splint in use on the mandible.

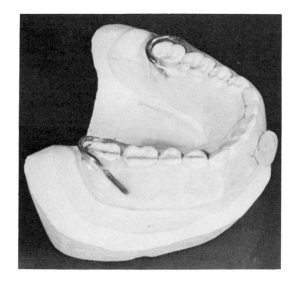

FIG. 5–31. Winged sectional splint. The buccal portion is divided through the button. Subsequent tension around the button tends to seat the splint firmly.

a chrome-cobalt alloy, can be tedious and time consuming.

To prevent inferior displacment of lingual splints, rests may be placed onto the occlusal surfaces of the bicuspid or molar teeth, or a superior margin of the splint may be designed over the lingual cusps of the posterior teeth.

Buccal Cast Splints

The buccal splint can either cover all of the buccal surface or be fitted to the gingival margins of the teeth (Fig. 5–34). It is wired to the teeth and is frequently used when problems with oral hygiene during treatment are anticipated. Buccal lugs, which are used for either elastic anchorage or interdental tie wires, are cast onto the splint.

Cast Cap Splints

The cast cap splint is designed to cover all the surfaces of the teeth (Fig. 5–35). It is retained by cement, which may be supple-

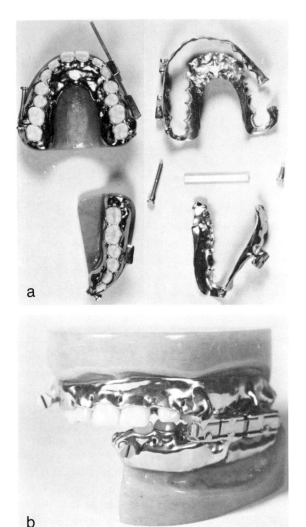

a

b

FIG. 5–32. Winged sectional and screw lock splints. **a,** Winged sectional maxillary splint is secured by a screw lock on the patient's right. The mandibular splint is secured to the mandibular teeth with a screw lock. **b,** In this patient who lost the right side of his mandible as a result of a gunshot injury, the two splints are locked together with a key in slot.

mented by intradental wires. Anchor lugs can be cast or soldered to the buccal face of the splint. Prerequisite to the construction of a cast cap splint are making an accurate impression and establishing centric occlusion by articulating the model casts of the fragments. The models must be mounted on an articulator and the vertical dimension opened to allow for metal coverage on the occlusal surfaces of the teeth. A cast cap splint is strong and resistant to stress, hygienic, and partic-

ularly useful in treating children and patients with avulsive gunshot wounds of the maxillofacial skeleton. It is very useful for repositioning grossly distracted fragments whenever teeth are available for use within the splint. Although at times determining proper occlusion can be difficult using a cast cap splint, occlusal problems can be managed using a modification of the splint, a buccal-lingual splint, that leaves the occlusal surfaces free of metal at the cost of slightly less rigidity.

Screw Lock Splints

The screw lock sectional splint is used in the treatment of multiple fractures associated with severe displacement of the fragments (Figs. 5–32 and 5–36). This type of splint is also indicated when long-term treatment is contemplated and fragments must be held prior to grafting. Gunshot wounds and complex injuries to the mandible are examples of fractures that use this type of splint. Impressions are taken, either in sections or the total arch at one time, the models are prepared, and the casts are cut and reassembled in proper alignment. A tap and die kit is necessary when fabricating sectional splints, as the locking plates must be fitted to the appliance after the splint is inserted in the mouth.

Expansion Splints

These splints are buccal-lingual or cast cap splints with extension bars soldered to the buccal segments to allow traction in an outward direction and to reverse the muscle pull of collapsed fragments (Fig. 5–37). Expansion of the collapsed mandible may be necessary prior to fixating the fracture or placing a bone graft. Movement of the fragments usually is rapid after application of elastic traction. After occlusion is established, a plaster index may be made and the splint removed from the mouth and reassembled on a cast. The expansion arms are removed and a rigid splint is made by soldering the two segments together. This procedure must be done without delay, because a delay of even a few hours may allow the segments to recollapse.

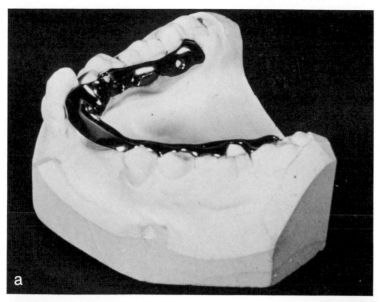

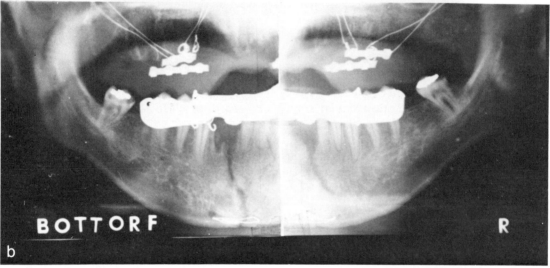

FIG. 5–33. Lingual splint. **a,** A cast-metal lingual splint on a model. **b,** Radiograph of a lingual splint stabilizing the superior aspect of the mandible following a symphyseal fracture. (The apparent two fracture lines are due to the type of view projected by the panoramic radiographic equipment.)

INTERNAL SKELETAL SUSPENSION

Le Fort fractures of the maxilla and midface are frequently comminuted and may result in inadequate sound bone for direct wiring or bone plating of fractured segments. While rigid external cranial fixation with headframes, when available, provides excellent support of midfacial skeletal injuries, it may involve poor outpatient compliance. Also, plaster of Paris headcaps for supporting devices are not as efficacious as internal suspension techniques. Intermaxillary fixation to an intact mandible of severely comminuted midfacial fractures may be compromised by periosteal instability over the midfacial fracture lines, reducing resistance to yawning and opening movements.

Internal skeletal suspension (ISS), used in conjunction with supporting measures such as antral packing has advantages over external cranial fixation with headframes or plaster headcaps and usually provides adequate stability for repair. One objective of ISS is to provide additional support to the maxilla and

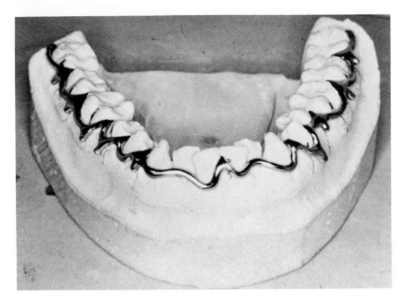

FIG. 5–34. A cast buccal splint may vary from a wire type, as illustrated, to nearly full coverage of the buccal and labial surfaces of the teeth.

midface by resisting opening vertical forces, which tend to lengthen the face, distracting the fractured bones. Another objective of ISS is to help prevent hypereruption of teeth from their alveoli when attached to arch appliances. The vertical opening forces without proper ISS can slowly extract teeth from their alveoli, which would be observed clinically as an anterior open bite with the posterior teeth in occlusion and radiographically as movement of the anterior teeth out of their alveoli.

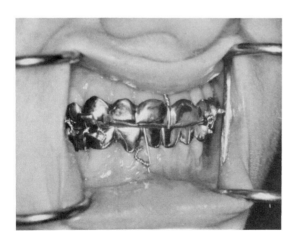

FIG. 5–35. A cast cap splint, in this patient, was secured by cementation and also by circummandibular and anterior nasal spine wiring. Note that lugs were provided for intermaxillary wire fixation.

Placement of ISS generally involves suspending the fractured segments to the nearest appropriate superiorly intact bone. The ISS is placed to provide as near vertical support as possible to the suspended segments, avoiding anteroposterior displacement vectors. Suspension wires can be attached to maxillary arch appliances or prostheses, mandibular arch appliances or prostheses, or circummandibular support wires, either directly or by an intermediate wire. Correct middle and lower facial height proportions should be observed when tightening suspension wires to avoid foreshortening the face (Fig. 5–38).

Malar Arch Suspension

The malar arch, also referred to as the jugal ridge, is a sturdy area for bone suspension or direct wiring (Fig. 5–39). A 1.5-cm incision is made in the depth of the vestibule and a mucoperiosteal flap is elevated to expose the root of the arch and the lateral wall of the maxillary antrum. The tissues are elevated superiorly along the zygomaticoalveolar crest to the region of the maxillozygomatic suture line. A bur hole is made in an anteroposterior direction, and a wire is passed through the hole. Both ends are brought out through the incision and are attached to the maxillary splint,

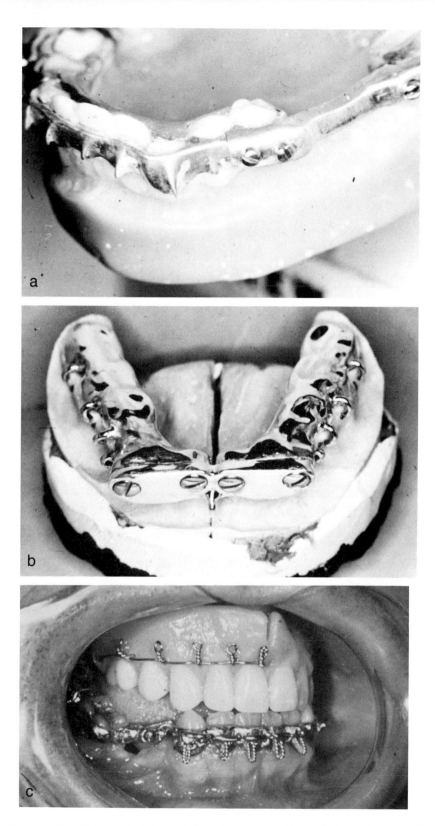

FIG. 5–36.   Screw lock splints. **a,** Splint consisting of lingual and buccal elements secured by screws. **b,** Full cast cap splints are placed on the left and right sides of the mandible, after expansion of a midline defect, and are secured with screws engaging a locking plate. **c,** Mandibular splint over a right midbody fracture site, secured by screws and wiring. Note the use of T lugs on the mandibular splint and the continuous loop wiring on the maxillary denture.

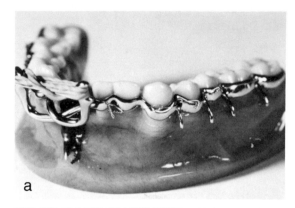

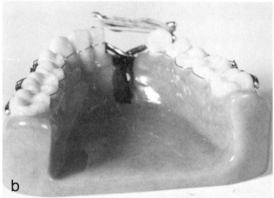

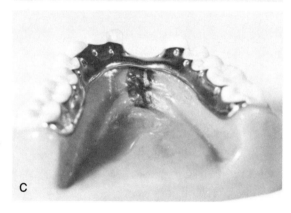

FIG. 5–37. Expansion splint. **a** and **b,** Gentle, steady rubber band traction will usually produce an expansion of an avulsive loss and collapse of the anterior mandible. **c,** The expansion, maintained by a lingual splint, permits a bone graft reconstruction to be performed.

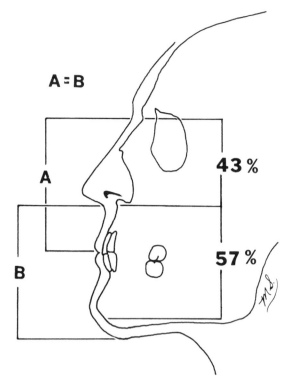

FIG. 5–38. Many formulas are available to determine correct facial proportions. This illustration is of a formula that has served well in the emergency rooms and during urgent operations.

and the incision is closed with interrupted sutures. The short span of wire provides for a stable suspension.

Nasal Piriform Suspension

A stable wire may be placed in the rim of the nasal orifice. Placement of this wire may be combined with another suspending technique (Fig. 5–39). A horizontal incision is made in the vestibule, medial to the canine fossa, and the mucoperiosteum is elevated to expose the piriform fossa on the medial border of the maxilla. The nasal mucosa is elevated and a bur hole placed in the piriform fossa. A wire is threaded through the hole around the edge of the fossa and both ends are attached to the splint or arch appliance.

Anterior Nasal Spine Suspension

A vertical incision is made over the area of the maxillary midline and the mucoperiosteum is elevated, exposing the anterior nasal spine (Fig. 5–40). A horizontal transosseous hole is made at the root of the spine, and a wire is threaded through and attached to the arch appliance or splint near the midline. This method also stabilizes the fractured anterior

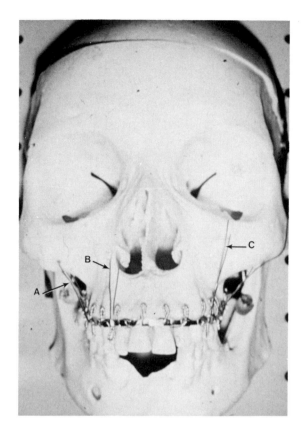

FIG. 5–39.   Various suspension points. Jugal ridge (A). Piriform aperture (B). Infraorbital rim (C).

maxilla or allows attachment of a maxillary prosthesis to the anterior maxilla.

Infraorbital Suspension

A 3- to 5-cm horizontal vestibular incision is placed approximately 1 cm above the mucogingival line between the cuspid eminence and the midline (Figs. 5–39 and 5–41). The mucoperiosteum is elevated from the anterior maxilla, allowing identification of the infraorbital foramen and nerve and exposing the rim lateral to the nerve. The dissection is carried slightly posterior to the rim and a retractor is placed into the anterior orbital floor to protect the eye. A hole is drilled through the rim to the retractor and a wire passed through both ends brought inferiorly to be attached to arch appliances or splints. The incision is closed with a continuous suture.

Circumzygomatic Arch Suspension

Circumzygomatic wiring is a simple and effective method of suspending arch bars or splints (Fig. 5–42). Because of the span from the arch to the splint and because of the posterior to anterior direction of the wires, however, circumzygomatic wiring usually should be combined with other supports such as anterior nasal spine or piriform rim wiring.

Numerous instruments are advocated for passing circumzygomatic wires—autopsy needles, spinal needles with the hubs removed, intravenous plastic cannula needles, various awls, and sewing needles (Fig. 5–43).

After the skin over the zygomatic arch is prepared, a small stab incision is made with a no. 11 Bard-Parker scalpel just superior to the arch and posterior to the frontal process of the zygomatic bone. The needle is inserted through the incision to contact the superior border of the arch. Then, with contact with the arch being maintained, the needle is guided into the mouth medially to the arch, adjacent to the maxillary first molar. The path of insertion into the mouth is guided by the forefinger of the surgeon's other hand. A length of stainless steel wire is attached to the needle. The needle is grasped with a needle holder and pulled through into the mouth, thus bringing one strand of wire into the oral cavity from a sterile field to an unsterile field. Another needle is attached to the opposite end of the wire and is passed into the incision to contact the superior border of the arch. The needle is then directed laterally to the arch, inferiorly and medially into the mouth through the same oral wound through which the medial wire passed. Both ends of the wire are grasped with needle holders and a slight sawing motion is used to bring the wire down onto the arch, eliminating dimpling of the skin. Both ends of the wire can then be attached to upper or lower arch appliances or circummandibular wires by primary means or using intermediate wires (Fig. 5–44). Intermediate wires are especially useful when crossing the bite plane for fixation to the mandible; they allow the fixation to be cut without risking destruction of the suspension wires themselves. This method of wire fixation reduces the possibility of passing the oral flora

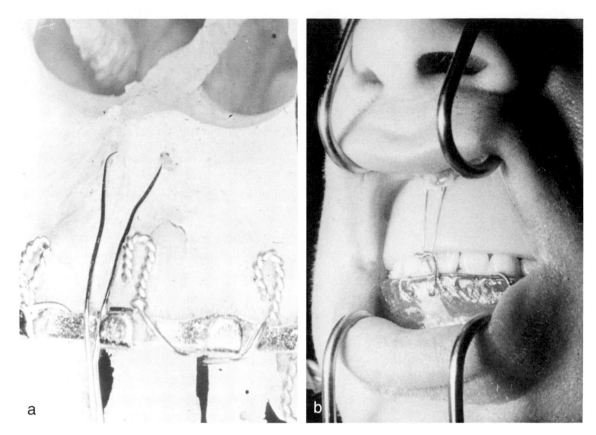

FIG. 5–40.   Anterior nasal spine suspension **a,** If the spine is not well developed, V-shaped drill holes, rather than a horizontal hole, may be placed to provide a stable suspension area. **b,** Anterior nasal spine wire passing over a maxillary splint and engaging an intermediate wire fastened to the mandibular labial splint.

into the infratemporal space, as may occur when an awl is used or when the same needle is used for more than one passage of wire.

The technique for using an awl is the same as that described above for the needle approach, except that the awl is used from above to pass both ends of the wire into the mouth. Another method is to pass the awl laterally to the arch into the mouth at the level of the first molar tooth and attach the wire through the eyelet intraorally. With one motion the tip and the wire are withdrawn superiorly and the awl redirected medially into the mouth through the same opening. The wire can then be attached to arch appliances or fixation devices in the way previously mentioned.

Frontal Bone Suspension

In midfacial fractures involving one or both zygomas, the most immediate superiorly in-

tact bone is the frontal bone (Fig. 5–45). Assuming that the patient has not incurred fractures of the frontal bone, a suspension wire may be placed through a transosseous hole in the zygomatic process of the frontal bone; because the wire can be difficult to remove after the fractures are repaired, a pull-out wire can be used to aid in its removal. Pull-out capability is incorporated into the suspension wire by creating an eyelet and a twist in the center of the suspension wire; this is done by folding a 35-cm length of appropriately sized wire in half and around a 1- or 2-mm-wide instrument and making a 2-cm twist (Fig. 5–46). One transosseous hole is then drilled through a lateral brow incision in the zygomatic process above the fracture from the anterior surface to the temporal fossa surface. One end of the suspension wire is then placed through the drill hole and both wires are

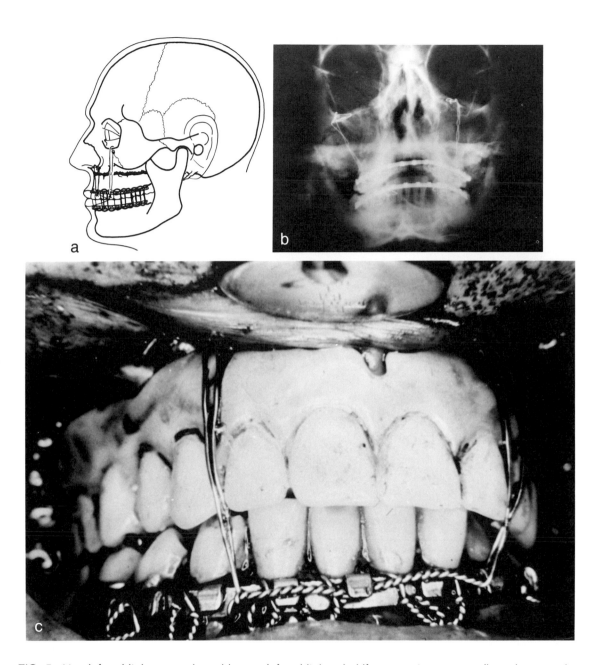

FIG. 5–41.   Infraorbital suspension wiring. **a,** Infraorbital and piriform aperture suspending wires passing to the maxillary arch bar. (Courtesy of U.S. Army.) **b,** Radiograph of infraorbital wires passing to the maxillary arch bar. Extensive comminution of the midface made the use of bone plates unfeasible. (Courtesy of U.S. Army.) **c,** Infraorbital wires passing over the dentition to the mandibular arch bar.

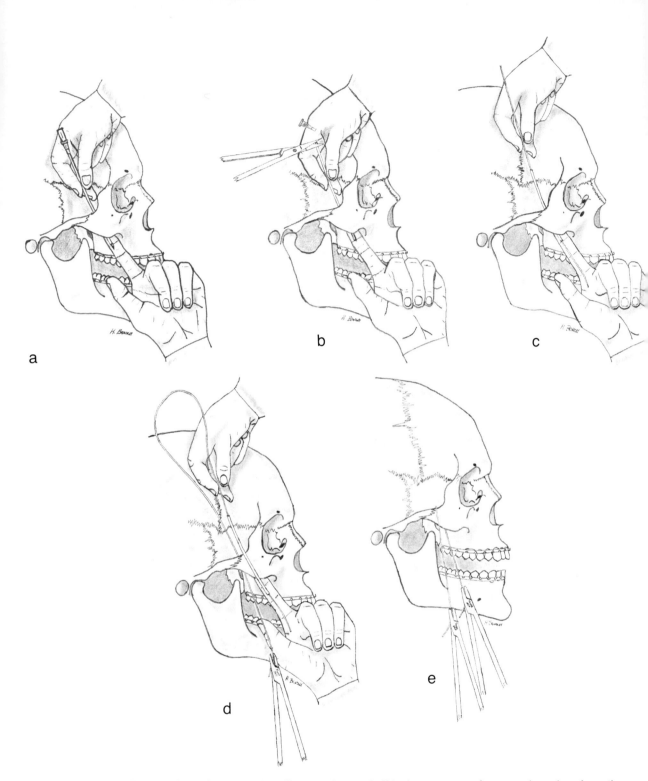

FIG. 5–42. Zygomatic arch suspension. Illustrated on a skull is the passage of suspension wires from the zygomatic arch to the oral cavity using intravenous catheter devices. **a,** The catheter is passed with its stylet in place. With all techniques, considerable pressure is exerted with the palpating finger to provide a target for the needle or awl; the pressure also compacts the soft tissue and thus shortens the distance that must be transversed in the soft tissue. Care is exercised to keep the point of the instrument on or near bone and to protect the parotid duct. **b,** The stylet is withdrawn and the hub of the catheter is removed. **c,** A wire is passed through the catheter and the catheter is drawn inferiorly and out of the mouth. **d,** The procedure is repeated on the lateral side of the arch. **e,** The wire is firmly seated.

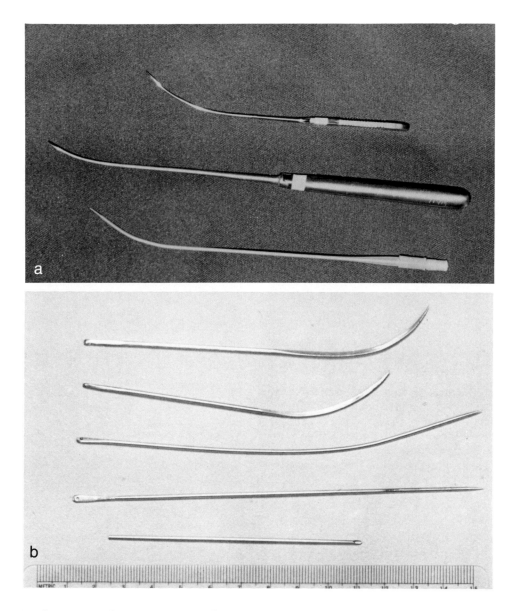

FIG. 5–43.   Instruments for passing suspending wires. **a,** Two types of awls and the intravascular catheter. **b,** Autopsy needle, straight and curved needles, and metallic cannula.

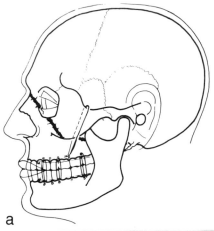

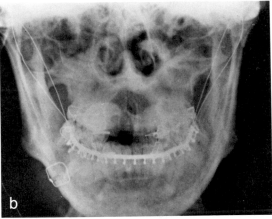

FIG. 5–44. Zygomatic arch suspension wires. **a,** Wires in place in a diagram of a Le Fort II fracture. (Courtesy of U.S. Army.) **b,** Radiograph of extreme comminution of the midfacial skeleton. The zygomatic arch suspending wires pass to the mandible, and the midface is supported by intrasinal contouring and packing.

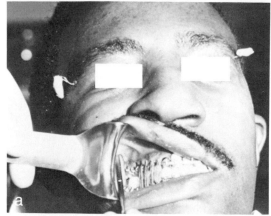

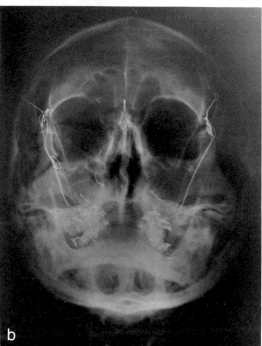

FIG. 5–45. Frontal bone suspension. **a,** Wires extend from the zygomatic process of the frontal bones to the arch bar in the oral cavity. Pull-out wires are identified with the white tape. (Courtesy of U.S. Army.) **b,** Multiple facial fractures treated with open reductions, intrasinal and intranasal packing, and support of a maxillary splint by frontal craniofacial suspension wires.

passed simultaneously or separately into the mouth posterior to the frontal process of the zygoma. The ends of the wire are then secured with intermediate or direct fixation wires to the upper appliance directly, or to lower appliances or circummandibular wires. When used in conjunction with an open reduction of the zygoma with transosseous wiring at the frontozygomatic suture fracture site, the superior drill hole for the transosseous wire will usually suffice for the pull-out suspension wire, with the twist of wire resting on the lateral surface of the process. (Care must be taken that the suspension wire is not trapped under the transosseous wire.) Prior

to closure of the incision with interrupted sutures, the external wire twist and eyelet are bent close to the skin to avoid being caught in clothing. The area should be cleaned daily with a solution of 1 part hydrogen peroxide and 2 parts water. Antibiotic petroleum ointment can be used around the pull-out twist

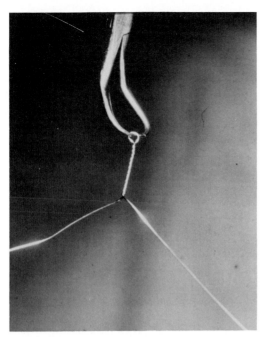

FIG. 5–46. The twist on frontal suspension wire. will extend out of the incision line and be used during the removal of the wire, as described in the text.

of wires to help prevent infection, with due regard for possible secondary cutaneous problems that may result from the ointment (Fig. 5–47).

The suspension wire can be removed by either of two methods. The first requires thorough preparation of the mouth and wires with antiseptic solution. The ends of the wires are cut below the mucosa and the wires removed by pulling the eyelet at the lateral brow. The other method is to cut the wires in

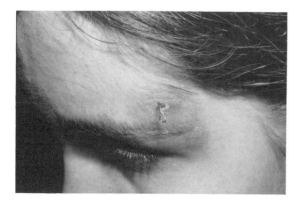

FIG. 5–47. Topical antibiotic reaction. Erythma secondary to use of topical antibiotics around a pull-out wire.

the oral cavity, taking care to firmly attach hemostats to the cut ends. The lateral brow site is thoroughly prepared and the wire is pulled superiorly until the two wires are visualized below the twists. Both are cut below the twist and the wires are removed by pulling the ends down through the mouth. The advantage of the latter method is that it avoids contamination, but care must be taken to cut well below the twist, or exploration of the lateral brow to retrieve wire ends will be necessary. The key to avoiding infection with either approach is thorough preparation of the cutaneous and oral areas and administration of antibiotics for 2 days after removal.

INTERNAL SKELETAL FIXATION

Direct reduction and fixation of midfacial skeletal fractures may be achieved by direct wiring and by small bone plates.

Access to the more superior fracture sites, the naso-orbital, ethmoidal, nasal, and ZMC areas, may be through coronal, hemicoronal, nasion, lateral brow, and infraorbital incisions. Access to the more inferior fracture sites, the infraorbital, sinal, and lower lateral nasal areas, may be through transoral incisions. Of course, lacerations incurred during trauma may provide access to any of the fracture sites.

Transosseous wiring will firmly immobilize fracture lines located in rims, pillars, and buttresses of bone. The objective of transosseous wiring of fractures of the anterior sinal walls is to orient, not necessarily immobilize, the bony fragments. Transosseous wires placed through small bony fragments, as on the anterior sinal walls, may pull through the delicate bone when twisting forces are applied. Wiring will not be as effective as bone plates in preventing superior intrusion of midfacial fracture sites when craniofacial suspension devices are placed.

For the superior fracture sites, small bone plates, as finger plates and miniplates, provide positive and sometimes compressive reductions. However, the plates are bulkier than direct wiring. For the inferior fracture sites, the plates are useful in areas where there is dense bone and where positive alignment of fractured segments is possible. The plates must be accurately contoured to prevent displacements that cannot be corrected by intermaxillary traction. When used with midfacial suspension devices and techniques, the plates will prevent superior intrusions of fracture sites of the facial skeleton.

When placing wires or plates on small bone segments, the surgeon must take care to maintain mucoperiosteal and periosteal attachments. In general, these vital attachments should not be lost in order to place a bone plate or transosseous wiring.

MIDFACIAL SUPPORT DEVICES

In the management of comminuted midfacial fractures, direct bone wiring and suspension wiring may not prevent intrusion of the free segments when the patient swallows or bites. Support devices of various types are frequently used not only to provide additional vertical support but also to maintain the internal shape of various cavities of the midface.

Nasal Splints

Nasal complex fractures involve fracture of the nasal pyramid, the nasal bones, and the nasal process of the maxilla. The fractured bones tend to splay, causing a wider than normal superior nasal bridge. External nasal splints are frequently needed following the reduction of the fractures to maintain the position of the fractured segments. Metallic lead plates can be molded easily to the shape of the area and secured by a horizontal mattress transnasal wire to provide rigidity and retention. Padded prefabricated nasal bridge splints can be adapted to maintain the shape of the nasal bridge. Tincture of benzoin and paper tape covering the skin underneath the splint prevent pressure breakdown. The preadapted splint is secured by several long pieces of paper tape crossing the splint in a cruciate fashion and attaching to the forehead and infraorbital skin. Similarly, plaster of Paris nasal splints can be fashioned and secured to provide support during healing.

Internal splints are also helpful in securing comminuted nasal fractures or when the soft tissues of the nose have been significantly disrupted. Endotracheal tubes or nasal airways in such circumstances can serve as stents not only to provide an adequate airway after healing but also to allow healing of the nasal mucosa without significant stenosis. The disadvantage of these stents is that they tend to widen the alae abnormally and render a less than desirable cosmetic result. Anterior nasal packing following reduction of nasal fractures stabilizes internal fractures and is frequently used in conjunction with external splinting. Packing is usually performed with ribbon gauze. Septal splints made from contoured radiographic film that fits against the nasal septum on both sides of the nose can be transfixed with nylon sutures to provide vertical support to a traumatically deviated cartilaginous septum.

Intrasinal Support

Maxillary antral support devices are the most common means of midfacial support. Intrasinal supports should be used for lateral reduction and retention of medially displaced antrum walls and ZMC fractures, and in cases in which bone at the infraorbital rim is inadequate and the lateral antral wall is comminuted in medially displaced unstable zygomas. Intrasinal supports should also be used to retain the integrity of the antrum by maintaining patency and not allowing loose fragments to compartmentalize the antrum with inadequate or no drainage; to resist superior displacement of Le Fort fractures of the mid-face and the foreshortening that could result; and to provide hemostasis and prevent large clots from forming that could lead to infection and residual sinus disease. Finally, with blow-out fractures, intrasinal support is used to restore and support the integrity of the orbital floor.

The devices used to provide intrasinal support are antral balloons, Foley catheters, and gauze packing. Antral balloons and Foley catheters are inflated, usually with normal saline, and thus support fractured sinal walls. Because support is directed in all directions equally, however, it is possible to displace weak areas such as the floor of the orbit if too much pressure is used, which can lead to entrapment of the inferior rectus and oblique eye muscles, as well as to proptosis.

Antral gauze packing is used most frequently. One-half inch gauze packing can be saturated with a variety of substances, such as balsam of Peru and antibiotic petroleum ointments to reduce bacterial growth and unfavorable odors and to improve tissue tolerance when packing is used for long periods of time. Petroleum antibiotic mixtures are readily available and provide excellent results but should be avoided in patients with poor laryngeal protection because of the possibility of a persistent pneumonitis from aspiration of the oily antibiotic mixture. Antral packing may be removed in 24 to 48 hrs if used for hemostasis only. When the pack is needed for support, it is kept in place for 10 to 14 days, at which time early fibrosis will probably have stabilized the fracture segments.

Antral packing is usually performed through a 3- to 4-cm horizontal Caldwell-Luc incision. When orbital floor comminution is severe, it is sometimes helpful to do the packing while observing the floor through a subtarsal infraorbital incision to prevent superior displacement of the fragments from the floor of the orbit and the resulting proptosis or inferior rectus muscle entrapment. Packing should begin posteriorly and should be placed in layers toward the anterior aspect of the antrum. It is helpful in unstable zygoma fractures to hold the malar bone laterally and anteriorly from inside the antrum while packing laterally to ensure proper positioning. Periodic compression of the gauze with the tip of the finger to remove excess packing medium further adds to the density of the pack and improves the support (Fig. 5–48). After the antrum is fully packed, future pack removal can be provided for in one of three ways: the pack can be left beneath the incision at its anterior extent and removed later by opening the incision with a hemostat and pulling the pack out through the mouth; the pack can be sutured at the anterior extent of the oral incision with a nonresorbable suture and can be removed at the desired time simply by removing the retaining suture and pulling the pack into the mouth; or the pack can be brought out through a nasal-antral window and sutured to the columella or nasal septum with a 2-0 nylon suture.

The first two alternatives for pack removal have a higher incidence of oral-antral fistulae than the third method. Care must be taken not to suture the packing to the intraoral incision closure. Another precaution is to use one continuous length of gauze and to avoid the need to lengthen the pack by tying knots that would make pack removal in an outpatient extremely difficult and painful. The patient should be kept on antibiotic coverage and decongestants to maintain drainage while being supported with antral packing.

DIRECT FRACTURE FIXATION TECHNIQUES

Techniques that provide fixation of bone segments by attaching directly to bone are direct fixation techniques. The two major categories of direct fixation techniques are external and internal direct fixation devices.

EXTERNAL DIRECT FIXATION DEVICES

External devices provide fixation or support for the fractured segments extraorally.

Zygomatic Arch Support

The isolated zygomatic arch fracture usually maintains its position following elevation. If the fracture tends to return medially and is unstable, support and lateral traction may be necessary to maintain a corrected arch position.

A stainless steel 24-gauge wire is placed around the circumference of the zygomatic arch with a small aneurysm needle and is brought through the skin above and below the arch. In addition to generalized traction support devices such as headcaps and headframes, localized isolated traction and support can be accomplished using several devices. A trapeze device as described by Allen is made from a contoured acrylic doughnut with an embedded heavy iron wire trapeze that can be attached to the circumferential arch wire either directly or by elastic bands[18] (Fig. 5–49). Alternatively, a finger fracture splint may be contoured and cushioned to rest on the solid bone of the zygomatic arch anterior and posterior to the fracture. The cir-

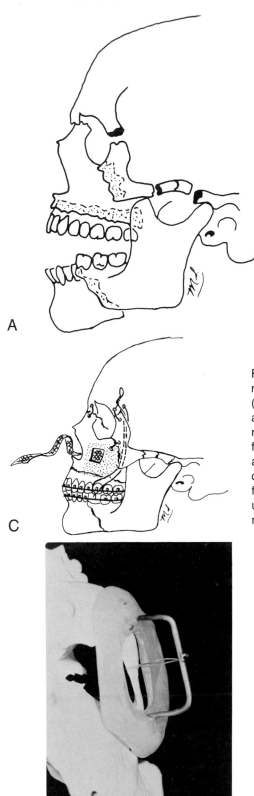

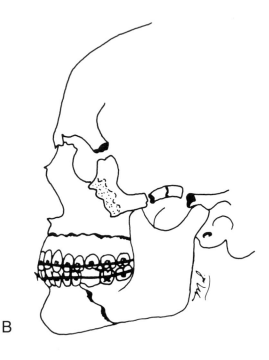

FIG. 5–48.   Multiple facial fractures. **a,** The fractures include mandibular, Le Fort I and II, ZMC, nasal-orbital-ethmoidal (NOE), and zygomatic arch. **b,** The mandible is reduced first and guides the lower midfacial segments to an anatomic relationship. **c,** Illustrated are open reductions of the ZMC fracture at the frontal and maxillary area, the NOE fracture and suspension from the frontal bones. Excessive reduction of the midfacial fractures and hence foreshortening of the facies are prevented by intrasinal packing. This packing is usually necessary to support the comminuted fractures of the midface, including the orbital floor.

FIG. 5–49.   Allen's zygomatic arch trapeze. Support for an unstable depressed zygomatic arch fracture is provided by the suspending wires.

cumferential arch wire is attached by elastic traction to the supporting frame. This apparatus, simple to use and maintain, can easily be detached for cleaning and reapplied. Finally, a Fox eye patch can be used by directly attaching the circumferential arch wires to the perforated metallic dome-shaped grid, providing outward traction using the cushioned rim as support. Adequate hygiene and skin care around the wires under the device is difficult to achieve because of its occlusive nature.

All of these devices have satisfactory patient acceptance, although they are somewhat bulky and unsightly. They are more acceptable in the management of isolated unstable arch fractures than are cranially supported traction devices such as headcaps and headframes.

Plaster Headcap

A plaster headcap provides support for external direct fixation devices. Its primary application is to provide superior support for midfacial fractures through rigid attachments from the headcap directly to bone, through suspension wiring, or through traction devices applied by elastics, using the headcap attachments as anchorage (Fig. 5–50). The major advantage of using the headcap is that pins for support need not be placed against the outer cortex of the cranium. The major disadvantages are its mobility resulting from movement of cutaneous tissues over bone, painful pressure sores and ulcerations, and inability to maintain scalp hygiene.

The following materials are needed to apply a plaster headcap: a piece of 30-inch-long stockinette of a large enough diameter to pull snugly over the entire head; several packs of 3- or 4-inch quick-setting plaster bandage; a large pair of bandage scissors; metal struts and attachments for securing appliances; supply of cold water and mixing bowls; and a pair of pliers for bending the wire attachments.

The plaster bandages are cut into 12- to 15-inch lengths and placed on a nearby dry working surface. The stockinette is placed over the entire head to the angle of the mandible and tied in a small knot at the top of the head. The excess beyond the knot is cut and discarded, with care taken during the procedure not to allow the stockinette to creep upward. The plaster bandage is moistened in cold water and placed around the circumference of the head over the stockinette, with the first circular pass made from below the occiput and high on the forehead. The second pass should be made from above the occiput and low on the forehead. Care should be taken to adapt these first rows of bandage tightly and to avoid folding the stockinette, which would produce a loose-fitting headcap. The inferior application of bandage should extend to a point 2 cm above the supraorbital rim anteriorly, above the ears laterally, posteriorly to allow adaptation to the three occipital retention points between the insertion of the right and left trapezius and sternocleidomastoid muscles and the opisthion, and

medially between the trapezius muscles. Pressure should be placed periodically against the three posterior retention points while the bandage sets to ensure stability. A thin layer of material is usually placed over the top of the head to prevent settling and ulceration of the supraorbital rim, with most of the material resting laterally around the circumference of the head. An opening can be left superiorly to provide ventilation. After 0.75 to 1.0 cm of material has been applied, metal attachments are adapted to the contour of the head. At least one angled bend for anchorage should be made in the part of the metal attachment incorporated in the substance of the headcap. Attachments may be made commercially or fabricated from heavy wires such as coat hangers. Several more pre-cut layers of plaster bandage are then applied and the metallic attachments secured. Before the outer layers are completely set, the stockinette is trimmed with scissors to within 1 inch of the inferior and superior aspect of the bandage, and the cut end is rolled over the wet plaster laterally. Another layer of bandages is then placed over the cut edge of the stockinette and the entire outer surface of the headcap smoothed with hand pressure and slight moisture before the plaster sets. A roll of stockinette at the inferior aspect of the headcap is made in this fashion to resist irritation to adjacent soft tissues.

Whenever possible headcaps should be made from newer, light-weight casting materials, using the same basic technique of application. These materials consist of knitted fiberglass tapes saturated with polyurethane resin that becomes rigid when activated by water. Compared with plaster of Paris, these materials are stronger, lighter, radiolucent, porous, and nondegradable by moisture. Gloves should be worn when applying the material to avoid fiberglass cuts on the fingers and because the stickier material is more easily smoothed with a gloved hand.

External Skeletal Fixation Devices

External pin or screw devices, which may be monophasic or biphasic, have numerous applications, particularly in situations requiring long-term fixation of segments without

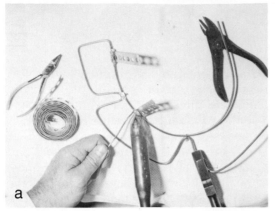

FIG. 5–50. Application of a plaster headcap. **a,** The metallic superstructure is prepared. **b,** The stockinette is trimmed. **c,** The plaster bandages are placed below the occiput and low on the forehead. **d** and **e,** The metallic superstructure is incorporated into the plaster bandages. **f,** Various suspending devices are placed on the superstructure.

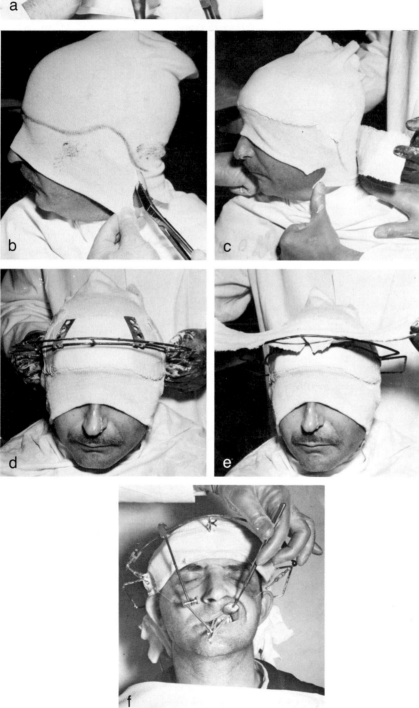

intermaxillary fixation. They can be used for comminuted (bag-of-bones) fractures for which arch alignment is difficult to maintain; for continuity defects such as gunshot wounds or resected tumors; for fractures in patients who are unreliable and may remove intermaxillary fixation devices; as an adjunct to stabilize bone grafts; in edentulous fractures when unfavorable muscle pull may cause displacement, and intraoral splints are either ineffective or not available at the time of surgery; and for midfacial fractures when combining external craniofacial support with direct control of the mandible is indicated.

The disadvantage of external pin or screw fixation is the difficulty in cleaning beneath the connecting bar, especially in male patients in whom facial hair growth is a problem. The potential for infection, especially where external pins or screws are used to stabilize free bone grafts, is also of concern. Infection can generally be minimized by maintaining adequate hygiene, avoiding wetting external pins or screws while bathing, and applying solutions around the pin to retard infection. Pediatric triple sulfa oral suspension with methylene blue mixed to make a 1% solution is particularly helpful in preventing pin or screw infection, except for those allergic to sulfa. Petroleum antibiotic ointments usually can be used only for 10 to 14 days before a skin reaction occurs, requiring cessation of use.

Monophasic Pin Fixation Device

The monophasic pin fixation device is simple and easy to apply.[19] The pins used in the device are 1/8-inch- or 9/64-inch-diameter threaded Steinmann's pins that are placed with a drill. The disadvantage of using the monophase system is that the fracture must be held manually in a reduced position until the acrylic base is fully set and rigid. For this reason, and because the threaded pins tend to be tangled in soft tissue, pins should be applied prior to closure of incisions if the device is used in conjunction with open reduction or bone grafting procedures. A minimum of three pins should be placed, two on one side of the fracture and at least one on the opposite side. In comminuted fractures, pins should be placed in the most proximal stable

bone and the appliance bar used to span the comminuted portion. As a rule, the larger the continuity defect or comminution to be spanned by a bar, the more pins needed in the proximal segments to provide stability. When pins are placed through soft tissue, a trocar must be used to prevent the threaded pins from becoming engaged in soft tissue.

Before the monophase pin device is placed, the skin is prepared with an antiseptic scrub and solution (Fig. 5–51). A no. 15 scalpel blade is used to make a stab incision through the soft tissue down to bone. The soft-tissue opening is enlarged with blunt dissection using a curved hemostat to accommodate the metallic trocar. A drill trocar with obturator is inserted through the wound down to bone. The obturator is removed and the sawtooth trocar edge seated firmly on bone. (The trocar that is used is frequently the same as that used in compression bone plate kits for placing lag screws in the ramus.) A threaded Steinmann's pin is placed against the bone perpendicularly and the pin is drilled through the mandible until the point exits the medial cortex. This process is continued until all pins have been placed in as straight a line as possible and the pins are equally cut to an appropriate length. The fracture should be manually reduced and held in position at this time if direct transosseous wiring or plating have not been used. A no. 10 plastic endotracheal tube is used as the external bar former after the endotracheal tube balloon is removed with a pair of scissors. If the endotracheal tube is not long enough to attach to all pins, an appropriate length of large flexible plastic tubing can be used. Holes are made in the inside plastic tubing with a no. 15 Bard-Parker blade to allow the pins to penetrate into the lumen without displacing the fracture. Acrylic monomer and polymer are mixed together and are placed into a tapered 60-cc irrigation syringe; the syringe is used to inject the mixture the full length of the tubing. The fracture is held in a reduced position until the acrylic has set.

A modification of the monophasic pin device is used to stabilize the mandible against the fractured midface (Fig. 5–52). Threaded Steinmann's pins are placed into the intact body of the zygomas bilaterally and mandib-

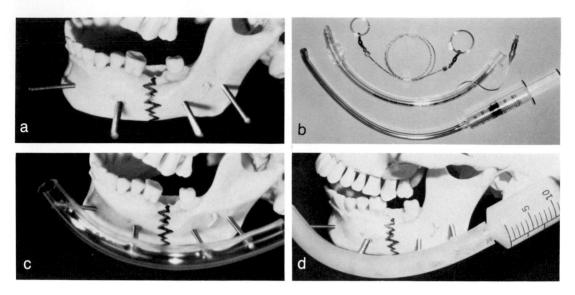

FIG. 5–51.   Placement of a monophasic pin device. **a,** Threaded Steinmann's pins are placed on both sides of fracture, engaging both cortices. **b,** A large-bore plastic tubing or a no. 10 endotracheal tube is used as the bar former. A survival saw, similar to a Gigli's wire saw, is used to section the bar at the time of removal. **c,** Small holes are made on the inside of the large plastic tube, and the tube is placed over the threaded pins. **d,** A 60-ml catheter-tipped syringe is used to inject the acrylic solution into the tubing.

ular pins are placed as previously mentioned. The tube is placed on the mandibular pins as described but is bent to allow attachment of the zygoma pins. A small wedge excision in the plastic tubing may be necessary to allow the pins to be adapted and the tube to remain patent at the bend. A small amount of ½-inch plastic tape can be placed over the bend after the removal of the wedge to seal the opening and facilitate flow of acrylic beyond the bend. If the acrylic mixture cannot be forced far enough from one end, acrylic may need to be injected from the opposite end of the tubing before a wedge cut is made, and the opposite end is placed over the zygoma pin. The remaining tube from the wedge cut superiorly can be filled easily after the tubing is in place. This modification provides excellent stability, although care must be taken, when placing the tubing over the zygoma pins, that proper facial proportions are maintained to avoid elongation or foreshortening of the face.

Biphasic Screw Fixation Device

Dr. Joe H. Morris developed and described in 1951 a biphasic screw fixation device that uses predrilled holes with bone-embedding screws and a nonyielding connecting stabilizer bar of quick-cured acrylic (Fig. 5–53). Dr. Merle Hale and his associates modified this type of device by developing it in stainless steel rather than cobalt-chromium alloy, giving the screws sharper lags that better engage the bone. This method of screw fixation has many advantages over skeletal pin techniques. Retention in bone is better than with pin devices. The bone-embedding screw increases the time that the screws remain rigidly integrated to bone.

Also, this device permits the fragments to be adjusted prior to placement of the acrylic stabilizing bar, thereby allowing the timing of surgery to be more flexible. In addition, because there are no friction-holding clamps in the final acrylic phase, there is less chance of displacement after surgery. The equipment is uncomplicated to use, and no special preoperative preparation of special splints is necessary. The device is lightweight and sufficiently strong to furnish adequate stabilization. Also, bone screws designed to reach a limited depth are available.

Placing the biphasic pin device consists of several steps (Fig. 5–54). The sites for the screws are marked on the skin, usually with

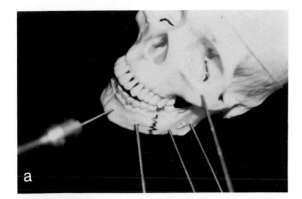

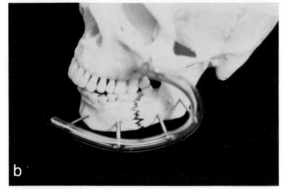

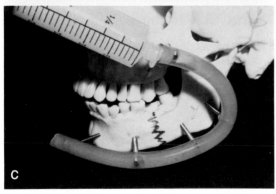

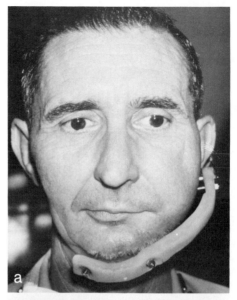

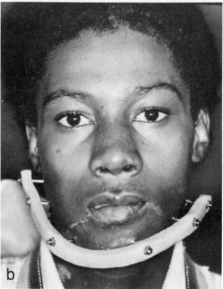

FIG. 5–52. Monophase pin fixation device between the mandible and midface. **a,** Threaded pins are placed in the stable body of the zygoma as well as the mandible. The pins should be as parallel as possible. **b,** The large plastic tube is placed over the threaded pins through small perforations in the tubing wall. **c,** A 60-ml catheter-tipped syringe is used to inject the acrylic mixture into the plastic tubing. Care must be taken when placing this device to ensure proper facial proportions.

FIG. 5–53. Biphasic pin fixation device. **a,** A second-phase acrylic bar stabilizes a left mandibular defect. **b,** Bilateral application may be necessary for larger defects.

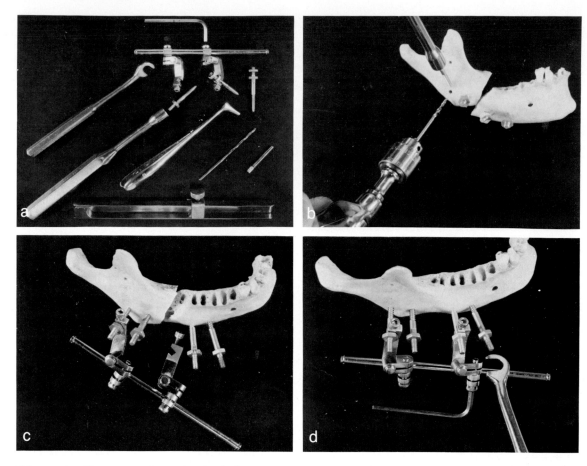

FIG. 5–54.   Placement of a biphasic pin fixation device. **a,** Equipment: first-phase fixation bar and devices that attach to the bone pins, holding wrench, pin socket driver, nasal speculum, trocar, bone pins, pilot drill, drill guide, adjustable acrylic tray former. **b,** Holes are drilled in the mandible on both sides of the surgical site and pins are inserted to engage both cortices. **c,** The first-phase holding attachment is secured to a pin on both sides of the surgical site. **d,** The fracture is reduced and the first-phase device tightened.

methylene blue. When indicated, local anesthesia may be used for screw placement. Whenever possible, two screws should be placed in major segments of the mandible with care taken to avoid the inferior alveolar neurovascular bundle and the dentition. A skin incision approximately 1 cm in length is made. The incision is located just superior to the inferior border of the mandible and at an estimated distance of 1.5 cm or more from the fracture site. The bone is exposed by blunt dissection down to the periosteum. The periosteum is sharply incised and elevated. After the periosteum has been elevated from the bone, a small nasal speculum or drill trocar may be used as a tissue retractor. The length of the speculum blades should be reduced

and the ends serrated to ensure a nonslipping bone contact.

A 3/32-inch drill bit in a hand drill or a motorized power drill is used to pierce the lateral and medial cortical plates of the mandible. Tissue retraction with the speculum prevents soft tissue from becoming entangled in the drill and facilitates locating the hole when the bone screw is placed.

With the self-retaining driving wrench, the bone screws are inserted so that both the lateral and medial cortical plates are engaged by the bone screw lags. The screws may be provided with a varying number of lags that terminate in a flat plane. When the plane comes to rest on the lateral cortical bone, the inward movement of the screw will cease. If the

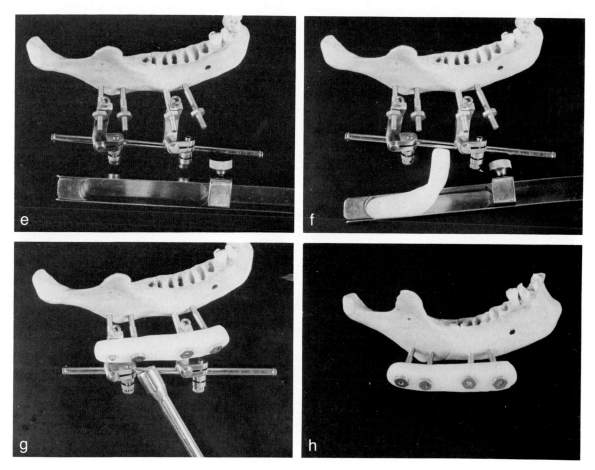

FIG. 5–54 (continued). **e,** The tray former is adjusted to the proper size. **f,** The former bar is removed from the tray. **g,** The second-phase acrylic bar is placed over the pins and taps are placed. Note the tap imprinted in the acrylic bar to lock the bar firmly. **h,** The first-phase retaining device is removed.

screws do not have a flat plane, in order to ensure engaging both cortices the screw should be turned four times in the ramus, six to eight times in the body, and eight to ten times in the parasymphysis area.

To control the fracture, flat facets just below the hexagonal table on the bone screws are turned either superiorly or inferiorly. If the screws are supplied with the Hale's modification of multiple facets, the inferior and superior positioning of the facets is not necessary. The facets are used for locking the primary connecting bar to the bone screws. In case of bone grafting or open reduction of comminuted fractures, the primary connecting bar should be positioned above the screws to give greater surgical access to the inferior border of the mandible. Placement of the screws prior to the soft-tissue dissection at the surgical site may severely restrict access, however.

The bar clamps of the primary connector are then locked to the bone screws; the set screw in the clamp locks against a facet. The bar clamps of the primary connector are left slightly loose so that the fragments can be manipulated without hindrance. When the primary metal connector is attached to the bone screws, one may manipulate the fragments and adjust the arch alignment and occlusion to effect a reduction of the fractures.

When a satisfactory fragment alignment is obtained, either by manipulation or by surgery, the connector bar clamps are secured thus locking the fragments in position. An antitorque wrench will stabilize the appliance and ensure that no torque is introduced to displace the alignment.

A choice of procedures is now available. Radiographic inspection of the fragments may be performed in the operating room and the nonyielding connecting stabilizer bar of quick-cured acrylic applied immediately. Alternatively, the patient may leave the operating room with the first-phase metallic connector bar in place. The radiographs may be made following the patient's recovery from general anesthesia and the second-phase plastic connector placed if satisfactory alignment has been achieved. If reduction is not satisfactory, the connecting stabilizer bar can be loosened and manipulated again until the desired position is obtained. The acrylic bar may then be applied in the usual manner.

To fabricate the acrylic bar, a series of steps are followed. The distance between the end screws is measured; for each 2.5 cm of acrylic bar desired using a commonly supplied rapid-curing acrylic, 1 cc of monomer and 1 U of polymer are required. Thus, a 7.5-cm bar will require approximately 3 cc of liquid and 3 U of powder of the rapid-curing acrylic.

After being mixed, the material is allowed to stand for several minutes, at which time it may be removed in a dry but rubbery consistency, rolled into a tube form, and pressed into a two-piece adjustable mold, which had been set at the proper length and lightly lubricated with petroleum jelly or mineral oil.

The excess acrylic is discarded and the mold is opened. The bar thus formed is pliable and is adapted over the screws. A variation for forming the acrylic bar is to use a plastic tubing similar to that mentioned in the monophase pin device.

The acrylic bar is adapted to the screw so that a negative impression of the hexagonal table is imprinted on the underside of the connector bar and a locknut is turned down on top of the bar until it is securely seated into the acrylic. This metal and acrylic interlock produces an extremely stable union between the plastic bar and the bone screws.

During polymerization of the acrylic, cracked ice in gauzes, gloves, or both are applied to the first-phase metal connecting bar to dissipate the heat that would be conducted through the bone screws to the mandible. Care should be taken to prevent the acrylic bar from contacting the soft tissues, because the heat of polymerizaton may be sufficient to cause a skin burn.

When the bar has cooled to room temperature, the first-phase metal connectors may be removed by loosening the screws and clamps holding the metallic connector bar to the bone screws.

Finally, an antibiotic ointment dressing is applied to the base of the screws and a fluff pressure dressing is placed around the screw wounds. Occasionally, sutures may be needed at the site of the screws to obtain adequate soft-tissue closure.

Occasionally, placement of the screws produces tension at the soft-tissue margins, causing a puckering effect. Puckering is relieved by extending the incision in the direction of the soft-tissue buildup to allow passive positioning of the soft tissue against the screw.

Removal of the acrylic bar can be accomplished by cutting with a small coping or bow saw, using a round blade. A faster method is to use a survival saw while stabilizing the appliance with hand pressure. The survival saw is similar in design and function to a Gigli's wire saw and is used to cut between the screws. Removal of the pins that are still attached to an acrylic segment is usually accomplished without the need for any anesthetic.

Frontal Fixation Pin

Frontal bone fixation pins provide a means of attaching to the frontal bone devices that provide support for midfacial fractures. One pin is placed in the zygomatic process of the frontal bone and another is placed in the frontal bone just above the supraorbital rim. The pins are placed so that their shafts nearly intersect each other. An adjustable locking device attached to the pins secures the pins and gives the appliance rigidity. Supporting buccal wires attached to either a maxillary splint or a mandibular arch appliance can be attached from the appliance, which protrudes from the skin approximately 1 inch.

Headframes

The use of a headframe with a three-point fixation device to stabilize complex midfacial fractures was first advocated by Crawford in

1943. Headframes have been refined and improved during the intervening years (Fig. 5–55). In 1966, Crewe developed pins that would engage only the outer table of skull; the device produced, however, was a complete halo with limited flexibility for pin location and placement and for apparatus attachment.[22] Irby developed a modified headframe device that consisted of two thirds of a halo frame with four-point skull fixation attached to a parallel accessory attachment bar and a coronal connecting bar.[23] This modification gave greater flexibility for attachment

of stabilization appliances and eliminated the discomfort of the halo behind the head for the patient lying supine. Morris developed a lightweight adaptable two-thirds halo frame with a single bar that served to attach both skull pins and apparatus for stabilization.[24] It was also designed to be integrated with the biphasic external skeletal pin apparatus.

When compared with plaster of Paris headcaps, headframes have several advantages. They can be modified to provide shoulder support for cervical fractures; also, unlike headcaps, headframes can be used in skull

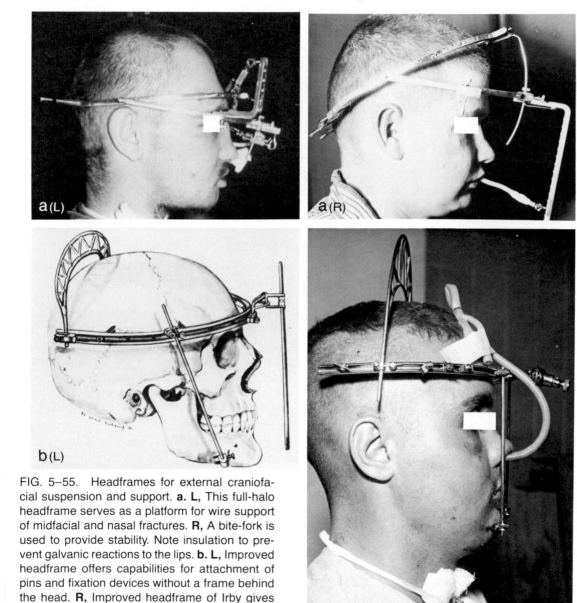

FIG. 5–55.   Headframes for external craniofacial suspension and support. **a. L,** This full-halo headframe serves as a platform for wire support of midfacial and nasal fractures. **R,** A bite-fork is used to provide stability. Note insulation to prevent galvanic reactions to the lips. **b. L,** Improved headframe offers capabilities for attachment of pins and fixation devices without a frame behind the head. **R,** Improved headframe of Irby gives vertical stability to multiple midfacial fractures. The overhead truss rather than a halo design provides rigidity to the frame.

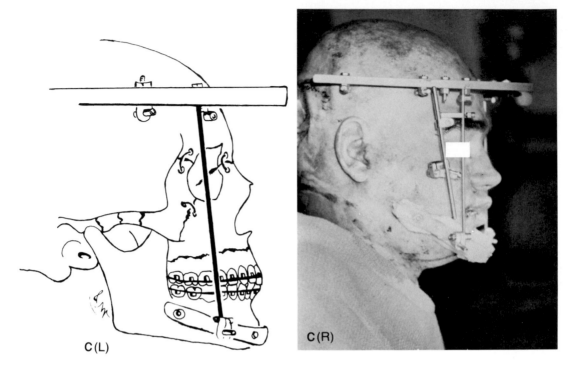

C(L)   C(R)

FIG. 5–55 (continued). **c. L,** Headframe designed by Dr. J.H. Morris can be used in conjunction with the biphasic external pin devices. **R,** The illustrated patient had his head shaven for other reasons than the application of the headframe. In most cases, surgical soap shampoos and removal of hair at the site of the pin punctures is all that is necessary. The pins pass through a small cutaneous incision and engage the outer cortex of the skull.

fractures by prudent placement of pins. Headframes are easily applied to an unconscious patient or a patient with cervical fractures. They provide better comfort and cleanliness. Also, headframes have an unmatched ability to retain in an anterior direction unstable depressed fractures of the maxillofacial area.

Headframe pins must be kept clean to avoid infection. Coating the pins daily with applications of a 1% methylene blue and pediatric triple sulfa oral solution following cleaning with hydrogen peroxide diluted one half in water reduces the problems associated with infection but must be avoided in those allergic to sulfa. The pins should be kept as dry as possible.

Headframe application begins with selecting the apparatus. Both the Irby and Morris frames are used frequently in the U.S. The devices used with the Morris headframe system are compatible with the Morris mandibular biphasic external screw devices. After the

apparatus is selected, tufts of hair are shaved and the areas of pin placement prepared with an antiseptic scrub solution. Generally, two pins are placed bilaterally in the parietal and two in the frontotemporal areas, allowing for cranial fractures if present. The pins' axes are oriented perpendicular to the tangent of the outer table of the skull at the point of application. The frame is located superior-inferiorly at approximately the level of greatest diameter of the skull to allow pin placement in the most desirable location. When the frame is placed, the skull pins should be tightened initially to just clear the scalp, and the frame halo should be equidistant from the scalp in all directions. Minor tightening of the screws can then indent the skin slightly to locate the entry points for the pins, or the entry points can be marked with methylene blue. The scalp is then injected with local anesthetic solutions, preferably with vasoconstrictors for hemostasis if compatible with the anesthetic chosen and the patient's cardiovascular status. A stab incision is made over the entry point of the pins into the scalp and widened with minimal blunt dissection to accommodate the skull pins. With the frame in position, opposite pins in the sequence are tightened in an equal number of turns to prevent the apparatus from sliding or rotating. Tightening of the skull pins should continue until the apparatus is firmly secured to the outer table of the skull. Additional tightening of one half to one complete turn will be necessary in 1 to 2 days to prevent loosening of the apparatus, but further tightening of the skull pins should not be necessary. The outer skull should be engaged by the pins but not penetrated by the entire pin diameter.

After the frame is applied to the cranium, devices may be attached to stabilize the facial fractures. For example, nasal and nasoethmoid fractures that have been displaced posteriorly can be stabilized by a transnasal horizontal mattress wire attached to the lateral nasal plates or by wires placed in the medial wall of the orbits; a connecting wire is attached to the midline of a vertical support rod from the headframe using either elastic traction or direct wiring following surgical evaluation. Unstable ZMC fractures can be stabilized by attaching a transcutaneous screw placed in the body of the zygoma to a lateral vertical rod supported superiorly from the headframe using direct wiring or elastic traction. Transcutaneous Kirschner wires of appropriate diameter can be placed in the body of the zygoma and secured to attachments sliding over the lateral vertical rod.

Midfacial fractures can be stabilized and the vertical proportions of the face can be maintained with a headframe apparatus in three ways. In the first, the upper and lower dental arch appliances can be attached directly to the headframe by transcutaneous wires that penetrate the buccal tissues in a direct line from the headframe to the inferior attachment. The point of penetration of the wire through the skin is usually on a vertical line below a line extending inferiorly from the outer canthus of the eye. The wire should be placed so that it is as passive as possible in soft tissue to prevent its migration through the soft tissues with resultant scarring. Cheek wires are usu-

ally less comfortable than other methods of support fixation.

The second method for stabilizing midfacial fractures is to use a bite-fork fused with an intermediate occlusal wafer or splint connected directly to a midline vertical support rod that is attached superiorly to the frame. Still another variation is to attach traction wire to an upper arch appliance and the vertical midline rod. The former provides more rigid support but interferes more with speech. The lip should be protected from ulceration caused by galvanic irritation by placing an insulating washer.

The third method for stabilizing midfacial fractures is to drive a transcutaneous Kirschner rod through the anterior mandibular parasymphyseal area horizontally below the apices of the teeth, allowing enough of the rod to protrude on both sides to provide attachment to bilateral vertical support rods that are attached superiorly to the headframe. The Kirschner rod can be placed to utilize a single through-and-through Kirschner wire or two separate wires on each side tied together with a connecting device such as that used in the Irby appliance. An alternative method of attaching mandibular fixation to a headframe is to substitute comparable threaded Steinmann's pins for the smooth vertical support rods and attach the acrylic bar of a biphasic pin device to the threaded support rod by means of a small amount of self-curing acrylic.

INTERNAL DIRECT FIXATION METHODS AND DEVICES

Direct Transosseous Wiring

A reliable means of providing direct internal fixation of facial skeletal fractures is by transosseous wiring. The wires should not be stretched prior to use. In order to compress the fracture line firmly when the transosseous wires are secured, the wires should be placed either perpendicular or at a slight angle to the fracture line to nullify secondary displacements by muscular forces (Fig. 5–56). In oblique fractures of the mandible, a horizontal mattress wire placed at right angles to the

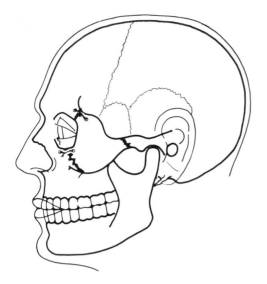

FIG. 5–56. Direct transosseous wiring of a ZMC fracture. Compressive wires are placed at right angles to the general line of the fractures. Miniplates (as used in midfacial orthognathic surgery) in these locations may be used. (Courtesy of U.S. Army.)

fracture will firmly hold the fracture in position (Fig. 5–57).

Transosseous holes for wire should be drilled with fluted or wire-passing burs instead of crosscut or tapered burs, which tend to bind in bone and may break. Wire-passing burs are seldom used for retrieving wires because the tip to the bur may break in removal. Holes are generally placed through the full thickness from outer cortex to inner cortex. When holes are drilled with an engine driven bur, the bur should be irrigated with a lavage of saline.

Wire used for transosseous fixation in the mandible is generally 24 gauge in diameter and in the maxilla, infraorbital rims, and frontozygomatic area is 24 to 26 gauge. When, in placing transosseous wires on the mandible, passing ends of the wire from the medial surface is awkward and difficult, a smaller gauge pull-through wire can be folded and the loop passed from outside and retrieved medially (Fig. 5–58). The end of the medial larger wire is then placed through the loop of the smaller wire and folded tightly against itself 1 to 1.5 cm from the loop. The loop of smaller wire is then used to pull through the larger wire from the medial surface.

Double Transosseous Compression Wiring

The double compression wiring technique of Alling consists of passing two wires through the same two transosseous wire drill holes (Fig. 5–58). The drill holes are placed and the wires passed to provide single direction reduction and fixation of the fracture. Drill holes may be placed to compensate for secondary muscular vector displacements; for example, in right-angle mandible fractures, the posterior hole may be slightly higher and the anterior hole slightly lower than at a right angle to the fracture line. One wire is twisted adjacent to the anterior drill hole and the other adjacent to the posterior drill hole. The wires are tightened alternately to slowly re-

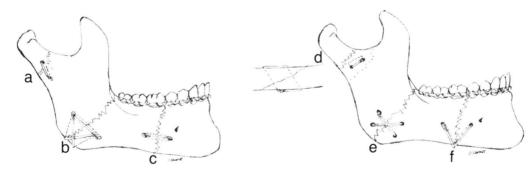

FIG. 5–57. Various methods of transosseous wiring. Direct transosseous wire properly placed in a subcondylar fracture of the mandible (a). A figure-of-8 wire used in conjunction with a direct transosseous wire to retain an angle of the mandible fracture (b). A double wire compression fixation to stabilize a body of the mandible fracture (c). A horizontal mattress wire from two views placed to stabilize an oblique subcondylar fracture of the mandible (d). A high-low cruciate wire to stabilize an angle of the mandible fracture (e). A figure-of-8 wire used to stabilize a body of the mandible fracture (f).

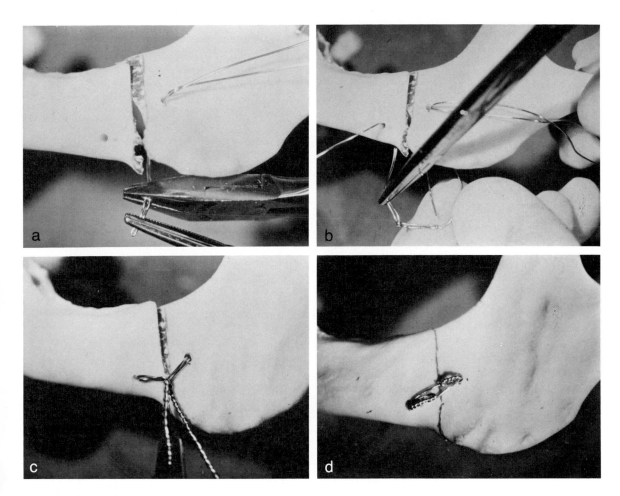

FIG. 5–58.   Pull-through wire to facilitate placement of double wire compression fixation. **a,** A folded strand of 24-gauge wire is passed through the proximal fragment and retrieved inferiorly from the medial surface. **b,** The 24-gauge wire is cut into two strands. One end is passed through the loop of a 26-gauge folded pull-through wire, crimped for ease of passage. The 26-gauge segment pull-through wire with attached 24-gauge wire is withdrawn by winding the double-strand 26-gauge wire around the head of a wire twister. **c,** The double wire compression fixation is tightened. Care is taken to ensure that the ends being twisted together belong to the same strand. **d,** The cut twisted ends are turned clockwise and tucked into a drill hole. Note the slight angle of the wire alignment with reference to the line of the fracture. This alignment counteracts the upward muscle vectors acting on the posterior segment of bone.

duce the fracture with compression and without unduly work hardening the wires. If one wire should break, however, the other is sufficient to retain the fracture in its compressed, reduced state. The wire ends are cut and tucked into the nearest available drill hole.

High-Low Wiring

The high-low cruciate technique requires four transosseous wire holes placed through both cortices. The wires are passed in a high-low fashion, forming an "x" over the fracture site, each at a 45° angle to the line of fracture. The wires are tightened alternately providing even control of both fracture segments. The ends of the cut wires are placed into the nearest available transosseous wire hole (Fig. 5–57). This technique must be used carefully to prevent displacement of the segments. It has minimal or no application in oblique fractures.

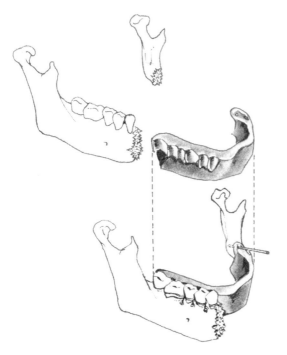

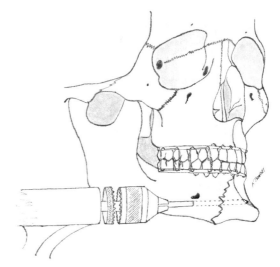

FIG. 5–60.   Intramedullary pin for fracture stabilization. An intramedullary pin at the inferior border of a symphyseal fracture provides reduction and fixation.

FIG. 5–59.   Intramedullary pin to stabilize a splint. A mandibular splint is stabilized to the mandibular ramus following an avulsive injury.

Intramedullary Pins

Intramedullary pins in the ramus or posterior body areas have little use except to attach stabilization splints in continuity defects (Fig. 5–59). Fractures in the anterior curved portion of the mandible can be fixated using Kirschner intramedullary pins. Condylar head fractures can also be stabilized with intramedullary pins, although this direct fixation means is usually used in conjunction with labial arch bars or lingual splints to provide superior support.

Through an external incision, the pin is directed into the outer cortex of one segment, then into the medullary space and across the fracture site to firmly engage, but not penetrate, the opposite outer cortex. The fracture is kept reduced while the wire rod is drilled into position. The pin is cut close to the mandible with a steel diamond wheel (Fig. 5–60).

To add to the retention, fluted Steinmann's pins can be used instead of smooth Kirschner pins. Steinmann's pins can be used in the same way as Kirschner pins or as internal matrix support for continuity defects. In situations such as gunshot wounds and tumor resections, in which stability is needed for grafting, intramedullary Steinmann's pins can be placed in the opposite segments for support.

Figure-of-8 Wiring

The figure-of-8 wiring technique consists of passing a single transosseous wire through one of the transosseous wire holes from the lateral to the medial aspect of the mandible. The end of the wire on the medial side is then retrieved and brought laterally to the mandible across the inferior border and is passed through the other transosseous hole in the smae fashion. The medial end of the wire is again retrieved and is passed across the inferior mandibular border to join and tie to the other end of the wire on the lateral surface (Fig. 5–57). Care should be taken to place the wires at the inferior border of the mandible so that they do not pull into the line of fracture. This wiring technique is helpful to stabilize small free segments at the inferior border. It is also helpful to provide additional stability when atrophy is severe or mandibular height is limited. A second wire may be passed between the drill holes as a direct transosseous wire.

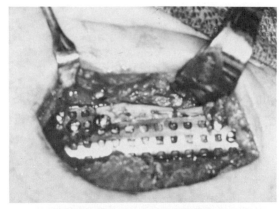

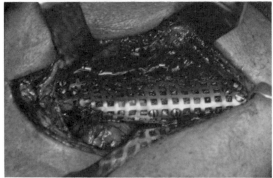

FIG. 5–61. Titanium trays are used to provide fixation and to hold cancellous bone grafts for management of fractures of atrophic mandibles.

Wire Mesh Stabilization

Wire mesh of a cobalt-chromium alloy or titanium trays can provide stability in the fixation of mandibular fractures when superior-inferior body height is limited, as in severely atrophic mandibular fractures; in some cases, the addition of autogenous cancellous bone grafting is the primary repair procedure (Fig. 5–61). Wire mesh is used to hold cancellous bone when using grafts to repair continuity defects secondary to comminution with avulsion, to bone loss from infection, or following resection of neoplasms. Acrylic can be added to the mesh frame to form a condyle for holding a functional alignment of the mandible following an avulsive injury or for resection of a neoplasm when the condyle as well as the ramus of the mandible is lost and primary grafting is to be delayed.

One disadvantage of using wire mesh trays is that more soft-tissue reactions occur than with smaller appliances, although tissue tolerance is generally good; surface corrosion of the tray can result from interaction with tissue fluids, causing fracture of the tray. Also, special instruments made of the same type of metal are required for manipulation and bending of the trays to avoid galvanic response in tissue. The trays usually need to be removed after several years because remolding of the bone may cause the cutaneous or mucosal surface to dehisce over the tray. Also, trays are more difficult to handle than other rigid fixation devices. After the tray is adapted, it should be autoclaved to pacify the surface of the metal to improve its corrosion resistance.[25]

Trays are applied through an external incision generous enough to allow the tray to overlap the proximal and distal segments by 1.5 to 2.5 cm; this overlap provides ample grid openings for screw fixation. Superiorly, the metal should not extend high enough to risk intraoral ulceration through the mucosa. The inferior portion of the tray is bent to form a J shape, with the lip of the bend to be placed medially. Prefabricated trays need only to be trimmed to the appropriate length and height. When grafting continuity defects with autogenous cancellous bone, using a millipore filter attached to the tray may be indicated to retard graft dissolution, especially in areas exhibiting infection. The metal should be pacified by autoclaving before the device is secured to bone to reduce corrosion and the likelihood of metal fatigue's causing fracture of the appliance. The appliance is secured to bone using appropriately placed self-tapping screws made of the same material to avoid galvanic corrosion. If attached wires are used in composite bone grafts, they should be of the same metal to avoid galvanic response. Composite block grafts should be placed prior to the placement of the tray, though cancellous marrow grafting should be placed after the tray is fixed to bone. The tray and graft usually provide excellent stability.

Bone Plate Stabilization

Rigid bone plates of varying designs have been used for many years in both orthopedic and oral and maxillofacial surgery. Plates may be used to provide internal fixation in comminuted fractures where segments are missing or when stripping the periosteal covering of bone for wiring is contraindicated because of the danger of sequestration. Plates can also be applied when condylar injuries are present and an early mobilization is required to reduce the likelihood of ankylosis. Plates are used to stabilize bone grafts when repairing continuity defects. Mandibular bone plates are indicated for stabilization of reconstructive procedures; resected areas or avulsed areas prior to reconstruction; mandibles weakened by disease (to prevent fractures); mandibles when intermaxillary fixation is contraindicated because of medical risk; fractured mandibles in uncooperative patients who are likely to remove intermaxillary fixation against medical advice; and fractured mandibles to provide immediate or early mobilization.

Plate fixation has many advantages, including such effective stabilization of fracture segments that intermaxillary fixation may not be needed. Another advantage is the ease of intraoral application, which may be easier than intraoral transosseous wiring because it does not require stripping the medial periosteum and retrieving wires from the medial surface of the mandible.

The disadvantages of plate fixation are slight in view of the advantages. Because plates are extremely rigid and inflexible, care must be taken to properly adapt the plates to a reduced fracture keeping teeth lightly in occlusion to prevent malalignment and malocclusion. Whereas transosseous wiring of bone allows enough flexibility that elastic traction intermaxillary fixation can correct slight discrepancies in occlusion after open reduction procedures, this accommodation is not possible with rigid plate fixation. One of the problems is that a bone plate may produce an adequate lateral cortex reduction at surgery, but postoperative radiographs may reveal a gaping displacement on the medial cortex. This malalignment in the ramus area could result in malocclusion and increased intracondylar distance and temporomandibular joint pain and dysfunction. For all the above reasons, using plates requires more exacting technique, with more attention paid to three-dimensional reduction. Another slight disadvantage is the bulkiness of some systems, which occasionally causes undesirable facial fullness in individuals with limited soft-tissue coverage. Use of plates is severely limited in children because of the difficulty of placing screws to avoid impinging on or blocking tooth formation and eruption.

Static Bone Plates

Bone plates of varying sizes and descriptions have been used for many years as adjuncts of direct internal fixation of fractures of osseous defects.[26] Since the advent of dynamic compression plates, the tendency has been to incorrectly group plates into compression and noncompression systems. However, all bone plates work by compression. Static bone plate systems work by compression of the bone plate against the outer cortex of the bone. As the screws engage the bone, the plate is compressed between the screwhead and the cortex of the bone, providing the rigidity and stability needed for fracture repair. These systems generally use self-tapping screws. The earliest screws were made with flutes similar to sheet metal screws, with little difference between the core diameter and thread diameter of the screw shaft. In addition, the flutes were closer together, which gave the screws limited retentive ability. Later versions used screws more like wood screws, with wide flutes and larger thread diameters compared to the core diameters. Although this design improves screw retention, the screws loosen quickly because of the lateral compression against bone.

Sherman plates are relatively thick orthopedic plates used to provide maxillofacial fixation (Fig. 5–62). Other, less rigid plating systems incorporate a semi-rigid plate that is more easily bent and adapted with screws, providing excellent retention. Plates of this nature are available in varying lengths and sizes and are easily trimmed to a desired length with heavy-gauge wire cutters. They are generally not rigid enough to be used without adjunctive intermaxillary fixation but do allow for some minor movement to correct discrepancies in occlusion.

The inlay or L plate modification gives three-dimensional stability to plate fixation.

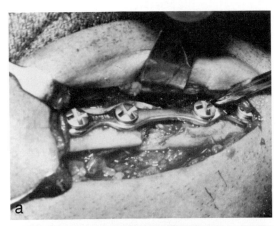

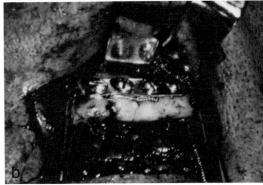

FIG. 5–62. Static bone plates, **a,** Orthopedic (Sherman) plate. **b,** Semi-rigid, easily contoured bone plate.

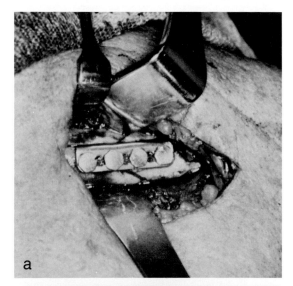

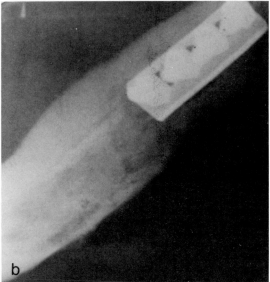

FIG. 5–63. L plate static fixation. **a,** A groove is created in the outer cortex to accommodate the L extension of the inferior plate margin. **b,** Proper compensatory bending of the plate yields solid reduction and fixation of the fracture.

This plate can be used in either axial compression or static systems by adding a short, 90° flange to one edge of the plate. After the plate is adapted to the outer surface of the mandible, a linear cut is made in the outer mandible to accommodate the recessed flange. The flange is frequently notched to allow room for even bending of the plate without interference. When secured, this flange, if tightly adapted to bone, will help resist rotational forces and reduce stress applied to the plate, which can loosen screws and cause metal fatigue and fracture of the plate (Fig. 5–63). Small plates, miniplates, and finger plates are used in maxillary or midfacial fractures as well as in subcondylar fractures or atrophic mandibular fractures (Fig. 5–64).

The technique for applying bone plates does not vary a great deal whether an intraoral or extraoral approach is used. The overlying soft tissue is prepared with antiseptic solutions in the usual manner. Ample access must be obtained for either approach with an incision long enough to allow application of the apparatus without excessive tension on the soft-tissue margins. With the teeth in light occlusion using intermaxillary elastics, the fracture is reduced and held in position. Occasionally, arch appliances must be sectioned across the fracture to allow manip-

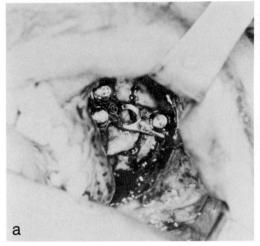
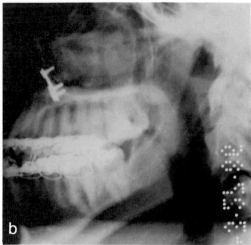
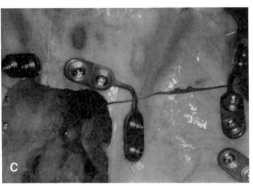

FIG. 5–64.   Miniplates for static fixation of mid-facial fractures. Where possible, when there is no comminution of fracture lines, the T- or L-shaped linear plane miniplates provide excellent resistance to rotational displacement of Le Fort I fractures. In some cases, one may elect to use the self-tapping screws of one system with the flexible miniplates of another. **a,** Miniplate systems are excellent for providing support and stability of fractures at the jugal ridges, and **b,** on the piriform rim. **c,** Easily adapted miniplate system. (Courtesy of Hall Reconstructive Systems.)

ulation of the fracture into a reduced position. The plate is bent to conform passively in all dimensions to the lateral surface of the mandible or maxilla. Thinner plates can be bent with wire twisters, forceps, or pliers. Thicker plates must be bent or adapted with special bending tools or with bending machines (Fig. 5–65). The plate is held in position with an appropriate instrument during hole and screw placement. Using a twist drill with the core diameter of the screw shaft, holes are placed full thickness, through both cortices, into the bone at right angles to the outer cortex. A depth gauge is used to determine the length of screw necessary to slightly penetrate the medial cortex. A length of wire with a small angled bend can be used for this purpose if a depth gauge is not available. Screws are inserted into their predrilled holes and the plate secured. Self-tapping screws should not be removed because they are likely to strip out when reinserted.

Dynamic Compression Plates (DCP)

Paramount in the correct placement of a dynamic compression plate is a basic under-standing of the forces affecting mandibular stabilization under functional loading.[27,28] The functional loading of the mandible tends to create zones of compression toward the inferior border and zones of tension toward the alveolar process or superior aspect of the mandible. Thus, the tendency for a fracture of the mandible under function is to gap open at the superior margin and to compress or overlap at the inferior border (Fig. 5–66). In addition, placement of a DCP at the inferior border may result in gapping of the superior margin of the mandible. These two tendencies may be compensated for in various ways, including arch bars or lingual splints in the midbody and symphyseal areas.

In the angle of the mandible area through an impacted third molar following the removal of the impacted tooth, an intraorally placed transosseous wire can suffice to prevent gapping. Because placement of this wire does not provide for compression at the superior margin or alveolar process, however, the advantages of primary bone healing may be lost. A small two-hole compression plate

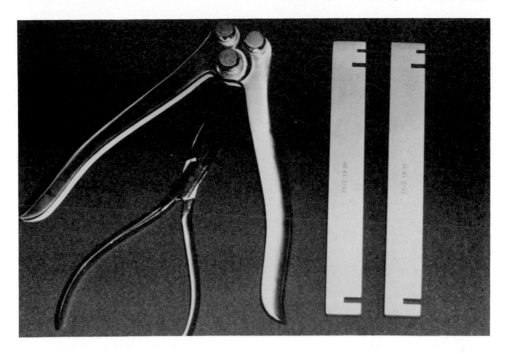

FIG. 5–65.   Contouring instruments. Small plates can be adapted using pliers. Thicker plates will require the use of bending instruments.

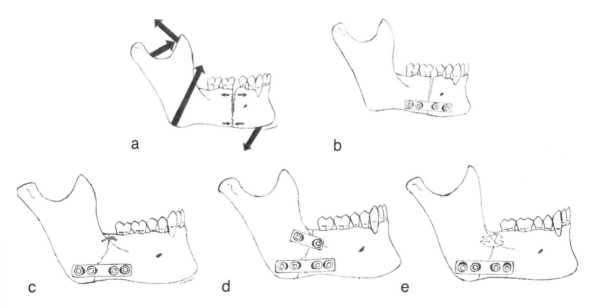

FIG. 5–66.   Details in the placement of bone plates. **a,** Muscular vectors cause compression at the inferior border of the fracture site and distraction at the superior margin. **b,** Gapping at the superior margin results from lack of compensation for tension created by placing a dynamic compression plate (DCP) at the inferior border of the mandible. **c,** Transosseous wiring is used to prevent gapping at the superior margin of an angle of the mandible fracture when a DCP is used to provide axial compression at the inferior border. **d,** A DCP can be used at the superior margin to prevent tension band gapping created by DCP axial compression at the inferior border. **e,** A single eccentric DCP (EDCP) plate placed at the inferior border can provide both axial compression at the inferior border and rotational compression at the superior margin.

can be placed near the external oblique line to provide for compression in this area. This plate, used in combination with a DCP at the inferior border, ensures greater stability of the angle fracture.

Still another alternative is a multidirectional compression system called the eccentric dynamic compression plate (EDCP), as described by Schmoker. The EDCP uses transversely positioned compression slots oriented between 45 and 90° to the plane of horizontal axial compression that, when the screws are tightened, will result in rotation around the already-placed horizontal compression screws to cause compression of the superior margin. Where horizontal compression screws are in danger of being too close to the line of fracture and pulling through bone, a modified EDCP has been advocated in which the slots closest to the fracture are rotational transverse slots and the distal slots are horizontal compression slots. This design produces less compression at the superior margin, however, because of a shorter fulcrum of rotation. The orientation of the transverse slots and the direction of movement of the screw must be 180° to the previously mentioned EDCP plate to produce the same compression at the superior bony margin (Fig. 5–67). The medial surface of the mandible should be observed to determine if gapping has occurred. A compensatory bend in the plate used in conjunction with the transverse rotational slot will also compress the fracture on the medial surface.

In the posterior or midbody of the mandible, a similar approach is taken, except that the tension band plate is eliminated because the roots of teeth prevent safe screw placement. Arch bars or wire functioning as a tension band can be used with either DCP or EDCP for stabilization. The EDCP yields more-uniform compression and stability than the DCP in this situation (Fig. 5–68).

In the symphyseal area, DCP is preferable to EDCP to prevent the thin alveolar bone from overriding under compression. In addition, an arch bar, wire, or lingual splint should be used where possible to provide a tension band support (Fig. 5–69).

For the fracture to remain stable, the plate and screws must remain tightly in place. Ori-enting the drill hole in the center of the slot is important to avoid static forces that can oppose the functional forces. This misalignment of the forces results in a back-and-forth action on the screw, causing it to loosen. Stability can also be improved by using a longer plate.

The plates used can be straight* (Fig. 5–70), those of varying angles especially adaptable to the ramus of the mandible, and with a slight sloping bend for use in the symphyseal area.

The plates of one system differ from another system in their lack of rotational slots and the presence of sliding noncompression slots adjacent to the fracture. In some systems, the varying distances between these slots adjacent to the fracture are particularly helpful in oblique fractures. The compression slots in some systems are smaller, which makes lag screwing of oblique fractures through the plate more difficult.

Synthes has a system available that is compatible with the Swiss Association for the Study of Internal Fixation (ASIF) system and can accommodate a metallic condyle. The plating is notched segmentally to allow for easier bending in the long axis of the plate.

In addition to the plates, the screws used in these systems are designed and placed to maximize retention and minimize the effect of screw loosening. The screw flutes are spaced like wood screws to provide excellent bone contact. The holes are tapped prior to screw placement to minimize lateral compression against the bone, which causes screws to loosen with time (Fig. 5–71). In addition, the holes can be drilled to function as either regular or lag screws. The total integration of the system of DCP and screw technology provides a flexible system that allows adaptation, when indicated, to virtually any existing fracture situation.

The dynamic compression bone plating system as used by ASIF and reported in their official bulletin for the treatment of fractures of the facial skeleton is an outgrowth of the

---

*Many plating systems are available. The above observations are of just a few systems and are neither inclusive nor exclusive of the splendid systems on the international markets. The purpose of the discussion is to orient the reader regarding principles and applications.

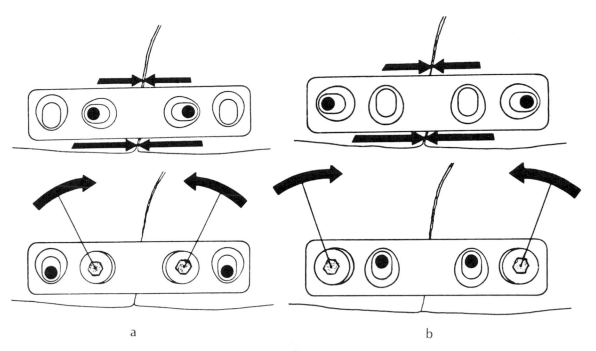

a

b

FIG. 5–67.   Rotational compression by the EDCP system. **a,** Illustrated is a system that pivots the rotational compression around the axial compression screws adjacent to the fracture. **b,** The EDCP system is designed to be used when proximity of the fracture to the screws could cause the inside axial compression screws to pull through the bone. Note that the eccentric compression slots are 180°, as opposed to those in Figure 5–67a.

work by Müller, which set forth principles and techniques of osteosynthesis.[30] With this technique of applying axial compression, fractures are repaired by primary bone healing in a shorter period of time.[31]

Perren described the use of gliding holes in plates, which allows for axial compression of fractures as well as compression of the plate

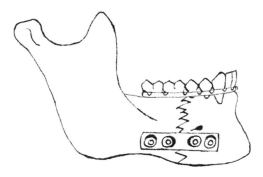

FIG. 5–68.   Arch bars in conjunction with bone plates. In tooth-bearing areas, arch bars can provide tension band protection when used with either DCP or EDCP plating sytems.

against the outer cortex of bone.[32] The hemispherical screwheads are tightened into the plate at the distal ends of the hole, and the holes are fabricated with inclined plane surfaces to direct the screwheads toward the center of the plate, thus forcing together the attached bone with resulting interfragmentary pressure (Fig. 5–72).

Preparing, exposing, and reducing the fracture for applying DCP follows the same procedure as for applying static bone plates. A plate that is shaped appropriately to provide horizontal axial compression in the area of the fracture is selected. With the plate held in position, the number and dimensions of the compensatory bands necessary to accomplish passive adaptation of the plate to the lateral cortex is estimated. Any gapping on the medial or lingual side should be observed prior to bending and compensated for in the bending process. With the adapted plate held in position by an appropriate instrument, drill holes are placed in the plate slots to either activate compression or position the screw

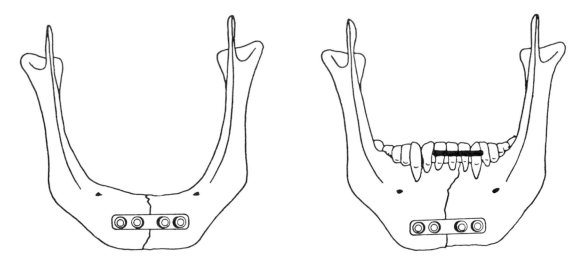

FIG. 5–69.   Fractures in the symphyseal area. In the symphyseal area, DCP is preferred to the EDCP system to prevent overriding of the thin alveolar process. Tension band protection with arch bars is desirable if teeth are present.

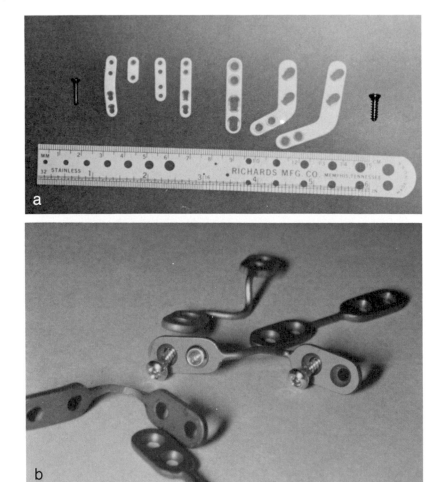

FIG. 5–70.   An example of plates in an osteosynthesis system. **a,** Various sizes and shapes of miniplates and standard plates in the Richards system. **b,** Adaptable miniplates in the Hall Reconstructive Systems that use spline recessed screws.

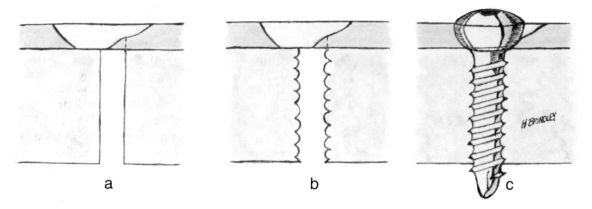

FIG. 5–71.   Steps in placing an osteosynthesis screw. To provide compression, the holes are drilled to place the screw head on the slope of the slot. **a,** Pilot drill hole of small diameter. **b,** Tapping the pilot hole. **c,** Insertion of the screw.

statically. A drill guide will properly orient the drill hole within the slot. The size of the drill corresponds to the core diameter of the screw shaft. The hole is tapped so that the tapping device just penetrates the medial cortex, and a depth gauge is used to measure the length of screw necessary to engage and slightly penetrate the medial cortex. The proximal screws are placed, moving from the proximal to the distal end of the plate, then tightened loosely. The horizontal compression screws are tightened first, then the transverse compression screws, and finally the neutral or sliding-slot screws (Fig. 5–73). It is important not to leave in place any loose or stripped-out screws, for they could be the nidus of an infection; these screws should be left out entirely or replaced with an emergency screw that has a slightly larger thread diameter.

A universally encountered problem with the application of any bone plate is the accurate retention of the fracture in a reduced position long enough to apply the fracture plates. Oblique fractures can be retained with a large penetrating towel clip or transosseous

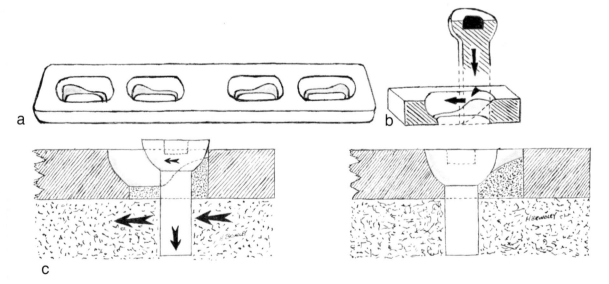

FIG. 5–72.   The mechanism of a DCP. **a,** The Synthes DCP with four compression slots. **b,** The slots are designed to produce an inclined plane surface that with tightening directs a screw head toward the apex. **c,** As the hemispherical screw is tightened, the attached bone moves in the same direction as the screw, thus compressing the fracture site.

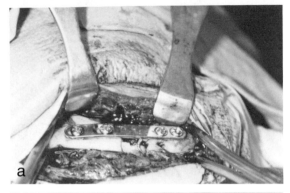

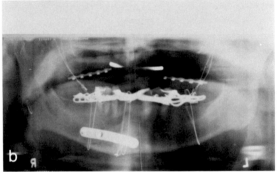

FIG. 5–73. Application of a compression plate to a comminuted midbody mandibular fracture. **a,** Direct transosseous wires or lag screws can help unite comminuted segments; however, excessive elevation of the periosteum must be avoided lest the segments become devitalized. **b,** Tension band protection is produced when the patient's removable partial denture is used as a splint.

wiring with the teeth in light fixation elastics. Occasionally, a single lag screw can be placed to stabilize the oblique fracture long enough to apply a bone plate inferiorly to the lag screw. One system employs a modified bone-holding forceps with a locking bar attachment that adequately holds the fracture segments in position (Fig. 5–74). This system is not applicable for intraoral application of plates, however. Synthes uses reduction compression pliers, which screw into the outer cortex of both segments. Preloading compression is applied to the fracture using tightening clamp and lateral pressure rollers, which further enhances the adaptation and stability (Fig. 5–74). This device can be used with either intraoral or extraoral approaches.

Synthes adopted the ASIF philosophy that advocates the removal of all devices after the fracture has healed. Any advantages of DCP or EDCP would be offset by the need for two operations, one for the placement of the device and another for its removal. In the U.S., most maxillofacial bone plates are not removed. It is safe to assume that the larger the device, the more likely that it must be removed to prevent interference with dentures, dehiscence, remodeling of the bone, and infection. Certainly, when the appliance is close to the oral mucosa and hence the likelihood of intraoral inflammation is increased, removal of the appliance should be considered. If such devices are left in place, the patient should be informed that the removal of the appliance may be necessary at some time in the future. Overall, whether the appliances should or must be removed is still a matter of the surgeon's judgment.

Lag Screws

Lag screw osteosynthesis is designed to produce a stable junction of two bone fragments under compression with the aid of screws under tension.[33] Screws can be used alone for stabilization of a fracture or in conjunction with a compression plate system. It should be emphasized that lag screw osteosynthesis is a concept, rather than a specific device, because either osteosynthesis screws or special "lag" screws can be used to accomplish lag screw osteosynthesis. It is even conceivable that, if properly sized drill bits were available, any screw could be used to achieve lag screw osteosynthesis to secure fractures.

To achieve compression using lag screw technique, only the medial or deep segment must be engaged by the flutes of the screw. The portion of the screw toward the head and superficial or lateral to the fracture site does not engage the bone, thus allowing the medial segment, with tightening, to pull against the head of the screw on the outer cortex. Placing two or more lag screws in this manner not only compresses the segments tightly together but prevents rotational instability. The stability achieved may be adequate to preclude intermaxillary fixation.

To better understand the principle of lag screw osteosynthesis it is helpful to consider the structure of screws. A screw consists of a head that has a straight slot, a Phillips, or a

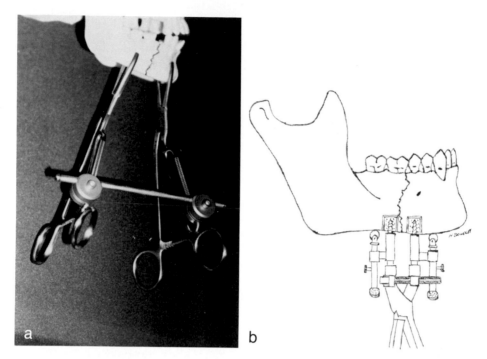

FIG. 5–74.   Reduction of fractures to aid in placing bone plates. **a,** In the Richards system, a modified bone forceps with locking bar attachments may be used. **b,** In the Synthes system, compression pliers may be employed.

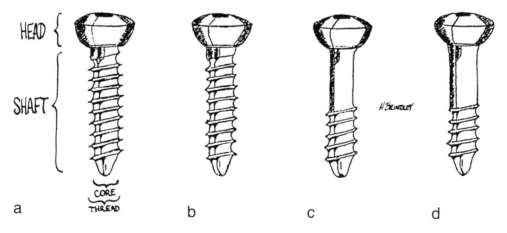

FIG. 5–75.   Details of lag screw utilization. **a,** Component parts of a bone screw. There is a larger difference in the core and thread diameters with osteosynthesis screws. **b,** A standard osteosynthesis screw requires that the outer segment of the fracture site be drilled to the thread diameter before it is used as a lag screw. **c,** Lag screws have a threadless core on the shaft below the head, which eliminates the need for drilling the outer segment of the fracture site to the thread diameter. **d,** A standard hardware lag screw has the upper shaft of the thread diameter, unlike the surgical screws discussed in this chapter.

hexagonal or other recess to accommodate a screw driver. The shaft of the screw consists of a core and threads (Fig. 5–75). Because the lag screws engage only the medial or inner segment, special lag screws are available with the upper shaft adjacent to the head devoid of threads.

In the osteosynthesis system, a pilot drill hole the size of the diameter of the shaft core is made (Fig. 5–76). Tapping the hole allows the screw to pass through the bone without lateral compression, thus preventing the early loosening that is seen in self-tapping screws. In comparison to self-tapping systems, lag osteosynthesis systems, which require tapping, reduce the likelihood of wedging apart at the fracture site if osteosynthesis screws are used. Screws that require tapping also reduce the likelihood of the breaking of fracture margins, as may occur with self-tapping screws. The thread diameter of the shaft of the screw is the same diameter as the gliding hole that is drilled in the outer segment to allow the screw threads to slide through without engaging the bone. The outer segment must remain aligned with the inner to avoid displacement when the screw of fixation is placed. A bevel is placed in the outer cortex for the head of the screw. The bevel is more important with less oblique fractures, as it tends to reduce pressure points in the cortex that can cause fracture. Placement of the screws follows the same basic principles as that of horizontal

mattress wiring in oblique fractures—the screw is oriented as nearly as possible at right angles to the fracture site. This orientation reduces the likelihood of fracturing the thin edges of the segments and prevents displacement as compression is achieved.

The preliminary preparation and the making of either intraoral or extraoral incisions are the same as for any open procedure. Using an open reduction approach, the fracture segments are reduced and retained in position. A core diameter drill hole is placed through the mandible at right angles to the line of fracture. The entire hole is then tapped until the tip of the tapping device perforates the medial cortex. The depth of the path of the tapping instrument should be measured, because there may be very little digital sensation of when it has passed through the medial cortical bone (Fig. 5–77).

If lag screws are to be used, an additional observation needs to be made; if the unthreaded portion of the shaft screw adjacent to the head is the same as the thread diameter, no additional change is necessary. If, however, the smooth shaft diameter is less than the threaded diameter (the core diameter), the outer segment hole should not be drilled out to form a gliding hole, because doing so would allow the outer segment to move while the screws were being seated. If the outer segment hole is not enlarged, the threads of the screws must not be engaged in the outer

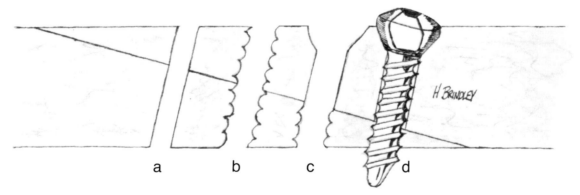

a   b   c   d

FIG. 7–76. Placement of osteosynthesis screw in a lag fashion. **a,** A pilot hole of the core diameter is placed as nearly perpendicular to the fracture as possible and is drilled through both segments. **b,** The entire hole is tapped to provide grooves in the bone exactly corresponding to the screw threads. **c,** The outer segment is drilled to the thread diameter to prevent wedging apart at the fracture interface. The external hole is countersunk to prevent fracturing from uneven pressures. **d,** The screw is placed, causing compression of the bone between the screw threads and the screw head.

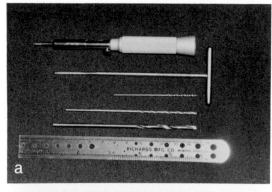

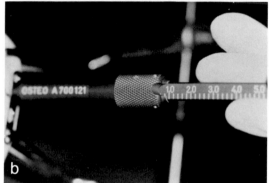

FIG. 5–77.   Devices used to place osteosynthesis screws. **a,** Various tapping instruments and pilot drills for screws. **b,** Depth gauge for determining proper screw length.

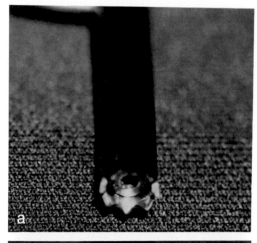

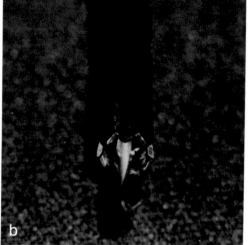

FIG. 5–79.   Protective trocars for percutaneous screw placement. **a,** Trocar with drill sleeve in place. **b,** Drilling through the trocar protects the soft tissue, prevents eccentric drill holes, and reduces the chances of the drill bit's fracturing.

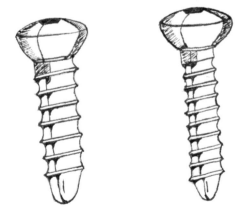

FIG. 5–78.   Emergency screw. The emergency screw (on the left) is compared to a standard osteosynthesis screw (on the right) for use as a self-tapping replacement of stripped-out bone screws.

segment or no compression will occur with tightening. This problem can be prevented by measuring the depth of the outer segment down to the fracture and comparing that measurement to the distance from the screw-head to the end of the unthreaded portion of the screw shaft. The distance of the screw should be equal to or greater than the outer bone segment width. If a gliding hole is indicated, it is prepared in the cortex down to the fracture site with a drill the size of the thread diameter. The entire hole is measured with a depth gauge to determine the length of the screw required to penetrate the medial cortex. Using a countersink-recessing tool, the outer cortex adjacent to the gliding hole is beveled in the long axis of the hole to allow the head of the screw to rest evenly on bone on all sides when seated. After all preparatory procedures are completed, the screw is inserted and tightened into the position.

Occasionally, if the tapping device penetrates too far past the medial cortex or if screws are overtightened, they can strip out the hole, causing loss of retention and compression. In such instances so-called emergency screws are available in some systems with slightly larger core and thread diameters with flutes or threads that are wider apart (Fig. 5–78). These can be inserted as self-tapping screws to provide stability. Also, intermaxillary fixation and a direct transosseous wiring type of procedure could be substituted.

The most widely used application for lag screw osteosynthesis is in oblique fractures of the mandible. Generally, the more oblique the fracture, the easier it is to use lag screws without the need of compression plating. Similarly, the less oblique the fracture is, the more likely the need for compression plates. Lag screws can be used in comminuted fractures to join fragments into larger fragments that can be stabilized by compression plates. Lag screws can be employed from an intraoral approach to stabilize posterior body or anterior ramus fractures that are accessible intraorally, or, when necessary, extraorally. A percutaneous approach may be used through small skin incisions and protective trocars inserted to accommodate the passage of instruments (Fig. 5–79).

REFERENCES

1. Rosenberg, F.A., DiStefano, J.F., and Byers, S.S.: Adhesive bonding of arch bars for maxillomandibular fixation. J Oral Surg 34:651, 1976.
2. Thoma, K.H.: Treatment of jaw fractures, past and present. J Oral Surg 17:5, 1959.
3. Oliver, R.T.: A method of treating mandibular fractures. JAMA 54:1187, 1910.
4. Lemons, J.E., and Alling, C.C. Considerations on prestretching metallic wires. J Oral Surg 35:237, 1977.
5. Lemons, J.E.: Personal communications, 1979 and 1986.
6. Gilmer, T.L.: A case of fracture of the lower jaw with remarks on treatment. Arch Dent 4:388, 1887.
7. Eby, J.D.: Intermaxillary wiring. Nat Dent Assoc J 7:771, 1920.
8. Ivy, R.H., and Curtis, L.: Fractures of the Jaws. Philadelphia, Lea & Febiger, 1938, p.60.
9. Stout, R.A.: Intramaxillary wiring and intermaxillary elastic traction and fixation. In Manual of Standard Practice of Plastic and Maxillofacial Surgery. Military Surgical Manuals, I. Philadelphia, W.B. Saunders, 1943, p.272.
10. Rowe, N.I., and Killey, H.C.: Fractures of the Facial Skeleton. Baltimore, Williams and Wilkins, 1955, p.83.
11. Risdon, F.: The treatment of fractures of the jaws. Can Med Assoc J 20:260, 1929.
12. Kazanjian, V.H.: Treatment of automobile injuries of the face and jaws. J Am Dent Assoc 20:757, 1933.
13. Schwartz, L.L. The development of the treatment of jaw fractures. Oral Surg 2:193, 1944.
14. Schwartz, L.L.: James Baxton Bean (1834–1870). Ann Dent 4:167, 1946.
15. Gunning, T.B.: The treatment of fractures of the lower jaw by interdental splints. NY Med J 3:433, 1866–67.
16. Wessberg, G.A., and Epker, B.N.: Intraoral skeletal fixation appliance. J Oral Maxillofac Surg 40:827, 1982.
17. DalPont, G.: A new method of intermaxillary bone fixation. In Oral Surgery. Edited by E. Husted and E. Hjørting-Hansen, Trnas. 2nd Congress of the International Association of Oral Surgeons. Copenhagen, Munksgaard, 1967, p.325.
18. Allen, N.: Personal communications, 1969 through 1986.
19. Wessbeg, G.A., Schendel, S.A., and Epker, B.N.: Monophase extraskeletal fixation. J Oral Surg 37:892, 1979.
20. Morris, J.H.: Biphasic connector, external skeletal splint for reduction and fixation of mandibular fractures. Oral Surg 2:1382, 1949.
21. Crawford, M.J.: Appliances and attachments for treatment of upper jaw fractures. Nav Med Bul 41:1151, 1943.
22. Crewe, T.C.: A halo frame for facial injuries. Br J Oral Surg 4:147, 1966.
23. Irby, W.B.: Extracranial fixation of the facial skeleton. J Oral Surg 27:900, 1969.
24. Morris, J.H.: Surgical roundtable. Am Assoc of Oral and Maxillofac Surgeons, Annual Scientific Sessions, 1981.
25. Recommended practices for surface preparation and marking of metallic surgical implants. Am Soc for Testing Materials, Annual Book of Standards. Philadelphia. ASTMF 86–75, 13.01: 16–16.
26. Winter, L.: Operative oral surgery. St. Louis, C.V. Mosby, 1947, p.724.
27. Spiessl, B.: New concepts in maxillofacial bone surgery. New York, Springer-Verlag, 1976.
28. Schwimmer, A.M., and Greenberg, A.M.: Management of mandibular trauma with rigid internal fixation. Oral Surg 62:630, 1986.
29. Schmoker, R., von Allman, G., and Tschopp, H.M.: Application of functionally stable fixation in maxil-

lofacial surgery according to the ASIF principles. J Oral Maxillofac Surg 40:457, 1982.

30. Müller, M.E., Allgöwer, M., and Willenegger, W.: Handbook of Osteosynthesis. Berlin, Springer-Verlag, 1969.

31. Schilli, W.: Compression plate osteosynthesis through the ASIF system. *In* Oral and Maxillofacial Traumatology. Edited by K. Kruger and W. Schilli.

Chicago, Quintessence Publishing Co., Inc., 1982, p.349.

32. Perren, S.M., et al.: A dynamic compression plate. Acta Orthop Scand (Suppl) 125:29, 1969.

33. Neiderdellmann, J.: Rigid internal fixation by means of lag screws. *In* Oral and Maxillofacial Traumatology. Edited by E. Kruger and W. Schilli. Chicago, Quintessence Publishing Co., Inc., 1982, p.371.

6

MANDIBULAR FRACTURES

CHARLES C. ALLING III

ETIOLOGY

Fractures of the mandible occur more frequently than fractures of the other facial bones, making up approximately two thirds of all maxillofacial fractures. Although the mandible is dense and strong, because it occupies the prominent peripheral position around the lower third of the facial skeleton it is exposed to frequent trauma. The majority of mandibular fractures are the result of external violence—altercations, vehicular accidents, gunshot and missile wounds, industrial accidents, and sports trauma. A few fractures of the mandible are secondary to surgical procedures such as third molar surgery.[1] Central lesions in the mandible, for example, odontogenic cysts and tumors, mandibular manifestations of general systemic diseases, and osteomyelitic destruction of segments of the mandible, predispose to fracture.

The dynamic forces that cause injuries may vary in intensity and direction. The intensity of the blow determines the severity and the degree of displacement of the fractures; the direction of the blow and the surface area of the traumatizing object influence the location of the fracture sites.

Many factors intrinsic to the mandible determine its reaction to the dynamic forces. The state of contraction or relaxation and the vectors of the major and accessory muscles of mastication and other factors influence the production of a fracture and the displacement of the segments. The susceptibility to fracture may vary with the age of the individual; a child may experience severe trauma with little resultant injury, whereas an older individual may incur severe fractures from relatively minor trauma. The presence of teeth, especially impacted teeth, reduces the density of bone in an area and increases the possibility of fracture. Fractures may occur owing to weakening of the bone by pathologic conditions and systemic diseases such as the reticuloendothelial diseases, Paget's disease, osteomalacia, and osteogenesis imperfecta, as well as local disorders such as fibrous dysplasia, tumors, cysts, osteomyelitis, and osteoradionecrosis. Areas of intrinsic anatomic weaknesses are classified in the following section.

The type of mandibular fractures incurred in any group is influenced by variables such as the conditions in which the population group lives and the group's socioeconomic background. For example, the facial injuries incurred by a primitive agrarian population would be quite different from those in a mobile industrial group, and both would be different from the injuries incurred in the military; further, troops in training would be expected to have different fracture patterns than those in combat.[2,3]

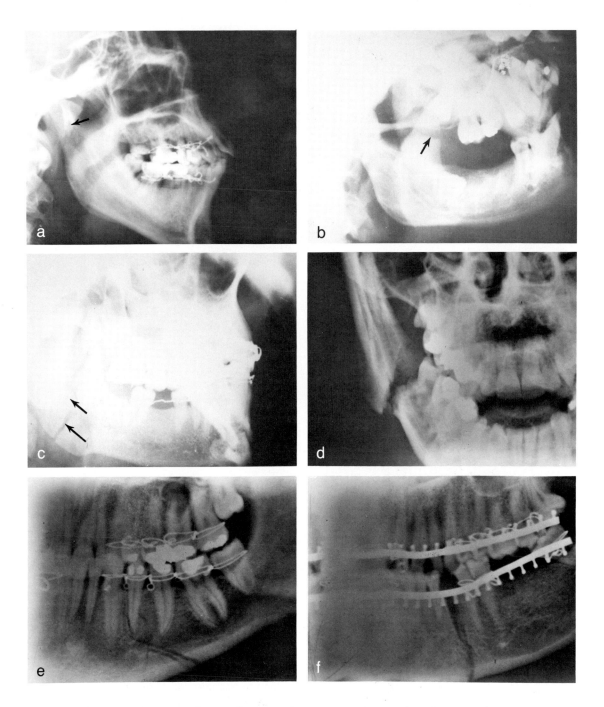

FIG. 6–1. Fractures of the mandible. **a,** Fracture of condylar neck (arrow). **b,** Fracture of coronoid process (arrow). **c,** Fracture of ramus of mandible (arrows). **d,** Fracture of angle of mandible. **e,** Fracture of body of mandible. **f,** Fracture of parasymphysis area of mandible.

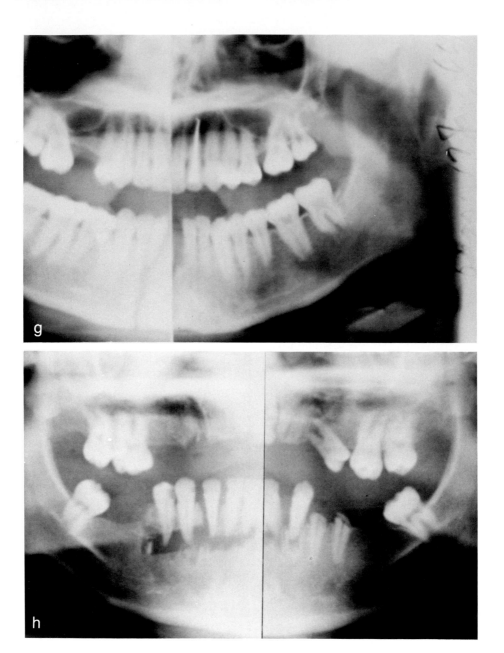

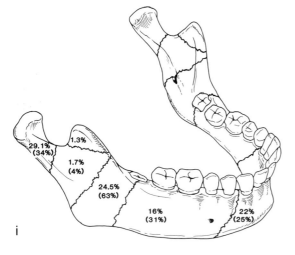

FIG. 6–1 (continued).   **g,** Fracture of symphyseal area of mandible (arrow). **h,** Fracture of alveolar process of mandible as well as dental fractures and avulsion of teeth. **i,** Diagram of anatomic distribution of fractures. The distribution of fractures for a civilian population is contrasted with those, in parentheses, of a military population. The civilian group had 3.0% of the fractures in the alveolar process. The military group does not include patients with fractures incurred by missiles. (Modified from Olson, R.A. et al.[1] and Chipps, J.E., et al.[2])

CLASSIFICATION

LOCATION

The logical classification of mandibular fractures is based on the anatomic location of the fracture (Fig. 6–1). This classification includes fractures, singly or in combinations, of the condyle, condylar neck, condylar process, ramus of the mandible, angle of the mandible, coronoid process, body of the mandible, area of the canine tooth, symphysis area, and alveolar process.

Condylar fractures are fractures of either the condyle or the most superior aspect of the condylar neck and are confined to the intracapsular area. In condylar neck fractures, the fracture line extends posteriorly from various locations on the condylar neck and crosses at the posterior border of the mandible at a location above the general level at the inferior alveolar foramen. In condylar process fractures, the fracture line passes from the mandibular (sigmoid) notch and extends posteriorly or posteroinferiorly. In ramus of the mandible fractures, the fracture extends from the anterior border of the ramus posteriorly to areas at or superior to the gonial angle of the mandible. In angle of the mandible fractures, the fracture extends from the second or third molar tooth area to the base of the mandible between the angle and the premasseteric notch. In body of the mandible fractures, the fracture occurs between the premasseteric notch and the region of the canine (cuspid) tooth. In fractures of the symphysis area, the fracture occurs in the area between the mandibular canine teeth. In fractures of the alveolar process, the fracture involves the bony structures above the general level of the mental foramina.

SEVERITY

Fractures may also be classified according to their severity (Fig. 6–2). In closed or simple fractures, the fracture is complete and the soft tissues may be damaged, but there is no open wound contiguous to the cutaneous surfaces or to the oral cavity. In open or compound fractures a break in the covering soft tissues produces an extraoral or intraoral wound continuous with the fracture line. All mandibular fractures that occur in the region of the teeth are compounded, or open, into the oral cavity. The fracture may occur through a tooth alveolus or extend from the apex of the socket to the base of the mandible.

In comminuted fractures the bone is splintered or crushed and more than one fracture line exists. These fractures may be closed or open. In greenstick fractures, one side of the cortex is broken and the other bent. This fracture often occurs in the neck of the condyle. In complex fractures, bony injuries may be complicated by fractures of teeth, injury of the neurovascular structures of the mandible and oral cavity, or severe trauma to the contiguous oral or facial soft tissues. Nerve injury is a frequent complication. Injury of blood vessels may cause hemorrhage and hematomas between the bony fragments. Infection is a threat in complex fractures and may result in an acute or chronic osteomyelitis. Fractures in children may be complicated by the presence of mixed deciduous and developing permanent teeth.

Finally, in impacted or compression fractures, the fragments of the fracture are driven firmly together in close interdigitation.

SECONDARY DISPLACEMENT

Fry and his associates classified fractures of the mandible as favorable or unfavorable depending on the probability of secondary displacement as influenced by the angulation of the fracture and the anticipated displacement resulting form muscular pull.[4] This classification is useful in helping to determine details of treatment planning.

ANATOMIC CONSIDERATIONS

BONES

The body of the mandible, usually a strong bone with a heavy cortical inferior rim, has certain areas of weakness that tend to fracture more readily. The ramus of the mandible has two thin plates of cortical bone that are separated by a narrow portion of cancellous bone of varying thickness; in some areas only one

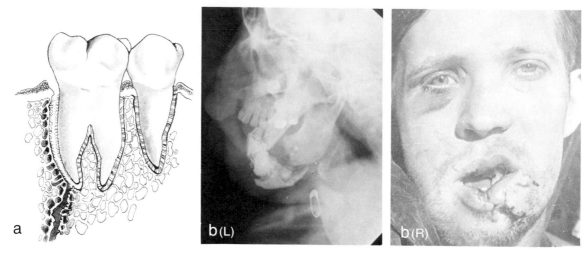

FIG. 6–2. Types of mandibular fractures. **a,** Diagram of fracture through an alveolus. **b L** and **R,** Compound, comminuted, complex fractures of the mandible. (Fig. 6–2b L courtesy of Letterman General Hospital Photographic Laboratory.) **c,** Closed fracture of mandible. **d,** Impending fracture caused by unstable implant device.

sheet of cortical bone and no cancellous bone is present. Because the body of the mandible is considerably thicker than the ramus, the junction of body and ramus is structurally weak, especially when a third molar is present. The alveolus is weaker than the rest of the mandible and may fracture independently from the body of the mandible. Other areas of weakness are the symphyseal region medial to canine teeth and the thin neck of the mandibular condyle.

MUSCLES (Fig. 6–3)

Understanding the function of the intricate musculature attached to the mandible is important in the diagnosis and treatment of fractures of this bone. The movement of the mandible depends primarily on three groups of muscles: the elevating, the depressing, and the rotating groups of muscles. Generally, the mandible is influenced by the depressing as well as the secondary rotating groups of muscles; the ramus is influenced by the elevating and primary rotating groups of muscles.

Elevating Muscles

The masseter muscle extends from the zygomatic arch to the lateral surface and angle of the mandibular ramus. Deep and superfi-

cial portions have the deeper fibers running vertically and the superficial fibers passing inferiorly and posteriorly. The masseter muscle is a main force in closing or elevating the mandible.

The temporalis muscle arises in a fan shape from the inferior temporal line of the temporal bone, descends medially to the zygomatic arch, and inserts on the lateral and medial surface of the coronoid process. The temporalis muscle retracts and rotates the mandible in addition to elevating it.

The medial pterygoid muscle originates from the pterygoid fossa of the sphenoid bone, the pyramidal process of the palatine bone, and adjacent parts of the maxillary tuberosity; it inserts on the medial surface of the ramus and the angle of the mandible, protruding and elevating the mandible.

Rotating Muscles

The lateral pterygoid muscle has at least two origins: the upper head, attached to the wing of the sphenoid bone, and the lower head, attached to the outer surface of the lateral plate of the pterygoid process and to the posterior tuberosity area of the maxilla. The fibers insert onto the anterior surface of the neck of the mandibular condyle. Functioning together, the left and right lateral pterygoid

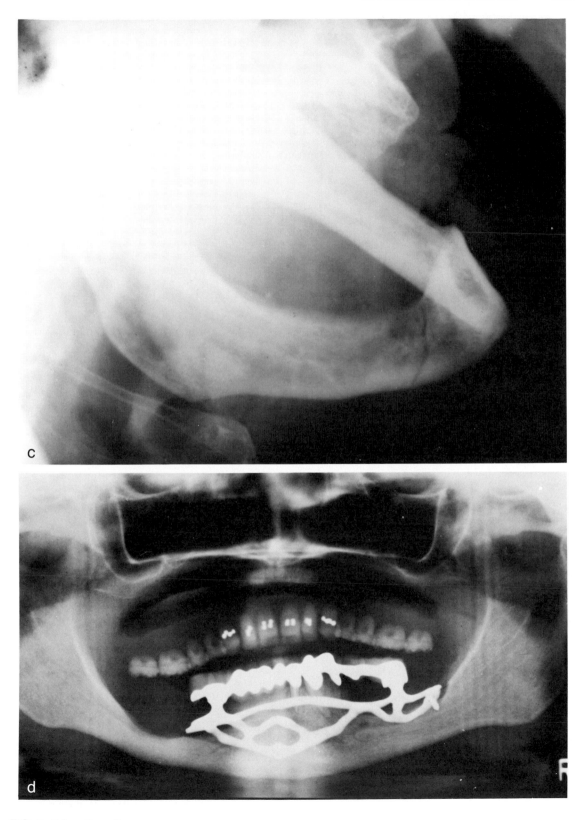

FIG. 6–2 (continued).

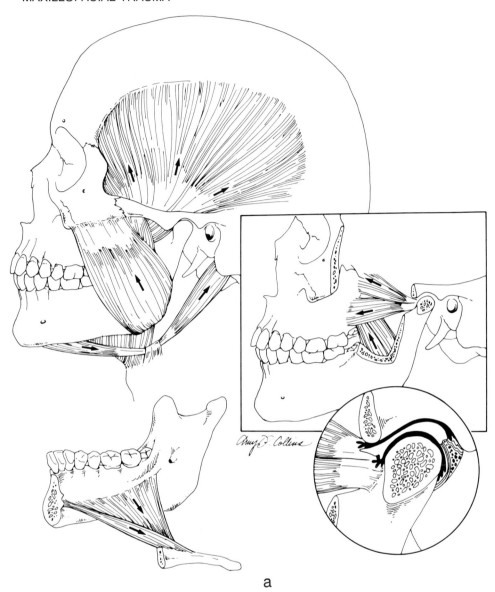

a

FIG. 6–3. Influence of muscles of masticaton on mandibular fracture displacement. **a,** Diagrams of the major and some of the accessory muscles of mastication.

muscles protrude the mandible, and functioning unilaterally they rotate the mandible. A portion of the upper head, the sphenomeniscus muscle, inserts into the articular disc of the temporomandibular joint and stabilizes the meniscus in opposition to the posterior meniscus bilaminar zone fibers during the sliding, translatory, and rotating movements of the condylar head.

The second mandibular rotating muscle, the temporalis muscle, works using its horizontal fibers.

By understanding the muscular vectors, one may predict the displacements of unfa-

vorable fractures. For example, with a fracture of the third molar region, a secondary displacement of the ramus may occur; the masseter, medial pterygoid, and temporal muscles will pull the proximal fragment upward, while the lateral pterygoid muscle will move the ramus forward and, in combination with the medial pterygoid muscle, cause an inward displacement.

Depressing Muscles and the Genioglossus Muscle

The muscles originating from the inner aspect of the mandible, the geniohyoid, the di-

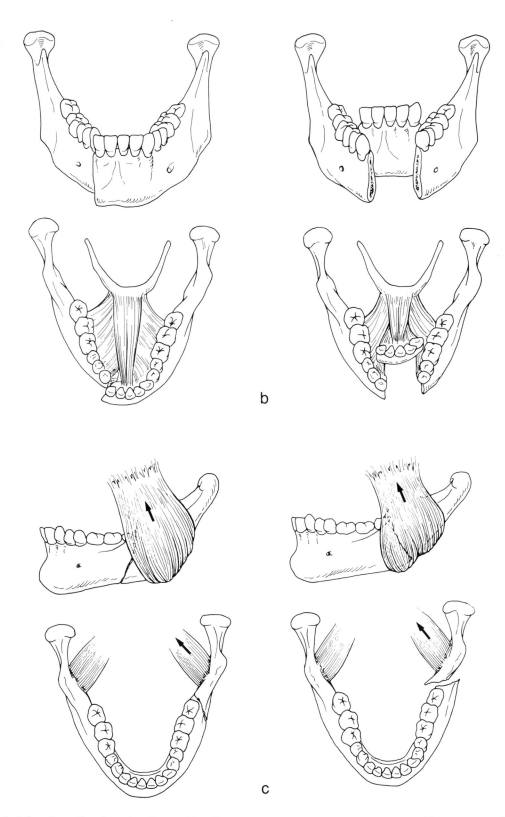

FIG. 6–3 (continued).   **b** and **c,** Favorable alignments and unfavorable alignments of fractures as affected by possible secondary displacements by muscles of mastication.

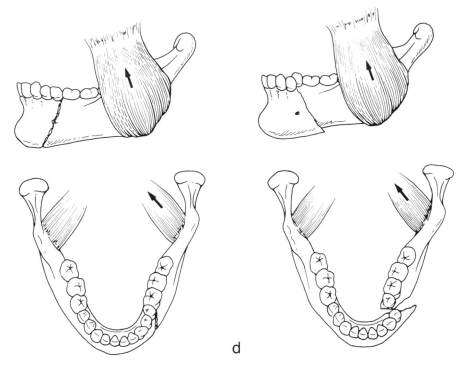

d

FIG. 6–3 (continued). **d,** Favorable alignments and unfavorable alignments of fractures as affected by possible secondary displacements by muscles of mastication.

gastric, the genioglossus, and the mylohyoid, exert a centripetal effect and tend to cause anterior segments to collapse in a posterior or medial direction. The group of muscles exerts a downward and posterior force that, in most cases, is a weaker force than that produced by the elevator muscles.

The geniohyoid muscle arises from the inner anterior border of the mandible at the inferior genial tubercle and inserts into the body of the hyoid bone.

The digastric muscle consists of two parts: an anterior belly and a posterior belly. The posterior belly arises form the mastoid notch, medial to the mastoid process, and passes downward and forward, forming an obtuse angle with the anterior belly through a fascial sling above the hyoid bone. The intermediate tendon between the anterior and posterior bellies slides through the fascial sling. The anterior belly arises from the intermediate tendon and inserts into the digastric fossa of the mandible at its lower border, close to the midline. The digastric muscles, acting independently, help rotate the mandible.

The mylohyoid muscle supports the floor of the mouth and elevates the tongue. Also, in combination with the other depressor muscles, it may effect the downward and inward pull of lateral segments when the hyoid bone is fixed by the infrahyoid group of muscles.

The genioglossus muscle arises from the superior genial tubercle on the inner anterior border of the mandible and passes posteriorly to become the major extrinsic muscle of the tongue. If bilateral parasymphyseal fractures occur, the tongue may fall posteriorly, obstructing the upper airway.

TEETH

Teeth, particularly the cuspid and the third molar teeth, may be a source of weakness and predispose an area to fracture; furthermore, impacted or unerupted third molar teeth increase the structural weakness of the mandible. Because using the teeth to support fracture appliances and align the maxillofacial skeleton is a fundamental consideration in the treatment of maxillofacial injuries, careful examination should include the number of teeth present and their relationship to fracture lines; whether the teeth are firmly attached or were loosened by the injury; the presence or absence of periodontal disease; the presence or absence of periapical lesions; and the general integrity of the coronal portions.

Perfect articulation is not present in all individuals, a crossbite relationship, prognathism, micrognathism, retrognathism, apertognathism, (open bite), or other unusual articulations may be normal for particular patients. The wear facets of the teeth can aid in establishing the proper articulation. The occlusion that is normal for the patient must be established, because an error in reduction may lead to serious derangement of the occlusion of the teeth with a corresponding impairment of masticatory efficiency and a progressive cycle of deterioration of the delicate neuromuscular and skeletal balances necessary for health of the maxillofacial area. *The return of function*, and not simply the union of the fragments, is the basic objective of treatment.

PERIOSTEUM

The mandible is covered with periosteum and mucoperiosteum. An intact periosteum usually decreases secondary displacement of fragments. Tearing of the periosteum or mucoperiosteum usually results in either ecchymosis in the buccal sulcus or a sublingual hematoma.

DIAGNOSIS

The possibility of mandibular fracture should be considered in every patient who has suffered an injury to the head or face. Not unusually, a fracture of the mandible remains undetected for a period of hours or days while attention is directed to injury in some other area of the body. The oral surgeon must consider the overall condition of the patient and not concentrate on the fracture of the mandible to the exclusion of the patient as a whole. (See Chapter 2.) A systematic, organized approach includes noting the patient's condition on admission, taking a history of the injury, performing a physical examination

and selected medical laboratory tests, and obtaining indicated radiographic examinations.

CONDITION ON ADMISSION

The immediate condition of the patient and the presence or absence of serious injuries are of prime concern. Detailed examination should be deferred until the patency of the airway and control of hemorrhage are assured. Present or impending shock should be assessed, and treated. The patient's mental condition should be classified as clear, confused, or disoriented. The level of consciousness should be assessed as stuporous (the patient is capable of being aroused but lapses into unconsciousness); comatose (the patient is incapable of being aroused); or declining.

During this phase the most qualified person should perform a thorough medical examination, including assessment for neurologic, abdominal, and orthopedic injuries. An audiogram may be indicated to establish if the ossicles of the ear or other auditory structures have been damaged.

HISTORY

A detailed history should be obtained from the patient or a responsible individual and be recorded as soon as possible. If the patient is rational and cooperative, the history can be obtained while the general condition is being evaluated. If the patient is unable to give the history, a relative, friend, or reliable witness should be used. Details of the accidents should be noted, i.e., the date and time of injury, the injuring agent, the direction of the force, and the condition and level of consciousness of the patient before and after the injury, with special regard to use of alcohol, drugs, and medicine that may have altered the sensorium. If the injury resulted from an automobile accident, it may be useful to know the position of the patient and whether air bags, seat belts, and shoulder belts were used.

Information should be obtained regarding the degree and duration of the loss of consciousness, which may indicate the severity of cerebral damage. The occurrence of vomiting, hemorrhage, and subjective symptoms should be noted. If the patient has been admitted or treated at another hospital, treatment and medications should be noted and recorded. If possible, a history to determine past illnesses, current medical therapy, or the presence of allergies and drug sensitivities should be obtained at this time.

DIRECTION OF FORCE

The direction and force of a blow to the mandible determines the type and location of the fracture or fractures. A direct blow to one side of the mandible often produces a fracture on the opposite side; for example, a blow to the mental area on one side may result in a fracture at the site of the trauma and also, when the mandible is forced toward the opposite side, a second fracture at the opposite angle or in the condylar area. Because the lingual plate of bone is thin in the angle region and there is a divergence of the ramus from the body, the mandible tends to be driven backward and medially, with a fracture through the lingual plate extending anteriorly and laterally to pass behind or around the alveolus of the third molar.

Crushing of the mandible from the side may occasionally cause a compression fracture in the symphysis because of tension of the outer plate. A direct blow to the symphysis from the anterior may force the angles outward, thereby placing the inner plate of the bone under tension, resulting in fracture at the symphysis and fractures of the necks of the condyle or the angles of the mandible.

PHYSICAL EXAMINATION

Depending on the degree and extent of injury, the initial clinical findings in fractures of the mandible may vary considerably. The examination should be performed systematically by dividing the techniques of examination into extraoral and intraoral phases.

Inspection

Inspection is made for edema, ecchymosis, and deformity in the region of the fracture. The escape of blood into the soft tissue adjacent to the fracture results in swelling and facial asymmetry. The overlying tissues become red or bluish because of hemorrhage and the formation of the hematoma near the site of the fracture. The overall symmetry of the face may be deformed because of displacement of mandibular fragments, and depending on the degree of the displacement, the appearance of the lower face may be radically changed. The patient may drool bloody saliva as a result of stimulation of salivary glands from pain and foreign materials and the inability of the patient to swallow the excess saliva.

The intraoral examination may reveal a number of conditions that will aid in the diagnosis of fracture of the mandible. For instance, the patient may have offensive breath from the multiplication of pathogenic and saprophytic organisms thriving in putrified food, blood clots, and mucus. The buccal and lingual sulci are inspected for the presence of ecchymosis, tears in the mucosa, and hemorrhage. A malalignment of the teeth with step defects of the occlusal plane may indicate fractured fragments. Because overriding of fragments is likely to occur in the regions of the symphysis and the angle of the mandible, the displacement may be in a horizontal or vertical direction. All remaining teeth and alveolar ridges should be inspected and palpated to determine if fractures, extensive caries, or periodontal disease is present. If the patient exhibits an abnormal occlusion, the facets of the teeth are inspected carefully to determine the occlusion prior to the injury. Because there may be considerable bloody saliva or dried blood on the teeth, irrigation and suctioning may be necessary to complete this portion of the examination.

Palpation

The areas of the face overlying the mandible should be palpated bimanually, beginning with the condylar area and proceeding down over the mandible, noting any areas of tenderness or abnormal contour. The patient should open and close the mouth, and any pain from this movement should be noted, as should pain accompanying speaking or swallowing. Abnormal mobility may be present if a fracture is unilateral; the mandible will shift toward the fracture side when the patient attempts to open the mouth. This mobility becomes more pronounced on protrusive motions, with the mandible shifting to the side of the injury. During these movements, crepitation may be present, with a cracking or grinding sound or sensation as the fragments move in contact.

Because a fracture of the body of the mandible breaks the continuity of the bone, it results in rupture or damage to the inferior alveolar neurovascular bundle contained within the inferior alveolar canal. This damage usually causes anesthesia of the mental distribution over the lower lip. The buccal and lingual sulci should be palpated to determine any discrepancxy or areas of tenderness. If no displacement is obvious, the doctor can examine the patient manually by placing the forefingers of each hand on the mandibular teeth and the thumbs below the jaw. Starting in either retromolar area, the fingers, kept 4 or 5 teeth apart, are moved around the arch, and an alternate up-and-down motion with each hand is used to ascertain any abnormal movements or crepitus. The anterior border of the ramus and the coronoid process are palpated intraorally.

Damage to the teeth may occur in conjunction with fractures of the mandible, with the anterior teeth involved most commonly. (See Chapter 11.) The cusps of premolar and molar teeth are often sheared off, with resultant pulp exposure that may cause considerable discomfort to the patient during the period of immobilization; therefore, a pulp exposure should be capped with a protective dressing, the pulp should be extirpated and palliative endodontia instituted, or the tooth should be removed prior to fixation. Whenever possible, fragments of teeth should be removed at the time of reduction unless this removal will result in the extensive loss of alveolar bone. Teeth in the line of fracture may aid in the stabilization of the fragments; for example, maintenance of a tooth or portion of a tooth may prevent dislocation of a proximal fragment and obviate the need for open reduction. If, however, the oral and maxillofacial surgeon judges a tooth in or near a line of fracture likely to cause a complication, the tooth should be removed.

RADIOGRAPHIC EXAMINATION

A variety of radiographic views, including periapical, occlusal, extraoral, and panoramic, are used singly or in combination to make a radiographic diagnosis of a mandibular fracture (Fig. 6–4). Computed tomographic (CT) surveys may be helpful for assessing intracapsular condylar fractures. A panoramic radiograph, if available, can be used as an initial screening film, and specific radiographs can be ordered as needed. Panoramic radiographs are laminagraphic, however, and, as in the case of a shearing fracture, the cortical fracture lines may be in a plane that will not be displayed.

After a tentative diagnosis of a fracture has been made, radiographs should be obtained in two planes—a projection for viewing inferior and superior displacement, and a projection for viewing medial and lateral displacement.

Fractures of the Symphysis Area

When a fracture in the symphysis area of the mandible is suspected, the most reliably diagnostic films are occlusal radiographs. One occlusal film should be taken at a 55° angle to the occlusal plane, and a second film should be taken with the central ray directly perpendicular to the film. In PA views of the mandible, fracture lines in the symphysis area may not be clear because of superimposition of the cervical vertebrae; a slight rotation of the head, however, will move the symphysis lateral to the spinal column and permit a diagnostic projection. Because the usual lateral oblique films hence show a distorted view of the symphysis area, a modification of the lateral oblique view, an anterior body of the mandible projection, should be obtained. Periapical films may not show the inferior border of the mandible but will be useful for detailed examinations of the relation of fracture line to the dentition.

Fractures of the Body, Angle, and Ramus

Panoramic radiographs are useful as an initial film and, often, for definitive interpretation of body of the mandible fractures; their

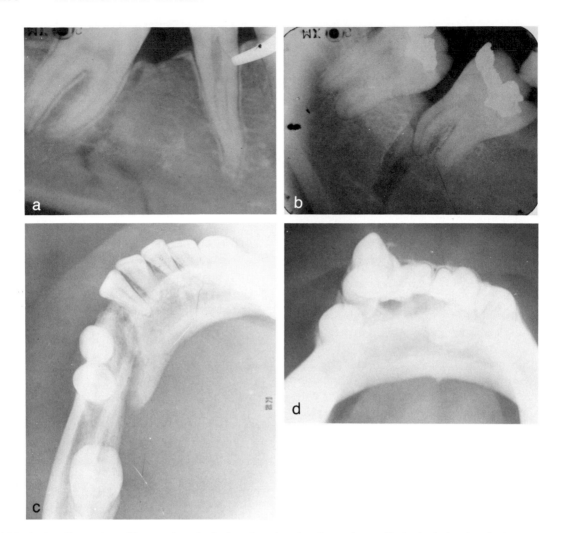

FIG. 6–4.   Examples of intraoral periapical and occlusal radiographs. **a,** Periapical view in which the molar tooth is not involved in the fracture line. **b,** Periapical view in which the tooth is clearly involved in the line of fracture. **c,** Occlusal radiograph displaying the posterior displacement of the anterior portion of the mandible caused by the suprahyoid musculature. **d,** Occlusal radiograph displaying an alveolar process fracture.

laminagraphic nature, however, may produce a thin view that, as in the case of a tangential fracture line, may not clearly demonstrate the fracture. Lateral oblique radiographs may show the fracture lines more clearly than panoramic radiographs. Occasionally, a single fracture may produce two discontinuity radiographic images as a result of breaks in the medial and lateral cortices. An occlusal film or PA film will clarify whether there are two fractures or whether a single fracture is being registered on the film. Also, occlusal views will show medial and lateral displacements of the fractured segments. Periapical radiographs are useful in determining the details of involvement of teeth in the lines of fracture.

Fractures of the Condylar Region

Fractures through the head of the condyle (intracapsular fractures) may be difficult to interpret with radiographs. Laminagraphs from a lateral projection and CT studies are helpful for viewing this region. These views will show the head of the condyle and its relationship to the glenoid fossa or the cranial fossa with great clarity.

Fractures through the neck of the condyle (extracapsular fractures) are quite common and unless suspected by history and clinical examination are sometimes not diagnosed. Generally, PA skull films obscure the condyle because the overlap of the mastoid process makes fractures difficult to visualize. Radiographs of diagnostic value for frontal or posterior views of fractures of the neck of the condyle are the Towne's AP and PA projections. For lateral views, in many patients, panoramic radiographs with special adjustments to show the temporomandibular joint area will disclose details of the condylar area. The usual lateral oblique films may produce a superimposition of the cervical vertebrae and structures of the neck, which can be partially avoided by extending the mandible forward. The lateral oblique projection may be modified to emphasize the ramus to show the neck of the condyle fractures. Transpharyngeal views, mouth open and closed, are extremely helpful for visualizing fracture lines of the ramus and the condylar necks although the injuries may limit mandibular movements. Temporomandibular joint series that are often used to assess the characteristics of the condylar head in degenerative arthritis and similar conditions may not be diagnostic for the fractures of the condylar head and neck, because the angle of the central ray may not pass through the fracture line and the diameter of the area exposed may be too small to include the fracture lines in the neck of the mandible.

Special views to depict concomitant injuries will be ordered by appropriate members of the total team; fractures of the cervical spine must be considered.

Commonly Used Views

The Periapical Views. The small dental intraoral films deliver high-definition views and are of particular value in assessing the condition of the dentition and the relationship of the fracture lines to the dental alveoli. These views are important in deciding whether teeth are involved in the fracture line and de-

termining the extent of periapical pathology that existed prior to the injury.

The Occlusal Views. These are extremely useful in fractures of the symphysis and body of the mandible areas to determine the degree of overriding and displacement. Occlusal views may also be taken in various angulations to exaggerate a fracture line that may exhibit minimal displacement on the 90° occlusal view.

The Panoramic View. This view displays the mandible in its entirety on one film. Special radiographic equipment in addition to the ability of the patient to sit up without danger are necessary with most types of current equipment. This view, with modifications, will depict the mandible from condyle to condyle and the maxillae including the lower portions of the maxillary antra. Because panoramic radiographic views are laminagrams with only one plane, however, the plane of the cut may not demonstrate the fracture. The principal registration on the radiographic film plate is the cortical bone; if the plane of the bone that is displayed is through the medullary bone, the fracture line may be clearly registered on the film.

Lateral Oblique Views. The mandible is visualized from the first premolar to the condyle region in the lateral oblique views. By varying the position of the head, one can more clearly demonstrate a specific area in the anterior body, midbody, and ramus regions. Modifications of the lateral views that can be taken with dental or general medical radiographic equipment include views of the anterior body of the mandible, body of the mandible, posterior body and ramus of the mandible, and ramus or transpharynx.

Temporomandibular Articulation Views. The temporomandibular joint views that may be taken with dental or general medical radiographic equipment demonstrate the relationship of the head of the condyle to the articular surfaces of the glenoid fossa.

Posteroanterior View. The PA and AP views demonstrate the outline of the mandible, although the zygomatic bones and the mastoid processes may make distinguishing the condylar region difficult. The lateral orbital rim, in the area of the zygomatic frontal suture, must not be interpreted as the neck of the condyle. The lateral orbital rim may be mistakenly diagnosed as a medial displacement of the neck of the condyle.

The Towne's View. The Towne's view is used in suspected fractures of the condylar head and neck in which satisfactory definition cannot be obtained form the PA view. This view, however, falsely elongates the ascending ramus and the condylar neck.

Laminagrams. Laminagraphic projections will demonstrate the details of overriding, compression, and complex fracture and are useful in visualizing the details of the head and neck of the mandibular condyle.

Cervical Radiographs. Cervical radiographs should be ordered to examine the patient for damage incurred to the vertebral structures when the mandibular portion of the maxillofacial skeleton received the impact.

Computed Tomography. CT is especially indicated to visualize the details of injuries to the condyle, the glenoid fossa, and the cranial fossa superior to the temporomandibular joint.

PRELIMINARY TREATMENT

GENERAL CONDITION

The primary consideration of the preliminary treatment in cases of mandibular fracture is to determine and treat the general condition of the patient. (See Chapter 2.) Because the general condition will vary, depending on the extent of the injuries, early treatment of fractures of the mandible consists of life-supporting first aid until the extent of all of the injuries has been evaluated and adequate facilities and personnel are available for definitive treatment. If definitive treatment must be delayed in a severely injured patient, temporary immobilization by head bandages or intraoral stabilizing devices may be performed.

Maintenance of the airway is of immediate importance. If the airway is not patent, the tongue should be grasped with fingers or a towel clip and pulled forward. The mouth should be inspected using adequate light and suction, and foreign bodies, broken teeth, and segments of dentures removed. If in an unconscious patient the tongue falls back against the posterior pharyngeal wall, for support a suture should be placed *horizontally* through the midline of the tongue and tied to the clothing or other external support, and a nasal or oral airway should be placed. If these maneuvers are not successful, an endotracheal tube should be inserted; if necessary, a tracheostomy should be performed.

Hemorrhage is usually not a life-threatening complication in mandibular fractures, even if the inferior alveolar vessels are severed. If soft-tissue wounds involving the major vessels of the neck and their main branches are associated, hemorrhage may threaten the patient's life by causing hypovolemic shock, exsanguination, or accumulation of blood in the airway. Locally applied pressure and suctioning are indicated until the bleeding vessel can be located and controlled.

Shock is not a prominent feature in the usual isolated mandibular fracture. If it is present, the patient is placed in the shock position with due regard for the airway, with the head, thorax, and abdomen level and the legs raised by a pillow or other support. The patient is kept warm and evaluated for possible blood loss.

To prevent infection in cases of soft-tissue injuries contaminated by dirt or debris, tetanus antitoxin is given (after a sensitivity test is performed) if the patient has not been previously immunized; if the patient has been immunized, tetanus toxoid is given. Generally, administration of prophylactic antibiotics is indicated in compound, complex fractures.

Pain can be relieved most readily by immobilization of the fracture segments. If intracranial damage or embarrassment of the respiration are possibilities, narcotics should not be administered.

METHODS OF IMMOBILIZATION

Permanent reduction and immobilization of fractures of the mandible should be performed within hours after injury, if practical. Immobilization makes the patient more comfortable and limits reflex spasm of the muscles and production of edema, which complicate

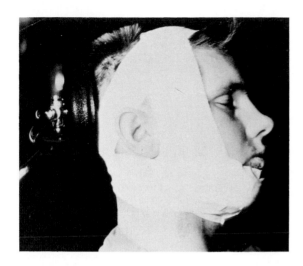

FIG. 6–5. Bartton head bandage supporting the fractured mandible of the patient during evacuation for definitive care. (Courtesy of the U.S. Army.)

the reduction procedures. If early definitive treatment is not possible, temporary stabilization should be employed. A head bandage is the most simple form of fixation, and several types are available (Fig. 6–5). Extreme care should be exercised in placing these bandages to prevent backward displacement of the fragments of the mandible, which may tend to obstruct the respiration.

Often, a simple intraoral appliance, an arch bar, dentures, or wires to immobilize the fragments are satisfactory for temporary stabilization. One intermaxillary wire placed on teeth near the midline between an intact symphysis and maxilla serves as excellent temporary stabilizing fixation; also, wiring around teeth adjacent to the fracture site, arch bars spanning the fractured area, construction of lingual splints from self-curing acrylic or vacuum-forming vinyls, and circumferentially wiring dentures provide stabilization of fractured segments.

DEFINITIVE TREATMENT

The principles for treating fractures of the mandible are the same as those for treating fractures in other parts of the body—to reduce the displacement of the fracture, immobilize the fracture segments, prevent infection, maintain immobilization for a sufficient pe-

riod to permit bone repair, provide appropriate local hygienic and other measures, and provide appropriate general supportive measures. The primary objectives in treatment of fractures are to restore normal function, to prevent disfigurement and asymmetry, and to allow the patient to return quickly to a useful life.

Numerous methods are available to treat fractures of the mandible, and the surgeon's selection will depend on careful evaluation of the type and location of fracture, the condition of the patient's mouth, the age and general condition of the patient, and the facilities and materials available. Regardless of the method selected, the treatment is directed toward placing the ends of the bone in anatomically acceptable contact and the maintaining of the position until healing occurs.

A time-honored mnemonic that summarizes fracture management is recalled as the four Rs: recognition, reduction, retention, and rehabilitation. To these we add resourcefulness based firmly on training and experience.

CLOSED REDUCTION

The various methods of closed reduction and immobilization of mandibular fractures usually depend on correct alignment of natural or artifical dentition into the position that existed prior to injury, thereby producing an anatomic realignment of the fractured segments. Most maxillofacial injuries that consist primarily or solely of a fractured mandible can be managed by closed reduction. One method of closed reduction depends on splints or bars that bridge the fracture site and hold the involved fragments in position until repair occurs. (See Chapter 5.) Examples of this method are the full cast-metal splints that cover the coronal portions of the teeth; sectional splints that rely on undercuts in the dental arches for stability; lingual or labial splints that are wired to the dentition; manufactured labial arch bars; bars formed by wiring techniques, using stainless steel wire; dentures or denture-like splints for circumferential wiring in the edentulous patient; and various external pin and screw fixation devices.

Another method of closed reduction depends on appliances equipped with lugs or wires that form loops and hooks for intermaxillary elastic treation or wire fixation. Examples are the single and multiple loop wiring techniques; manufactured labial arch bars; and plastic or metal splints, cast for the individual case.

Of course, combinations of the various methods are used as indicated by the requirements of each case.

CIRCUMMANDIBULAR WIRING

Circummandibular wiring consists of inserting wires or sutures around the mandible to secure a splint or a mandibular denture placed over the alveolar ridge. This method is used most often for fractures of edentulous mandibles. Optimal control of the fragments is achieved when the fracture is situated in the anterior portion of the mandible or within the area covered by the denture or splint base. This type of fixation is also indicated in fractures of children, which may be treated by constructing a splint over partially erupted and incompletely formed teeth, or over dentulous sections of the jaw where the teeth are periodontally unstable. Splints may also be used to treat comminuted fractures of the mandible that are split into longitudinal fragments, and comminuted fractures with shattered fragments, which may be held in position by wires placed to cradle the fragments. (See Chapter 5.)

In all of the circummandibular wiring techniques, the ends of the wire are grasped with the hemostat and sawed back and forth several times in order to move the wire through the tissues to the inferior border of the mandible. A dimple should not remain in the overlying skin. The splint or denture is placed over the alveolar ridge, and the lingual and buccal wires are twisted over the device. Usually three circummandibular wires are placed to stabilize the splint or denture, one each near the posterior ends on each side and one in the area of the midline.

EXTRAORAL SKELETAL PIN FIXATION

There have been many variations of external skeletal fixation devices, many of which

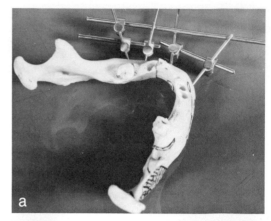

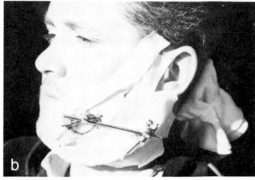

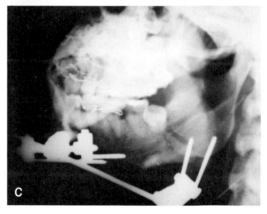

FIG. 6–6. **a,** Roger-Anderson fracture fixation device displayed on a dried specimen. **b,** The device on a patient who incurred a fracture of the angle, and **c,** As seen in the radiograph.

were developed from bone plates and pins used for fixation of long bones in the body. Fixation of the connecting bars of these appliances, usually included elbow and joint units, which were secured by friction clamps and set screws (Fig. 6–6). Some indications for the use of extraoral skeletal pin procedures include loss of bone substance (i.e., gunshot

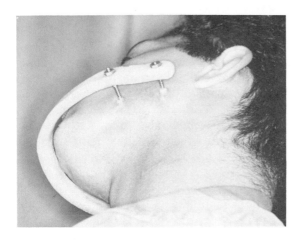

FIG. 6–7. Biphasic fracture fixation device (Dr. Joe H. Morris device). Illustrated is a modification of the biphasic device as designed at the University of Iowa under the direction of Merle Hale, D.D.S. The device is supporting fractures of the mandible that were repaired with intraoral open reduction techniques.

wound); comminuted fractures with multiple small fragments and unfavorable displacement forces; edentulous fractures with unfavorable displacement tendencies when intraoral splints are either ineffective or not available at the time of surgery; and situations in which a graft to the mandible is necessary and the relationship of the graft to the jaw is difficult to maintain.

Dr. Joe H. Morris described an extraskeletal appliance in 1951 that utilizes predrilled holes with bone-embedding screws and a nonyielding connecting stabilizer bar of quick-cured acrylic[5] (Fig. 6–7). This method (see Chapter 5) has many advantages over other skeletal pin techniques. Retention in bone is improved compared to pin devices in which the stabilizing pins are drilled into the bone. The Morris device uses a bone-embedded screw in a predrilled hole rather than the multiple friction-holding pins used in some of the other appliances. The Morris appliance permits a first phase of adjusting and manipulating fragments prior to the second phase placement of the stabilizing bar; this versatile device is known as the biphasic skeletal fixation device. Another advantage of the Morris appliance is that because there are no friction-holding clamps in the appliance, there is less chance of displacement after surgery. In ad-

dition, the equipment is uncomplicated to use, can be available at the time of surgery because no preparation of special splints is necessary, and is lightweight but sufficiently strong to furnish adequate stabilization. Also, the device may be effective over long periods of time. (I have kept the same device on a patient with complex fractures for 15 months. Other surgeons have mentioned even longer periods of use.)

OPEN REDUCTION

Open reduction and direct interosseous fixation of fragments has been used for decades. The advent of antibiosis and the introduction of tantalum, cobalt-chromium alloy, stainless steel, and titanium in the form of bars, screws, wires, and trays made open operations routine. Thus, open reduction, through either an intraoral or extraoral approach, has become an important adjunct for treating mandibular fractures. Rigid fixation by bone plates and lag screws, when feasible and available, often make open reduction the treatment of choice.

Lag screws and compression bone plates provide extremely close and absolute immobilizing approximation of the fractured segments and hence rapid repair. In many cases, the mandible can be mobilized immediately after reduction because of the stabilization of the segments, and primary repair of bone occurs without intermediate endosteal callus formation.[6] Lag screws are especially applicable in vertical fractures of the mandible that pass obliquely between the cortical plates.

Bone plate fixation, which was used for decades, in recent years has been termed rigid osteosynthesis. These techniques can be used in edentulous areas, in patients who cannot have the mandible immobilized, and in all cases in which an open approach, either intra- or extraoral, is the treatment of choice.[7,8]

Certain problems should be considered when using bone plate fixation and lag screw immobilization of mandible fractures. These operations are technique sensitive; that is, the procedures are relatively unforgiving in that segments could be locked into a position that may be incorrect by a few millimeters, resulting in occlusal disharmony or a challenge to the temporomandibular joint. In contrast, intermaxillary traction and wiring may guide segments to correct occlusal anatomic positions. Also, bone plate fixation techniques rely on expensive instruments compared to other open reduction procedures. A relative problem is the perceived need to remove all of the devices after bone repair either to prevent a possible stress shielding or to eliminate an area for shelter of hematogenous or locally induced bacterial invasion. Indeed, removing metallic appliances, especially bone plates, is often necessary because of contiguous soft-tissue irritation as the bone remodels away from the device. This problem occurs with all devices, including transosseous wire fixation. Another problem with bone plate fixation and lag screws is that when pressure from the screws is applied, crazing of the main fracture line may produce shattering at the margin of the fracture line. Bone plates, including finger plates adapted from orthopedic surgical instruments, have been useful adjuncts in fracture management, and the modern designs and the outstanding clinical research of the Swiss Association for the Study of Internal Fixation (ASIF) have assured their place among the options.[6] Lag screw reduction and fixation is an eminently practical concept in cases in which accurate approximation of fractures with the fracture lines free of marginal comminution and in which reasonable access are possible.

Advantages

Open reduction with direct transosseous wiring, plating or lag screw procedures combined with intraoral stabilization is the most accurate method of reducing and immobilizing fragments. Open reduction permits direct visualization of the fracture sites and allows displaced fragments to be rapidly returned to proper position and maintained with great security. The surgical procedure is relatively short, and the accurate reduction of the fragments with intimate bony contacts, especially under pressures of double wire compression, osteosynthesis bone plate fracture devices, or lag screws hastens bony repair. After the fragments are reduced and stabilized and the wound closed, the patient is comfortable.

Indications

In several situations, open reduction and either direct transosseous wiring or stabilization with a rigid bar, mesh, or screw may be considered the method of choice. Open reduction is indicated in fractures occurring at the gonial angle or posterior to the natural dentition, in which adequate reduction cannot be obtained except through either intraoral splints or skeletal fixation devices. Open reduction should be used in the edentulous mandible with displaced fragments, in which intraoral controls using either dentures or splints or using external skeletal fixation devices are not feasible. Another use is in patients who are completely edentulous or have insufficient teeth to allow for intermaxillary fixation without prescription of splints. Also, when treatment has been delayed for various causes or when soft tissue has become interposed between the fragments, open reduction is the best method for accurately freshening the bone ends and correcting the malposition.

In fractures of the mandible and midfacial bones, it is necessary to establish a base of normal occlusion as a foundation for reducing midfacial fractures. Direct visualization, alignment, and stabilization of the mandibular fragments permit restoration of the continuity of the midfacial bones.

Open reduction, often with bone grafting, usually is the treatment of choice when nonunion has resulted from other methods of treatment. When malunion has resulted from lack of treatment or inadequate treatment, open reduction provides access to the fracture site to permit reconstruction of the fracture.

In young children, open reduction and direct fixation is used to manage displaced fracture fragments that on rare occasions are difficult to control

Contraindications

Open reduction is not necessary if the fragments can be reduced and maintained in satisfactory position and alignment by techniques that do not require the surgical exposure of bone. Open reduction is contraindicated in comminuted fractures presenting many small fragments of bone when stripping of the periosteum would jeopardize the vitality of the fragments. Obviously, patients who are poor surgical risks because of overriding concomitant injuries, systemic disorders, or debilitating diseases should be evaluated by the head of the surgical team to determine the relative risks of general anesthetic and surgical procedures necessary to carry out open reductions.

The need to make incisions in cutaneous tissues could be considered a slight contraindication to extraoral open reduction procedures; however, with deft, delicate, and accurate management of the tissues, the incision line will be barely discernible and probably will disappear within a year. Intraoral compounding of the fracture is not a contraindication to open reduction.

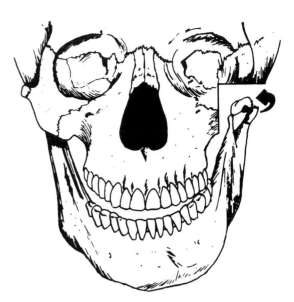

FIG. 6–8. Unilateral fracture of the condylar process. The mandible shifts towards the fractured area, resulting in a unilateral open crossbite relationship of the teeth.

CONSIDERATIONS IN TREATMENT OF FRACTURES OF THE VARIOUS REGIONS OF THE MANDIBLE

FRACTURES OF THE CONDYLAR PROCESS

The neck of the condylar process is usually quite thin and therefore susceptible to fractures, espcially from a blow to the symphysis area of the mandible. The lateral pterygoid muscle is attached to the anterior surface of the mandibular neck and exerts an anterior, inferior, and medial force. Fractures that occur above the lateral pterygoid muscle insertion are within the capsule of the joint and usually demonstrate only slight bony displacement. When the fracture occurs below the muscle attachment, however, displacement of the condyle is common in the direction of the pull of the muscle.

Diagnosis

The clinical findings of condylar fractures include asymmetry of the face resulting from edema over the area of the joint and from a shifting of the mandible posteriorly and laterally toward the fractured side (Fig. 6–8). The teeth on the fractured side will contact prematurely, resulting in an open bite on the opposite side. Palpating over the fractured

area elicits pain. Likewise, percussing an otherwise intact mandible in the symphysis may produce pain in the area of the fracture of the condylar process. With considerable displacement, laceration of the external auditory canal with bleeding may occur. Patients with bilateral condylar process fractures have an anterior open bite with difficulty or inability to protrude the mandible. Although displacement of the mandible with high intracapsular fractures is minimal, the patient often complains of pain and tenderness over the temporomandibular joint with inability to occlude the posterior teeth on the fractured side because of intracapsular edema.

Treatment

Prior to the mid-twentieth century, fractures of the condylar processes were usually treated by closed reduction, using intermaxillary fixation; the actual objective of the treatment was to return the occlusion to a normal relationship, not necessarily to return the fractured site to an anatomic alignment. A classic study reported by the Chalmers J. Lyons Academy in 1947 involved a review of the postoperative results of 120 cases of fractures of the mandibular condyle.[9] The study concluded that fractures treated by closed reduction healed satisfactorily without accurate alignment of the proximal and distal fragments; that ankylosis occurred infrequently; and that intraoral fixation methods were simple and effective.

A treatment philosophy that embraces the present capabilities for direct surgical reduction and retention of fractures pays due regard to the displacement of the superior fragment, the location of the fracture, and the objective of treatment. Bilateral condylar process fractures have the same considerations as unilateral fractures and a greater potential for disability.

The superior fragment is classified as being not too minimally displaced, meaning that the condyle is within its usual location in the glenoid fossa; as being displaced, meaning that the condyle is within range of its normal movements; or as being dislocated, meaning that the condyle is outside of its normal movements (Fig. 6–9a). The fracture may be a condylar (intracapsular) fracture; it may be located at the level of the condylar neck (below the condyle and above the mandibular [sigmoid] notch); or it may be located in the subcondylar base of the condylar process (the fracture line beginning at the level of the sigmoid notch and passing posteriorly or posteroinferiorly) (Fig. 6–9b). The objective of treatment may be correlated with any level or degree of displacement. The mandible may be returned to function by either producing a flail joint or training the mandible to move in its excursions with a malunion; the objective of achieving bony union implies an anatomic alignment.

Table 6-1 shows these relationships between displacement, level of fracture, and the effect on treatment. Correlations between the level of fracture and the amount of movement of the proximal segment are given as suggested guides toward treatment planning. If bony union is the objective of the treatment, immobilization of the parts is necessary either by immobilizing the mandible for 4 to 6 weeks or by using a rigid-type fixation (bone plates, screws, or pins). If the objective of treatment is to have function of the mandible but to accept a displaced or dislocated proximal seg-

ment, physiotherapeutic movement is indicated.

In cases of bilateral and unilateral condylar fractures in which restoration of function is the objective of treatment, intermaxillary immobilization in centric occlusion is used as briefly as possible, just long enough to relieve the patient of pain, after which the jaws are mobilized for trial excursions. The immobilization may last for a few days to two weeks. When the patient can return to centric position without pain, physical therapy of guiding traction and exercises are instituted to restore the excursions of the mandible. The longer the immobilization persists, the more difficult it will be for the patient to learn to control the mandible whose integrity has been affected by the fracture.

In some cases it is possible to place an occlusal wafer between the immobilized jaws and effect a return of a temporomandibular joint fracture to a normal alignment. The wafer is designed to open the bite 2 or 3 mm posteriorly. After the condyle has returned to its normal position, the wafer is removed and the immobilization is continued for 4 weeks to achieve bony union (Fig. 6–10).

In cases of bilateral and unilateral fractures in which the objective of treament is bony union, the intermaxillary immobilization is used for 4 to 6 weeks.

The level of the fracture line, the displacement of the fragments, and the age of the patient are important criteria in considering open reduction. A low fracture with dislocation is more amenable to surgery than a high fracture and, in children, is another indication for use of open reduction to preserve the growth potential. Open reduction of condylar process fractures may be indicated in cases of massive facial trauma. The mandible, especially the condylar process and the subcondylar areas, must be reconstructed to serve as a guide for occlusion, which produces a stabilizing platform for the skeleton of the middle face. The same criteria are true for cases of edentulism, when it is not possible to accurately orient the mandible to the maxilla.

If the trauma has resulted in a compound, comminuted fracture with severe and complex destruction of the integrity of the condylar process, as occurs in a gunshot wound,

TMJ FRACTURES

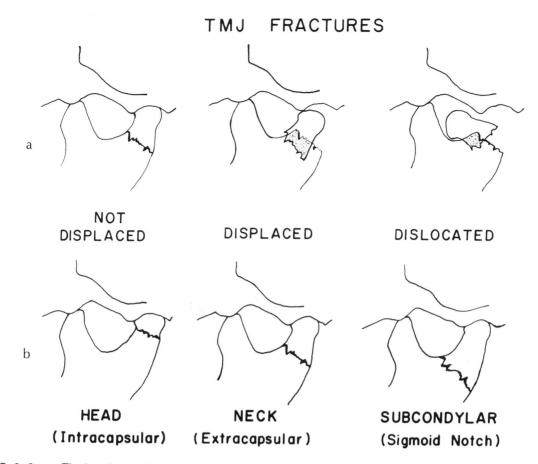

FIG. 6–9. **a,** The locations of fractures are correlated with the amount of movement of the proximal segment. In a displaced fracture, the fracture displacement is within the usual range of motion of the condylar head. In a dislocated fracture, the proximal segment has moved the head of the condyle beyond its normal ranges of motion. **b,** Depicted are locations of fractures of the condylar process of the mandible—fractures of the head, neck, and subcondylar areas. In this series of three, there is no to minimal displacement of the fractured proximal segment.

Table 6–1. Temporomandibular Joint Fractures

Displacement	Head (Intracapsular)	Neck (Extracapsular)	Subcondylar (Sigmoid notch)
Not displaced	Function movement*	Bony union (immobilization)	Bony union (immobilization)
Displaced	Function movement*	Bony union (manipulation, then immobilization) or Function movement*	Bony union (manipulation, then immobilization or open reduction)
Dislocated	Function movement* or excision	Function movement* or Bony union (open reduction)	Bony union (open reduction)

*Initial immobilization to relieve pain

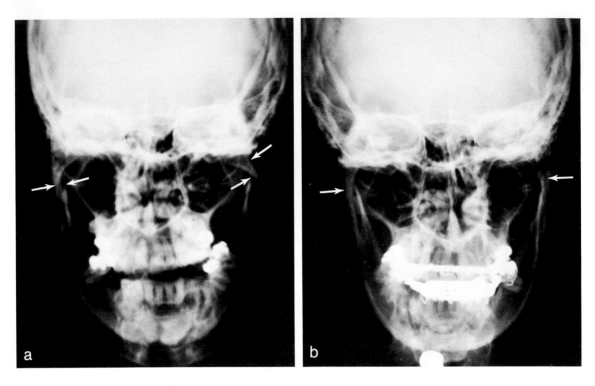

FIG. 6–10.   Closed manipulation, reduction, and retention of condylar neck fractures. **a,** Bilateral condylar neck fractures of the mandible with dislocation on one side and a marked displacement, probably a dislocation, on the other. **b,** The patient was treated with an occlusal splint placed between the teeth. The splint was designed to open the bite in the posterior approximately 2 or 3 mm, which permitted a physiologic and spontaneous reduction of the condylar fractures over a 5- to 7-day period. After the condylar head was repositioned in the glenoid fossa, the splint was removed and the mandible was immobilized for 6 weeks to achieve bony union. (Courtesy of Dr. Donald B. Osbon.)

the bone structures should be treated by wet debridement, closed reduction, and soft-tissue closure with drains. The oral and maxillofacial surgeon should be alert for necrotic and osteomyelitic changes, which require removal of the affected parts.

Technique for Open Reduction

The approach for reducing fractures of the condylar process, depends on the fracture's location. The preauricular approach is used less frequently than the submandibular[10] (Fig. 6–11).

If the fracture is high in the condylar neck, and providing an open reduction is indicated a preauricular approach is used. The primary consideration in planning the preauricular approach is to prevent damage to CN VII. The hair in the temporal area is shaved to provide access to the preauricular area; a small margin

of hair is left at the anterior aspect of the temporal area for orientation. The incision is placed in the skin crease, usually adjacent to the anterior helix, and is carried downward along the anterior margin of the ear to the superior attachment of the lobe, and the dissection exposes the fascia parotideomasseterica and temporal fascia. The tissues are reflected forward, and the branches of the superficial temporal artery and vein are identified and ligated if necessary. The branches of CN VII, which may be at the anterior border of the incision, are identified with the nerve stimulator and protected. The fascia is incised horizontally over the zygomatic process of the temporal bone and is extended downward along the posterior margin of the condyle. Extreme care must be exercised medial to the condyle to avoid the possibility of involving the maxillary artery and its branches and the auriculotemporal nerve. If

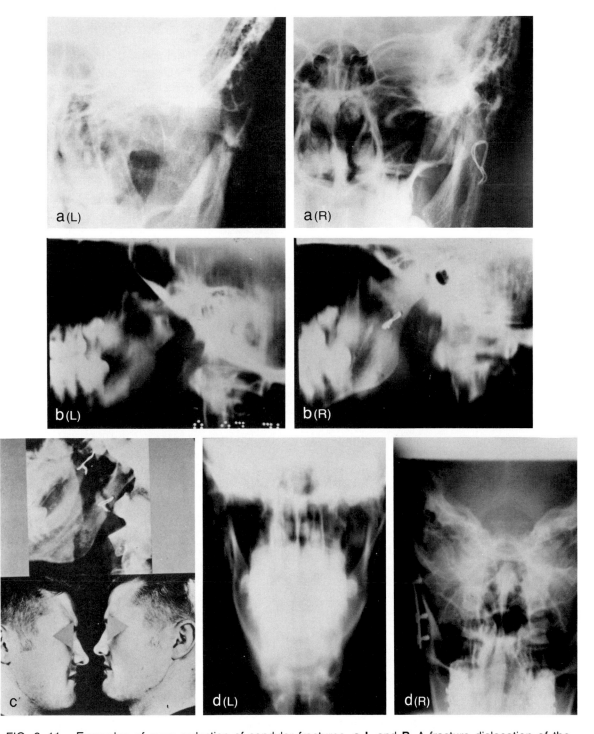

FIG. 6–11.   Examples of open reduction of condylar fractures. **a L** and **R,** A fracture dislocation of the condylar neck was managed by an open reduction with double wire compression to return the condylar head to an anatomic alignment. The patient's mandible was immobilized for 3 weeks and the patient was placed on a soft diet for an additional 3 weeks. **b L** and **R,** Laminagraphic pre- and postoperative studies of a unilateral subcondylar fracture on an 11-year-old child. The fracture was stabilized by the double wire compression technique via a gonial angle approach. **c,** Bilateral subcondylar fracture reduced and stabilized by direct transosseous fixation. **d L** and **R,** Open reduction of a comminuted fracture of the condylar neck with stabilization with an osteosynthesis pressure plate. (Courtesy of Dr. Hugh P. Brindley.)

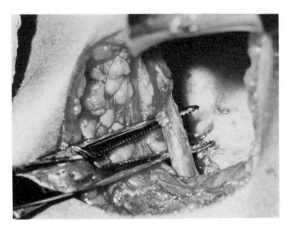

FIG. 6–12.   The posterior facial vein is displayed at the posterolateral aspect of the mandibular ramus during a gonial angle surgical approach to the mandible.

the condyle is displaced from the fossa, it is returned to position and immobilized with transosseous stainless steel wires, bone miniplates, lag screws, or other techniques. Distracting the fracture line may be necessary to provide more surgical access at the fracture site by creating traction at the gonial angle. The surgical site is closed by approximating the capsular tissues and parotideomasseteric fascia followed by subcutaneous and skin closure.

If the fracture is in the middle or lower part of the condylar neck, the submandibular approach is recommended. A 4- to 5-cm incision is placed approximately 1 cm below and behind the angle of the mandible. The dissection to the mandible is carried through the subcutaneous tissue and platysma muscle to the parotideomasseteric fascia. The dissection is accompanied by nerve stimulation to identify and protect branches of the facial nerve. The incision is made through the periosteum, along the inferior border of the mandible, and upward along the posterior border approximately to the level of the sigmoid notch. Care is taken to avoid or protect the posterior facial vein, which may be in the area (Fig. 6–12). The insertion of the masseter muscle and periosteum are elevated from the lateral aspect of the mandible upward to the site of the fracture. The transosseous mode of reduction and retention include transosseous wiring and in-

sertion of a metal fracture plate and a pin in the superior segment.

Transosseous wiring will compress the fracture line but may be relatively unstable if the direction of the fracture line is oblique. A metallic plate, preferably a compression plate, screwed to the lateral cortical bone provides rigid support but may require slightly greater surgical access (sometimes including a preauricular or postauricular incision) than a transosseous wire. A pin placed in the medullary portion of the superior fragment and then secured to the ramus provides accurate and rigid retention, but the surgical techniques require a longer perior of time, manipulation, and greater surgical field access than direct plating or wiring.[11,12] In our practice, transosseous wiring is the most direct and versatile method; however, plating will decrease from weeks to a matter of days the time needed for intermaxillary fixation.

If transosseous wires are being placed, a hole is drilled through the angle of the mandible and stainless steel wire passed through it, both ends grasped with a large needle holder so that the distal fragment may be retracted downward to aid reduction of the fracture. Army-Navy retractors, a laryngoscope, or a ramus soft-tissue retractor that is used for elective osteotomies (as in surgery to correct developmental deformities) are used to expose the fracture site. It may be necessary to administer a muscle relaxant to permit greater exposure of the fracture site. If the drilling of the holes is difficult from a direct lateral approach, a small stab incision is made in the skin, the drill point is forced through the tissue, and the holes are drilled at a right angle to the lateral surface of the bone. During the drilling procedure, metal retractors should be placed on the medial side of the mandible. If a transverse fracture with one cortex longer than the other is present, the fracture site may be reduced and retained while one hole is drilled through both fragments and the fragments are reduced by a transosseous wire. (A small L-shaped metal plate, bone plates, metallic meshes, and lag screws may be used for the reduction instead of transosseous wires.) Following reduction, the wound is closed in layers, ensuring that the fascia of the masseter muscle is sutured to the fascia of the medial pterygoid muscle along the lower border of the mandible. Placement of drains is not necessary.

Other Considerations of Neck Fractures

The higher the fracture on the condylar neck, the greater the problems in surgical and physiotherapeutic management. The lower the fracture, the greater the indications for open reductions to avoid disabilities and the greater the surgical access.

The proximal porton of a fracture of the condylar neck of the mandible, especially of high, dislocated fractures, may be easily displaced out of the body by the surgeon during the operation. This displacement is not surprising considering that a dislocated fracture of the mandibular condyle is accompanied by lacerations of the periosteum and the capsule, and the few fibers of the external pterygoid muscle that remain may not withstand much manipulation. If the proximal segment should be displaced out of the surgical site, its sterility should be preserved. While it is out of the surgical site, either drill holes for wires or tap holes for screws may be placed. Obviously, the time out of the body should be kept to a minimum.

The formation of a second head of the condyle that is positioned correctly on the fractured distal stump has been observed. This formation represents an osteogenesis of the periosteal sheath that enclosed the original condyle as it was dislocated at the time of injury and was stripped out of its periosteum. The patient eventually may produce some version of a bifid condyle, the original and secondary, on the mandible.

An idiopathic loss of the condyle may occur following trauma. The condyle receives its blood supply from the lateral pterygoid muscle and the medulllary channels from the condylar neck of the mandible. The manipulation that may accompany fracture reduction procedures or the trauma itself may produce an ischemic loss of the condylar head.

FRACTURES OF THE CONDYLE

Fractures of the condyle within the capsule are uncommon (Fig. 6–13).

Treatment should entail movement of the mandible as early and as extensively as possible. Even if movement is uncomfortable to the patient, functional demands must be placed on the condyle to decrease the possibility of an ankylosis.

Because the central portion of the condyle is richly endowed with vascular medullary bone and the articulating surface is a thin shield of cortical bone, intracapsular fractures will cause hemorrhage into the capsule space. If the coagulation of blood produces fibrous connective tissue in the capsular space, a severe limitation of motion of the head of the condyle known as a false ankylosis, could result. A true ankylosis, a bony union between the condyle and the temporal bone, may arise if a coagulum of extravasated blood in the joint space produces a scaffolding for the abundant osteoblasts originating from the medullary portion of the condyle.

Although the intracapsular fractures may exhibit only minimal displacement, the patient often complains of pain and tenderness over the temporomandibular joint with inability to close the posterior teeth on the fractured side usually caused by intracapsular edema and treatable with physical therapy.

If the fracture displacement precludes reasonable function, the condyle is visualized using a preauricular or a postauricular incision, and the displaced bony segment is either reduced and stabilized with a transosseous wire or suture, or removed. Repair and repositioning of the meniscus is performed, as indicated. If the meniscus is so badly damaged that it must be removed, a dermal or a fascial graft or the use of a glenoid fossa prosthesis may be considered, or no material or device may be considered.

FRACTURES OF THE CORONOID PROCESS

Fractures of the coronoid process occur in a small percentage of mandibular fractures and often are not treated if there is little or no displacement. These fractures usually occur in conjunction with other fractures of the mandible, unless they are the result of a gunshot wound. The masseter muscle and the low attachment of the tendons of the temporal muscle tend to splint the fractured cor-

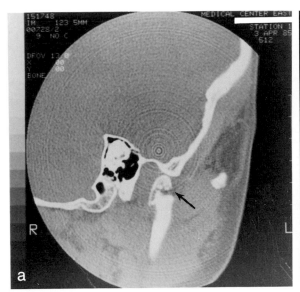

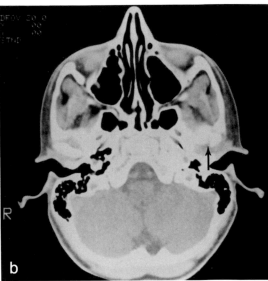

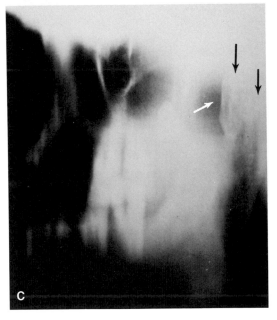

FIG. 6–13. Condyle fractures. **a,** A displaced fracture of the condyle is displayed on a CT study. The patient was treated by immobilization of the mandible to relieve pain and then by physiotherapeutic functioning exercises. **b,** On the left, a sagittal fracture is noted in the condyle. The unstable segment was removed. **c,** Condyle fracture resulted in an infusion of blood into the joint space. Subsequent fibrosis and osteogenesis produced an osseous malformation that required removal using a gonial angle approach to restore normal mandibular function. (Courtesy of Dr. Nicholas Pieroni.)

onoid process. If considerable upward displacement does occur, reduction procedures are performed using an intraoral approach through an incision along the anterior border of the ramus. The incision is carried through the buccinator muscle and the attachment of the temporal muscle, down to the bone. Elevation and reflection of the muscle tissues will expose the fracture. Holes are drilled in the anterior aspect of the ascending ramus and coronoid process. The limiting factor is surgical access, especially if the patient has trismus, a small mouth, or a flaring tuberosity. Usually there are no major vessels or nerves in the surgical field anterior to the ascending ramus. Through this approach it is also possible to remove the fractured process to prevent impingement of mandibular movement. Postoperative care must provide for movement and physiotherapy to prevent an ossification of a coagulum that could unite the coronoid process to the zygomatic arch.

FRACTURES OF THE RAMUS OF THE MANDIBLE

This rare fracture extends from either the sigmoid notch or the anterior border of the mandibular ramus to the angle of the mandible. Because of splinting action of the overlying fibers of the masseter muscle and the medial pterygoid muscle, very little secondary displacement occurs. Fractures of the region often are associated with fractures of the angle or of the body of the mandible on the opposite side. Fractures of the ramus are usually treated by closed reduction with intermaxillary fixation (Fig. 6–14).

FRACTURES OF THE ANGLE OF THE MANDIBLE

Fractures of the angle region are common. Surgically speaking, this area extends from the third molar area to the posterior attachments of the masseter muscle (Fig. 6–15). Although the overlying muscles afford some splinting action to angle fractures, displacement of the proximal fragment is common. This displacement may be either medial or lateral, depending on the plane and angle of the fracture and the direction of the force in-

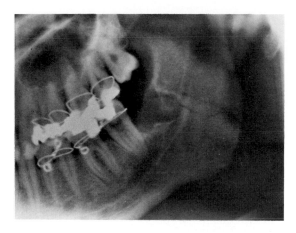

FIG. 6–14. A fracture of the ramus of the mandible. The stabilizing effect of the attachments of the masseter and the internal pterygoid muscles stabilized the fracture and prevented a secondary unfavorable displacement.

volved. Fractures of the angle are often associated with subcondylar, body, and mental region fractures of the opposite side of the mandible. If displacement is minimal, the angle fracture may be treated successfully by closed reduction with intermaxillary immobilization.

Open Reduction, Extraoral Approach

When displacement of an angle fracture is present, open reduction is usually necessary. The patient's head is turned and the neck extended to expose the proposed surgical site, and an incision is made through the skin and subcutaneous fascia, approximately 3 to 5 cm in length. The surface of the platysma muscle is visualized and the subcutaneous fascia is separated from it in all directions by blunt dissection to permit closure of the cutaneous and subcutaneous tissues without tension. The platysma muscle is incised and dissection proceeds to the lower border of the mandible, using blunt and sharp dissection. In the area of the posterior body of the mandible it is usually necessary to isolate and ligate the facial artery and vein to permit access to the mandible, and it is also important to avoid the mandibular branch of the facial nerve.

Dingman and Grabb found that the course of the mandibular branch of the facial nerve can be divided into an anterior and a posterior

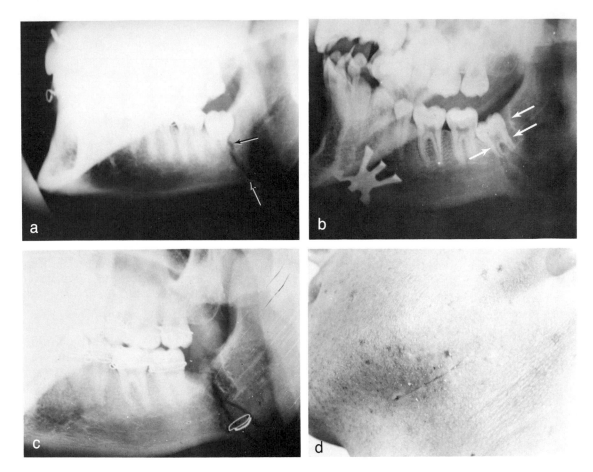

FIG. 6–15.   Fractures of the angle of the mandible. **a,** Fracture of the angle of mandible stabilized by the presence of the impacted third molar. Removal of this tooth would necessitate an open reduction. Hence, it is occasionally reasonable to leave teeth in the line of fracture, although close follow-up is necessary and usually the tooth should be removed after the fracture has been repaired because its vitality is jeopardized. **b** and **c,** Fracture of the angle of mandible that is an unfavorable alignment. The apparent two lines of fracture (arrows) represent a single fracture with separate radiographic images of the medial and lateral cortices of the mandible. (Courtesy of the U.S. Army.) **d,** The open reduction was performed through the incision line, which is shown 7 days postoperatively. **e,** Fracture of the left angle of the mandible was incurred during the removal of the mandibular third molar tooth. **f,** The mandible was immediately immobilized using continuous loop and eyelet wiring. Normal repair of both the fracture and the third molar surgical site occurred.

portion.[3] In dissecting 100 facial halves, they noted in 81% of the specimens that posterior to the facial artery the mandibular branch passed above the inferior border of the mandible; in the other 19% of the specimens, the mandibular branch or one or more of its branches passed 1 cm or less below the inferior border of the mandible. Anterior to the facial artery, 100% of the branches of the specimens passed above the inferior border of the mandible.

Dingman and Grabb also found an identi-

fiable and demonstrable trunk of the facial nerve to the inferior lip beneath the platysma muscle, below the base of the mandible, in the first bicuspid area. If dissection is carried inferior to the submandibular lymph node of Stahr, the facial nerve usually is safely retracted in the superior flap.

The facial artery and vein may be encountered at the anterior end of the premasseteric notch; the artery is usually located anterior and medial to the vein, and these vessels are tied and severed to gain access. The perios-

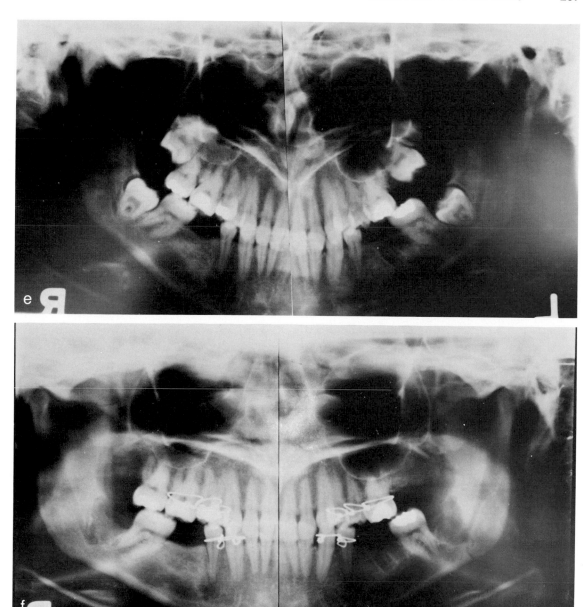

FIG. 6–15 (continued).

teum and overlying muscles of the mandible are incised along the inferior border, exposing the bone and its fracture. The periosteum is elevated on the outer surface to completely expose the fracture segments so that all interposed tissue, unattached bone spicules, clots, and foreign bodies may be removed. The lingual periosteum is reflected to expose the sites for using bone-holding forceps and making drill holes to receive transosseous wires, bone plates, or screws. Bone forceps are used to grasp the larger fragments and manipulate them into position.

If transosseous wires are to be used, a flat retractor is placed on the medial side of the bone from an inferior approach to protect the adjacent soft-tissue structures. Holes are drilled anteriorly and posteriorly approximately 1 cm on both sides of the fracture site and *at right angles* to the fracture line. With machine-powered drills, irrigation and aspiration should be used to prevent burning of the bone. One 20-cm length of 26-gauge stainless steel wire is doubled and then passed through the holes on both sides of the fracture so that the free ends of the doubled wire are brought to the outer surface of the mandible. Alternatively, one wire may be placed rather than two. Usually, a wire is doubled and the loop end is passed to assist in drawing one end of the immobilizing wires from the medial to the lateral side through one of the drill holes. The doubled wire is cut, providing two transosseous wires across the fracture site. If properly placed, either two drill holes, one in each fragment, or one drill hole, passing through the lateral and medial cortices of an oblique fracture, will suffice. One well-placed wire is sufficient for most fractures; however, if two wires are placed, they may be tightened alternately to exert pressure on the fracture site. Also, if one wire should break, the other will be in place to complete the immobilization. The placement of the drill holes will directly influence the efficiency of the immobilized single or double wire.

The twisted ends of the wires are cut long enough to permit the ends of the wire to be bent and inserted in one of the drill holes so that it will not irritate the overlying soft tissues. Different surgeons use many variations of the placement and number of drill holes. Primarily, however, the type of fracture and the position of the fracture segments will determine the wiring technique in each case. The bone forceps are removed and the operative site irrigated with normal saline.

Various transosseous metallic devices are available to reduce and immobilize fracture segments. Among the most effective are the osteosynthesis fracture plates. These are so firm that often intermaxillary fixation is not necessary, except to assist in aligning the segments. One technique is to stabilize the segments using intermaxillary fixation and to place the mandible in occlusion prior to placing a fracture plate or lag screw. An open approach to the lateral surface of the mandible is made and the fracture identified. A transosseous wire is placed to help stabilize the segments and may be removed after the plate is placed.

The soft tissue should be closed in layers, using 3-0 chromic catgut or polyglycolic material sutures to approximate the periosteum over the lower border of the mandible and to close the fasica and the platysma muscle. Inverted subcutaneous interrupted sutures using 4-0 plain catgut or other absorbable material are placed. Skin may be closed using several different methods, including 5-0 or 6-0 interrupted or mattress sutures and continuous cutaneous techniques using silk, cotton, nylon, or wire sutures. Subcutaneous techniques with polyethylene materials are aesthetically rewarding.

Open Reduction, Intraoral Approach

Intraoral approach to fractures of the third molar area should use an incision that begins over the external oblique ridge lateral and posterior to the third molar area. The incision should extend anteriorly to an area lateral to the first molar. This is essentially the same incision used for sagittal splitting osteotomies of the mandible. Elevation of tissues medial and lateral to the fracture line is usually fairly easy because the trauma will have caused a distraction of the periosteal attachments. A coronoid process soft-tissue retractor, as used in orthognathic surgical procedures, raises the soft tissues superiorly, thus preventing herniation of the bothersome buccal fat pad into the oral cavity. The third molar, if present, is usually removed as in sagittal split osteotomies; it may be left in place if still developing and potentially useful. Transosseous wires are placed, often only in the lateral cortical plates, or lag screws may be used. Soft-tissue closure is performed and the mandible is immobilized with intermaxillary fixation.

FRACTURES OF THE BODY OF THE MANDIBLE

The region of the body of the mandible, surgically speaking, extends from the mandibular cuspid to the anterior border of the masseter muscle. Fractures in the area of the body are usually either intraoral or extraoral compound fractures, exhibiting anesthesia of the lower lip caused by injury of the inferior alveolar nerve and at times demonstrating considerable displacement, depending on the type and direction of force and the resultant muscle pull on the fragments (Fig. 6–16). If teeth are present on both sides of the fracture line, minimal displacement results; however, if no teeth are present on the proximal segment, usually the segment will be displaced superiorly and medially until it impinges against the maxillary teeth or the alveolar ridge. If the fracture is bilateral through the body of the mandible, the anterior fragment will be displaced posteriorly and inferiorly, while the proximal fragments are displaced superiorly and medially.

If sound natural or artificial teeth are present on both sides of the fracture line, the fracture can be handled by intermaxillary fixation for immobilization and reduction. If teeth are missing, especially on the proximal fragment, or if the fractures are comminuted, managing the fracture by intermaxillary fixation alone may not be possible, and an open reducton will be necessary. It may be necessary to secure artificial teeth to the mandible with circumferential wiring, transalveolar process pins, or other techniques to gain stable points for the intermaxillary immobilization.

If the patient has bilateral body of the mandible fractures, especially anterior body of the mandible fractures, airway patency must be ensured. The genial muscles and the anterior bellies of the digastric muscles will displace the anterior fragment posteriorly, and the patient may have severe problems controlling the tongue and keeping it forward out of the oropharynx. Medial tipping of the mandible resulting from the vectors of the medial mandibular musculature may be expected, and a lingual splint may be the best device to stabilize the fragments. With multiple comminutions, external pin fixation may provide excellent accessory support.

Open Reduction, Extraoral Approach

To approach the body of the mandible, a submandibular incision is made at least one finger's breadth beneath the inferior surface of the mandible, following its contour. Cau-

tion is necessary to prevent damage to the anatomic structures beneath the platysma muscle after the skin and fascia have been exposed. Although the marginal mandibular branch of the facial nerve is usually well above the base of the mandible in this area, inspecting the soft tissues superficial and deep to the platysma muscle prior to incising is prudent. Pulsation of the facial artery may be palpated at the anterior end of the mandibular notch. Two other palpable landmarks for the artery are the anterior border of the masseter muscle and the second molar area.

When fractures of the mandible occur in the premolar and first molar area, the anterior facial artery and vein may be retracted and usually do not have to be clamped, sectioned, and ligated. The mandibular branch of the facial nerve, usually located above the inferior border of the mandible in this region, is not encountered. When the mandible posterior to the second molar must be exposed, however, the facial nerve and vessels can be in the field, and every effort should be made to identify them before the dissection proceeds.

Transosseous wiring (single-strand or, preferably, double-strand), lag screws (especially if the fracture line is oblique), and osteosynthesis plates are used for reduction and retention.

Open Reduction, Intraoral Approach

If a tooth must be removed from a displaced fragment, while the area is exposed a hole may be drilled in each fragment to hold a transosseous wire to maintain the fragments in an anatomic position. The fracture lines are often so situated that passing the wire through only the buccal cortical plate will ensure reduction. When necessary, however, the wire can be passed through the full thickness of the bone. With a more generous elevation of the mucoperiosteum, a lag screw or a metal plate can be placed.

Fractures of edentulous segments are especially amenable to treatment by intraoral open reduction. Exposure is relatively simple, and holes for screws, plates, and wires may be drilled using a hand drill or burs in a handpiece.

As in extraoral open reduction, when using

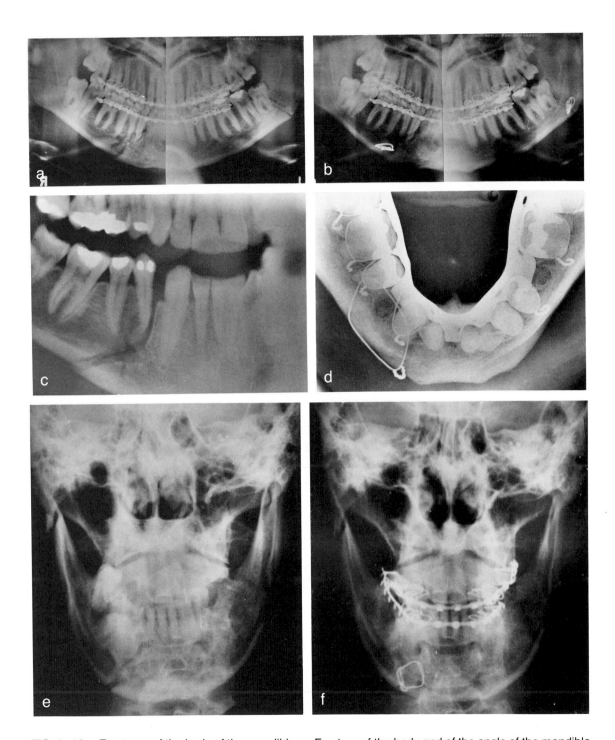

FIG. 6–16. Fractures of the body of the mandible. **a,** Fracture of the body and of the angle of the mandible. **b,** The fracture sites were treated by open reduction utilizing double wire compression fixation. **c,** Fracture of the body of the mandible, **d,** Fracture treated by a lingual splint and an intraoral open reduction with transosseous wire fixation. **e,** Fracture of the anterior body of the mandible. **f,** Fracture was managed by intermaxillary fixation and open reduction, via an intraoral approach, using double wire compression fixation.

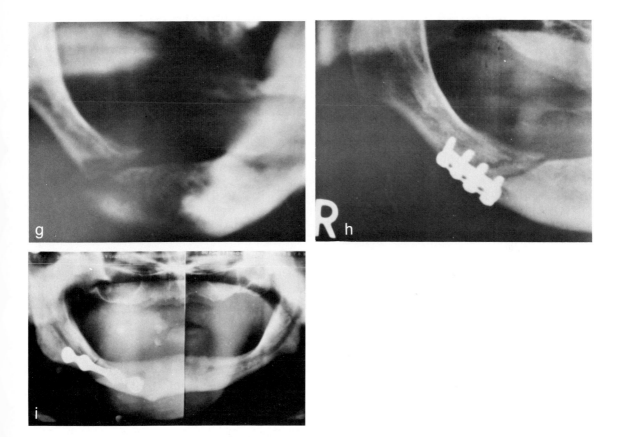

FIG. 6–16 (continued).   **g,** Anterior body of the mandible fracture in an edentulous patient treated with an "L" bone plate. This plate has a right angle flange along its length. **h,** A groove is made in the proximal and distal segments to receive the flange, which adds to the plate's horizontal stabilizing of the fracture segments. As with the majority of patients treated with bone plates, the time of intermaxillary immobilization of the mandible is reduced or, as in this case, eliminated. **i,** Body of the mandible fracture in an edentulous patient treated by a bone plate without intermaxillary immobilization. Stress shielding is usually not a problem in managing fractures of the mandible without a continuity defect, because both cortices do not undergo equal weight-bearing stress and also because the medial surface has generous musculature supporting areas of attachment.

transosseous wiring, additional immobilization should be provided by either intermaxillary immobilization or another method, for example, extraoral skeletal fixation. One should not depend on the interosseous wires for complete immobilization. Lag screws and fracture plates usually provide rigid fixation with little or no reliance on secondary immobilizing methods.

Wires placed using an intraoral approach usually must be removed, in a minor procedure, after bone healing; their position, relatively high on the alveolar ridge, sometimes causes irritation or interferes with a subsequent prosthesis.

Compared to an extraoral approach, intraoral transosseous fixation is advantageous in that it creates no extraoral incision, it provides no challenge to the facial nerve, and often it may be performed on an outpatient under sedation and local anesthesia. Major disadvantages are less control for manipulating and reducing the fragments and less access for controlling the rare hemorrhage from the inferior alveolar vessels.

FRACTURES OF THE SYMPHYSIS OF THE MANDIBLE

The symphysis region, surgically speaking, extends from one cuspid tooth to the other. Fractures in the mandibular midline are rare; most fracture lines extend posteriorly and laterally, the segments telescoping because of the musculature attached to the inner surface of the mandible (Fig. 6–17). Symphysis fractures are usually quite obvious clinically, with displacement on inspection and with swelling and ecchymosis of the floor of the mouth and in the submental region. A symphyseal fracture is often associated with either unilateral or bilateral subcondylar fractures.

Closed Reduction

If the dentition is adequate and a stable occlusion can be established, minimally displaced symphyseal fractures can be reduced and immobilized with intermaxillary fixation or splints. A horizontal wire placed across the fracture site aids in the reduction at the alveolar crest but may produce a separation at the inferior border. If this separation is minimal and the alignment of the dentition is satisfactory, healing will be uncomplicated.

Open Reduction

If separation at the lower border is wide or displacement is considerable, open reduction is indicated. Symphyseal fractures are slow to repair because of the great torquing forces to which the symphysis is subjected. After being immobilized for 5 to 6 weeks the patient may need to wear a lingual splint for an additional 4 to 6 weeks. Lag screw immobilization is especially indicated for symphyseal and parasymphyseal fractures and should be combined with a second immobilization method such as a splint or intermaxillary fixation because of torquing forces.

To approach the mandible in the symphysis area from the skin surface, an incision is made 1 to 1.5 cm beneath the inferior surface of the mandible, following the general contour of the mandible. Hyperextending the mandible and tilting the head backward will allow the incision to be well hidden after a few months of healing. Sharp dissection through skin, underlying fascia, and platysma muscle will expose the inferior surface of the mandible. The periosteum is incised and elevated and the depressor anguli oris (triangularis), depressor labii inferioris (quadratus labii inferioris), and mentales muscles may be elevated from their bony origin. On the medial surface of the mandible, depending on the location of the fracture, the surgeon may encounter the anterior belly of the digastric, mylohyoid, geniohyoid, and genioglossus muscles. In the event that all of the genial muscles, the digastric muscles, and both mylohyoid muscles are detached, either by injury or surgery, provision should be made to control tongue and the airway.

No major arteries or veins are encountered in this area; bleeding is usually minimal and can be controlled by clamping small bleeders or using electric coagulation for hemostasis. No major motor nerves are encountered in this surgical approach because the marginal mandibular nerve is well above the skin incision and the cervical branch of the facial

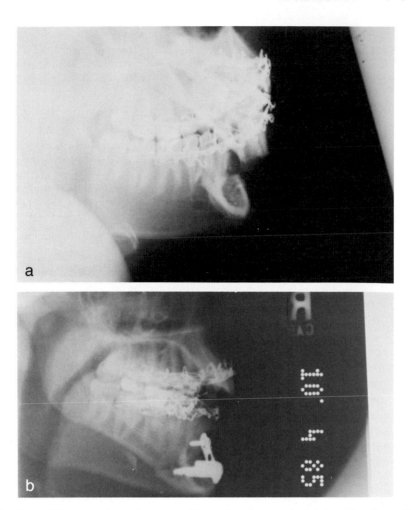

FIG. 6–17.   Fracture of the symphyseal area. **a,** The patient incurred a bilateral fracture of the base of the mandible anterior to the cuspid teeth, as well as a shattering of the alveolar process. This multiple-systems–injured patient was bedridden for several months. **b,** The surgical approach to this mandible fracture included intermaxillary fixation and placement, via an intraoral approach, of osteosynthesis plates to stabilize the severely displaced symphyseal segment.

nerve is below. The anterior cutaneous nerve provides the sensory innervation of this area.

Intraoral open reduction of symphyseal-area fractures is direct and rapid. Combined with intermaxillary fixation, splints, or external pin fixation, the intraoral approach ensures accurately reduced fractures. The operation may be performed on an outpatient under local anesthesia. Depending on the anatomic height of the alveolar process, the incision may be made either in the gingival crest or at the junction of the mucoperiosteum of the alveolar ridge and the mucosa of the vestibule; due regard for the mental nerves will influence the elevations of soft tissues. The incisions may extend bilaterally to the first molar regions, and the entire anterior mandible may be degloved. Transosseous wiring wires may be passed either in converging drill holes in the lateral cortex of the fragment or in drill holes through both the medial and lateral cortices. The access and exposure is adequate for the placement of lag screws or bones plates for rigid fixation.

A lingual splint is a valuable adjunct in the treatment of symphyseal and body of the mandible fractures. A plaster cast of the mandible can be sectioned and reassembled into a proper occlusion against a maxillary cast. The splint is then constructed on the repositioned model.

FRACTURES OF THE EDENTULOUS MANDIBLE

Fractures of the edentulous mandible may require adaptation of one or more of the techniques previously described. If the patient is wearing serviceable dentures, either full or partial, the problem is markedly reduced (Fig. 6–18). In order for the dentures to offer adequate support when used as splints, all the fragments of the fracture must be covered by the denture base. The mandibular denture (or, in the absence of a denture, a splint) may then be secured to the mandible by circumferential wires.

Generally, three wires give satisfactory support if they are placed in the bicuspid areas bilaterally and near the midline. Before the dentures or splints are used, they should be adapted for intermaxillary fixation by attachment of wire loops, metallic lugs, or segments of arch bars. One may remove the anterior incisor teeth to provide an opening for feeding and for an additional airway space.

Fractures of the edentulous mandible are well managed by bone plates or, if an oblique fracture is present (when viewed from a superior or inferior orientation) by lag screws.

The edentulous mandibular fractures that may be the greatest challenge to treatment are those that occur in mandibles that have undergone atrophy of the entire alveolar ridge as well as resorptive loss of the base of the mandible. I have observed this phenomenon in both sexes at ages ranging from the third decade of life onward, not only in aged osteoporetic individuals. The bone in the severely atrophied area has a different tactile quality when holes are drilled or when other bony procedures are performed, providing a sensation similar to the nonresilient sensation of operating in a very dense cartilage rather than to the feeling of resiliency noted when operating on normal bone. Trephine biopsies of the atrophied bone have disclosed a normal trabecular pattern but few to no osteocytes in the lacunae. Similar biopsies in adjacent symphyseal or ramal bone, where muscle attachment activity influences the life of the bone, appear normal. Hence, repair of the atrophied bone can be impaired because of the decrease in vitality. This premise has lead to the routine placing of an autogenous bone graft to augment an open reduction of fractures of the severely atrophied mandible. These grafts have included the sandwiching of the fractured site between split ribs; the use of me-

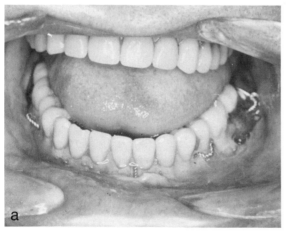
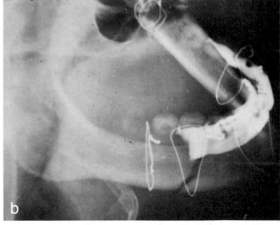

FIG. 6–18.   Fractures of the edentulous mandible. **a,** Fracture of the body of the mandible in an edentulous patient. **b,** Circumferential wiring was used to stabilize the vulcanite denture. (The metal-containing coloring material that was used in these early dentures is seen as a radiopaque band.)

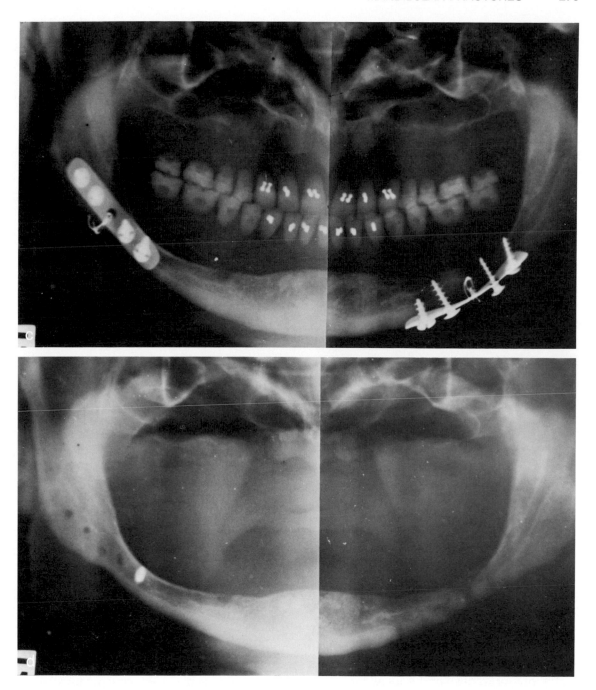

FIG. 6–18 (continued).   **c,** Fractures in an edentulous individual were stabilized with bone plates. The plate on the left was placed on the inferior border of the mandible and the one of the right in the usual lateral position. **d,** The bony plates were removed because of interferences with the flanges of dentures. One of the screws was fractured during the removal and was retained in the right body of the mandible.

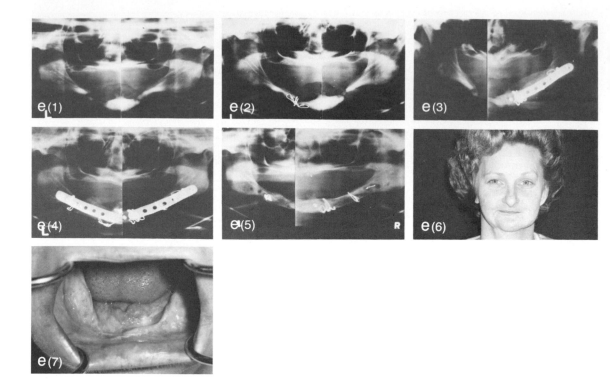

FIG. 6–18 (continued).   **e,** Radiographic series depicting the management of a patient with fractures in a severely atrophied mandible. The treatment consisted of two phase bone-graft reconstructions. **(1),** Bilateral body of the mandible fractures in a female patient with advanced atrophy of the mandible. **(2),** Wires from a previously attempted reduction and fixation procedure were removed. **(3),** 6 weeks later, a unilateral bone graft from the ilium was placed on the medial side of the mandible with a lateral fracture bar for stabilization. **(4),** 4 months later, a second bone graft was placed. **(5),** 4 months later, the bone plates were removed. **(6)** and **(7),** Clinical appearance of the patient. Note the ridges provided by the bone grafts for receipt of dentures. Only bone grafting, alloplastic augmentation, or implant denture devices for the area is further indicated.

tallic cribs screwed to the recipient sites and carrying autogenous cancellous bone marrow; and the placement of cortical-cancellous grafts on the medial surface of the fractured mandible with bone plate stabilization on either the lateral surface, if it is broad enough, or the inferior surface of the mandible.

If bilateral fractures of the severely atrophied mandible are present and are being repaired by bone grafts, one must take into account the effect of the unequal torquing forces on the bilateral fracture sites. The bilateral grafts may be placed at the same time the fractures are stabilized, when the bone plates are placed to unite the mandible. Intraoral splints have not been stable enough for the long-term treatment that is necessary and usually will not reach far enough posteriorly to provide firm fixation of the proximal segments. Also, pressure necrosis from the circumferential wire of splints may produce an additional fracture. If the ramal bone and the symphyseal bone are of a sufficient density and quantity to be solid recipients for screws, external biphasic (or monophasic) devices may be considered.

The most reliable method in my practice has been a two-phase operation. In the first extraoral procedure, one fracture site is directly wired for orientation and a cortical-cancellous graft from the inner crest of the ilium from the same side is placed on the medial aspect of the mandible. Care is taken to provide a generous overlap of the symphyseal

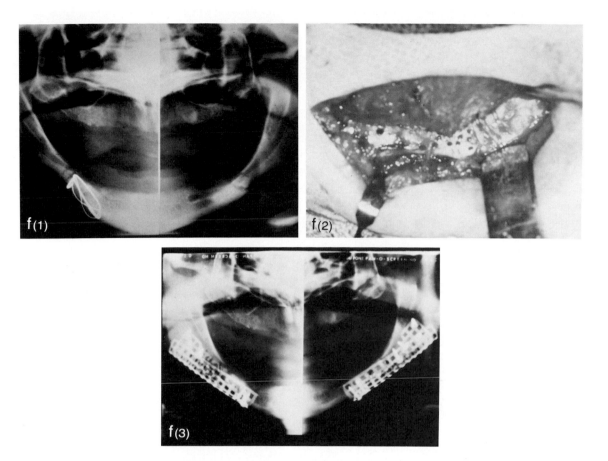

FIG. 6–18 (continued). **f,** Bilateral body of the mandible fractures in a 35-year-old male patient with advanced atrophy of the mandible. **(1),** Preoperative radiograph demonstrates wiring from a previously attempted reduction and fixation prior to referral to me. **(2),** Intraoperative view of the atrophied mandible. **(3),** Postoperative radiographic views. In time the metallic trays were removed and the mandible was stable. The patient was lost to follow-up 2 years postoperatively.

and the ramus recipient area. A bone plate is placed on the lateral or inferior surface and the bone graft and the symphysis are cantilevered from the ramus. No intermaxillary fixation, no circumferentially stabilized splints, and no external fixation devices are placed; the patient is maintained on a soft to liquid diet for 4 to 6 months. At the second phase of the surgical management, the procedure is repeated on the opposite side of the mandible, thus restoring the contour of the lower jaw; the superior crest of the iliac grafts produce processes for the eventual prescription of artificial dentures.

MANDIBULAR FRACTURES IN CHILDREN

In the child with deciduous teeth or a mixed dentition, immobilization of the jaws may be technically difficult (Fig. 6–19). Deciduous and developing permanent teeth may not retain a fracture appliance because their root structures may be shortened. Furthermore, the structure of the crowns of deciduous teeth may make for a tenuous retention of wires. Usually, however, eyelet loops, using 28- or 26-gauge wire, may provide an adaptable, secure, and well-tolerated means of closed reduction.

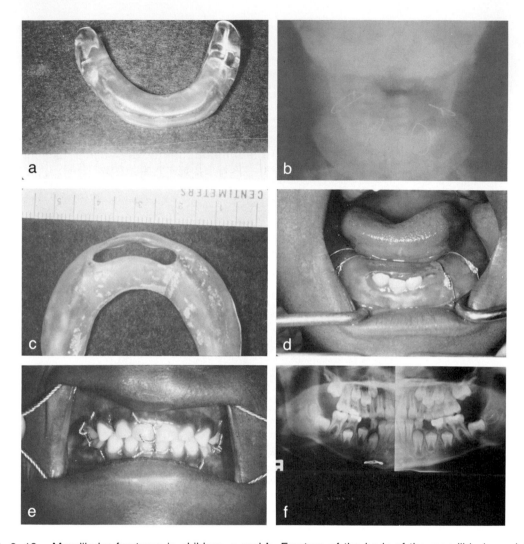

FIG. 6–19.   Mandibular fractures in children. **a** and **b,** Fracture of the body of the mandible in an infant that was treated by placement of an overlying splint for 2 to 3 weeks. **c** and **d,** Mandibular fracture in a 1-year-old child treated with an overlay splint for 3 weeks. **e,** Closed reduction of a fracture in a child. **f,** Fracture of the parasymphyseal area of a child. The fracture was treated by a double wire compression via a transoral approach. The patient was placed on a soft diet, and no other immobilization was indicated.

In body of the mandible fractures through the tooth-bearing area containing many unerupted teeth, closed reduction offers the least disturbance to the normal eruptive pattern of the permanent teeth. In fractures with considerable malposition, open reduction may be indicated in addition to the maxillary immobilization.

The developing and resorbing deciduous dentition may be so unsteady that there will not be sufficient points of fixation for fracture appliances. In these cases, the surgeon may design overlying occlusal splints that are either circumferentially attached to the mandible or cemented to the teeth. Of course, comparable maxillary splints may be necessary.

The management of fractures of the condylar neck in children is generally influenced by the considerations discussed earlier. One must also consider the factor of possible disturbance of the growth potential of a portion of the mandible. Several guidelines may be used. In nondisplaced fractures of the condylar neck that result in minimal pain and allow the patient to close the teeth in proper occlusion, immobilization is not necessary. Treatment consists of immediate and controlled use of the mandible with follow-up supervision by the surgeon. In fractures of the condylar neck with minimal displacement in which the patient exhibits pain and is unable to occlude the teeth properly, however, immobilization is required. After 2 weeks, functional movements are instituted to assist the soft-tissue matrix influence the final form of the bony matrix. In low fractures of the condylar neck with dislocation, open reduction may be the treatment of choice.

Beekler and Walker found that children show a definite propensity to reform the cartilaginous growth center on the condylar head, although the capacity varies with the level of the fracture site on the neck of the condyle.[14] Those fractures occurring near the growth center tend to repair and form a new growth center. In the low condylar fractures, however, there is less chance of reformation of the growth center on the condylar stump.

In all cases, children who have incurred severe mandibular trauma, with and without fracture, should be re-examined annually to assess possible growth aberrations.

COMMINUTED FRACTURES

Shell fragments, missiles, bullets, assault and battery, and high-speed vehicular accidents may cause an extreme comminution of the mandible. Two different concepts can direct management of comminuted fractures of the mandible. These concepts can be expressed as, first, a purposeful exposure and multiple open reductions, and second, closed reduction and control.

Principles of Care

The bone is the central subject in a skeletal injury, and its positions and repair are influenced by contiguous hard and soft tissues. The periodontal areas around teeth provide paths of infection into the body of the mandible. Devitalization of the teeth by any method may lead to periapical inflammations that will cause nonunion. The muscular influences may either distract or impact fractured segments. The inelastic periosteum, though torn, will support fractured segments; and, most importantly, the periosteum will be a key source for the osteogenesis of repair (Fig. 6–20).[15,16]

The principles of care of the shattered mandible are based on the same precepts as for the management of a bone graft. These are immobilization of the parts, contact between the parts, freedom or protection from infection, and vascularization.

Immobilization

A shattered mandible may be immobilized using immobilization of the mandible to the maxillae, intraoral splints, extraoral splinting, direct wiring of the segments, or bone plates over the segments. Combinations of methods are used whenever possible because, comminuted fractures require stabilization for longer periods than usual fractures do and back-up and supporting systems of control ensure that immobilization will be effective for several months, if necessary.

The mandible may be immobilized to the maxilla using fixation points in splints, the application of custom-made or commercial labial arch bars, or the placement of one of the many types of interdental wiring, i.e., Stout's continuous loop wiring, eyelet single loops, or Essig wiring.

Intraoral splints are advantageous because they guide fractured segments into a functional relationship and provide splints for intraoral immobilizations. With modern techniques, splints may be tailored to the patients' needs and fabricated rapidly. Intraoral splints may be stabilized by attachments to teeth and by circumferential wiring.

Extraoral splints, using the specially designed bone screws discussed under the biphasic skeletal fracture devices, can control major segments of the mandible for several months.

Direct wiring is useful for approximating, but not for immobilizing, shattered segments. A major disadvantage is the necessity to lift or detach the periosteum from the fragments

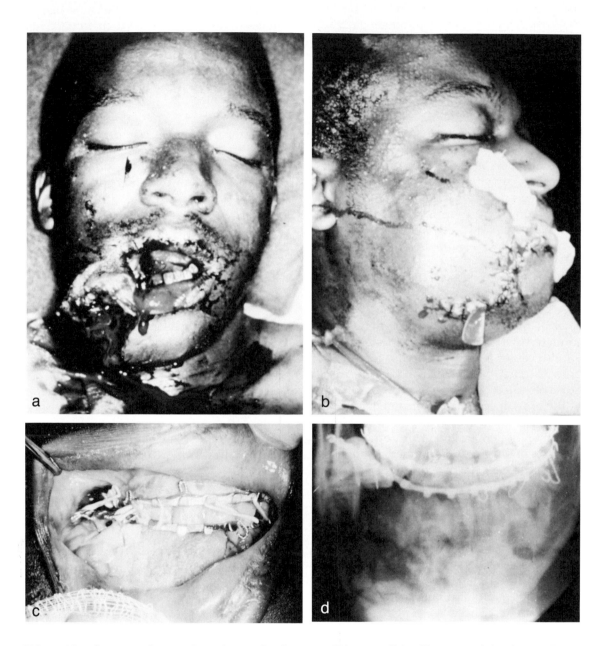

FIG. 6–20.   Compound, comminuted, complex fracture of the mandible. (Courtesy of the Armed Forces Institute of Pathology.) **a,** The appearance of the patient upon admission following a combat injury in Vietnam. **b,** The appearance of the patient following early surgical repair by a U.S. Army oral and maxillofacial surgeon in the combat zone. (Courtesy of Dr. Calvin Thompson.) **c,** The intraoral condition, and **d,** Radiographic view of the patient 1 week after early surgical repair and following aircraft ambulance evacuation from Vietnam to Walter Reed General Hospital, Washington, D.C. Although the segments were not aligned anatomically, they were stabilized.

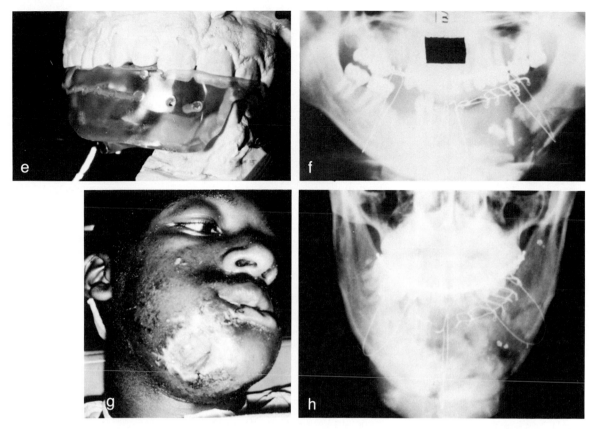

FIG. 6–20 (continued).   **e,** A splint was prepared that would provide support for circumferential wires that would encircle and support comminuted fractures in the right mandible. **f,** Panoramic radiograph of the stabilization of the mandible. **g,** A severe dehiscence over the fracture site at about 6 weeks postinjury was treated by the intraoral closure of the soft tissues and the application of a cyanoacrylate to the mucosal tissues. **h,** Anterior-posterior mandible radiograph as the repair of the comminution progressed.

to place drill holes. Bone plates can stabilize major segments of bone but require extraoral surgical exposure, which could challenge the periosteal attachments and blood supply to the shattered segments of bone.

Contact Between the Parts

In purposeful exposure and multiple direct open reductions of shattered fragments, close contact is achieved and visually confirmed at time of surgery. In this approach, it is necessary to dissect, expose, and control the segments so that holes may be drilled. This surgery requires the lifting of periosteal and musculofascial attachments from the fragments, a procedure that may convert the fragments to the equivalent of multiple autoge-

nous grafted segments. Surgery is concluded with sutured apposition of soft tissue to the bone and application of pressure dressings (Fig. 6–20).

When managing extreme comminution of the mandible using closed reductions, the fragments must be either in closed apposition or controlled by circumferential, nonreactive sutures.

Freedom from Infection

It is a clinical fact that the soft tissues in the vicinity of the oral cavity seem to be well protected from infections that might arise from the intraoral environment. However, the maxillofacial skeleton is susceptible to infections identified with extraoral sources. Acute

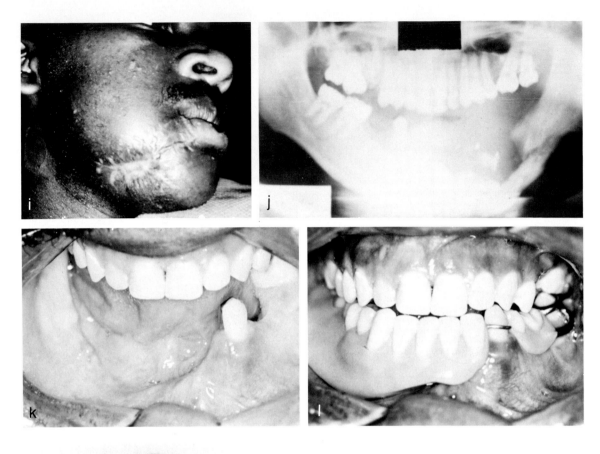

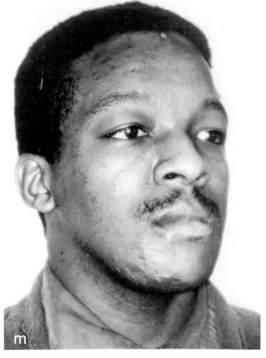

FIG. 6–20 (continued).   **i,** The closure of the dehiscence following the intraoral watertight repair and the use of the cyanoacrylate. **j,** The panoramic x-ray view reveals the bony union of the body of the mandible. Plans were made for bone graft augmentation of the area of bony loss at a later date. **k, l** and **m,** Clinical view of the patient's oral cavity, facies, and temporary prosthesis.

inflammations are seen when intraoral lacerations are not closed over muscular, glandular, and bony parts. Also, when teeth are devitalized by surgical techniques, caries, or trauma, an acute inflammatory process that will militate against repair of the facial skeleton and contiguous soft tissues is likely to occur.

Thus, prinicples of sterility, drainage, and supporting antibiosis are important to prevent a sabotaging infection.

Vascularization

If shattered bone fragments are purposefully dissected and exposed, and if their periosteal attachments are elevated, treatment becomes the management of multiple small autogenous bone grafts rather than the reduction and immobilization of a comminuted fracture. Revascularization of the bone grafts is critical before the shattered segments are lost by inflammation and exfoliation. If, on the other hand, the shattered fragments are permitted to keep their periosteal attachments, even though these attachments may be lacerated, the repair and osteogenesis can proceed as with fracture repair rather than as with multiple bone grafts.

TRAUMATIC INJURIES INVOLVING THE TEMPOROMANDIBULAR ARTICULATION

Acute traumatic injuries of the temporomandibular joint occur with or without an associated fracture of the mandible. The resultant signs and symptoms of meniscus subluxation (clicking) and dislocation (locking) as well as bursitis and capsulitis may occur from many causes other than acute trauma. These include psychological stress, clenching and grinding the teeth, malocclusal relationships, and facial skeletal deformities. Acute trauma imposed on conditions similar to these causes may aggravate dysfunctions of the temporomandibular joint and the associated musculature, or the trauma may be erroneously cited as the cause. As in all injuries, an empathetic and strong doctor-patient relationship should be established. The patient participates in his own care by un-

derstanding the problem, the therapy, and the desired results.

Acute Traumatic Arthritis

Acute arthritis or a sprain of the temporomandibular joint, as in other joints, usually is a reversible injury, and complete function returns following symptomatic treatment with mild analgesics, cold packs, and a short period of decreased function. Rest of the joint for 2 or 3 days may be achieved with the aid of soft and liquid diets, head bandages, and intermaxillary immobilization.

Anterior Condylar Dislocations

Excessive force such as yawning or shouting may produce a forward dislocation of the head of condyle. The condyle may be held forward by a contraction of the lateral pterygoid muscle and may seem to lock anterior to the articular eminence of the temporal bone. Return of the condylar head to the articulating fossa may be impossible without assistance.

This forward dislocation may tear the capsular attachments to the temporal bone and to the mandibular condyle. The meniscus could be detached, perhaps permanently, from its lateral and medial attachments to the condyle. The discomfort and pain associated with the dislocation, the resultant hemorrhage and inflammation, and the psychological effect on the patient may upset the entire neuromuscular balance of the mandible, so that the dislocation will be exceedingly difficult or impossible for the patient to reduce without professional assistance.

To replace the mandible in the glenoid fossa when no fracture is present, the surgeon should apply to the mandible in the molar region a downward and then a posterior and upward force (Fig. 6–21). If the surgeon uses his fingers for this maneuver, they should be lateral to the teeth so that they will not be injured by the occluding of the dentition; if he uses an instrument, he should consider using wooden tongue blades to avoid injuring the teeth.

In some instances of long-standing dislocation, especially if there is a psychologic

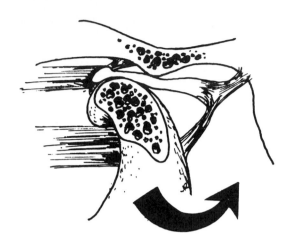

FIG. 6–21. Mandibular condylar dislocation. Direction of movement of the usual force to be transmitted to the condyle to reduce a dislocation.

overlay or extreme spasm of the external pterygoid muscle, the reduction technique may vary: the patient is seated in an upright position with the head against firm restraint; the mandible is grasped, as above, and a steady posterior pressure is applied with a rhythmic side-to-side rocking motion; after a period of several minutes, up to 15 or 20, the patient's muscles will fatigue and the mandibular dislocation will be reduced.

To control the patient's pain during these maneuvers, several adjuncts are considered: a local anesthetic may be injected into the joint and/or through the sigmoid notch into the lateral pterygoid muscle to relieve pain and spasm; Either 100 to 150 mg of sodium pentobarbital as a sedative and mild hypnotic, or 5 to 10 mg of diazepam as a tranquilizer and muscle relaxant may be administered intravenously to overcome the psychological blocks to cooperation. In an extremely resistant case when the maneuver cannot be accomplished even with the preceding pharmacotherapeutic aides, a general anesthetic may be required to reduce the dislocation; in very rare instances, it may be necessary to reduce the dislocation with a direct surgical approach. The operation is performed through a preauricular incision and metal instruments may be required as levers to place the head of the condyle back to the fossa.

Postoperative pain control can vary from a

regular course of 500 mg of aspirin every 2 hrs to the use of other analgesics. In all cases, early but controlled movement of the mandible is exceedingly important to avoid a possible ankylosis that could arise from hemorrhage in the capsular space.

Generally recurrence of dislocations is easier to manage because the patient knows what to expect and is able to cooperate more effectively. Further, stretching of the capsular ligament could result in some elongation that would permit easier reduction of the dislocation.

If the dislocation recurs frequently and self-reduction is not possible, the surgeon should consider surgical removal of the lateral $\frac{1}{3}$ of the articular eminence, which permits the head of the condyle to return to the fossa with less osseous impediment. This procedure is performed outside of the joint space; a by-product of all surgery is fibrosis, which, in this case, will further restrict mandibular movements. Prior to reduction of the articular eminence, laminagraphic radiologic or CT studies should be performed to assess surgical hazards that may be created by the proximity of the cranical vault and by extensions of the mastoid air cells.

An excellent method to control dislocation, as described by Terry, is to attach a metal miniplate to the zygomatic arch with a right angle extension in a coronal direction to provide a mechanical block to forward movements of the condyle.[17] Other mechanical blocks to forward movements of the mandible may be considered, such as laying silicone rubber or bone into slots prepared in the articular eminence of the temporal bone.

Another method to restrain movement of the condylar head is to fibrose the capsule by introducing a sclerosing solution into the capsular space. For example, under local anesthesia, 0.25 to 0.5 cc of 5% sodium psylliate may be used.

Surgical measures that are currently not recommended include condyloplasty, which shortens the condylar process as well as scarring and fibrosis of the capsule and adjacent tissues, thus further restraining the mandible. The surgeon may consider placing nonabsorbable sutures of plastic and metals through the condylar head and into the posterior temporal buttress of the zygomatic arch.

Other Dislocations

With or without fracturing of the head or neck, the condylar head may be dislocated posteriorly, damaging the auditory system,[18] or superiorly, through the mandibular fossa of the temporal bone.[19]

The usual auditory system injury is either a tear of the external auditory meatus or a fracture of the tympanic plate. In these instances, immobilizing the mandible with the condyle returned to its appropriate anatomic location, closing or dressing of lacerations, and manually replacing the tympanic plate are the usual extents of treatment. In all cases of mandibular trauma, and most especially when trauma directed toward the symphyseal area of the mandible is evident, damage to the auditory apparatus should be considered.

A superior dislocation of the condylar head through the thin mandibular (glenoid) fossa of the temporal bone can be lethal. In patients with this unusual finding (which has occurred in my practice only in two children), the treatment is directed toward immobilizing the mandible in its correct anatomic relation to the maxilla, which returns the condyle to its normal level with reference to the glenoid fossa. The fractured temporal bone may follow the condyle and thus reform the fossa. All degrees of injury are possible, of course, and a concurrent intracranial neurosurgical approach may be necessary. CT studies are especially helpful in diagnosing and planning treatment with neurosurgical colleagues.

Meniscus Injuries

External facial trauma may involve the meniscus, capsule, and associated ligaments and results in sequelae ranging from inflammation, to complete or partial severing of the meniscus from its attachments, to tearing or fracturing of the meniscus itself. These occurrences are rare, however. Inflammation of the temporomandibular joint structures may manifest as an acute arthritis of sudden onset and directly related to traumatic etiology.

Following a major acute trauma to the temporomandibular joint, the mandible will deviate to the affected side on protrusion, a crepitation may or may not be evident on auscultation, pain will be present on palpation, and recovery from the inflammation follows a decreased use of the mandible for 2 or 3 weeks. Intense pain can be relieved by immobilizing the mandible against the maxilla or by a *one time* injection of a steroid, for example, 5 to 25 mg of hydrocortisone, into the joint capsular space.

The meniscus will be dislocated if it becomes detached from any of its four major areas of attachment: the medial and lateral poles of the condyle, anterior muscular attachments, and posterior bilaminar fibrous attachments. The dislocation will result in blockages in excursions of the mandible. The use of nonsurgical methods of intraoral splint therapy and physical therapy may reseat the meniscus. If nonsurgical approaches are not successful and if a dislocation of the meniscus is diagnosed within a few weeks following injury, the treatment may be surgical reattachment or reconstruction of the meniscus. If the diagnosis is made months after injury, the treatment may be a meniscectomy if the cartilage has degenerated; a glenoid fossa dermal or fascial graft or prosthesis can be indicated following meniscectomy. The surgical site would be approached using a variation of either a preauricular or a postauricular incision.

REFERENCES

1. Olson, R.A., Fonseca, R.J., Zeitler, D.L., and Osbon, D.B.: Fractures of the mandible, review of 580 cases. J Oral Maxillofac Surg 40:23, 1982.
2. Chipps, J.E., Canham, R.G., and Makel, H.P.: Intermediate treatment of maxillofacial injuries. U.S. Armed Forces Med J 4:951, 1953.
3. Bochlogyros, P.N.: A retrospective study of 1,521 mandibular fractures. J Oral Maxillofac Surg 43:597, 1985.
4. Fry, W.K., Shepherd, P.R., McLeod, A.C., and Parfitt, G.J.: The Dental Management of Maxillofacial Injuries. American Edition. Philadelphia and Montreal; J.B. Lippincott Co., 1942, pp.12–14.
5. Morris, J.H.: Biphasic connector, external skeletal splint for reduction and fixation of mandibular fractures. Oral Surg 2:1382, 1949.

6. Spiessl, B.: Principles of rigid internal fixation in fractures of the lower jaw. *In* New Concepts of Maxillofacial Bone Surgery. Edited by B. Spiessel. New York, Springer Verlag, 1976.

7. Kahnberg, D.E., and Ridell, A.: Bone plate fixation of mandibular fractures. Int J Oral Surg *9*:267, 1980.

8. Tu, H.K., and Tenhulzen, D.: Compression osteosynthesis of mandibular fractures. J Oral Maxillofac Surg *43*:585, 1985.

9. Members of the Chalmers J. Lyons Club. (Prepared by Hayward, J.R.): Fractures involving the mandibular condyle. A posttreatment survey of 120 cases. J Oral Surg *5*:45, 1947.

10. Zide, M.F., and Kent, J.N.: Indications for open reduction of mandibular condyle fractures. J Oral Maxillofac Surg *41*:89, 1983.

11. Petzel, J.: Functionally stable traction-screw osteosynthesis of condylar fractures. J Oral and Maxillofac Surg *40*:108, 1982.

12. Wennogle, C.,F., and Delo, R.I.: A pin-in-grove technique for reduction of displaced subcondylar fractures of the mandible. J Oral and Maxillofac Surg *43*:659, 1985.

13. Dingman, R.O., and Grabb, W.C.: Surgical anatomy of the mandibular ramus of the facial nerve based on dissection of 100 facial halves. Plast Reconstr Surg *29*:266, 1962.

14. Beekler, D.M., and Walker, R.V.: Condyle fractures. J Oral Surg *27*:563, 1969.

15. Alling, C.C., and Davis, R.P., Jr.: Compound comminuted complex maxillofacial fractures. J Oral Surg *32*:415, 1974.

16. Shuker, S.: Management of comminuted mandibular war injuries with multiple circumferential wires. J Oral Maxillofac Surg *44*:152, 1986.

17. Terry, B.C.: Personal communication, 1986.

18. Conover, G.L., and Crammond, R.J.: Tympanic plate fracture from mandibular trauma. J Oral Maxillofac Surg *43*:292, 1982.

19. Copenhaver, R.H., et al.: Fracture of the glenoid fossa with dislocation of the condyle into the middle cranial fossa. J Oral Maxillofac Surg *43*:974, 1985.

7

MAXILLARY FRACTURES

KENNETH K. KEMPF

ETIOLOGY

By its position in the middle third of the face, the maxilla is somewhat protected by the more prominent mandible, zygomas, nasal bones, and frontal bone. Hence, it is not surprising that fractures of the mandible and zygomatic complex are more common than those of the maxilla.

Interpersonal violence accounts for most mandibular, zygomaticomaxillary complex, and nasal fractures, whereas motor vehicle accidents account most commonly for maxillary fractures.[1] In a review of 403 patients with facial fractures, Neal et al. found that 71% of maxillary fractures were associated with motor vehicle accidents.[1] Similarly Turvey reported on 593 patients with many types of midfacial fractures of which 69% were zygomaticomaxillary complex, 32% nasal, 21% Le Fort type, 9% zygomatic arch, 5% maxillary alveolar, and 4% blow-out fractures;[2] Again, almost 50% of the fractures in this series were the result of motor vehicle accidents.

The small number of maxillary fractures caused by interpersonal violence typically are closed fractures involving one or several facial bones with minimal soft-tissue disruption (Fig. 7–1). Motor vehicle accidents, on the other hand, produce a vast array of complex injuries. Rapid deceleration throws the face against a dash or steering wheel, creating complex, comminuted fractures involving the whole of the midface (Fig. 7–2). Broken glass and metal will cause avulsive soft-tissue injuries of the face and oral cavity, setting the stage for airway obstruction. Concomitant injuries of the skull, limbs, chest, abdomen, eye, and cervical spine are associated with injuries caused by motor vehicle accidents more than by other forms of trauma. By contrast, gunshot wounds of the maxilla that are the result of suicide attempts, civilian violence, and military confrontations, typically produce penetrating, avulsive, through-and-through injuries with the loss of bone and soft tissue (Fig. 7–3). Whatever the cause, maxillary fractures occur more frequently in the young, mobile segment of our population, with greatest incidence in the 20- to 30-year age group. Men are the victims three times more frequently than women.

Maxillary fractures in children are uncommon before the age of 12 because the maxilla of the child is more elastic, less pneumatized, and more protected by the mandible and frontal bone. Also, the child's lighter weight produces less inertial force when the head hits an object. The most common causes of maxillary fractures in the child are motor vehicle accidents, falls, and physical abuse.

Maxillary fractures in elderly individuals occur less frequently than in younger people and are most often the result of falls. A higher

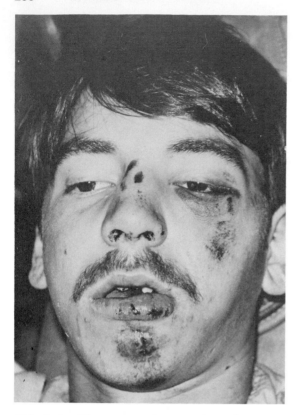

FIG. 7–1.   Blunt trauma from an altercation.

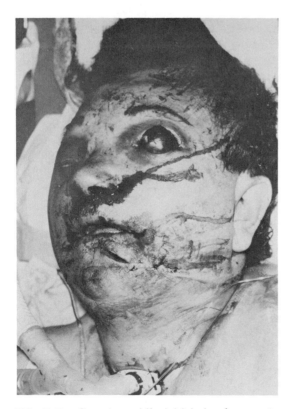

FIG. 7–2.   Complex midfacial injuries from motor vehicle accident. Note ocular injury.

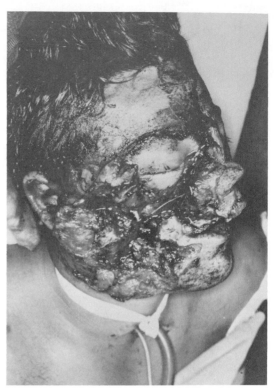

FIG. 7–3.   High-velocity gunshot wound.

percentage of fractured maxillas in the elderly are edentulous, thereby complicating intermaxillary fixation.

CLASSIFICATION

An accurate clinical and radiographic appraisal of all the bones involved in midfacial fractures is often difficult. One method of classifying fractures of the midface defines areas of the facial skeleton as stable and not stable.

Rene Le Fort of Paris reported in 1901 his classic experiment producing fractures of the maxilla on a series of cadavers.[3] By varying the degree and direction of blows to the maxilla, Le Fort found that fractures could generally be classified according to the highest level of fracture.

LE FORT I—HORIZONTAL FRACTURE
(Fig. 7–4)

The Le Fort I is the most common type of maxillary fracture. It begins at the lateral pyr-

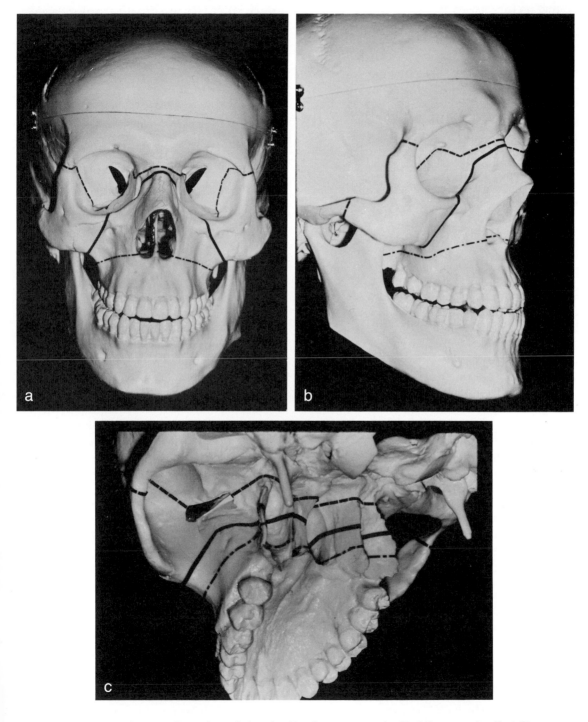

FIG. 7–4.   **a,** Le Fort fracture lines, frontal view. Le Fort I — · — · —; Le Fort II ———; Le Fort III — — — — . **b,** Le Fort fracture lines, lateral view. **c,** Le Fort fracture lines, posterior view.

iform rim, runs horizontally above the apices of the teeth, passes below the zygomatico-maxillary junction, crosses the pterygomaxillary junction, and passes through both pterygoid plates, usually at or below the pterygomaxillary fissure. Intranasally, the cartilaginous nasal septum is separated from the nasal spine and anterior palate and a fracture extends through the base of the vomer. In individuals with high palatal vaults and alveolar vertical excess, the fracture may begin under the nasal spine and pyriform rim and then proceed posteriorly as described previously.

LE FORT II—PYRAMIDAL FRACTURE
(Fig. 7–4)

The geometric pattern formed by the lines of this fracture resembles a pyramid. The fracture begins at a weaker portion of the nasal bridge just below or at the frontonasal sutures and passes bilaterally through the frontal process of the maxillae, across the lacrimal bones to the anterior crest of the nasolacrimal canal. The fracture line then passes downward, laterally and anteriorly across the most anterior aspect of the orbital floor and across the inferior orbital rim through or near the infraorbital foramen and then inferiorly along the anterior wall of the antrum. From here it runs under the zygoma, as does the Le Fort I fracture, and then extends along the tuberosity across the pterygomaxillary fissure and through the pterygoid plates at a higher level than does the Le Fort I fracture. Intranasally, the fracture runs through the upper third of the nasal septum, passing through the perpendicular plate of the ethmoid and across the middle of the vomer.

LE FORT III—TRANSVERSE FRACTURE
(Fig. 7–4)

A complete craniofacial dysjunction is produced by the Le Fort III fracture. The fracture begins at the frontonasal and frontomaxillary junctions, passes bilaterally through the uppermost aspect of the nasolacrimal groove, and extends posteriorly along the ethmoid to a point just anterior to the optic foramen. Because the sphenoid bone surrounding the op-tic foramen is considerably thicker, the incidence of fracture into the optic canal is reduced. The fracture then descends to the most posterior extent of the infraorbital canal and from there extends to the sphenopalatine fossa and then high across the pterygoid plates.

From within the orbit, a second fracture line passes anteriorly along the inferior orbital fissure and then extends superiorly along the lateral orbital wall at the junction of the zygoma and greater wing of the sphenoid bone. It then passes through the zygomaticofrontal suture. A fracture through the zygomatic arches completes the extranasal course of the Le Fort III fracture.

Within the nose, the fracture line passes through the base of the perpendicular plate of the ethmoid, usually causing a disruption and comminution of the cribriform plate. The fracture line finally passes through the connection of the vomer with the sphenoid bone, thus completing the dysjunction of the midface from its cranial connection.

The Le Fort description provides a basis with which to identify and classify maxillary fractures. Though the fractures frequently occur as recognizable entities, combinations are also produced, and all three types of maxillary fractures can be present in the same patient either bilaterally or unilaterally. Fractures that split the maxilla and palate in a sagittal direction are less common but can be seen singly or in combination with other maxillary fractures. When combined with other fractures, the sagittal fracture adds to the instability of the other maxillary fractures and the continuity of the palatal buttress must be reestablished to maintain correct dental occlusion. The adjacent facial bones are commonly involved in maxillary fractures.

Displacement of midfacial fractures is a result of the direction and degree of the traumatic force. A frontal force of moderate degree such as from a fall will often produce a maxillary alveolar fracture or a Le Fort I fracture. A frontal force of greater degree such as from a deceleration injury in a motor vehicle accident will often result in a Le Fort II or III fracture and a sagittal palatal fracture. A frontal force from a superior direction such as from a club or stick will often result in a Le

Fort III fracture in addition to nasoethmoid fractures. Most frontal forces will produce a backward and downward dislocation or impaction of the maxilla. Blows to the midface from a lateral direction tend to produce bilateral zygoma fractures and a rotation of the maxilla to the contralateral side.

Muscle pull plays a dominant role in distracting mandibular fractures but only a minor role in distracting maxillary fractures. Fractures through the pterygoid plates will allow the pterygoid muscles to distract the fractured maxilla distally and inferiorly, causing premature contact of the molars and the typical open bite. The posterior displacement of the maxilla manifests as a midfacial depression (dish-face), and the downward displacement results in facial elongation (Fig. 7–5).

ANATOMIC CONSIDERATIONS

The maxilla and associated facial bones are collectively called the midface or middle one-third of the facial skeleton. This complex area is bounded above by a transverse line passing through the zygomaticofrontal, frontomaxillary and frontonasal junctions, below by the occlusal table, and posteriorly by the sphenoethmoid junction above and the pterygoid processes below. The middle third of the facial skeleton is composed of the paired nasal, lacrimal, zygomatic, inferior nasal conchae, palatine, and maxilla bones, and the unpaired vomer, ethmoid, and sphenoid bones.

The maxilla is the principal bone of the midface, contributing to the structure of the orbit, nasal cavity, paranasal sinuses, and the hard palate. It consists of a body and four processes—frontal, zygomatic, palatine, and alveolar. The body is hollowed by the pyramid shaped maxillary sinus, with its base formed by the lateral nasal wall and its apex extending into the body of the zygoma. At birth the maxillary sinus is no larger than a marble; it attains its adult size at about 15 years of age. The maxilla articulates medially with the nasal bone, superiorly with the frontal bone at the frontomaxillary suture, laterally with the zygoma, and posteriorly with the vertical and horizontal plates of the palatine bone. The maxilla joins the vertical plate of the palatine bone to complete the pterygopalatine canal and with the horizontal plate of the palatine bone to form the posterior part of the hard palate.

The maxilla can best be described as a four-sided pyramid with its base forming the lateral nasal wall. The anterior wall is thinned in the area of canine fossa and thickened laterally at its junction with the zygoma. The posterior wall, which is formed by the maxillary tuberosity, faces the infratemporal space and forms the anterior boundary of the pterygopalatine fossa. The superior wall forms the greater portion of the anterior floor of the orbit and is transversed by the infraorbital groove containing the infraorbital nerve and vessels. The inferior wall of the maxilla is formed by the alveolar process containing the maxillary teeth.[4]

The middle facial skeleton, designed to resist the vertical forces of mastication, is reinforced by six vertical pillars, three on each side (Fig. 7–6). These pillars, the canine, zygomatic, and pterygoid pillars, transmit the vertical forces from the teeth and distribute those forces over a broad area of the cranial base. The canine pillar originates from the canine eminence of the alveolar process, passes superiorly, reinforcing the lateral pyriform rim, and then continues through the frontal process of the maxilla to the supraorbital rim. The zygomatic pillar begins at the zygomaticoalveolar crest and extends upward into the zygoma, where it divides into two limbs. The anterior limb ascends along the lateral orbital rim to the lateral half of the supraorbital rim, and the posterior limb courses along the zygomatic arch to the temporal bone. The pterygoid pillar is formed by the pterygoid process, which is attached to the maxilla by the intervening palatine bone. These pillars are further reinforced superiorly by the superior and inferior orbital rims and inferiorly by the palatine and alveolar processes.[5]

Traumatic forces applied to the maxilla are distributed to the base of the skull through these pillars. Although these pillars are effective in resisting a traumatic force exerted in a vertical direction, shear forces directed perpendicularly to the vertical pillars produce dysjunctions of the maxilla.

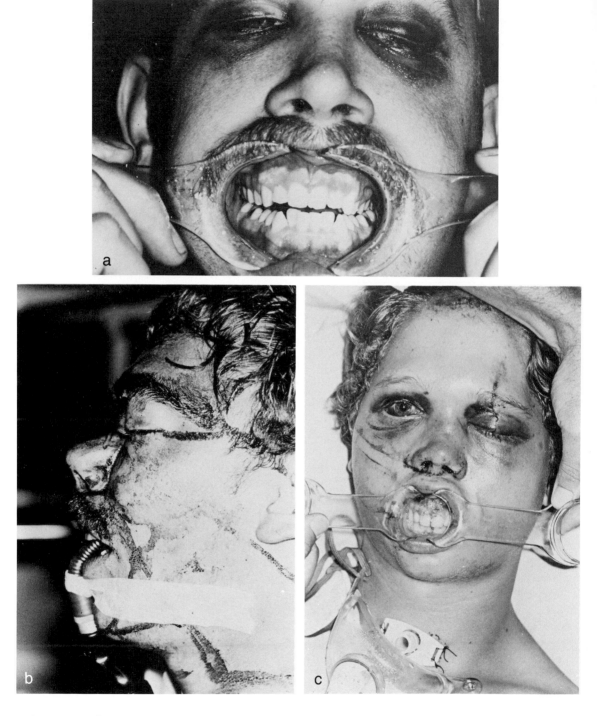

FIG. 7–5.   **a,** Open bite, Le Fort I fracture. **b,** Midfacial depression, Le Fort II fracture. **c,** Facial elongation, Le Fort III fracture.

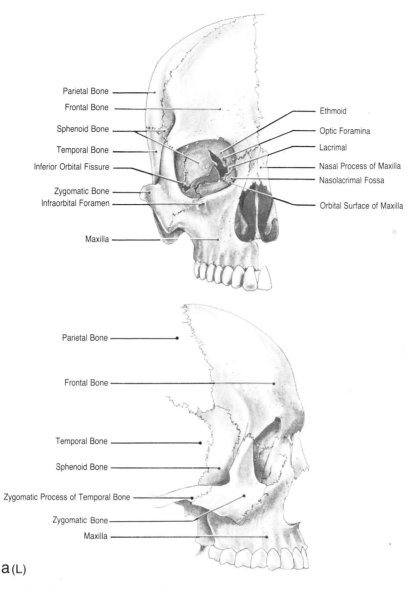

Parietal Bone
Frontal Bone
Sphenoid Bone
Temporal Bone
Inferior Orbital Fissure
Zygomatic Bone
Infraorbital Foramen
Maxilla

Ethmoid
Optic Foramina
Lacrimal
Nasal Process of Maxilla
Nasolacrimal Fossa
Orbital Surface of Maxilla

Parietal Bone
Frontal Bone
Temporal Bone
Sphenoid Bone
Zygomatic Process of Temporal Bone
Zygomatic Bone
Maxilla

a(L)

FIG. 7–6.   **a L** and **R,** Osteology of the maxilla.

ASSOCIATED INJURIES

The surgeon treating facial fractures must be aware that patients with midfacial injuries frequently have concomitant injuries to other regions of the body involving many organ systems. Injuries to the cranium, cervical spine, orbit, trachea, and chest must be rapidly and sequentially identified and managed before definitive treatment of the facial fractures is initiated.

Studies conducted at various trauma centers have consistently shown that the frequency of complex maxillofacial, cranial, tho-

racic, and abdominal injuries is two to three times greater in high-velocity, high-impact trauma, as in motor vehicle accidents, than in low-velocity, low-impact trauma, as in interpersonal violence, falls, or sports injuries.[6]

Of 270 consecutive patients with midfacial injuries treated at the University of Iowa, 96 (nearly 36%) had associated body injuries. Table 7–1 summarizes the percentage of associated body injuries in these patients.

Other injuries frequently associated with midfacial fractures include other facial fractures, facial lacerations, and orthopedic injuries. Turvey found that of the 9 patients that

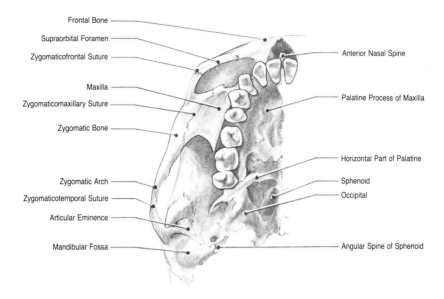

Frontal Bone

Supraorbital Foramen

Zygomaticofrontal Suture

Maxilla

Zygomaticomaxillary Suture

Zygomatic Bone

Zygomatic Arch

Zygomaticotemporal Suture

Articular Eminence

Mandibular Fossa

Anterior Nasal Spine

Palatine Process of Maxilla

Horizontal Part of Palatine

Sphenoid

Occipital

Angular Spine of Sphenoid

Lateral View

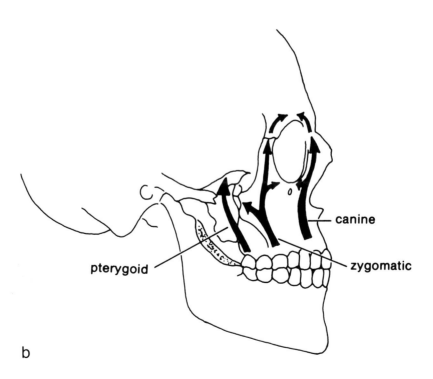

canine

pterygoid

zygomatic

b

FIG. 7–6 (continued).   **b,** Structural pillars protect the maxilla from vertical forces.

Table 7–1. Body Injuries Associated with Midfacial Trauma*

Associated Injury	Low-Velocity Trauma	High-Velocity Trauma
Cerebrospinal	12%	36%
Thoracic	9.1%	19.4%
Abdominal	4%	11%
Ocular	2.7% overall	

*Data from 270 consecutive patients at the University of Iowa

died out of 593 patients with midfacial fractures, none of these deaths was due to the facial injury, but rather to the associated injuries or complications of those associated injuries.[2]

Although midfacial fractures in themselves are seldom life-threatening, other than by causing acute airway obstruction or hemorrhage, life-threatening injuries are not infrequently associated with midfacial fractures. Hence, the most significant management priority is finding or ruling out these potentially lethal or permanently disfiguring injuries; definitive management of the fractures can be delayed until the patient's overall condition is stabilized. Because of the frequency of associated injuries, the patient with facial trauma should primarily be under the care of a trauma team capable of the diagnosis and emergency management of these associated injuries.

In addition to the oral and maxillofacial surgeon, who is responsible for treating facial skeletal injuries that involve occlusion of the teeth and function of the oral cavity, other specialists are also concerned with midfacial trauma. The team approach, possible in medical centers where specialists in the various disciplines are available, is desirable for the most comprehensive care of the patient.

ORBITAL AND OCULAR INJURIES

These injuries are produced directly by trauma to the orbit or indirectly from maxillary and zygomatic fractures (Fig. 7–2). Although these injuries do not occur frequently, when they are unrecognized or not managed appropriately the results can be disastrous for the patient. The signs and symptoms of fractures of the orbit include periorbital edema, ecchymosis, subconjunctival hemorrhage,

ptosis of the lids, enophthalmos, exophthalmos, chemosis, and restriction of ocular motility. Ocular complications involving the globe include rupture of the globe, vitreous and anterior chamber hemorrhage, dislocated lens, choroid rupture, and late complications such as glaucoma and cataract formation.[7] Any injury that involves the globe demands a pretreatment ophthalmologic consultation.

Le Fort III and nasoethmoid fractures involve the orbit and are associated with the highest incidence of orbital and ocular injuries.[6] Le Fort III fractures disrupt the medial, lateral, and inferior orbital walls and may reach the orbital apex, producing several recognized syndromes.

Superior Orbital Fissure Syndrome

The superior orbital fissure syndrome is caused by pressure or disruption of the contents of the superior orbital fissure, namely, the oculomotor, trochlear, and abducent nerves, the three branches of the ophthalmic division of the trigeminal nerve, and sympathetic nerves from the cavernous plexus.[8] The most common cause for this syndrome is pressure at the apex within the muscular cone formed by the common tendinous ring, the pressure being the result of edema or hemorrhage. Less commonly, the fissure itself will be disrupted and fragments of bone will impinge on the contents of the fissure. The results of this injury include varying degrees of exophthalmos, ophthalmoplegia, retro-orbital pain, a fixed-dilated pupil, ptosis, and anesthesia over the distribution of the ophthalmic division of V, including loss of the corneal reflex.

Orbital Apex Syndrome

Fracture through the optic foramen and optic nerve injury is termed the orbital apex syndrome. Although the optic nerve is well protected by the body of the sphenoid bone, a fracture nevertheless may penetrate the foramen. Pressure from edema and hemorrhage may cause optic nerve damage without fracture. The results of optic nerve injury are neuritis, papilledema, or blindness.

Unilateral or bilateral loss of vision may accompany fractures of the frontonasal complex. On the rare occasion that unilateral vision loss occurs and fracture of the orbital apex on the opposite side is suspected, manipulation of the fractures should be delayed until fracture of the optic foramina is ruled out. Weymuller recommends that should there be loss of vision in one eye and fracture of the optic foramen in the other, the fractures of the midface should be stabilized but not reduced in order to prevent possible bilateral loss of vision.[9]

Diplopia

Diplopia, either monocular or binocular, is a common sign of an orbital fracture.[10] Monocular diplopia is caused by direct injury to the globe such as hemorrhage into the anterior chamber or a detached lens. Binocular diplopia is usually caused by restriction of extraocular muscles, as is seen in orbital floor fractures, medial wall fractures, and blow-out fractures. Hemorrhage and edema causing increased intraorbital pressure can cause a transient diplopia, whereas a decrease in volume of the orbital contents as seen with herniation of fat and muscle into the maxillary sinus can result in permanent diplopia unless treated.

CERVICAL SPINE INJURIES

Any force capable of producing facial bone fractures can cause injury to the cervical spine. Whereas less than 1% of isolated maxillary fractures are associated with cervical spine injuries, the incidence increases when maxillary and mandibular fractures are combined. The possibility of cervical spine injury should always be kept in mind even when the symptoms are slight or there are no neurologic findings. The articulation between the first and second cervical vertebrae is loose and mobile and hence most subject to injury.

A deceleration force causing a hyperflexion of the neck is the most common source of cervical spine injury. Tearing of the lateral and spinous ligaments can occur, as well as fracturing of the odontoid process of the second cervical vertebra. A hyperextension or whiplash force can have the same effect or injury as seen in hyperflexion of the neck.[11] Clinical findings of cervical spine injury include nuchal pain, which may be slight, and limitation of head motion. Involuntarily holding the head in an unnatural position is pathognomonic for dislocation. Cervical spine radiographs including a PA view to examine the odontoid should be taken routinely for all patients with moderate to severe midfacial injuries. Inattention to the possibility of cervical spine injury could lead to dislocation and compression of the spinal cord.

CEREBROSPINAL FLUID LEAKAGE

Le Fort III and nasoethmoid fractures can result in fracture and disruption of the cribriform plate of the ethmoid, leading to a dural tear followed by cerebrospinal rhinorrhea. If the patient is supine, the leakage may pass into the nasopharynx and not be detected. Cerebrospinal fluid otorrhea, mastoid ecchymosis (Fig. 7–7), and lateral scleral ecchymosis can also result from Le Fort III fractures associated with basilar skull fractures.

INTRACRANIAL INJURIES

The patient with displaced midfacial fractures may also have some degree of intracranial injury. The surgeon treating facial fractures must be competent to make a neurologic assessment. A history of loss of consciousness or amnesia of the traumatic event is indicative of significant intracranial trauma. The examiner must search for evidence of skull fracture and include in the examination AP and lateral radiographic films of the skull. Subdural hemorrhage may be reflected initially by headaches of varying intensity and a dilated pupil. A neurosurgical consultation is required

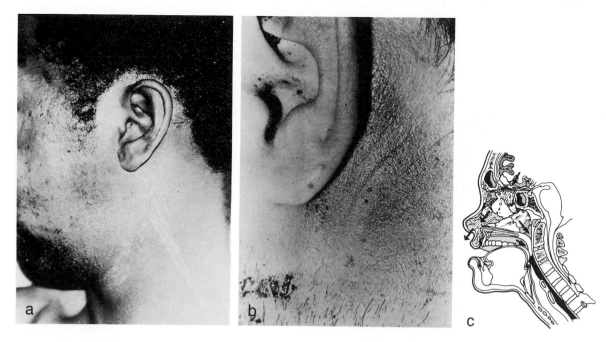

FIG. 7–7. **a,** Cerebrospinal fluid otorrhea. **b,** Mastoid ecchymosis (Battle's sign). **c,** Cerebrospinal fluid leakage through cribriform plate fracture (arrows).

when there is any indication of intracranial injury, no matter how slight.

DIAGNOSIS

Diagnosis of the type and extent of injuries sustained by the patient is obtained from the history, clinical examination, and radiographic evaluation. In the emergency situation, airway management and hemorrhage control take precedence. After the airway is established and hemorrhage is controlled, a brief history is taken to determine the cause and time of the injury and a rapid but thorough physical assessment is made to detect associated injuries that are potentially life-threatening. After the patient's condition is stabilized, a detailed history can be taken and clinical examination performed.

HISTORY

Information concerning the type of trauma and its intensity and direction is helpful in establishing a diagnosis. As mentioned earlier, a concentrated traumatic force such as from a fist or club would suggest a more lo-calized injury such as fractures of the teeth, alveolar process, nasal bones, or zygoma. High-velocity accidents produce greater displacement and comminution of facial bones and show a statistically greater incidence of intracranial, cervical spine, and other body injuries. A history of loss of consciousness or amnesia of the traumatic event suggests the possibility of intracranial injury.

CLINICAL EXAMINATION

The facial features of the patient who has sustained midfacial trauma are obscured by edema, ecchymosis, and hematoma. Soft-tissue edema forms quickly, especially in the periorbital regions where the subcutaneous tissues are loose (Fig. 7–8). Areas of ecchymosis, especially in the periorbital regions, strongly suggest underlying fracture.

The clinical examination should be detailed and systematic in order that no areas are overlooked. The necessary instruments are a good light, preferably a headlamp, suction, dental and laryngeal mirrors, tongue blade, small or medium nasal speculum, otoscope, and ophthalmoscope. The classic technique for examining the head and neck is observation fol-

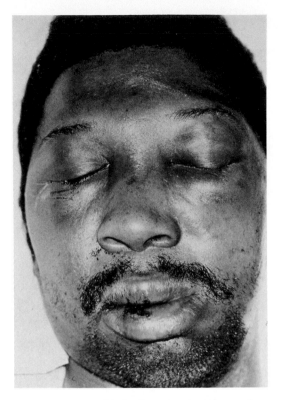

FIG. 7–8.   Periorbital edema and ecchymosis are suggestive of maxillary fracture.

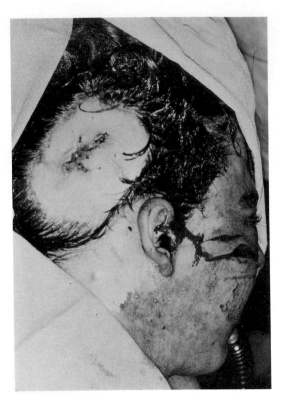

FIG. 7–9.   Scalp laceration associated with mid-facial injuries.

lowed by palpation. The examiner should closely observe the face, looking for asymmetry from the frontal and lateral views, as well as from the coronal view (that is, looking over the face from above). Although swelling may obscure the underlying discrepancies, the observer can still note depressed fractures of the maxilla, zygoma, and zygomatic arch, as well as orbital rim and nasal fractures. The patient should be examined for rhinorrhea, which either can be obscured by nasal bleeding or can escape into the nasopharynx when the patient is observed in the supine position.

The external ear is inspected for lacerations, otorrhagia, or otorrhea. The presence of retroauricular ecchymosis suggests basilar skull fracture.

After the initial observation of the head and face, the scalp and cranium must be inspected and palpated prior to any other manipulation. A hematoma containing a large volume of blood can form under the scalp, and scalp lacerations are notorious for continuing to bleed even under pressure dressings (Fig.

7–9). These findings indicate the possibility of a skull fracture.

Next, the cervical spine is palpated for tenderness, crepitus, and rigidity. If nuchal pain, abnormal head positioning, and range of motion limitation are present, suggesting cervical spine injury, further manipulation of the head other than for airway management should be avoided until cervical-spine injuries are ruled out by a radiographic survey. The temporary use of a soft collar or sand bags on either side of the head will help reduce the chance of further cervical spine or spinal cord injury during the examination.

The next priority is a systematic intraoral examination. Loose or broken dentures, bridges, crowns, and fillings should be carefully removed to avoid aspiration. Next, the base of the tongue and the parapharyngeal and retropharyngeal areas are examined for foreign objects and trapdoor lacerations, which can lead to airway obstruction. Careful observation of the floor of the mouth and buccal mucosa may reveal lacerations of the main

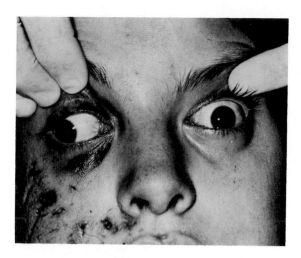

FIG. 7–10   Initial eye examination for foreign bodies, abrasions, lacerations, penetrating injuries, and ocular motility. Note palsy of the left oculomotor nerve.

salivary ducts. A thorough ophthalmologic examination should be performed at this stage prior to any manipulation or treatment to rule out any injury to the eye. A minimal eye exam at this time would include carefully retracting the lids to examine for conjunctival or scleral lacerations, foreign bodies, corneal abrasions, penetrating injuries of the globe, ocular movements, pupillary response, enophthalmos, proptosis, and diplopia and to evaluate gross visual acuity (Fig. 7–10). If edema and dried blood hamper the eye examination, gently retracting the lids with a lid retractor or moist cotton applicator wooden sticks and washing the eye with sterile water will clear the field for a more unobstructed examination. Should any injuries to the globe, orbit, or periorbita be detected, an immediate ophthalmologic consultation should be requested.

A detailed examination of the maxilla begins with the dentition (Fig. 7–11). Each tooth should be examined individually for fracture and mobility. A vertical alveolar or palatal fracture can be detected by manipulating the teeth. A tear in the palatal mucosa, a step deformity, or palatal ecchymosis may disclose a sagittal palatal fracture. Displaced and/or impacted maxillary fractures will produce a malocclusion. To detect maxillary tipping, the lips are retracted and the teeth brought into contact so that the occlusion can be examined from a frontal view. Most horizontal maxillary fractures result in an anterior open bite.

The examining finger is next moved along the anterior and lateral sinus walls to detect a step or discontinuity in the bone. Special attention should be directed to the junction of the zygoma and alveolar process, where a step or separation in the bone can be readily felt. The presence of vestibular ecchymosis suggests an underlying fracture.

Next, a bimanual palpation of the facial skeleton is carried out to detect the type and extent of the maxillary fractures. The head is stabilized with the one hand while the other hand attempts to move the maxilla. In Le Fort I fractures, the alveolar process of the maxilla and palate moves. With a sagittal fracture of the palate and alveolus, the two sides of the maxilla may move independently of one another. A finger placed in the vestibule while the maxilla is being manipulated will detect the fracture lines. If movement is noticed at the frontonasal junction as well as at the inferior orbital rims, a Le Fort II fracture is present. In a Le Fort III fracture, the entire midface is movable, and palpation will reveal separation and movement at the frontonasal and frontozygomatic junctions as well as movement over the zygomatic arches. These fractures are best detected with a second examiner stabilizing the head while the primary examiner manipulates the maxilla and simultaneously palpates the bony junctions. If a Le Fort III fracture is identified, further manipulation of the maxilla should be avoided until radiographs have ruled out a fracture into the orbital apex.

Although ecchymosis and swelling will obscure fractures about the face, the orbital rims can be palpated even with considerable swelling. Examination of the rims is facilitated by moistening the examining finger with water or petroleum jelly. The examination begins in the medial canthal regions and progresses over the inferior, lateral, and superior borders of the rim. Lack of integrity and displacement can be readily detected even when not apparent on radiographs. The medial canthal regions should be palpated for crepitus and movement. The intercanthal distance should be measured (normal is 33 to 35 mm); an in-

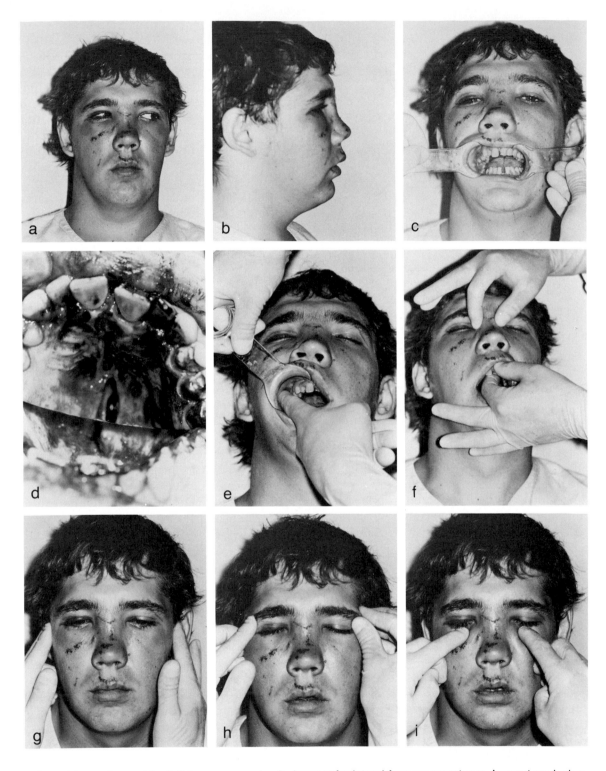

FIG. 7–11.   **a,** Inspect for full-face asymmetry. **b,** Inspect for lateral-face asymmetry. **c,** Inspect occlusion. **d,** Inspect for alveolar and palatal fractures. **e,** Palpate sinus walls. **f,** Test maxilla for mobility. **g,** Palpate zygomatic maxillary suture. **h,** Palpate supraorbital rims. **i,** Palpate infraorbital rims. **j,** Measure medial canthal distance. **k,** Palpate medial canthal ligaments and nasal bones. **l,** Inspect nasal septum. **m,** Examine for dysesthesia. **n,** Examine external ear.

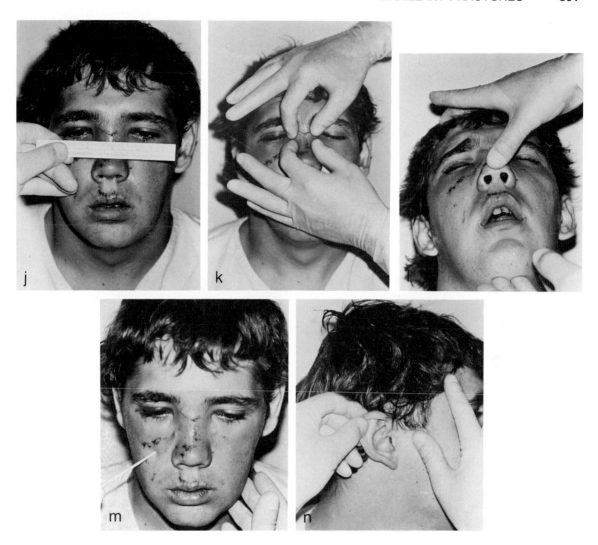

FIG. 7–11 (continued).

crease may be the result of a displaced fracture of the frontomaxillary and lacrimal bones or of a tearing loose of the medial canthal ligament from the anterior and posterior lacrimal crests. The lateral canthal ligament is attached to the frontal process of the zygoma. Inferior and medial displacement of the zygoma will cause a narrowing and inferior displacement of the lateral palpebral fissure. The orbital process of the maxilla forms the greater part of the anterior floor of the orbit. A displaced Le Fort II fracture will disrupt the floor and inferior orbital rim. When the floor of the orbit is disrupted, orbital fat may herniate into the antrum, carrying with it the inferior rectus muscle. Diplopia, enophthalmos, inferior rectus dysfunction, and infraorbital nerve hy-

poesthesia or anesthesia are cardinal signs of orbital floor fracture.

The zygomas are then examined visually and tactilely for asymmetry. A depressed zygoma can be readily appreciated by viewing the face from a coronal position. The surgeon can better appreciate an asymmetry by displacing the edematous tissues over the zygoma. Another method to detect zygoma displacement is to place a tongue blade so that it contacts the bridge of the nose and the most prominent point on the zygoma and to compare to the opposite side the angle that the tongue blade makes with the frontal plane of the face. Palpation of the zygomaticoalveolar junction will disclose the lack of continuity associated with the displaced zygoma. Displaced zygoma fractures can produce hypoesthesia or anesthesia over the infraorbital nerve and zygomaticofrontal and zygomaticotemporal nerve distributions.

To complete the midfacial examination, the nose is examined both externally and internally for nasal bone displacement, crepitation, obstruction, submucosal hematoma, septal displacement, and cerebrospinal fluid rhinorrhea. In maxillary fractures or in isolated nasal fractures, the septum is frequently displaced from the midline. The escape of cerebrospinal fluid through the nose might indicate the presence of a pyramidal or transverse facial fracture in addition to a fracture of the cribriform plate. Nasal discharge can be identified as mucus rather than cerebrospinal fluid if it starches a cloth when drying, or by medical laboratory evaluation.

RADIOGRAPHIC EXAMINATION

Radiographs, CT studies, or both are taken on all patients with suspected or known facial bone fractures to confirm the clinical examination.

In general, routine paranasal sinus (Waters) and lateral skull views are taken first, along with a lateral cervical spine film. If the neurologic and general status of the patient will permit, special views of the skull, face, and mandible may be taken. The Waters or stereo Waters view is the most informative film for maxillary fractures. The nasal septum, lateral nasal walls, lateral sinus walls, orbital rims, nasal bones, and frontozygomatic, frontomaxillary, and frontonasal junctions can be readily assessed from the Waters or stereo Waters views (Fig. 7–12). One should always compare one side of the facial skeleton film with the other and look for differences in densities, displacement and air-fluid levels in the frontal and maxillary sinuses.

Other useful standard radiographic views are the PA view of the maxilla, the lateral maxillary views, and lateral nasal views. The standard cephalometric view can be useful in detecting vertical displacement of the maxilla and is retaken later to check the post-treatment position of the maxilla.[12] The lateral maxillary view gives an excellent outline of the inner and outer tables of the skull, ante-

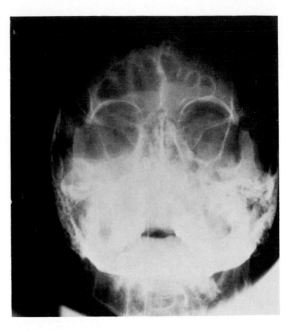

FIG. 7–12. Frontal view of maxilla: complex maxillary fracture and bilateral zygoma fractures. Note air-fluid levels in the frontal sinus.

rior and posterior walls of the frontal sinus, floor of the anterior cranial fossa, and cribriform plate (Fig. 7–13). When the condition of the patient permits, AP and lateral tomograms of the face will delineate more accurately the fracture lines, especially midsagittal fractures of the maxilla, orbital floor fractures,

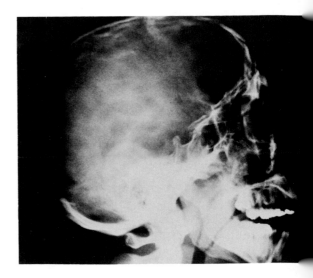

FIG. 7–13. Lateral skull radiograph: maxillary fractures (open bite) and fracture of frontal bone.

orbital apex fractures, and pterygoid plate fractures.

The use of computed tomography (CT) in clinical diagnosis was first described by Hounsfield in 1973.[13] Since then, CT has proven to be especially helpful in the assessment of midfacial injuries, fractures of the orbital walls, and potential airway obstruction caused by laryngeal edema.[14] Fractures of the midface are sometimes difficult to identify on conventional radiographs because of soft-tissue edema and the complex anatomy of this region. The bones are thin, lie in different planes, and may be superimposed on each other. CT clearly displays and differentiates hard and soft tissue and shows distortion and displacement of bone, cartilage, and muscle. Also, CT can be useful in examining the optic canals if there is clinical evidence of visual deficit. Manfredi, in a retrospective study of 379 patients who underwent repair of facial fractures, reported a 6% incidence of blindness in at least one eye.[15] He recommended that preoperative CT scan of the orbits be done on those patients who show evidence of fractures associated with hemorrhage into the ethmoid and sphenoid sinuses as seen on conventional films. Such a preoperative study might help identify those patients who could suffer optic nerve injury during reduction of the fractures.

Magnetic resonance imaging (MRI) is the latest advance in diagnostic cross-sectional depiction of the internal structures of the human body. Radiowaves, rather than ionizing radiation, are used to penetrate the tissues. MRI is sensitive to soft-tissue changes and shows good detail of fat and muscle planes. Excellent images of the orbits, paranasal sinuses, and cranial cavity are obtained from both sagittal and frontal planes. Currently the major drawbacks of using MRI in the traumatized patient are the length of time needed for the study and the absolute need for lack of motion during the imaging procedure.

The patient should never be sent to the radiograph area of the hospital without a well-trained attendant—one who is capable of monitoring the patient's level of consciousness, vital signs, and airway patency.

PRELIMINARY TREATMENT

Patients with maxillary fractures and other midfacial injuries are not likely to die from those injuries alone but can succumb to associated cervical spine, thoracic, abdominal, or extremity injuries. The complete spectrum of treatment encompasses emergency care, stabilization of body systems, and definitive fracture management. The principles of emergency care are to establish an airway, control hemorrhage, and treat associated injuries.

Establish an Airway. The maxilla forms a part of the nasal and oral airways. Hence, when the maxilla is fractured, the nasal airway can be compromised by displacement of the nasal septum and lateral nasal walls, hemorrhage into the nose, and mucosal edema. Likewise, the oral airway can be compromised by the posterior and inferior displacement of the maxilla, blood clots in the oropharynx, and edema of the soft palate and faucial pillars. If bilateral mandibular body or condylar fractures are also present, the tongue, having lost its skeletal support, may fall back against the oropharynx if the patient is in the supine position.

The first step in airway management is to suction the mouth and oropharynx with a high-volume suction. The mouth is quickly inspected for avulsed teeth and broken or displaced prosthetic devices, all of which must be removed to prevent aspiration. If the tongue is edematous and blocking the airway, it must be grasped with a sponge and pulled forward so that the oropharynx can be inspected for blood clots and lacerations at the base of the tongue. A towel clip or suture placed through the tip of the tongue will aid in keeping it forward. If cervical spine injuries are not evident, the patient can be rolled on his right side to keep the tongue from occluding the airway and to prevent blood and other debris from collecting in the oropharynx.

Once the oral airway is established, the nasal cavity should be suctioned with a soft, fine catheter. The nasal airway can be established with a lubricated soft-rubber nasopharyngeal tube passed along the floor of the nose (Fig. 7–14). If resistance felt at the posterior nasal

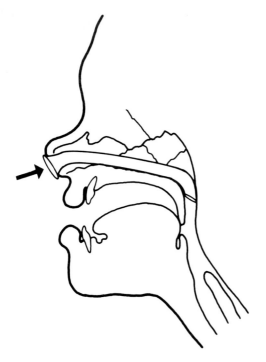

FIG. 7–14. Airway maintained with a nasopharyngeal tube (arrow).

opening is caused by a posteriorly displaced maxilla, a finger can be placed behind the soft palate and the maxilla pulled forward enough to allow for passage of the tube. Nasopharyngeal tubes are quickly blocked by mucus and blood and must be continuously monitored for patency. Passing a nasoendotracheal tube is the best way to maintain an airway and is necessary if the patient is unconscious or has otherwise lost protective pharyngeal and laryngeal reflexes, has severe combined midfacial and mandibular fractures, or has extensive soft-tissue injuries of the face with marked edema that encroaches on the airway. If extensive comminuted nasal fractures preclude the passing of a nasal tube, an oral endotracheal tube will ensure an airway until a tracheostomy can be performed over the endotracheal tube (Fig. 7–15).

Control Bleeding. Hemorrhage is usually not a problem with maxillary fractures. If bleeding is present, it usually comes from the nose and passes into the oral cavity via the nasopharynx. Slow, persistent bleeding can come from the nasal septal vessels or the anterior and posterior ethmoid vessels. Brisk nasal bleeding is usually caused by rupture of

the descending palatine or sphenopalatine branches of the maxillary artery.

The sources of bleeding should be ascertained with suction, a headlamp, and a nasal speculum. Placing soft-rubber nasopharyngeal tubes bilaterally will control most bleeding from the nose and will also maintain a nasal airway.

Persistent anterior nasal bleeding can be controlled by anterior packing (Fig. 7–16a). The nasal passages are suctioned and sprayed with 5% cocaine for topical anesthesia and vasoconstriction. A strip gauze ½ inch wide is packed in the anterior nasal cavity starting from the floor of the nose and layered upward (Fig. 7–16b). If the bleeding is brisk and uncontrolled by the anterior pack, a posterior nasal pack must also be placed. One temporary but quick and effective method is to insert a lubricated Foley catheter into the nasal cavity until the balloon is near the posterior nasal aperture. The balloon is blown up with air or 5 to 10 cc of sterile water. The tubing is then clamped and taped to the outside of the face. A second method is to place a catheter through the nose into the nasopharynx. The catheter tip is grasped with a sponge forceps or large hemostat in the nasopharynx and brought out through the mouth. The tip of the catheter is tied or sutured to a throat pack, sponge, or round tonsil pad with strings such as umbilical tape at both ends. The catheter is then pulled back out of the nose, thereby pulling the packing with it into the posterior nasal aperture (Fig. 7–16c). The catheter is removed and the nasal and oral strings are tied together or taped to the face. Anterior and posterior packs are placed bilaterally (Fig. 7–16d). The packs should be removed in 24 hrs so as not to encourage infection.

Rapid blood loss from the scalp lacerations can be controlled by wrapping the head with many layers of Esmarch's bandage. Hemorrhage from neck lacerations or puncture wounds is best managed by direct pressure over the common carotid artery until the neck can be explored. Concomitantly with the management of hemorrhage, a large-bore intravenous catheter is placed for fluid administration and blood is drawn for type and crossmatch. The intravenous line should not be inserted in an injured extremity or in a leg

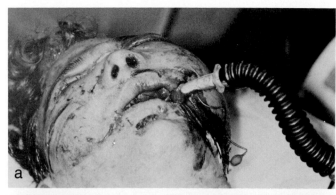

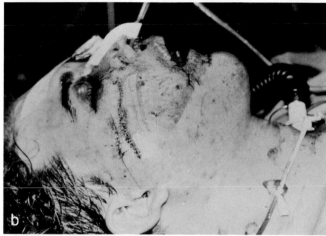

FIG. 7–15. **a,** Airway initially secured with an oral endotracheal tube. **b,** In the operating room, a tracheostomy is performed over the endotracheal tube.

vein if abdominal injuries are suspected. Two intravenous catheters should be placed in case one of the catheters becomes dislodged or if rapid fluid replacement becomes necessary.

Blood loss from midfacial injuries alone is usually not sufficient to induce hypovolemic shock unless the jugular venous system is disrupted or a basilar skull fracture is present. If shock occurs, the surgeon should look elsewhere for blood loss. Abdominal, thoracic, or major extremity injuries can easily hide several units of blood and be responsible for the patient's hypotensive state.

Treat Associated Injuries. Once airway and bleeding problems are reasonably controlled, attention should be directed toward determining if potentially life-threatening injuries exist elsewhere. Cranial and spinal cord injuries must be strongly suspected in the facial trauma patient and require that unnecessary manipulation of the head be avoided. The patient should not be subjected to extensive skull and facial radiographic procedures

until a lateral cervical spine film is shown to be negative. Treatment of midfacial injuries can and must be delayed until life-threatening injuries are stabilized. Facial laceration closure can be delayed 24 hrs[16] and facial fractures can be treated 7–10 days later without compromising the results of treatment. An exception, of course, is an eye injury; an injured eye should be gently patched and an ophthalmologic consultation sought immediately.

As soon as the patient's general condition permits, alginate impressions should be taken of both dental arches. Two sets of impressions are taken, or one set is duplicated, so that one set of casts can be cut and reassembled while the other set is used as a pretreatment record. Additionally, temporary intermaxillary fixation should be applied using local anesthesia. The benefits of temporary stabilization are increased patient comfort, hemorrhage control, reduced contamination of compounded fractures, and encouragement of early mucosal healing. The temporary fixation can be

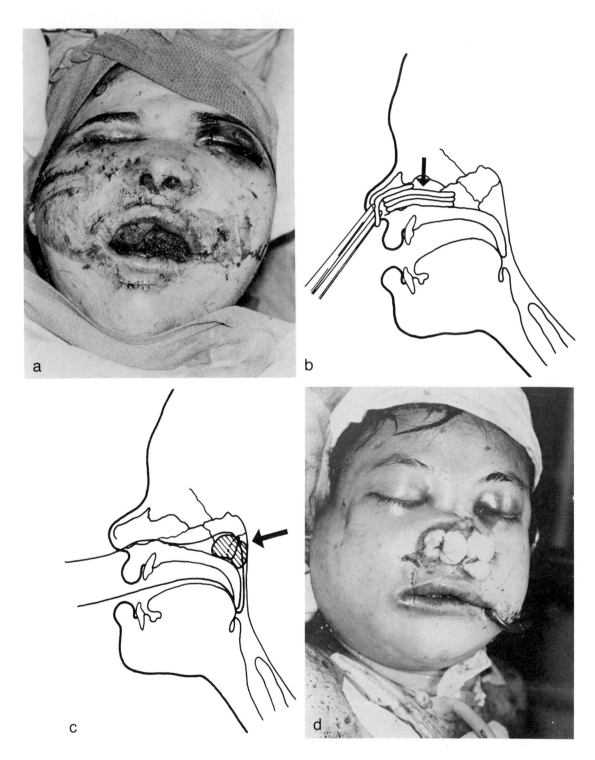

FIG. 7–16. **a,** Anterior nasal packing and tight oral packing to control hemorrhage associated with maxillary and nasal fractures. **b,** Gauze strip packed in anterior nasal cavity (arrow). **c,** Posterior nasal packing with tonsil pads (arrow). **d,** Anterior nasal packs tied to posterior nasal packing for control of nasal bleeding.

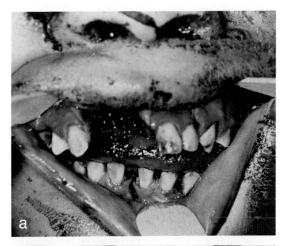

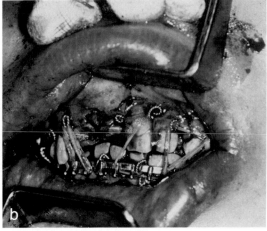

FIG. 7–17. **a,** Complex maxillary and mandibular fractures. **b,** Temporary stabilization using dental wires and elastics.

achieved by placing wire ligatures around several teeth in each quadrant or placing an eyelet loop in each posterior quadrant and anterior quadrant (Fig. 7–17). As the patient's condition permits, complete facial radiographs should be taken. The initial examination, dental casts, and radiographs are used to formulate a definitive treatment plan. Close communication with other interested services (such as orthopedics, general surgery, neurosurgery, and anesthesia) should be maintained so that treatment can be coordinated. Often, many body injuries can be treated during the same administration of anesthestic.

DEFINITIVE TREATMENT

The objectives in the treatment of maxillary fractures are the reestablishment of functions of the oral cavity with the teeth in normal occlusion and the correction of facial deformity. Returning the teeth to their preinjury occlusion is the key for reducing maxillary fractures; on the basis of this reduction, other midfacial fractures are reduced. The mandible is the structural pillar of the lower midface; it relates the midface to the cranium through the temporomandibular articulation. Bringing the maxillary teeth into occlusion with the intact mandible accurately establishes the maxillary position. If the mandible also is fractured, it must first be reduced and stabilized before treatment of maxillary and associated midfacial fractures can proceed. It cannot be over-emphasized that the key to establishing the position of the midface is the articulation of the teeth. When the patient's natural teeth are missing, dentures or surgical splints will act as the key to reduction and provide sufficient stabilization.

Because midfacial injuries produce a wide array of fracture patterns, no single treatment pattern or method can be applied to all patients. The principles of fracture treatment, however, are adequate reduction of the fragments, adequate immobilization of the fragments, and maintenance of the fragments in the immobilized position for sufficient time to allow the fracture to heal.[17] The preferred method of treatment is the simplest one that satisfies the principles of fracture reduction and produces the best results.

Minimally displaced Le Fort I and II fractures are amenable to treatment in an outpatient clinic with the patient under local anesthesia. Moderately displaced Le Fort I and II and all Le Fort III fractures are managed in the operating room with the patient under nasoendotracheal general anesthesia. When the passage of a nasoendotracheal tube is impossible because of nasal fractures, an oral endotracheal tube is placed first and either a tracheostomy is performed over the endotracheal tube or the fractures are treated, with final immobilization to the mandible delayed for a few days, when indicated. In the vast majority of midfacial fractures, however, a nasoendotracheal tube can be used.

The treatment of midfacial fractures, like other fractures of the face, involves several steps:

1. Cleansing and debriding the oral cavity and face
2. Making dental impressions and pouring stone casts
3. Removing fractured, nonrestorable teeth and temporarily protecting injured, restorable teeth
4. Closing all oral and oropharyngeal lacerations, including lacerated major salivary gland ducts
5. Applying interdental wire ligature or arch bars
6. Reducing dental arch fractures and ligating custom-made splints
7. Reducing maxillary fractures and applying intermaxillary fixation
8. Performing transoral open reductions and fixation with miniplates or intraosseous wiring, when indicated
9. Reducing and fixating zygomatic, nasoethmoid, orbital, and nasal fractures
10. Placing zygomatic, cranial, and extracranial suspension, if needed
11. Closing all facial incisions and lacerations

INITIAL WOUND CARE AND DEBRIDEMENT

Regardless of the extent or degree of injury, the oral cavity must first be inspected for loose teeth, prostheses, foreign bodies such as glass and metal fragments, avulsed bone, and lacerated soft tissues. The oral cavity is then cleansed by irrigation with copious amounts of sterile saline or an antiseptic solution (povidone-iodine, 5%) using a 30- to 50-cc plastic syringe and a blunted 18-gauge irrigating needle. The use of solutions containing hydrogen peroxide should be discouraged because they can cause subcutaneous emphysema. A toothbrush can be used to clean the teeth, gingiva, tongue, and hard palate of dried blood clots. Cotton applicator wooden sticks, cotton pliers, curettes, and small hemostats can be used to dislodge and remove embedded foreign material. If loose bone fragments are encountered, only those fragments that will become dislodged with irri-

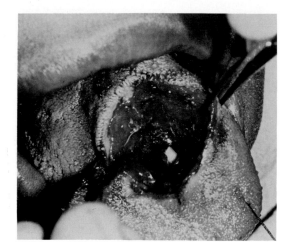

FIG. 7–18. Lacerated tongue with imbedded tooth fragment.

gation should be removed. All other bone fragments, no matter how minimally attached to soft tissue, must be retained. Likewise, all tissues must be retained unless they are obviously nonvital. The repair potential of the oral soft tissues is extraordinary; only crushed tissue or tissues without blood supply should be excised.

The tongue must be thoroughly examined on all surfaces for through-and-through lacerations as well as for embedded tooth fragments (Fig. 7–18). Brisk bleeding that occurs during this phase of treatment can be managed by pressure from gauze sponges or, occasionally, by clamping and tying of vessels.

Facial lacerations should likewise be cleansed, but closure should be delayed until the intraoral procedures are completed and the surgeon has determined that those facial lacerations will not be used for open reduction of fractures.

DENTAL IMPRESSIONS AND CASTS

Models poured in stone from alginate impressions should be obtained in each case if possible. Impressions should be taken before lacerations are closed so that sutured areas will not be disrupted. If the patient has trismus or is unwilling to open his mouth, local anesthesia should be given to block out the pain so that impressions can be taken.

When necessary, plastic disposable trays

can be modified with an acrylic bur and used when standard trays do not fit. Perforated trays are preferred. When the dental arches are greatly displaced, impressions can be taken more easily if an intra-arch wire ligature (bridle wire) is first placed around several of the teeth adjacent to the fracture to partially reduce and stabilize the fracture. The oropharyngeal airway must be packed when taking impressions on the unconscious patient. Two or more impressions of each dental arch should be taken in case multiple sectioning of models is needed to determine a difficult occlusal relationship or a model should be inadvertently broken or damaged. The stone or plaster models are sectioned and reassembled to determine the preinjury occlusion and used for the fabrication of splints and appliances if necessary (Fig. 7–19). A member of the treatment team can construct splints of clear acrylic using the cold-cure and pressure cooker technique while others proceed with the remainder of the treatment.

INJURED AND FRACTURED TEETH

Only those teeth that are fractured beyond repair or impacted teeth that are displaced in a fracture line should be removed. Sound, fully erupted, and functional teeth left in the line of fracture have not been shown to increase the incidence of infection or nonunion.[18] Exposed dentin should be protected with intermediate restorative materials, and exposed pulps should be partially or totally extirpated and the pulp chamber sealed. Teeth with nonrestorable caries that will not aid in intermaxillary fixation are best removed at this time.

CLOSURE OF ORAL LACERATIONS

A watertight seal of the oral mucosa is necessary to prevent continued contamination of underlying fractures. If a laceration can be used to gain access for an intraoral open reduction, its closure can be delayed until after fracture reduction and application of intermaxillary fixation. Gingival and mucosal lacerations are best closed with interrupted absorbable sutures such as 3-0 or 4-0 chromic gut. Lacerations of the tongue are closed before intermaxillary fixation is applied; all muscle layers of the tongue are closed with deep, widely placed absorbable sutures. If a laceration passed through the areas of the parotid and submandibular ducts, the ducts should be probed; if they are found to be severed, their ends should be identified and closed with 5-0 or 6-0 silk over a polyethylene tube with an inside diameter of at least 0.034 inches. The polyethylene tube is left in place for 2 weeks.

REDUCTION OF DENTAL ARCH FRACTURES AND INSERTION OF SPLINTS

Alveolar and palatal fractures are manually reduced and the splints trial-fitted. If the splints fit, arch bars, eyelet loops, Stout loops, or other types of dental ligatures are then applied prior to final placement of the splints. If arch bars are used, they should be ligated to the teeth loosely until the final occlusion is attained. The arch bar can also be split at the fracture site to allow for minor manipulation of the fracture. When the palate is fractured in two or more pieces, a palatal acrylic splint is essential (Fig. 7–20). The splint is ligated to all the maxillary teeth after the arch bars or dental ligatures are placed. If the teeth cannot be brought into maximum occlusion and the splint is suspected of being at fault, the splint must be removed, another maxillary impression taken, and the splint remade. If the splint cannot be remade at this time, intermaxillary fixation can be applied so that treatment can continue, and the remade splint can be inserted later as an outpatient procedure and the intermaxillary fixation then reapplied.

REDUCTION OF MAXILLARY FRACTURES AND INTERMAXILLARY FIXATION

When the maxillary arch and dentition have been stabilized, the maxilla is then reduced. Le Fort I fractures that are nondisplaced need only be placed in maxillomandibular fixation using 26-gauge stainless steel wires ligated to the previously placed maxillary and mandibular arch bars or interdental loops. The displaced maxilla can be brought into its proper position by manual manipulation. A wire

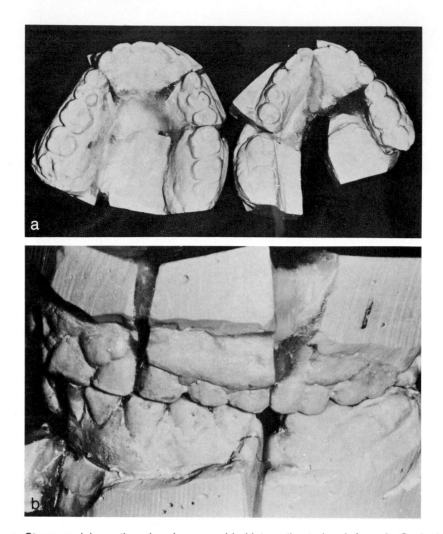

FIG. 7–19.   **a,** Stone models sectioned and reassembled into estimated arch form. **b,** Occlusion re-established on models.

placed around the arch bar near the midline can be used to pull the impacted maxilla forward and into occlusion. If complete reduction is not accomplished initially, intermaxillary elastics can be placed to counteract the direction of displacement and should bring the maxilla into its correct position within several hours (Fig. 7–21). If the maxilla is so impacted or displaced that it cannot be reduced by the previous methods, disimpaction forceps should be used to reduce the maxilla with the patient under a general anesthetic. The Rowe disimpaction forceps engages the palate bilaterally from the nasal and oral side and provides excellent leverage and control. The Tessier disimpaction forceps engages the tuberosity just below the fracture line and dis-

impacts the maxilla by rocking it slowly. At this point intermaxillary wires are applied and the anterior and lateral maxillary walls are palpated to confirm anatomic reduction. Sudden bleeding from the descending palatine or transeptal arteries may occur during this maneuver.

Le Fort II fractures are managed in a similar manner. The surgeon should manually reduce Le Fort II fractures with great care, remembering that the medial orbital wall and anterior orbital floor are fractures and that excessive manipulation could damage the nasolacrimal duct and inferior orbital nerve. After intermaxillary fixation is applied, the frontonasal junction and inferior orbital rims are palpated to confirm fracture reduction.

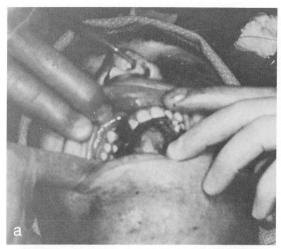

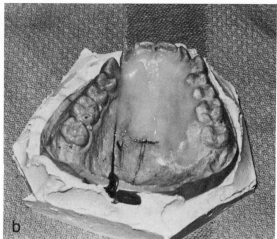

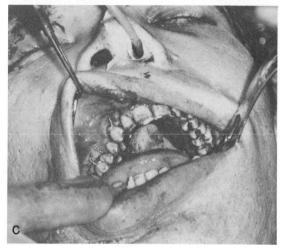

FIG. 7–20. **a,** Palatal fracture. **b,** Splint is made on sectioned model with self-curing acrylic. **c,** Fracture is reduced and splint is wired to teeth.

Ocular motility must be checked at this time to ensure that the inferior rectus has not been entrapped during the reduction procedure.

As with the Le Fort I and II fractures of the maxilla, the Le Fort III fracture is reduced by first placing the maxillary and mandibular teeth into occlusion and applying intermaxillary fixation. Disimpaction forceps may be needed to bring the fractured buttresses into anatomic position. As mentioned earlier in this chapter, the possibility of fracture into the optic foraminae should be ruled out before manipulating the midface. If there is any doubt about injury to the optic nerves, fracture reduction should be delayed. During manipulation of the midface the frontonasal and zygomaticofrontal junction should be palpated to confirm adequate mobilization and reduction. Nasal bleeding, if encountered, will usually stop once the midface is fully reduced and stabilized to the mandible.

SKELETAL FIXATION AND OPEN REDUCTION

Skeletal fixation of maxillary fractures can be achieved through the use of suspension wires, direct intraosseous wires, miniplates, or external cranial suspension devices. Skeletal fixation is indicated only when closed fracture reduction and intermaxillary fixation fail to reduce and stabilize the fractured maxilla.

In a review of the treatment of 112 maxillary fractures, Kuepper and Harrigan reported success using intermaxillary fixation alone in 100% of Le Fort I fractures, 89% of Le Fort II fractures, and 83% of Le Fort III fractures.[19]

The sites commonly used for placement of suspension wires, compression plates and miniplates, or intraosseous wires are the anterior nasal spine, lateral piriform rim, inferior orbital rim, zygomatic buttress, zygomatic arch, and frontomaxillary junction (Fig.

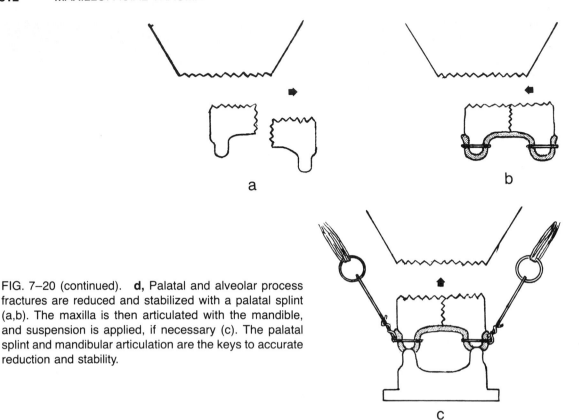

FIG. 7–20 (continued). **d,** Palatal and alveolar process fractures are reduced and stabilized with a palatal splint (a,b). The maxilla is then articulated with the mandible, and suspension is applied, if necessary (c). The palatal splint and mandibular articulation are the keys to accurate reduction and stability.

7–22). Suspension wires serve to prevent distraction of the maxilla in an inferior direction when the teeth are in occlusion. The surgeon must bear in mind, however, that suspension wires from the zygomatic arch and from the frontozygomatic junction when tightened are angled 30 to 45° from the vertical and exert a backward and upward pull on the maxilla, which tends to displace the maxilla superiorly and posteriorly. Great care must be exercised not to tighten the wires such that the midface is shortened; also, the wires must be placed with equal tension on both sides so as not to cant the maxilla.

The use of suspension wires is contraindicated in cases in which intermaxillary fixation cannot be applied, for example, in edentulous cases when splints or dentures are not available. Transosseous wires or bone plates, such as those used in orthognathic surgery, are used. A headframe for external craniofacial support should be considered in the following three examples: in midfacial fractures that require significant anterior traction for reduc-

tion and fixation; in midfacial fractures with concomitant bilateral, dislocated condylar process fractures that are not amenable to open reduction; and in severely comminuted midfacial fractures that do not provide the stable bone contacts at the fractured areas. In the latter example, in many cases one could use suspension wires in conjunction with intrasinal supports of packing or balloons via the Caldwell-Luc approach.

The first intact bone above the fracture site ordinarily serves for wire suspension, although wires may be suspended from higher sites (Fig. 7–23). If suspension wires are necessary for the treatment of a horizontal maxillary fracture (Le Fort I), the level of the fracture will influence the site used for suspension. The anterior nasal spine can be used only if the fracture is below this point. The lateral piriform rim and zygomatic arch can be used as points of suspension for high or low horizontal fractures. Circumzygomatic wiring can also serve in the suspension of a pyramidal (Le Fort II) fracture. Other sites of

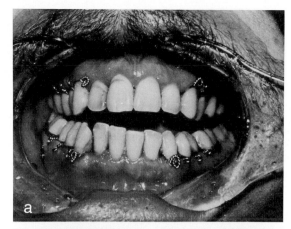

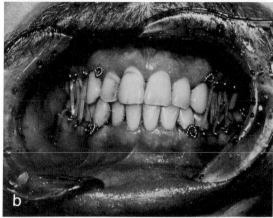

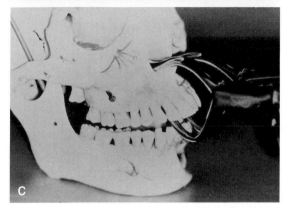

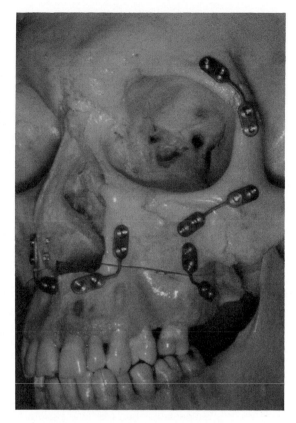

FIG. 7–22.   Miniplates, as used in orthognathic surgery, may be used for fixation of selected midfacial fractures. Avulsive injuries, comminution, and lack of available equipment may limit routine use of this approach. (Courtesy of Hall Reconstructive Systems, Santa Barbara, California.)

FIG. 7–21.   Reduction of Le Fort fractures. **a,** Reduction of impacted maxillary Le Fort I fracture with elastic traction. Anterior open bite, continuous loop wiring placed. **b,** Fracture reduction. **c,** Rowe disimpaction forceps.

suspension that can be used in the Le Fort II type fracture are the lateral infraorbital rims, in the absence of zygoma fractures, and the zygomatic processes of the frontal bone. Intraosseous wire fixation in the infraorbital area can be accomplished concurrently, although it is needed infrequently because reestablishment of the occlusion and wire suspension when indicated will usually restore orbital rim contour. Suspension of the transverse facial (Le Fort III) fracture is accomplished by means of direct intraosseous wiring of the zygomaticofrontal separation and concurrent placement of suspension wires from the zygomatic processes of the frontal bones; the suspension wires are introduced into the oral cavity with a zygomatic passing awl. Combinations of fractures, such as a Le Fort I on one side and Le Fort II on the other,

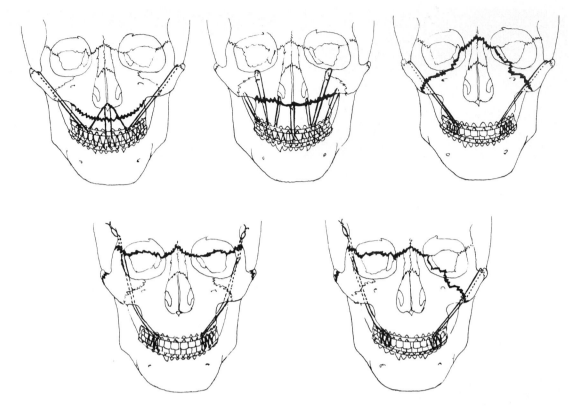

FIG. 7–23. Suspension wires. Midfacial skeletal fractures are usually comminuted, with unstable associated sections of bone. Suspending wires circumvent the fragmented fracture lines and preserve the nonyielding sling of the periosteal sheath and the periosteum attachments to bony fragments. Bone plates, used widely in midfacial orthognathic surgery in which surgical osteotomies are stabilized, have a more limited use in midfacial fractures. **a,** Le Fort I, zygomatic arch suspension. **b,** Le Fort I, infraorbital suspension. **c,** Le Fort II, zygomatic arch suspension. **d,** Le Fort III, frontal bone suspension.

may also require suspension. If so, the same suspension point should be used for both sides to avoid any difference in angulation or tension on the suspension wire.

Techniques for Placement of Suspension and Intraosseous Wires

Because all suspension wires communicate with the oral cavity, one might expect infection to be a complicating factor. Actually, infection occurs rarely, as the wires are usually placed and removed under antibiotic coverage and the oral cavity is sanitized.

Anterior Nasal Spine. The anterior nasal spine is approached through a 1.5-cm vertical mucoperiosteal incision directly over it. A sharp periosteum elevator or a large dental curette is used to expose the spine, after which a hole is drilled through the spine with a wire-passing bur. A length of 25- or 26-gauge stainless steel wire is threaded through the hole and the incision is closed around it.

Lateral Piriform Rim (Fig. 7–24). The lateral piriform rim is palpated and a vertical mucoperiosteal incision is made just lateral to it so as not to enter the nose. The periosteum is elevated laterally and the nasal mucosa is carefully elevated medially to allow insertion of a submucous elevator or a periosteum elevator under the nasal mucosa for protection from the bur. A bur hole is made from a lateral direction and placed at least 5 mm above the fracture and 5 mm lateral to the rim. A wire is then threaded through the hole and extended through the incision. The mucosa is closed around the wire. This wire provides strong, direct support to the anterior maxilla.

Infraorbital Rim (Fig. 7–25). The infraorbital rim is approached through a 2-cm-long

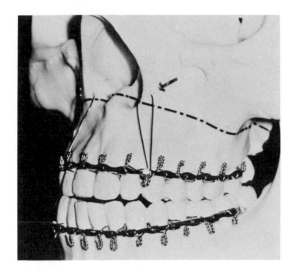

FIG. 7–24.   Lateral piriform rim suspension.

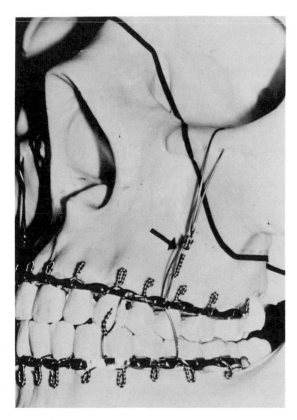

FIG. 7–25.   Infraorbital rim suspension. An intermediate wire (arrow) is placed between the suspension wire and arch bar to prevent breaking of the suspension wire.

horizontal incision made in the mucobuccal fold at the canine fossa. While a finger palpates the infraorbital rim externally, the mucoperiosteum is elevated lateral to the infraorbital foramen until the rim is reached. The periosteal reflection is then carried to the orbital side of the rim. An instrument protects the globe while a bur hole is started 3 to 5 mm below the rim, slanted superiorly, and carried until the bur perforates the anterior orbital floor and hits the protecting instrument. With the protecting instrument still in place, a length of wire is placed through the hole, grasped, and brought through the incision. The incision is closed around the wire.

The infraorbital wire provides direct support to the entire maxilla and avoids the posterior angulation seen with circumzygomatic wires. It can also be used in the pyramidal fracture, provided that the zygoma is intact and the wire is placed lateral to the infraorbital fracture.

Zygomatic Buttress (Fig. 7–26). The zygomatic buttress is approached through a horizontal mucoperiosteal incision placed in the buccal sulcus directly over the buttress. The buttress is exposed on both its anterior and posterior surfaces. A bur hole is made through the buttress, passing from anterior to posterior, and is placed at least 5 mm above the fracture line. A wire is then passed through both bur holes and brought through the incision. The mucosa is closed around the wire. The zygomatic buttress wire provides strong, direct suspension for the Le Fort I fracture when the zygoma is intact. In the edentulous patient it also provides a direct method of securing the denture or splint to the maxilla.

Zygomatic Arch. Circumzygomatic wires extend circumferentially from the temporal border of the zygoma into the oral cavity (Fig. 7–27). Several techniques are used for passing the wire, one of which is the use of a special passing awl with a hole at its tip. After both temporal regions are prepared in the usual manner, the zygoma is palpated along its temporal border until the curved junction of the body of the zygoma and the zygomatic arch is felt. The surgeon introduces the awl through the skin at this point and passes it along the medial surface of the zygomatic

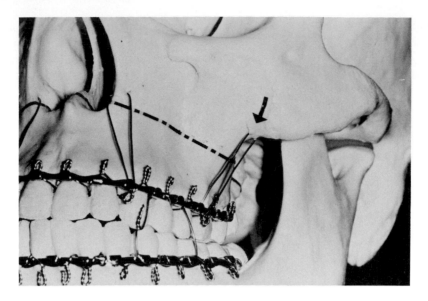

FIG. 7–26. Zygomatic buttress suspension wire (arrow).

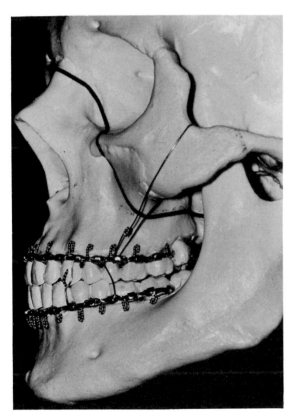

FIG. 7–27. Zygomatic suspension wire.

arch with the tip of the awl pointing buccally. With the other hand, the surgeon intraorally palpates the buccal sulcus opposite the first molar and locates the awl as it pierces the mucosa. The awl tip is brought into the mouth and a strand of 25-gauge wire is passed through the hole in the awl and twisted. The awl is slowly withdrawn until it is level with the superior surface of the zygomatic arch. The awl tip is then directed over the arch first laterally and then medially (Fig. 7–28). The awl pulls the wire over the arch and carries the wire intraorally through the previous tract. The wire is removed from the awl and the awl is withdrawn, and both ends of the wire are grasped with clamps intraorally and sawed back and forth until the wire is felt to be contacting the arch without the intervention of soft tissue. The suspension wire is then attached to the maxillary arch bar, dental wires, or splint in the area of the second bicuspid and first molar by an intermediate wire.

The second method of passing the suspension wire involves the use of a no. 18 spinal needle that has been slightly curved. The needle is passed medially to the zygomatic arch from the same point on the skin from which the awl is passed. After the needle enters the oral cavity a strand of wire is passed through the lumen of the needle into the mouth. The intraoral end of the wire is

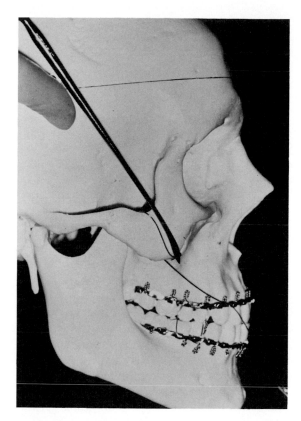

FIG. 7–28. Introducing wire over zygomatic arch with passing awl.

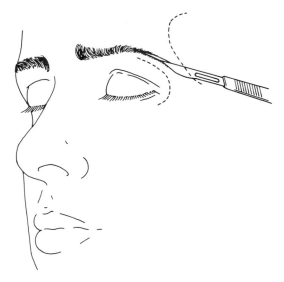

FIG. 7–29. Eyebrow approach to zygomaticofrontal suture. The incision is made over the lateral third of the eyebrow.

grasped with a hemostat and the needle is then withdrawn superiorly and passed laterally to the arch, directing the wire ahead of the needle. The wire is carried over the arch and into the mouth. The end of the wire in the needle is pulled out of the needle and the needle is removed inferiorly. Both ends of the suspension wire are grasped and a sawing motion is used to ensure that the wire is securely placed over the arch.

Among the many variations for passing circumzygomatic arch wires and other circumferential wires are the use of autopsy needles, no. 18 spinal needles, and intracatheter plastic cannulas. These may be introduced from a sterile cutaneous area into the oral cavity carrying the wire medially to the zygomatic arch, for example. The carrying instrument is discarded and a second, sterile carrying instrument is introduced into the same cutaneous puncture site and carries the other end of the wire into the oral cavity.

Zygomatic Process of the Frontal Bone.

The zygomaticofrontal suture is the landmark used to place a suspension wire from the frontal bone. The suture is not palpable unless it is separated. The suture is found directly under the lateral third of the eyebrow. The eyebrows are not shaved. Following the usual skin preparation, a skin incision 1.5 cm long is made through the lateral third of the eyebrow (Fig. 7–29). Because orbital twigs from the facial nerve may be encountered, the incision should not reach the outer canthus. The incision may be carried directly to bone. The periosteum is elevated to expose the zygomaticofrontal suture. A finger is placed along the orbital surface of the suture to protect the globe in case the periosteum elevator should slip. The temporal fascia is incised, and the temporal muscle must be elevated slightly and protected from the bur. A bur hole is made through the zygomatic process of the frontal bone obliquely from the facial to the temporal surface. The hole is placed 5 mm superiorly to the suture line. If the suture is separated, a second hole is placed inferiorly to the separation through the frontal process of the zygoma. A second wire, usually 26 gauge, is passed through both holes, tightened to reduce the separation, and twisted on the temporal surface of the frontal process of the zygoma. The suspension wire is then passed through the superior bone hole, and with a passing awl or other instrument both ends of the wires are carried medially to the zygomatic arch and under the zygoma into the oral cavity in the region of the first molar (Fig. 7–30). Before the craniofacial suspension wire is tightened it is inspected to make certain it is not under the transosseous wire, a condition that makes its removal difficult. The incision is left open until the contralateral wiring has been completed.

Extraoral Approach to the Inferior Orbital Rim. An extraoral approach to the inferior orbital rim will be necessary when there is a displaced fracture through the inferior orbital rim in a Le Fort II or zygoma fracture that is unstable or not reducible by closed methods of treatment; or when there is a fracture with disruption of the orbital floor.

A 5-0 nylon suture is passed through the skin of both eyelids and gently tied to protect the globe. The rim is palpated and an incision is planned to center over the fracture. The infraorbital incision is made in a skin crease of the lower lid just above the inferior orbital rim (Fig. 7–31). The incision, about 1 inch

long, is carried through the skin and subcutaneous layer. This layer is undermined to expose the fibers of the orbiculi oculi. The orbiculi oculi fibers are spread horizontally with a small scissors parallel to their line of orientation.

The periosteum is then sharply incised over the rim and gently elevated anteriorly to expose the fracture and identify the infraorbital foramen and nerve. Small fragments of bone that are encountered should not be freed from their periosteal attachment, but rather preserved and minimally repositioned. The periosteum is also carefully elevated from the anterior orbital floor. Great care must be taken not to perforate the periosteum or orbital septum, as perforation would result in the extravasation of orbital fat. The infraorbital fracture is reduced and bur holes are placed approximately 5 mm on each side of the fracture. The bur is directed from the facial surface of the rim diagonally posteriorly and superiorly to pass through the orbital side of the rim. The globe must be protected with an instrument during the drilling. A 28-gauge wire is then passed through both bur holes and

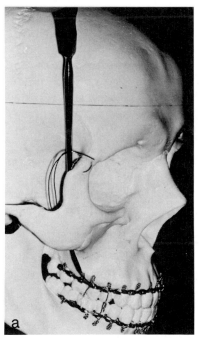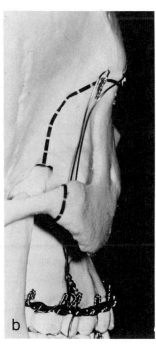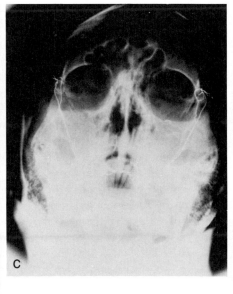

FIG. 7–30.   **a,** Frontal suspension wire. Passing awl carries wire behind and medial to the zygoma and into the oral cavity. **b,** Suspension wire attached to arch bar with the intermediate wire in the region of the maxillary first molar. **c,** Frontal suspension wires in Le Fort III fracture.

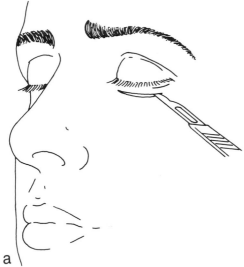

FIG. 7–31.   **a,** Approach to the infraorbital rim. Skin incision in the crease of the lower lid. **b,** Orbicularis oculi fibers spread to expose the periosteum. **c,** Infraorbital rim exposed and intraosseous wire placed across fracture. **d,** Infraorbital wire placement (arrow). **e,** Infraorbital incision 1 week postoperative.

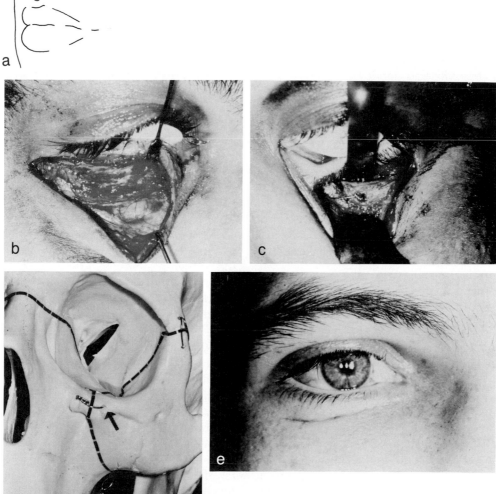

twisted on the facial side of the rim. If possible, the twisted end of the wire is placed into one of the holes so that it will not interfere with the orbiculis oculi function. The periosteum and muscle layers are closed separately and a subcutaneous running suture of 5-0 nylon is used for skin closure.

Open Reduction. Open reduction with fixation by plates or wires should not be attempted with severely comminuted fractures, because stripping periosteum away from small bone fragments will devitalize the fragments and increase chances of bone loss. Instead, the fragments should be molded into their approximate position and treated by intrasinal methods. The "bag of bones" concept allows the bone fragments to form the framework for repair and reduces the incidence of continuity defects seen with aggressive periosteal stripping and debridement.

As transosseous wires between fragments of midfacial skeletal fractures are tightened, the wires may pull through or displace small, thin fragments. Miniplates, either noncompressive or compressive, are simpler to place than transosseous wires, but their use is limited to fragments sufficiently thick to hold the screws and large enough to maintain periosteal attachments. Transosseous wires and miniplates are best employed on the pillars of the midfacial skeleton when the lines of fracture are not comminuted.

External Cranial Suspension

The use of halo-type and box type headframes has been well documented.[20–22] They provide a stable base well above the fractures of the midface and allow for anterior traction of the maxilla and mandible, which internal wire suspension cannot provide.

In several situations, external cranial suspension is strongly indicated. It should be used in severely comminuted midfacial fractures that lack a solid bone base from which to suspend the maxilla or to wire or plate directly; in displaced midfacial fractures associated with bilaterally displaced or dislocated mandibular condylar fractures; in a patient whose associated injuries will not permit lengthy fracture reduction and fixation procedures; and in delayed treatment of impacted maxillary fractures, which require continuous anterior traction for reduction. Because the need for a headframe may arise suddenly, the surgeon responsible for treating maxillofacial fractures should have a headframe set ready to use.

Numerous halo-type headframes are available. The Irby and Morris headframes can be adapted to any combination of facial fractures and allow patient comfort because they encircle only the anterior half of the cranium (Fig. 7–32). The frame may be applied under either local or general anesthesia. The scalp is cleansed and prepared in the usual fashion. The hair is not shaved. The frame is positioned so that the cranial thumbscrews contact the skull on a straight line beginning 3 cm above the external auditory canal, passing anteriorly over the glabella, and ending 3 cm above the external auditory canal on the opposite side. The points of screw contact are marked and infiltrated with local anesthetic. Incisions 5 mm in length are made through the skin to prevent crushing of the tissues by the screws. The screws are tightened until they firmly contact the cranial surface.

The maxilla is best stabilized by the use of an acrylic palatal splint into which has been embedded a specially designed rod or a flattened Steinmann[1] pin. A bite-fork can also be adapted for this purpose. The palatal splint rod is then attached to an anterior stabilization rod with a universal clamp. The maxilla is reduced, intermaxillary fixation is applied, and the clamps on the stabilizing bar are tightened. In cases with concomitant bilateral mandibular condylar or mandibular body fractures, using the biphasic appliance on the mandible in addition to rigid fixation to a headframe stabilizes the total facial skeleton by stabilizing the mandible to the cranium and immobilizing the maxillary fragments in between.[23]

A supraorbital pin system can also be used for rigid craniomaxillary fixation as long as the supraorbital ridge area is not fractured.[22] Pins are less cumbersome than the headframe. Before the pins are placed, a PA radiograph of the skull is taken to determine the lateral extent of the frontal sinus. The pins are placed just above the supraorbital ridges and lateral to the frontal sinus. A hand-op-

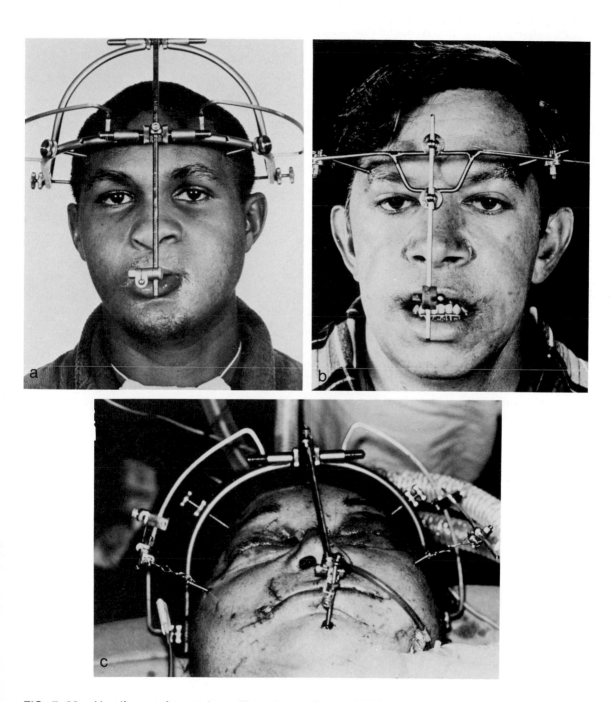

FIG. 7–32.   Headframes for craniomaxillary suspension. **a,** Irby headframe with central support rod to stabilize maxilla. **b,** Patient with multiple comminuted midfacial fractures. Rods are extended from headframe to support zygomas and mandible. **c,** Supraorbital pins with Levant frame to support fractured edentulous maxilla. The cental support rod connects to the maxillary splint.

erated drill, such as the Smedburg, is used to perforate the outer cortex. The bilateral pins are screwed into the frontal bone until the outer table is penetrated and the screw tip barely engages the inner table. A Levant frame is then attached to the pins with clamps, and an anterior stabilizing bar is clamped to the frame. The stabilizing bar is then attached to a maxillary palatal splint.

CONSIDERATIONS IN TREATMENT OF VARIOUS TYPES OF MAXILLARY FRACTURES

FRACTURES IN THE EDENTULOUS PATIENT

The absence of natural teeth reduces traumatic force on the maxilla, and an artificial denture absorbs traumatic force; these factors make the edentulous patient less susceptible to maxillary fractures than the dentulous patient. Fractures do occur in these patients, however, and the complexity of treatment varies directly with the degree of displacement and the absence or presence of artificial dentures.

If there is no displacement, no treatment is required other than restricting the diet to liquids for 1 week and to soft foods for an additional 2 weeks or until the patient can manage a regular diet. If the maxilla is mobile or displaced, reduction and fixation are necessary. A displaced maxillary fracture should not be allowed to heal in a malposition, because subsequent prosthetic restoration might be impossible or at best compromised, and the edentulous patient deserves the same accurate reduction and stabilization as the dentulous patient.

If the dentures are broken, they are first repaired and tried into the mouth to ensure accuracy of fit. If the patient does not object, the central incisors can be removed from the dentures to facilitate feeding. An arch bar, eyelet loops, or other techniques used to produce lugs are then applied to the dentures. The mandibular denture is secured to the mandible with three circumferential wires (Fig. 7–33).

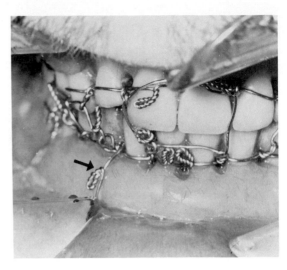

FIG. 7–33. Mandibular denture secured with circummandibular wires.

Methods of Securing Dentures or Splints to the Maxilla

The maxillary denture can be secured to the maxilla through the anterior nasal spine, though the zygomatic buttress, using perialveolar wiring, or using Kirschner wiring.

In the first technique, a 26-gauge wire is passed through the anterior nasal spine and through a hole drilled in the midline of the denture flange (Fig. 7–34a).

Alternatively, a wire passed through the zygomatic buttress in the first molar region can be tied to the maxillary denture through a hole in the buccal flange, passed through the arch wire or through an Ivy loop (Fig. 7–34b). This wire also provides adequate suspension for Le Fort I fractures.

To use perialveolar wire, holes are drilled bilaterally through the buccal flange and palate of the denture (Fig. 7–35). The holes must be large enough to accommodate an alveolar awl. The maxillary denture is seated and the awl is passed through the hole in the buccal flange, through the alveolus and palate, and through the hole on the palate side of the denture. A wire is threaded onto the awl and the awl is then withdrawn, pulling one end of the wire on through the buccal flange hole. The palatal end of the wire is then brought buccally over the teeth and both ends are twisted on the buccal surface of the denture.

In Kirschner wire fixation, the denture or

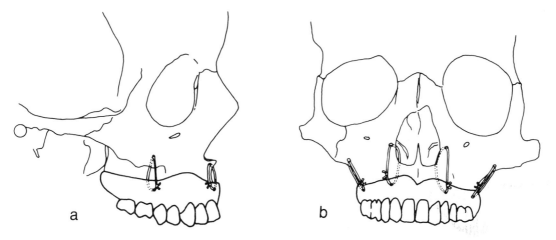

FIG. 7–34. **a,** Maxillary denture secured with nasal spine and zygomatic buttress wires. Used for Le Fort I fractures occurring below the nasal spine. **b,** Maxillary denture secured with lateral piriform rim and zygomatic buttress wires.

splint is pinned to the maxillary alveolus with Kirschner wires passing through the buccal flanges. Medium-gauge Kirschner wires are drilled through the flanges in the cuspid or first bicuspid areas, angulated downward toward the palate about 30°. With the denture firmly supported, the Kirschner wires are made to pass through the denture and alveolus. They are stopped just as the tip of the wire is palpated on the palatal side of the acrylic. The wires are cut on the lateral side close to the denture flanges (Fig. 7–36). A small amount of rapid-curing acrylic is placed over the cut ends of the wires to protect the mucosa. Once the denture is secured to the maxilla, the dentures are occluded and intermaxillary wires applied. If the occlusion does not lock, an acrylic interocclusal wafer is made to stabilize the occlusion. If suspension wires are necessary, they are applied as previously described for the dentulous fractures and secured to the maxillary denture.

If artificial dentures are not available, a modified Gunning-type splint is used (Fig. 7–37). Impressions are made and stone models poured. If displacement is slight, a bite is registered in the centric position and the models mounted on an articulator. If reduction is necessary, the models are mounted on an articulator with the intermaxillary distance and centric relation estimated. Clear acrylic bases are processed containing arch bar segments, hooks, or loops to receive in-

termaxillary and suspension wires. Bite rims are keyed with occlusal notches that articulate in centric position. A feeding hole can be placed in the anterior as well. The mandibular base is inserted and fixed in place with three circumferential wires. The maxillary base is secured to the maxilla and, by manipulation of the maxilla, the denture bases are made to articulate. The bases are ligated to each other by intermaxillary wires. If suspension wires are necessary, they are ligated to either the maxillary or the mandibular base.

Removal of Suspension Wires and Pins

Prior to their removal, intraoral pins and wires should be thoroughly cleansed with hydrogen peroxide solution and the patient placed on antibiotics to help prevent a wire or pin tract infection. Local anesthesia is injected along the wire tract. One strand of the suspension wires is cut as high in the buccal sulcus as possible, the other end grasped with a wire twister and withdrawn.

For the longer wires placed in the zygomatic processes of the frontal bones, the surgeon may place a 15-mm twist on a length of wire, pass one end of the wire through the bur hole and the other lateral to the process, and seat the base of the twist firmly on the bone; both ends of the wire are then passed from the sterile cutaneous area, usually through a metal cannula, into the oral cavity,

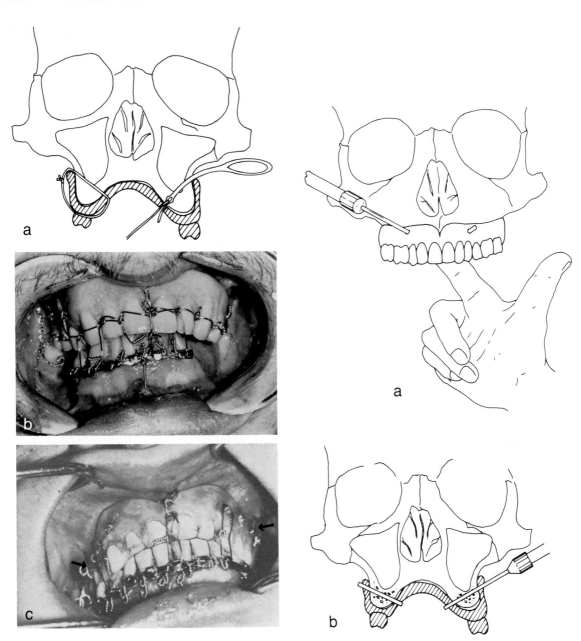

FIG. 7–35. **a,** Perialveolar wiring. The wire is passed bilaterally in the first bicuspid region with an alveolar awl. Holes are predrilled in the denture palate to allow for passage of the awl. **b,** Maxillary denture modified with Stout continuous loops and secured to the maxilla with a nasal spine wire and bilateral perialveolar wires. **c,** Maxillary denture with imbedded arch bar secured to maxilla with zygomatic buttress wires (arrows) and nasal spine wire.

FIG. 7–36. **a,** Kirschner wires used to stabilize maxillary denture or splint. The wire is drilled through the denture flange in the cuspid area. A finger palpates the palatal surface to detect where the end of the wire begins to perforate the denture on the palatal surface. **b,**The pins must pass through the buccal flange, alveolus, and palatal surface of the denture.

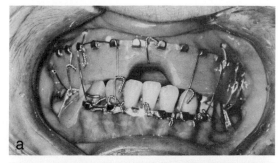
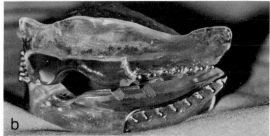
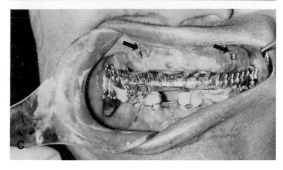

FIG. 7–37. **a,** Maxillary splint with arch bar imbedded on its labial surface is secured to maxilla with nasal spine and bilateral perialveolar wires. **b,** Gunning's splint. **c,** Maxillary splint secured to maxilla with Kirschner wires (arrows).

with the cannula being carried inferiorly and out of the oral cavity. When the wires are to be removed, both ends in the oral cavity are cut and individually grasped with wire twisters. The wires are then drawn superiorly into the sterile cutaneous area, the two vertical wires are cut just below the twist, and the two separated vertical wires are removed inferiorly out of the oral cavity.

FRACTURE INVOLVING THE MAXILLARY SINUS

Acute or chronic sinusitis seldom develops as a result of midfacial fractures involving the maxillary sinus. Although radiographs will often show an opacified sinus or an air-fluid level in the sinus initially, the sinus is usually clear on radiographs taken 5 to 6 weeks following the fracture. Special treatment of the sinus is usually not required apart from the reduction and fixation of the facial fracture. However, sinus exploration becomes necessary when teeth or foreign bodies are displaced into the sinus or in cases of herniation of orbital contents into the sinus, purulent sinusitis, or severe comminution of the sinal area.

Teeth or foreign objects such as metallic fragments should be removed from the sinus via a Caldwell-Luc approach. The sinus need not be explored merely because it is opacified or because there is an air-fluid level.

With a fracture of the orbital floor with clinical and radiographic evidence of herniation of orbital fat and muscle into the sinus, Killey suggests performing a Caldwell-Luc operation to ascertain the extent of the injury by directly inspecting the orbital floor.[24] If the bone fragments of the orbital floor can be manipulated back into place, the sinus can be gently packed with ½-inch-wide iodoform gauze saturated with bacitracin or other ointment. The free end of the pack can be left protruding from the Caldwell-Luc incision or from a nasal antrostomy and withdrawn in 2 weeks. If a continuity defect of the orbital floor is found, exploration of the orbital floor is necessary via a lower eyelid incision and the floor is supported with a 0.5-to-1 mm-thick sheet of alloplastic material cut to a triangular shape and large enough to be supported by the remaining bone of the orbital floor.

Should a purulent sinusitis develop following a midfacial fracture, the sinus should be opened via a Caldwell-Luc approach, irrigated, and debrided. A nasal antrostomy should be performed if drainage through the normal osteum is deemed inadequate. The area is irrigated daily through the osteum or antrostomy with normal saline until the purulent drainage ceases. Antibiotics are also necessary to combat the predominantly anaerobic organisms, and humidification is helpful to keep the nasal passages moist and patent.

COMPLICATIONS OF MAXILLARY FRACTURES

Complications occur seldom if midfacial fractures receive early and adequate treatment. Complications are usually the result of the injury itself but can also be secondary to delayed or improper treatment.

One must be constantly alert for delayed manifestations of cerebral injury. Steidler, in a review of 240 patients with facial fractures, found that 15% of those patients who experienced loss of consciousness at the time of injury had some form of residual cerebral disturbance, most commonly manifested as epilepsy or personality changes.[25] Cerebrospinal fluid rhinorrhea is not uncommon with Le Fort II and III fractures and usually resolves spontaneously after fracture reduction. Persistent rhinorrhea has been reported to last as long as 105 days, and in such cases craniotomy and dural repair are necessary.[26]

Cranial nerve injuries are common. The most common nerve injury is to the infraorbital nerve in Le Fort II and zygoma fractures. With proper fracture reduction, nerve dysfunction usually resolves within 2 months.

Most orbital complications are found in about 20% of facial injuries. Though most of these are due to direct injury to the globe itself, a few can be caused by manipulation of the fracture. The most disastrous complication is blindness secondary to optic nerve compression. Weymuller suggests that when unilateral loss of vision occurs and fracture through the orbital apex of the opposite side is suspected, midfacial fractures should not be reduced.[8] Other orbital complications include diplopia, enophthalmos, blurred vision, and telecanthus. Diplopia is commonly caused by untreated entrapment of the inferior rectus muscle or loss of integrity of the orbital floor with loss of orbital fat. Telecanthus results from not repairing a medial canthal ligament detachment or inadequately reducing nasal bone fractures.

Occlusal and maxillofacial deformities after trauma include dental malocclusion, facial asymmetry, and limited jaw opening.[27] These are almost exclusively the result of failure to restore proper dental occlusion at the time of initial fracture treatment and failure to ade-

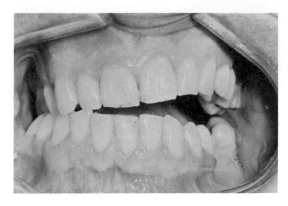

FIG. 7–38. Malocclusion from inadequately treated maxillary fracture.

quately reduce associated facial bone fractures (Fig. 7–38). If the dental occlusion is not restored to its preinjury condition, it is not possible to restore the face to its normal symmetry. These deformities can limit the patient's ability to chew, interfere with normal speech, and cause serious emotional and social problems. Malunions of facial bone fractures should be treated by osteotomy to restore normal form and function.

GUNSHOT WOUNDS OF THE MAXILLA

Missile wounds of the maxillofacial region accounted for approximately 15% of all wounds in the Vietnam conflict. Of these combat wounds, 38% were gunshot wounds, 52% were fragment wounds, and about 10% were other types.[28] Civilian missile wounds are most commonly gunshot wounds and are the result of homicide attempts, suicide attempts, and accidents. Most military gunshot wounds are produced by high-velocity bullets, whereas most civilian gunshot wounds are produced by low-velocity bullets. The capacity of a missile to injure depends on its kinetic energy on impact. The formula for kinetic energy, $KE = \frac{1}{2}$ mass $\times$ velocity^2, shows that as the velocity doubles, the kinetic energy quadruples. Low-velocity missiles (<1000 ft/sec) create smaller entrance and exit wounds, produce fewer fractures, and damage less soft tissue (Fig. 7–39). High-velocity missiles (>3000 ft/sec) create large exit wounds, produce extensive fracture and comminution of bone, and damage soft tissues

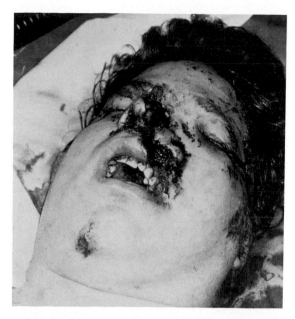

FIG. 7–39.   Low-velocity gunshot wound of maxilla. Missile entered the submental region, pierced the palate, and exited through the anterior nasal cavity. Note absence of bone and soft-tissue avulsion.

well beyond the missile tract (Fig. 7–40). Fractured teeth and bone themselves act as secondary missiles, creating even greater damage. A knowledge of the type and velocity of the weapon involved can aid the surgeon in estimating the extent of damage. Gunshot trauma typically produces wounds characterized by compound, comminuted fractures, extensive soft-tissue damage, and gross contamination.[29] The clinical and radiographic ex-

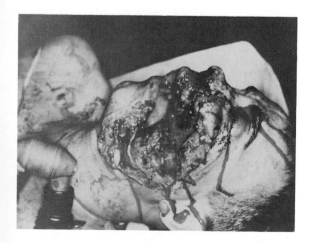

FIG. 7–40.   High-velocity gunshot exit wound with extensive bone and soft-tissue damage.

amination does not readily show the extent of the injury, and the viability of fractured bone and teeth is not easily evaluated. The true extent of damage is best determined at surgery.

Specifically, gunshot wounds of the maxilla produce fractures that rarely follow the classic Le Fort lines of fracture. Alveolar fracturing is common with associated oroantral and oronasal communication. The antrum, nose, eye, and ear are commonly injured. One should assume that the eye has been injured and obtain an ophthalmologic consultation prior to definitive treatment.

Preliminary Treatment

Initial treatment consists of airway management and hemorrhage control. To manage the airway, the surgeon must suction the oral cavity and look for fractured teeth, restorations, or a broken prosthesis; position patient on his side and pull tongue forward; and perform oral intubation if there is extensive palatal or floor of mouth damage. Fractures of the mandible and maxilla may necessitate a tracheostomy in the operating room.

To control hemorrhage, the surgeon must suction oral and nasal cavities and check for points of bleeding. Nasal bleeding can be managed by inserting soft-rubber nasopharyngeal tubes. Oral bleeding is usually from lacerated soft tissues and is managed by clamping vessels or applying direct pressure with gauze packing. If bleeding is not well controlled, intubation must be accomplished, followed by anterior and posterior nasal packing, oral packing, and antral packing, if necessary.

Once the airway is secured and bleeding controlled, a thorough clinical and radiographic examination is accomplished. A chest radiograph is taken to determine if any tooth fragments or restorations have been aspirated.

Because gunshot wounds are prone to tetanus, the patient's tetanus immunization record should be checked. If there is doubt as to the immunization status, 0.5 cc of tetanus toxoid must be administered intramuscularly.

Definitive Treatment

Definitive treatment of maxillary gunshot wounds is best done under general anesthesia and consists of debridement, management of fractured and partially avulsed teeth, reduction and fixation of fractures, and closure of mucosa and skin.

Debridement. To debride the wound, it is carefully explored for metallic fragments, broken prostheses, and tooth parts. The entire area is vigorously irrigated with saline. Only those bone fragments that wash away should be removed;[30] bone fragments that have even the smallest amount of periosteal attachments can be preserved by the excellent blood supply to the face. Soft tissue that appears somewhat discolored will usually survive; obviously nonvital soft tissue is sharply excised. The lateral margins of the wound should be bluntly probed with the finger to locate bone fragments pushed away by the force of the missile. Because all gunshot wounds are grossly contaminated, extensive irrigation with a syringe or pulsating water lavage must be meticulously carried out (Fig. 7–41).

Management of Fractured Teeth. Teeth with fractured roots or crowns that are nonrestorable should be removed. Fractured but restorable teeth should be retained, especially if they may aid in stabilization of a bone fragment. Exposed pulps should be extirpated and the canals sealed with calcium hydroxide.

Fracture Reduction and Fixation. Open reduction of comminuted maxillary fractures should be avoided; instead, the fragments are molded into position using the dental occlusion as a guide and held in place with the soft-tissue closure. Horizontal interdental wires, eyelet loops, or arch bars can be used to initially stabilize loose dentoalveolar fragments. In most instances the palate is fractured and an acrylic palatal splint is necessary to provide adequate fixation. Early in the treatment an alginate impression is taken of the maxillary and mandibular arches so that a self-curing acrylic palatal splint can be constructed. The dental plaster or stone models are sectioned and the best estimate of the occlusion is obtained. The splint should be made of clear acrylic to allow for the detection

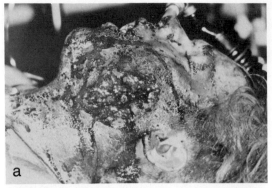

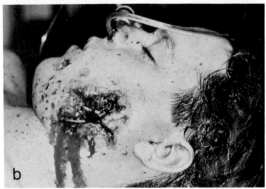

FIG. 7–41. **a,** Close-range gunshot wound contaminated with powder and metallic fragments. **b,** Same wound following cleansing, irrigation, and conservative debridement.

of pressure points upon insertion. Prior to insertion of the splint, palatal lacerations are closed with chromic gut suture. The palatal splint can then be wired to all remaining maxillary teeth (Fig. 7–42). If labial arch bars or wire loops are used, they are placed before the splint is placed. Intermaxillary fixation is then applied. Comminuted antral walls are supported with an antral packing of ½-inch gauze containing a topical antibiotic ointment; the free end of the packing can exit through either an oral mucosa incision or a nasal antrostomy, and the packing is left in place for 2 weeks. Suspension wires or a headframe may be used, if necessary, to support the maxilla.

Soft-Tissue Closure. Oral mucosal lacerations are closed to provide a watertight seal prior to skin closure.[31] The parotid duct should be probed if there is a possibility of ductal laceration. If a laceration of the duct is identified, it is repaired as described earlier.

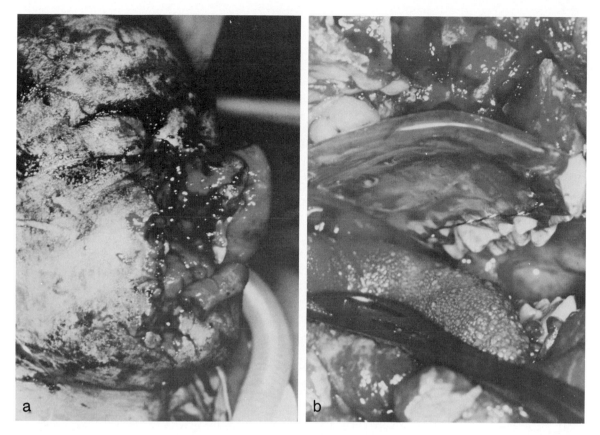

FIG. 7–42. **a,** High-velocity gunshot wound causing loss of mandibular symphysis and premaxilla with extensive oral and facial tissue damage. **b,** Acrylic palatal splint fabricated to stabilize loose maxillary dental-alveolar fragments.

Every attempt is made to close the mucosa primarily over antral and nasal communications. Widely undermining the mucosa will usually provide enough tissue for primary closure. If the communications cannot be closed, the cavities are packed open with ½-inch or 1-inch gauze containing a topical antibiotic ointment. All accessible nasal mucosal lacerations are likewise closed. If nasal bleeding persists, soft-rubber nasal tubes are placed or the nose is packed with ½-inch gauze containing a topical antibiotic ointment.

After all oral and nasal mucosal lacerations are closed, the skin is prepared and all facial lacerations are irrigated with saline. Nonvital tissue is conservatively excised and closed in layers. The skin can be widely undermined to achieve primary closure (Fig. 7–43). If gross loss of soft tissue prevents primary closure, the oral mucosa can be sutured directly to the skin (Fig. 7–44). Lacerations of the lips and oral commissures should be closed first and with great accuracy. Once the lips are reconstructed, the remainder of the lacerations can be closed. A pressure dressing made from gauze fluffs, roll bandage, and elastoplast is applied to support the soft tissues for several days.

Because most gunshot wounds are contam-

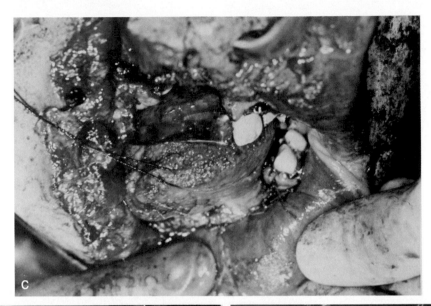

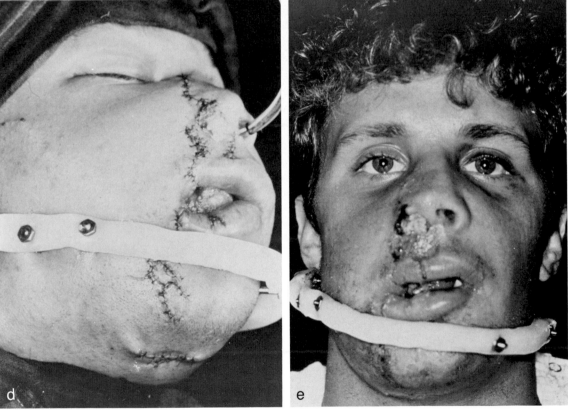

FIG. 7–42 (continued). **c,** Watertight closure of mucosal lacerations. **d,** Stabilization of mandible with biphase appliance, intermaxillary wire fixation with segmented arch bars, and meticulous closure of skin lacerations. **e,** Two weeks postinjury. Nasal packing in right nares to prevent constriction.

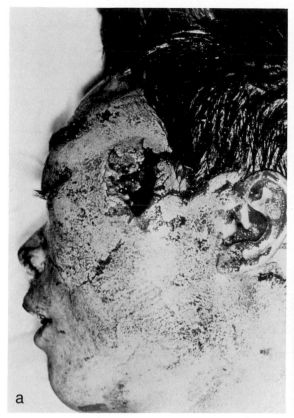 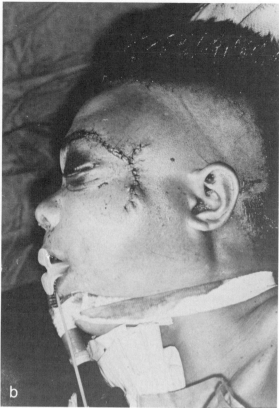

FIG. 7–43. **a,** Low-velocity missile exit wound. **b,** Soft tissue is conservatively excised. The skin is undermined and primary closure is performed.

inated from the ambient organisms on the oral mucosal and cutaneous surfaces, high-dose antibiotics should be started at the earliest possible opportunity after injury and continued for 7 to 10 days postoperatively. If wound breakdown occurs because of infection, gram-negative, anaerobic organisms should be suspected and a specimen for Gram's stain and aerobic and anaerobic cultures taken. The wound should be irrigated at least twice daily with saline[32] and dry fluff dressings applied loosely.

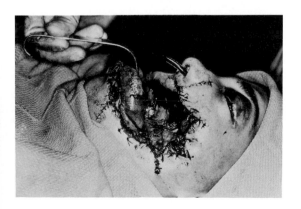

FIG. 7–44. Gross loss of soft tissue from high-velocity wound. Mucosa is sutured directly to skin.

REFERENCES

1. Neal, D.C., Wagner, W.F., Fiedler, L.D., and Alpert, B.: The epidemiology of facial fractures. J Med Assoc 275: 1978.
2. Turvey, T.: Midfacial fractures: A retrospective analysis of 593 cases. J Oral Surg 35:887, 1977.
3. Le Fort, R.: Etude experimental sur les fractures de la machoire superieure, Parts I, II, III. Rev Chir Paris 23:201, 1901.
4. Sicher, H.: Oral Anatomy. St. Louis, The C.V. Mosby Co., 1960.
5. Rowe, N.L., Killey, H.C.: Fractures of the Facial Skeleton. Baltimore, The Williams and Wilkins Co., 1968.
6. Luce, E.A., Tubb, T.D., and Moore, A.M.: Review

of 1,000 major facial fractures and associated injuries. Plast Reconstr Surg 63:26, 1979.

7. Smiler, D.G., Ling, A.M., and Wennogle, C.F.: Signs and symptoms of zygomaticomaxillary fractures involving the orbit. J Oral Surg 29:103, 1971.

8. Pogrel, M.A.: The superior orbital fissue syndrome. J Oral Surg 38:215, 1980.

9. Weymuller, E.A.: Blindness and LeFort III fractures. Ann Otol Rhinol Laryngol 93:2, 1984.

10. Trokel, S.L.: The orbit. Arch Ophthalmol 91:223, 1974.

11. Haisova, L., and Kramova, I.: Facial bone fractures associated with cervical spine injuries. Oral Surg 30:742, 1970.

12. Ferraro, J.W., and Berggren, R.B.: A precise method for determination of the displacement in fractures of the midface. Plast Reconstr Surg 50:447, 1972.

13. Hounsfield, G.H.: Computerized transverse axial scanning (tomography): Description of the system. Br J Radiol 46:1016, 1973.

14. Frame, J.W., and Wake, M.J.C.: Evaluation of maxillofacial injuries by use of computerized tomography. J Oral Maxillofac Surg 40:482, 1982.

15. Manfredi, S.J., et al.: Computerized tomographic scan findings in facial fractures associated with blindness. Plast Reconstr Surg 68:479, 1981.

16. Baker, S.P., and Schultz, R.C.: Recurrent problems in emergency room management of maxillofacial injuries. Clin Plast Surg 2:65, 1975.

17. Georgiode, N.G.: Plastic and Maxillofacial Trauma Symposium, Vol. I. St. Louis, The C.V. Mosby Co., 1969. p.57.

18. James, R.B., Fredrickson, C., and Kent, J.N.: Prospective study of mandibular fractures. J Oral Surg 39:275, 1981.

19. Kuepper, R.C., and Harrigan, W.F.: Treatment of midfacial fractures at Bellvue Hospital Center 1955–1976. J Oral Surg 35:420, 1977.

20. Irby, W.B., and Rast, W.C.: Extracranial fixation of the facial skeleton: Review and report of a case. Oral Surg 27:900, 1969.

21. Strauss, H.R., Morgan, M.J., and Hamilton, M.K.: External fixation of facial fractures. Am Surg 30:144–159, March 1979.

22. Banks, P.: Fixation of facial fractures. Br Dent J 138:129, 1975.

23. Gonty, A.A.: Combining the Irby head frame and the Morris external pin fixation set to stabilize midface fractures. J Oral Surg 41:410, 1983.

24. Killey, H.C., and Kay, L.W.: The Maxillary Sinus and Its Dental Implications. Bristol, John Wright and Sons, Ltd., 1975, pp.31–19.

25. Steidler, N.E., Cook, R.M., and Reade, P.C.: Residual complications in patients with major middle third facial fractures. Int J Oral Surg 9:259, 1980.

26. Leopard, P.: Dural tears in maxillo-facial injuries. Br J Oral Surg 8:222, 1970.

27. Walker, R.V.: Delayed occlusal and maxillofacial deformities after trauma. J Am Dent Assoc 82:858, 1971.

28. Rich, N.M.: Evaluation of missile wounds at the 2nd surgical hospital in Vietnam. Plastic and Maxillofacial Trauma Symposium. Vol. I. St. Louis, The C.V. Mosby Co., 1969, p.9.

29. Kelly, F.J.: Maxillofacial missile wounds. J Oral Surg 31:438, 1973.

30. Terry, B.C.: Facial injuries in military combat: Definitive care. J Oral Surg 27:551, 1969.

31. Osbon, D.B.: Early treatment of soft tissue injuries of the face. J Oral Surg 27:480, 1969.

32. Morgan, H.H., and Szmyd, L.: Maxillofacial war injuries. J Oral Surg 26:727, 1968.

8

FRACTURES OF THE ZYGOMATIC ARCH AND THE ZYGOMATICOMAXILLARY COMPLEX

CHARLES C. ALLING III

Both the zygomatic arch and the zygomaticomaxillary complex (ZMC) are fragile and, because of their positions, are exposed to direct trauma. When fractured, the arch usually undergoes a midportion medial depression and the complex undergoes a posterior and inferior displacement. Combined injuries of the two bones result from multiple trauma or are part of extensive facial skeletal injuries.

Common clinical signs of zygomatic arch and ZMC fractures may include flatness of the unusually rounded cheek area or zygomatic arch, which is best visualized by standing behind the patient and looking down over the head. Also, a displacement may be palpable over the zygomatic arch. Step defects along the infraorbital rim and at the zygomaticofrontal suture line are usually palpable if not obscured by edema and lacerations.

Limited mandibular movements may be present, caused by direct mechanical impingement of the coronoid process against a displaced ZMC or zygomatic arch or caused by myospasm of the temporal muscle. Another symptom is dysfunction of the sensory nerves to the cheek, ala of the nose, upper lip, and gingiva secondary to fracturing at the infraorbital foramen or posteriorly in the orbital floor. Also, diplopia, particularly in the upward-outward gaze, may result from lateral palpebral ligament displacement, usually inferiorly, and ocular muscle incarceration, usually of the inferior oblique and inferior rectus muscles.

If a blow-out fracture of the orbit occurs associated with a ZMC fracture, the patient may exhibit enophthalmos. Another sign is unilateral nosebleed from hemorrhage into the antrum, which drains into the nose via the maxillary ostium. Circumorbital and subconjunctival ecchymosis, particularly in the lateral conjunctiva, may also be present. Intraoral tenderness and uneveness may be evident on palpation of the sinal walls with ecchymosis in the upper buccal sulcus.

On rare occasions, ZMC fractures may be complicated by damage to the superior orbital fissure by actual disruption of the bony margins of the fissure, or by the formation of a hematoma or aneurysm within its boundaries. This syndrome is clinically characterized by ophthalmoplegia, ptosis of the upper lid, proptosis, and a fixed dilated pupil in addition to sensory disturbances over the distribution of the ophthalmic nerve with possible retro-orbital pain.

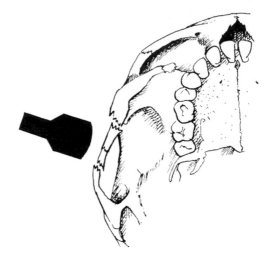

ZYGOMATIC ARCH FRACTURES

ETIOLOGY

Isolated zygomatic arch injuries are usually the result of acute, direct trauma to the side of the face that produces either a medially directed segmental displacement or a V-shaped deformity of the midportion of the arch (Fig. 8–1). Inferior displacement of the fractured arch by the masseter muscle is rare because of the superior support provided by the temporal fascia; likewise, superior displacement is rare because of the attachments of the masseter muscle. Inferior or superior displacements may be noted if either the temporal fascia or the masseter muscle are lacerated (Fig. 8–2). Zygomatic arch fractures may remain untreated if masked by edema. When a deformity is first noticed 2 or 3 weeks after injury, the patient may choose to forgo surgical correction and learn to live with the defect. If the medial depression of the arch is so severe that it impairs excursions of the mandible by impinging on the coronoid process, the patient will usually seek treatment.

Acute, direct trauma to the midportion of the arch is the most common cause of solitary zygomatic arch fractures. When a posteriorly displaced fracture of the ZMC occurs with a fracture of the zygomatic arch, the fracture in the arch may be either greenstick in nature or posteriorly impacted. The zygomatic arch may be comminuted when the patient has sustained massive facial trauma with multiple midface fractures.

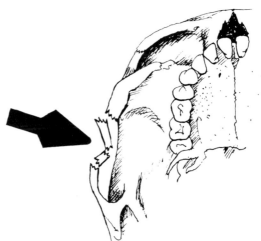

FIG. 8–1.   Typical zygomatic arch fractures.

ANATOMIC CONSIDERATIONS

The zygomatic arch is formed by the zygomatic processes of the temporal and the zygomatic bones. The arch provides attachment for the masseter muscle and the temporomandibular (lateral) ligaments of the joint. This frail arch receives sturdy superior support from the temporal fascia.

DIAGNOSIS

A positive sign of a depressed zygomatic arch fracture following trauma to the side of the face is dimpling over the region of the arch. Intraoral and extraoral palpation may elicit acute point tenderness indicative of a fracture. Impaired motions of the mandible,

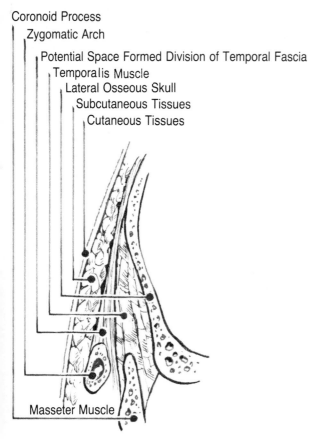

Coronoid Process
Zygomatic Arch
Potential Space Formed Division of Temporal Fascia
Temporalis Muscle
Lateral Osseous Skull
Subcutaneous Tissues
Cutaneous Tissues

Masseter Muscle

FIG. 8–2. Coronal cross section of zygomatic arch.

particularly lateral excursions to the affected side, may be diagnostic of a depressed fracture.[1]

Radiographic views usually will confirm clinical impressions of a zygomatic arch fracture. Radiographic examination may demonstrate an occult fracture that was obscured by either edema or body fat or is an extension of other fractures. The submentovertex view of the skull, sometimes called the jug handle view, is useful (Fig. 8–3). This view shows well the arches lateral to the skull in most individuals. When the affected part is masked, modified submentovertex views that emphasize the side of the skull with the affected arch may be employed. Also the Waters stereoparanasal sinal projection may be useful.

TREATMENT

Depressed fractures of the zygomatic arch are corrected by contouring and molding the arch laterally with an elevator using a transoral, temporal hairline, or lateral brow approach. In case of the V-type depression, both fragments must be brought up at the same time to avoid overlapping. Therefore, in all transoral and extraoral approaches, the tip of the instrument must be placed directly at the point of greatest depression so that both bony fragments will be engaged simultaneously (Fig. 8–4). From either a transoral or an extraoral approach, it is possible to elevate a depressed ZMC fracture as well as the zygomatic arch. If the arch and the ZMC have been fractured or elevated to an anatomic position, transosseous wiring or plating, usually at the lateral rim of the orbits and sometimes at the infraorbital rim, is indicated.

Transoral Approach

The transoral approach involves a 15-mm horizontal incision in the mucous membrane above the maxillary molar teeth overlying the jugal ridge buttress and just above the attached gingival mucoperiosteum. The underlying submucosal tissue is bluntly dissected subperiosteally to create a pathway for the elevating instrument. With the patient in the supine position and the head turned to the unaffected side, the elevating instrument is passed through the incision until the tip reaches the depressed portion on the medial surface of the arch. Care is taken to prevent the tip of the instrument from rotating medially and superiorly against the thin lateral wall of the orbit and to ensure that the tip of the instrument does not become positioned medial to the coronoid process of the mandible. Pressure is then exerted laterally and superiorly, without a lever action on the surface of the maxilla or teeth, to elevate the depressed bony fragments. The opposite hand is used for counterpressure with the palm placed on the parietal area of the skull and the fingers palpating the zygomatic arch to follow the progress of the reduction and alignment. When the bony fragments have been elevated and normal contour has been

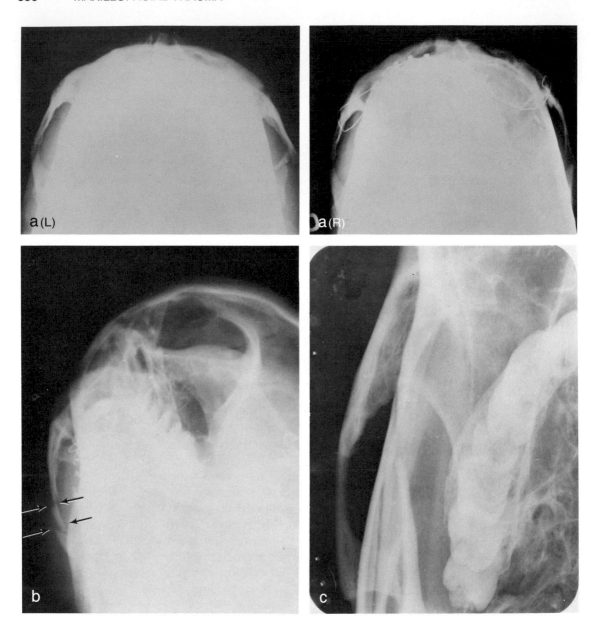

FIG. 8–3.   Jug handle radiologic views. **a L,** Standard preoperative view. **R,** Standard postoperative view. **b,** Modified extraoral view. (Courtesy of Dr. Cecil Albright.) **c,** Modified view with occlusal film. (Courtesy of Dr. Cecil Albright.)

restored as determined by palpation, the bony fragments usually will remain locked in position.

Temporal Approach

The temporal (Gillies') approach may be used primarily for elevating fractures of the zygomatic arch (Fig. 8–5).[2] Elevation of ZMC as well as arch fractures through the temporal approach was used commonly and was reported by Ellis and associates.[3] A 2-cm vertical incision is placed anterior and superior to the helix of the ear within the temporal hair, which may be shaved, and is carried through the subcutaneous tissues directly to the temporal fascia. An incision through the temporal fascia is made at an angle to the cutaneous and subcutaneous incisions to expose the belly of the temporal muscles because this

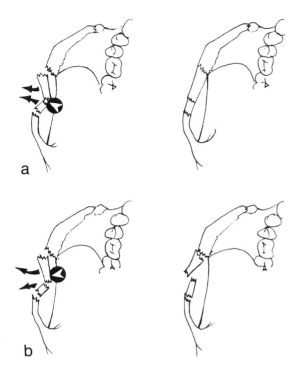

FIG. 8–4. **a,** Correct positioning of elevating instrument. **b,** Incorrect positioning of elevating instrument.

method uses divergent incision lines and places the superficial tissue on a base of intact fascia. The lines of repair where the fascia and skin incisions are closed will be less likely to cause a scar contracture. If the surgeon tries to introduce the elevator prior to penetrating the temporal fascia, the instrument will approach the lateral and superior surface of the arch rather than the medial surface. The elevating instrument must be passed anteriorly and inferiorly in the space between the temporal fascia and the muscle to the medial surface of the zygomatic arch. Following elevation of the depressed fragments, the surgical site is closed in layers.

Lateral Brow Approach

When a zygomatic arch fracture is present concurrently with a depressed ZMC fracture and a lateral brow surgical approach to the ZMC fracture is planned, the same surgical site usually may be used to elevate a depressed arch.

Other Approaches

In all of the elevating approaches, the belly of the temporal muscle will serve to maintain arch form. If the zygomatic arch is severely comminuted and will not maintain the contoured reduction, however, it may be stabilized by a trapeze device with cirumferential wiring. On occasion, an open reduction procedure through a horizontal transcutaneous incision just above the zygomatic arch or, preferably, through a hemicoronal flap may be indicated in order to visualize, align, and stabilize the bony fragments with a small bone plate or, preferably, with transosseous wiring. Even more rarely, molding the arch and stabilizing it in the desired contour can be performed with gauze or other material placed on the medial aspect of the arch. If the gauze were to be placed through the horizontal transcutaneous approach, the temporal fascial sling that supports the arch would be severed; introducing gauze via the transoral, temporal, or lateral brow routes would not violate the temporal fascia. In any case, the gauze or other material should be removed in 5 to 7 days.

COMPLICATIONS

Complications of zygomatic arch fractures include malunion in a medially depressed position and osteomyelitis. A depressed arch may interere with anterior and lateral excursions of the mandible because of impingement of the coronoid process. The condition may be corrected by refracturing and elevating the depressed fractures through a hemicoronal approach, a horizontal transcutaneous approach, a transoral approach, or a combination of approaches.

If refracturing and elevating the depressed zygomatic arch is not feasible, the function of the mandible may be improved by removing the coronoid process transorally via an incision through the mucous membrane overlying the anterior border of the ramus, and by sectioning the coronoid process (Fig. 8–6). The coronoid process need not be removed from the surgical site as it will be retracted by the temporal muscle and either be resorbed or become reattached by fibrous connective or osseous tissue.

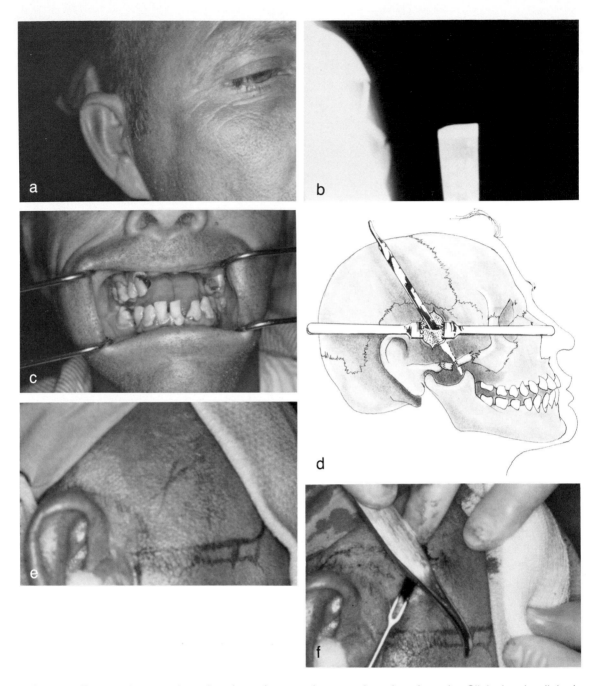

FIG. 8–5. Temporal approach to elevating a depressed zygomatic arch. **a, b,** and **c,** Clinical and radiologic views of depressed arch causing a limitation of mandibular movements. **d,** Diagram of placement of elevating instrument. **e, f,** and **g,** Surgical steps in elevating the arch: arch and incisional lines (skin and temporal fascia incisions) are marked on the skin; the incisions are completed and the elevating instrument is measured for correct placement; the elevating instrument in place. **h, i,** and **j,** Three-day postoperative clinical and radiologic views.

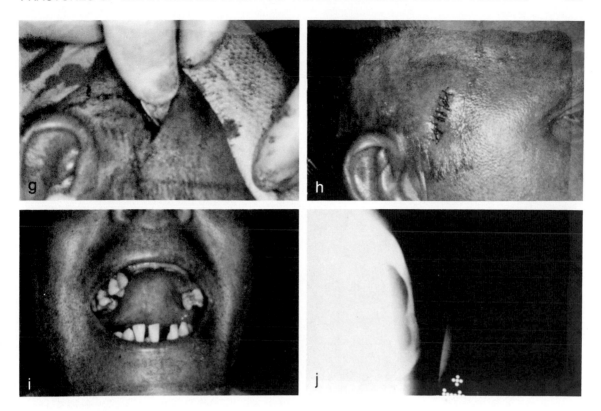

FIG. 8–5 (continued).

If the patient's mandibular function is adequate, normal contouring of the arch at the fracture site may be accomplished for aesthetic reasons by placing a graft of bone, cartilage, or one of the alloplastic materials as an overlay. A horizontal transcutaneous incision line approach could be used, although a hemicoronal flap will provide a better bed for the graft because it is not contiguous with the direct soft-tissue dissection, provides superior surgical access, and aesthetically is a more acceptable incision line (Fig. 8–7). The graft may be held in position by small notches at both ends of its lateral surface that accommodate circumferential or semicircumferential wires or sutures.

Beginning in the second half of the twentieth century, osteomyelitis became rare, but not unknown, with facial skeletal fractures. Recalled for this text is a case of an acutely infected inflammatory process of the zygoma and the zygomatic arch following a transoral elevation procedure for depressed fractures (Fig. 8–8). Review of the records of the referring source revealed that there was no pre-operative preparation of the oral cavity by drying and applying antiseptic solutions.

ZYGOMATICOMAXILLARY COMPLEX (ZMC) FRACTURES

ETIOLOGY

ZMC fracture lines usually are near the zygomaticomaxillary suture, involving the inferior orbital rim and floor of the orbit, and near the zygomaticofrontal suture line, involving the lateral orbital rim and the lateral synchondrosis of the orbital cavity. Fractures through the inferior rim of the bony orbit rarely are limited to the aforementioned suture line, instead extending to involve the anterior and lateral walls of the maxillary antrum and the thin orbital plate of the maxilla (Fig. 8–9). Such fracture lines usually course across the buttress of the maxilla and across the anterior and posterior walls of the maxillary antrum. The superior portion of the fracture line passes posteriorly and laterally

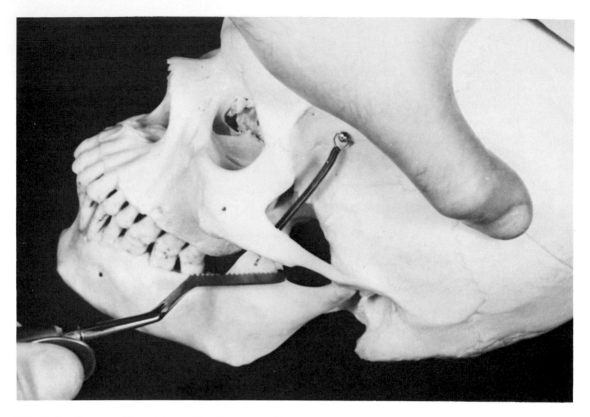

FIG. 8–6.   Saw positioned to section the coronoid process.

across the floor of the orbit, which forms the roof of the antrum, and joins the ascending fracture line in the posterior antral wall at the inferior orbital fissure. The line of fracture continues up the lateral wall of the bony orbit through the thin plates of the sphenoid bone to the zygomaticofrontal suture line; displacements of the zygoma usually will be a marked separation at this point. Fractures involving the zygoma usually involve a portion of the maxilla as well. Hence, the fractures are referred to as zygomaticomaxillary complex fractures.

ZMC fractures directly involve the contents of the orbital cavity, especially the periorbital tissue and the extraocular muscles. True blow-out fractures, involving only trauma to the orbit with resultant fracture of the bony floor or one of the walls and featuring herniation of the periorbital tissue, involve neither other facial bones nor the infraorbital rim.[4] Most blow-out fractures are modified, causing fracturing trauma also to the ZMC and the bony orbital rim. The blow-out feature results from a sudden increase in intraor-

bital pressure caused by trauma to the globe that is transmitted to the periorbital soft tissues. When the orbital contents are forcibly displaced, the pressures cause a blow-out at a weak area of the orbital wall, resulting in herniation of the periorbital tissues, most frequently into the maxillary antrum. This mechanism protects against significant injury to the globe.

ANATOMIC CONSIDERATIONS

The zygoma bone (the zygomatic or malar bone) is frequently involved in midfacial injuries because of its prominence as the cheek bone. The zygoma is quadrilateral and is located immediately inferior and somewhat lateral to the orbit (Fig. 8–10). It has an outer convex and two inner concave surfaces; the posterior surface forms part of the infratemporal fossa, while its superior surface forms the lateral half of the floor and the inferior half of the lateral wall of the bony orbit.

The zygoma has four processes that join with the maxillary, frontal, and temporal

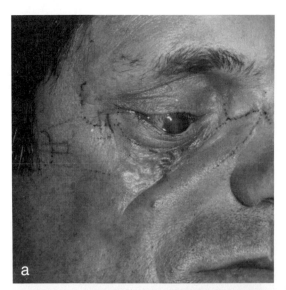

FIG. 8–7. Reconstruction of an anterior zygomatic arch and ZMC defect via a hemicoronal flap. The patient underwent excision of a tumor, type unknown, as a child. A surgical defect resulted, involving loss of the anterior zygomatic arch, the zygoma, the right maxilla, and the eye and producing an oral-nasal-antral opening. The patient was referred for the following surgery. **a,** Preoperative view. Skin markings in the periorbital regions are for planning purposes. **b,** At first surgery. The proposed line of incision for the hemicoronal flap, the anterior hairline, and the surgical defect in the lateral orbital rim are marked. **c,** Retractors are under the iliac graft that reconstructs the anterior zygomatic arch and lateral orbital rim.

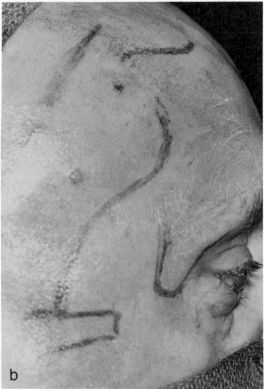

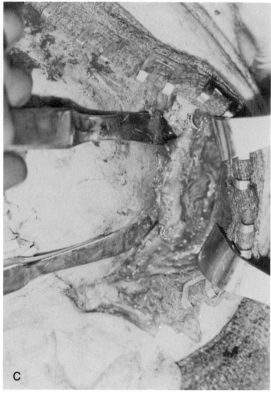

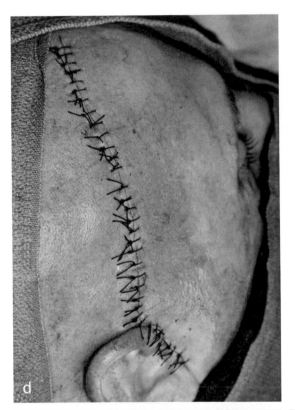

FIG. 8–7 (continued). **d,** Closure of the hemicoronal flap. **e,** At second surgery, 6 months later. Infraorbital incision made for placement of an iliac bone graft replacing the infraorbital rim, floor of the orbit, and anterior wall of the sinus. At this time, the referring ophthalmologist reconstructed the nasolacrimal duct. **f,** Closure of the infraorbital incision.

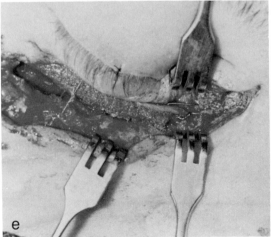

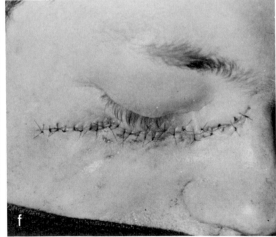

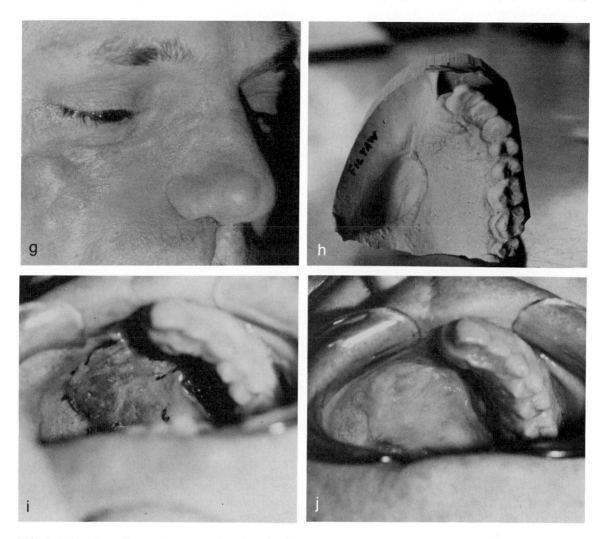

FIG. 8–7 (continued). **g,** Postoperative view. **h,** Cast of the oral-sinus-nasal opening. **i,** At third surgery, 4 months later. Posteriorly based full palatal pedicle flap covers the defect. **j,** Postoperative view of oral cavity. Surgery was followed by prescription of an intraoral maxillofacial prosthesis.

bones and the greater wing of the sphenoid. The maxillary process articulates with a triangular portion of the maxilla via irregular suture lines. This articulation forms a strong buttress on the lateral wall of the maxillary antrum, which reinforces the position of the zygoma and acts as a keystone for the facial contour. The frontal process articulates with the zygomatic synchondrosis of the bony orbit and forms the anterior inferior portion of the lateral wall and rim of the bony orbit. The temporal process is a long, narrow, triangular projection that articulates with the zygomatic process of the temporal bone; the temporal and zygomatic processes form the zygomatic arch. The sphenoidal or orbital process is a thin plate of bone that forms the major portion of the floor of the orbit and contains the inferior orbital fissure, which divides the process into a maxillary and sphenoidal portion.

The zygoma has three borders. The zygomatic border has a tubercle for the tendinous attachment of the anterior portion of the masseter muscle; the orbital border is concave and provides an attachment for the palpebral fascia, as well as forming the lateral border of the inferior rim of the orbit; the temporal border is sharply angled and provides for an attachment of the temporal fascia.

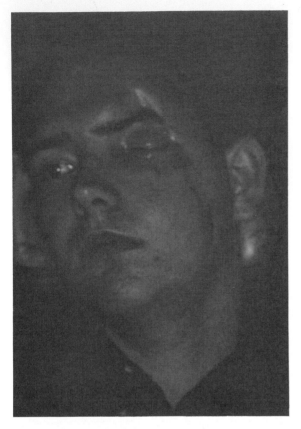

FIG. 8–8. Patient with osteomyelitis of the zygomatic arch and ZMC.

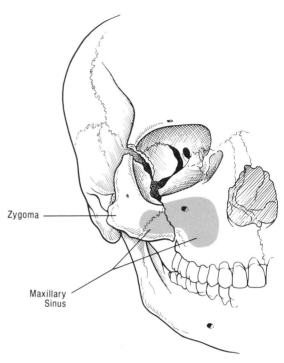

FIG. 8–9. ZMC fracture involving the maxillary antrum and the floor of the orbit.

The zygoma also serves as an attachment for the greater and lesser zygomatic muscles of facial expression. The zygomaticotemporal nerve, which provides sensory innervation to most of the anterior area of the temporal region, is transmitted by a small foramen located on the posterior, temporal fossa surface; the zygomaticofacial nerve, which provides innervation to the soft tissues of the skin lateral to the eye and overlying the cheek prominence, passes through by a small foramen located on the anterior surface of the bone.

The zygomatic bone with its various processes may be divided into an upper triangular half related to the orbital cavity and the temporal fossa, and a lower triangular half related to the facial aspect of the skull and the infratemporal fossa. The fully developed maxillary sinus resembles an irregular pyramid, its base formed by the lateral wall of the nose and its apex by the junction of the zygoma and maxillary bones, or actually formed within the body of the zygoma. Thus, the zygomatic bone helps to anchor the maxilla, gives origin to the masseter muscle, transmits masticatory forces from the maxilla to the cranium, and contains the maxillary sinus.

DIAGNOSIS

History and Clinical Examination

After obtaining a history from the patient or a sponsor, a physical examination is made of the structures of the face. Inspection, including viewing from above and below the face, may demonstrate asymmetries (Fig. 8–11).

Establishing an early and accurate diagnosis of ZMC fractures is desirable. Unless a patient is seen immediately following injury, the clinical signs may be obscured by edema, hematoma, and lacerations. Prior to the onset of edema, inspection may reveal flattening of the cheek prominence and a palpation disparity in the inferior and lateral rims of the

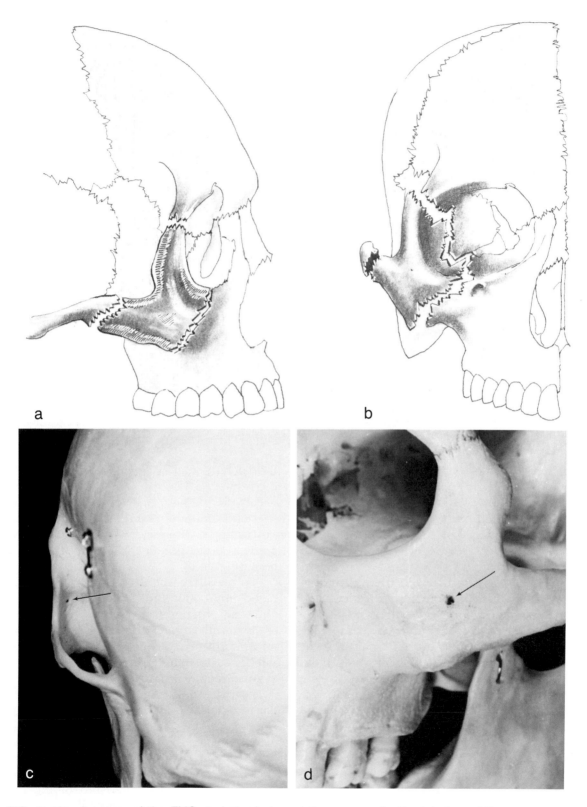

FIG. 8–10.   Anatomy of the ZMC. **a**, Lateral view of the zygoma. **b,** Frontal view of the zygoma. **c,** Zygomaticotemporal nerve foramen. **d,** Zygomaticofacial nerve foramen.

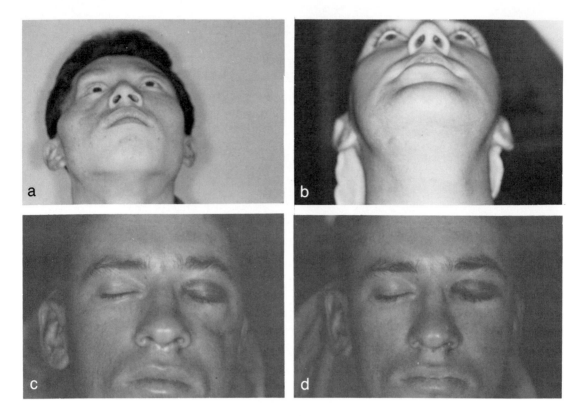

FIG. 8–11.   Preoperative facial asymmetry due to ZMC fracture and postoperative views following transoral elevation. **a,** Preoperative. **b,** Postoperative. **c,** Preoperative. **d,** Postoperative.

bony orbit. A marked deformity may be noticed if the lateral palpebral ligament is displaced inferiorly with the zygoma. The signs of skeletal deformity in ZMC fractures are often accompanied by subconjunctival edema over the sclera of the eye; enophthalmos; marked periorbital edema and ecchymosis; paresthesia or anesthesia in the distribution of the zygomaticotemporal, zygomaticofacial, and, especially, infraorbital nerves; epistaxis or nasal hematoma; impaired extraocular muscle function; and possibly, pain with or limitation of excursions of the mandible. If the ZMC floor is significantly displaced, the extraocular muscles, especially the inferior rectus, produce a clinically discernible diplopia primarily in the upward gaze (Fig. 8–12). Periorbital edema without muscle entrapment, which often results from ZMC fractures, may cause diplopia; however, in these cases the diplopia is usually in all fields of gaze and not limited to just the upward gaze. ZMC fractures also may cause a clinically obvious lowering of the outer canthus of the eye because

the lateral palpebral ligament is attached to the frontal process of the zygomatic bone.

Palpation is performed simultaneously bilaterally beginning with the orbital rims and proceeding to the zygomatic arches, the zygomatic bone prominences, and the nasal bone (Fig. 8–13).

The maxillary antral walls should be palpated intraorally and bilaterally, beginning with the anterior wall and proceeding laterally to rule out any disparities in the region of the buttress of the maxilla. The medial and inferior surfaces of the anterior portion of the zygomatic arches may be palpated intraorally.

The patient with a ZMC fracture usually has the subjective symptoms of regional pain, upper gaze diplopia, and a decrease in visual acuity. Fractures of the ZMC, which extend into the floor of the orbit, may form a defect or void in the orbital floor through which the periorbital tissue is herniated into the antrum, resulting in a clinical enophthalmos or hypotropia. If the fractures of the orbital floor are overlapping in a trapdoor fashion without

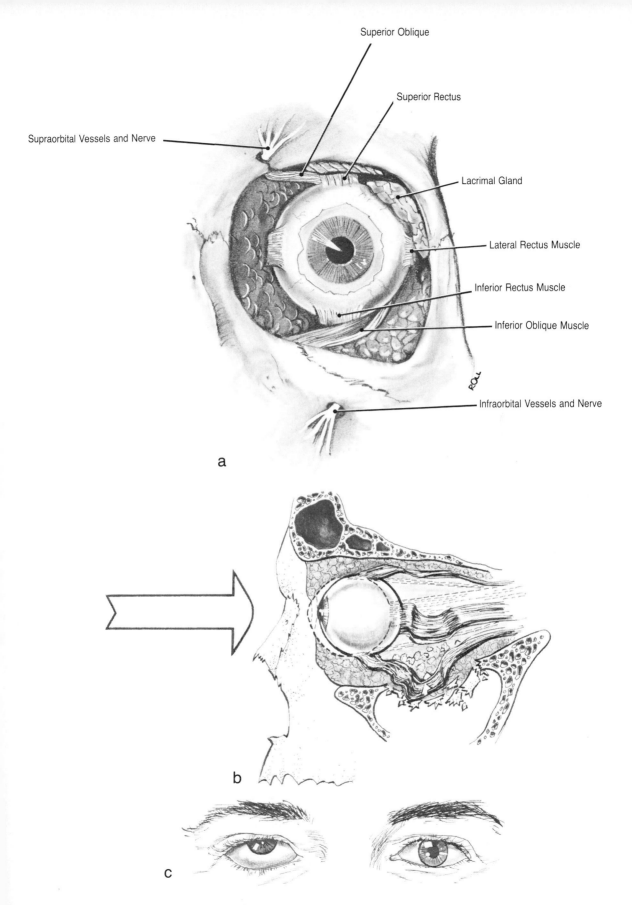

Superior Oblique

Superior Rectus

Supraorbital Vessels and Nerve

Lacrimal Gland

Lateral Rectus Muscle

Inferior Rectus Muscle

Inferior Oblique Muscle

Infraorbital Vessels and Nerve

a

b

c

FIG. 8–12.   Diplopia secondary to a blow-out fracture. **a,** Anterior view of the eye. **b,** Mechanism producing a blow-out fracture. **c,** Illustration of impeded upper gaze.

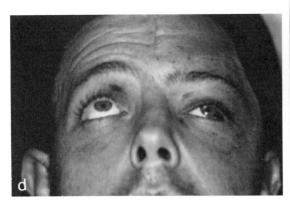
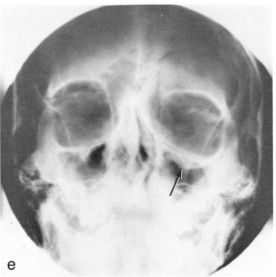

FIG. 8–12 (continued). **d,** Patient with impeded upper gaze. **e,** Paranasal sinus radiologic view of herniation into the sinus without concurrent ZMC fracturing.

a void in the bony floor, an entrapment of the inferior rectus muscle, the inferior oblique muscle, and Tenon's capsule may be present, with a resultant restriction in extraocular movements and an upper-gaze diplopia. These limitations reflect the anatomy of the origin of the inferior oblique muscle from the orbital floor near the lacrimal groove and its lateral margin. The inferior rectus muscle is situated directly beneath the globe and immediately above the infraorbital canal and may become impounded, resulting in restricted motion.

The optic nerve is rarely damaged, directly or indirectly, because of the unique bony anatomy of the optic foramen, which provides extra strength to the bony orbit in the region of the foramen. Fractures extending to the apex of the bony orbit rarely encroach on the optic foramen or canal but may endanger vision by involvement of the clinoid process or by pressure from vascular injuries secondary to fractures. These conditions, if not reversed, may lead to permanent loss of sight; with the aid of CT views of the optic foramen and route laminagraphy, however, early evaluation and correction by the ophthalmologist may avert irreversible damage to sight.

If vision is not impaired, evaluation of diplopia and enophthalmos includes the traction test. With the patient under general anesthesia and before surgical exploration, traction is applied to the tendon of the inferior rectus muscle to ascertain if upward free rotation of the globe can be achieved; if it cannot, incarceration of the inferior rectus muscle may exist. However, a positive forced traction *may be present without* entrapment of the inferior rectus muscle. If no entrapment of the inferior rectus is demonstrated by CT, the dipplopia will probably resolve.[5]

It is important that an ophthalmologist be involved in management of the ZMC fracture to verify the extent of injuries to assure, as far as possible, normal ocular function and visual acuity.

Concurrent fracturing of the maxilla may be demonstrated by grasping the maxillary alveolar processes with the thumb and index finger and attempting to rotate, rock, and move the maxilla or alveolar segments. If the mandible is intact, useful information regarding the extent of possible concurrent midfacial fractures can be obtained by having the patient close the mouth in centric occlusion and then attempt to move the midface by mandibular grinding movements. These procedures to determine associated transverse fractures of the maxillae, isolated fractures of the alveolar processes, and even occult midfacial

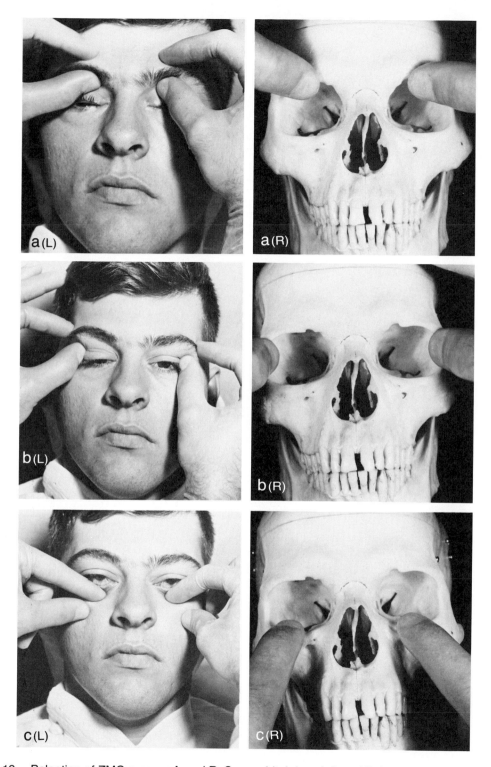

FIG. 8–13. Palpation of ZMC areas. **a L** and **R,** Supraorbital rims. **b L** and **R,** Lateral orbital rims. **c L** and **R,** Infraorbital rims.

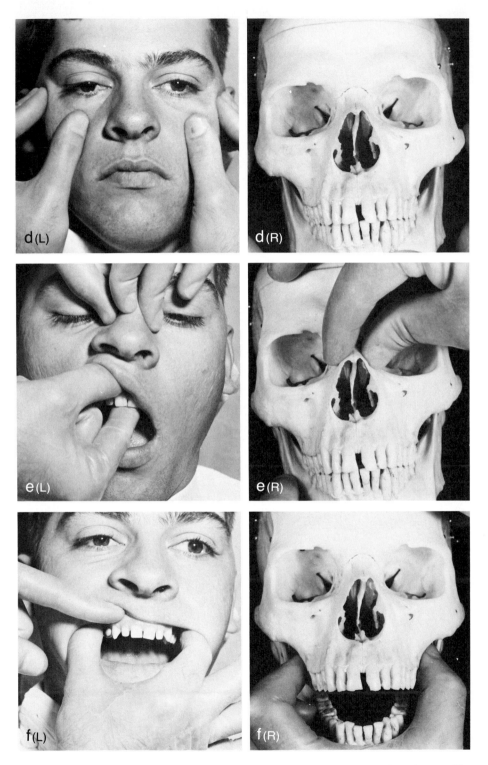

FIG. 8–13 (continued). **d L** and **R**, Zygoma and zygomatic arch. **e L** and **R**, Anterior maxilla and nasal bones. **f L** and **R**, Maxilla.

pyramidal fractures and craniofacial dysjunctions should be performed as part of the assessment of ZMC fractures that appear to be isolated. If other fractures are present as well, the management of the ZMC fracture will need to be scheduled with regard to the other injuries.

Radiographic Examination

The most useful imaging technique for confirming clinical impressions and establishing the extent of injuries is the CT scan.[4] CT will clearly display the orbit, ocular muscles, bone and bone fragment positions, and collections of hematomas. Widely available flat plane and stereoscopic paranasal sinal projections display the contours of the ZMC with only minimal superimposition of other structures. Opacification of the antrum, resulting from hemorrhage, may obscure evidence of a blow-out fracture, and displaced bony fragments on flat plane films may be indicative of fractures involving the antrum. When the floor of the bony orbit is determined to be involved, the extent and degree of fragmentation, as well as herniation from a blow-out fracture, may be evaluated by standard laminagraphy, stereoscopic paranasal projections, and CT scans. The flat plane submentovertex view is often useful in demonstrating the amount of posterior displacement of the ZMC, and this information is readily apparent on the transverse cuts of a CT scan.

Evidence of fragmentation of the orbital floor with or without displacement of the globe may be noted by medical imagery examinations, and herniation of the periorbital soft tissues into the maxillary sinus may be noted. Either of these findings, correlated with the clinical finding of diplopia in the upward gaze, is indicative of a blow-out fracture. However, neither the clinical nor the imagery findings alone should be relied on for definitive diagnosis.

TREATMENT

The treatment of ZMC fractures is determined by the clinical and radiographic findings, the type and extent of the fractures, the amount of comminution, the degree and direction of displacement of the bony fragments, the involvement of adjacent structures, the presence of concurrent injuries, and the general health of the patient. Immediate treatment of ZMC fractures is not indicated in patients with a history of brain injury. Whenever feasible, the maxillofacial surgical procedures should be accomplished concomitant to other surgical procedures requiring a general anesthetic. The best results for the ZMC fractures can be obtained if the treatment is performed within 10 days following injury.

Transoral Approach

Some of the uncomplicated ZMC fractures may be reduced by transoral, extra-antral elevation of the bony fragments to their normal position and alignment against adjacent bones (Fig. 8–11). The modified no. 22 urethral sound, which provides for the transmission of strong elevating and manipulating pressures, is one of the useful instruments for this procedure. Another effective instrument is the Seldin elevator which may be marked in centimeter lines for accurate placement; another of the many elevating instruments is a large curved hemostat (Fig. 8–14). A 15-mm horizontal incision is made in the vestibule, above the maxillary first and second molar teeth, overlying the jugal buttress and just above the attached gingival mucoperiosteum. If the incision is extended posteriorly and laterally, depending on individual anatomic variations, a bothersome herniation of the buccal fat pad into the surgical site may occur. The incision should be designed to permit an anterior extension if a sinusotomy becomes a necessary part of the procedure.

The tissue is bluntly dissected subperiosteally with a periosteal elevator or small curved hemostat to a position lateral to the wall of the maxillary antrum. The dissection is continued posteriorly and superiorly with a periosteum elevator or a large curved hemostat to a position beneath the zygomatic process of the maxilla and the body of the zygoma. Introducing the forceps with the beaks closed and withdrawing it with the beaks open will create a pathway for introducing an elevating instrument if the forceps

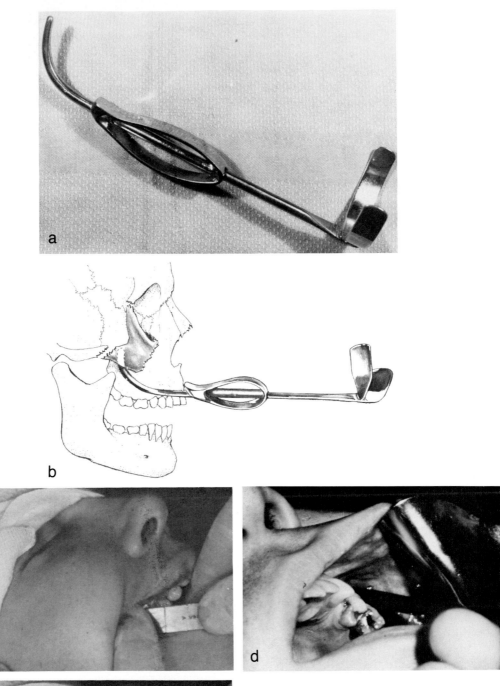

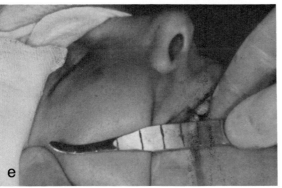

FIG. 8–14. Transoral elevation of ZMC fractures. **a,** Modified urethral sound. **b,** Sound in place for elevation. **c, d,** and **e,** Periosteum elevator measured and placed for elevation.

is not used for the elevation. The tip of the elevating instrument should not be allowed to rotate medially and superiorly against the thin wall of the bony orbit.

With the patient's head turned toward the unaffected side, the elevating instrument is positioned beneath the depressed ZMC. Pressure is exerted in a lateral and superior direction, without a lever action on the surface of the maxilla or teeth, to properly reposition the depressed ZMC. The opposite hand is used for counterpressure, with the heel and palm on the parietal area of the skull and the fingers sensing the reduction by palpating through the skin overlying the inferior and lateral orbital rim.

The repositioned ZMC may remain in position without fixation. In some cases, direct fixation of fractures at the anterior or lateral surfaces of the zygoma or of the orbital rim is necessary; this may be accomplished during a transoral approach either by transosseous wiring or by placing small bone plates (Fig. 8–15). The transoral approach permits visualization of fracture lines on the jugal ridge and the infraorbital rim. Miniplates of transosseous wires can stabilize a repositioned fracture of the ZMC as long as there is minimal to no comminution of the fracture lines. If considerable fragmentation is present, a combination of open reduction via a lateral brow approach and an intrasinal elevation with support by sinal packing or balloons may be in order.

Extraoral Open Reduction

Reduction with direct wiring or bone plating of the lateral rim and, when necessary, of the infraorbital rim of the orbit stabilizes the ZMC (Fig. 8–16). Although the open reduction of the lateral orbital rim may stabilize the ZMC, it may not eliminate the disparity of a fracture line in the inferior orbital rim, and an open reduction of the infraorbital rim with interosseous wiring or placing of a bone plate may be necessary. In many cases the entire inferior rim is comminuted and plating or transosseous wiring may not be possible. In these cases, an orbital floor autogenous or freeze-dried bone implant or an alloplastic biomaterial implant may be placed to form an artificial infraorbital rim. Another method is to suspend a cable, made by twisting 26-gauge stainless steel wire, across the defect and to wire or suture the bony fragments, with as much periosteum still attached as possible, to the cable.

The direct approach to fractures of the lateral rim begins with palpation to accurately locate the fracture. A normal osseous projection to which the temporal fascia is attached on the posterolateral surface of the frontal process of the zygoma may be mistaken for a fracture discrepancy. The frontozygomatic suture, a site for fracturing, is superior to this projection.

The eyebrow is *never* shaved when the surgical site is prepared. The incision bisects the

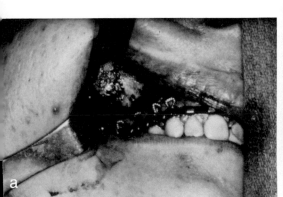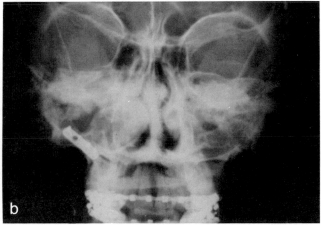

FIG. 8–15. **a,** Exposure of a ZMC fracture via a transoral approach. **b,** Radiograph of a miniplate for rigid fixation of a ZMC fracture.

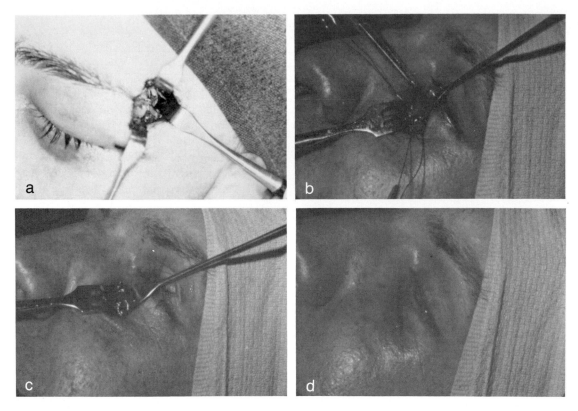

FIG. 8–16. Lateral and infraorbital rim reduction and fixation of ZMC fractures. **a,** Lateral rim surgical site. **b, c,** and **d,** Infraorbital rim wiring, following exploration of the orbital floor, and closure. The suture line demonstrates the usual placement of the incision.

line of fracture and is carried usually in three layers, down through the periosteum. Another incision is necessary to detach the temporal fascia from the posterolateral rim of the frontal process of the zygoma and from the zygomatic process of the frontal bone, and subperiosteal elevation exposes the concavity of the anterior aspect of the temporal fossa. The elevation of the periosteum of the temporal fossa opens a channel for the introduction of elevating instruments to the posterior surfaces of the ZMC and the medial surface of the zygomatic arch. Holes are drilled from the lateral surfaces, above and below the fracture line. The drill holes are directed posteriorly and medially to exit on the temporal fossa aspect of the processes. The ZMC is elevated into an anatomic alignment by placing an elevator firmly on the posterior surface of the zygoma and elevating laterally and superiorly. A wire placed in the drill hole of the fragment may be used to move the segment into an anatomic alignment, with great care

taken not to pull the fragment apart. Palpation at the infraorbital rim during these maneuvers helps to assure optimum positioning. A 26-gauge transosseous wire with the twist placed on the temporal fossa surface is used to immobilize the fragment. A small bone plate may be placed but is less versatile than wire for this particular application. The incision is closed in layers; plain gut is used subcutaneously, and polyethylene or nylon sutures are placed on the cutaneous surface.

Because occult fracture lines can be present radiating from the fracture on the lateral and infraorbital rims, drill holes or screws holes placed too close to the obvious major fracture may cause small comminutions into the fracture site. Therefore, the drill holes should be placed as far as is practical from the macroscopically obvious fracture line.

Intrasinal Approaches

ZMC fractures may be reduced and recontoured from within the maxillary antrum to provide support for a comminuted ZMC or to reduce a blow-out fracture. An intrasinal approach is usually contraindicated for non-comminuted and nonblow-out ZMC fractures. The recontouring and support consists of placing, through a Caldwell-Luc approach, gauze dressings carrying various medications, antral balloons, or Foley catheters (Fig. 8–17).

Blow-out fractures may be treated from the sinal approach. The inferiorly displaced orbital floor and orbital contents are elevated from within the sinus to a correct anatomic position. Thus, the orbital periosteum is not surgically dissected, and the bone fragments of the orbital floor maintain contact with their supportive periosteum.

The maxillary antrum is entered via an opening through the anterior wall of the sinus. This procedure is begun by exploring an existing laceration or by making a sharp curvilinear incision through the mucous membrane and periosteum from the region of the jugal ridge anteriorly to the vicinity of the pyriform fossa of the nose. The position of the incision immediately above the attached mucoperiosteal gingiva facilitates subsequent closure over intact bone. The flap usually is elevated to expose the infraorbital foramen and the inferior rim of the bony orbit. The jugal ridge serves as a landmark for the degree and direction of displacement of the ZMC.

At this stage of the operation, the medially displaced and rotated ZMC can be elevated extra-antrally. Access is gained into the antrum by elevating bony comminutions in the anterior wall or by making a circular opening through the bone, approximately 2.0 cm in diameter, using a chisel and mallet, a bone bur, or an end-biting rongeur. Frequently, fractured bone is elevated with the mucoperiosteum, which allows for adequate entrance into the antrum; these bony flakes are left attached to the mucoperiosteum and are replaced in a normal position at the conclusion of the operation.

The antrum is irrigated with copious amounts of normal saline or an antibiotic solution, and clotted blood and debris are re-

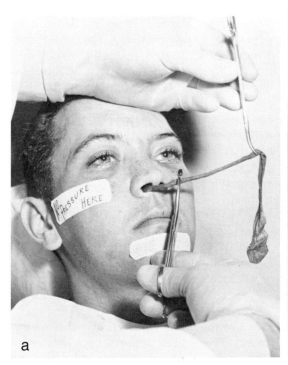
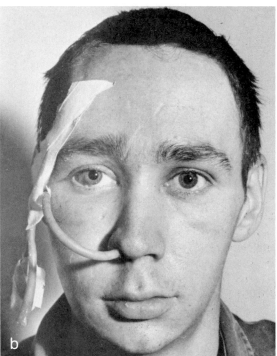

FIG. 8–17.   Intrasinal support of a ZMC fracture. **a,** Postoperative nasoantrostomy. **b,** Postoperative Foley catheter support.

moved by aspiration. A headlamp or fiber-optic retracting instruments facilitate visualization of the antrum and allow for evaluation of fracture lines and of a blow-out fracture into the sinus from the antral roof. Further antral exploration is performed by introducing palpating fingers through the sinusotomy. The type and extent of bony fragmentation of a blow-out fracture and involvement of the antral membrane may be such that continuity of the roof may be regained by manual manipulation.

Following reduction of the fractures, a 12- to 25-mm wide plain gauze strip approximately 1 m long carrying bacitracin ointment, balsam of Peru, or a similar product may be placed to support the ZMC. The gauze is placed so that an end extends through either the oral incisional line or the nostrils through a nasoantrostomy. If the latter approach is used, the nasoantrostomy may be made with a curved hemostat forceps entering orally and exiting from the anterior aspect of the sinus and from there out the nares. A 10 cm by 10 cm gauze is grasped with a forceps and drawn through the nares into the sinus and then out of the mouth; the gauze is moved back and forth to smooth and file the bony opening of the nasoantrostomy to assure ease in the eventual removal of the packing and is then discarded. One end of the gauze packing is then carried from the oral aspect, across the anterior sinus, and out through the nares. The other end is placed deep in the posterior aspect of the sinus after which enough of the remaining length of gauze is placed in layers over the end that is in the posterior aspect of the sinus to provide adequate retention and accurate support of the fracture. The oral incision is closed with absorbable sutures.

In anticipation of subsequent removal, only one length of gauze strip is used. The tail of the gauze may be permitted to remain completely in the sinus and will be retrieved through an intraoral incision line. Usually a tail of gauze is left in the oral incision line, or a nasal antrostomy is performed and the tail is brought through an opening below the anterior portion of the inferior turbinate and exits through the external nares. The decision regarding the positioning of the tail of the packing gauze includes the relatively minor consideration of endeavoring to reestablish anterior maxillary sinal wall bony fragments as autogenous grafts, in which the tail of the gauze should exit via a nasal antrostomy.

Although the ZMC fracture reduction is checked during the surgery, radiographs should be obtained 24 hrs after operation to evaluate maintenance of anatomic positioning and alignment of the fractured segments. The bony segments can be displaced by undue pressure on the cheek, which might occur while the patient is transported or might result from the patient's lying on the affected side of his face. A "No Pressure Here" sign on adhesive tape on a paper cup can be placed over the fractured ZMC. To further eliminate the possibility of displacement of the repositioned ZMC and to negate the pull of the masseter muscle, intermaxillary traction fixation can be applied. During the immediate postoperative period, the patient should be evaluated to rule out restricted movement of the globe, diplopia, and decreased visual acuity.

Gradual decompression of the antrum is begun on the tenth to fourteenth postoperative day by removing approximately one third of the gauze dressing. The next two thirds are removed on alternate days until the entire packing has been removed. Following gauze removal, the antrostomy will remain open from 2 to 3 weeks, after which it will be closed by a thin layer of fibrous connective tissue and epithelium. Actually, the longer the opening persists, the healthier the antrum will remain because of the continuous drainage that the opening provides.

Antral balloons and Foley catheters exert an equal force in all directions within the antrum, and they can exert too much pressure in weakened or fractured areas. This weakness considered, a 30-cc Foley catheter can be placed through a Caldwell-Luc incision into the antrum to position and support the fractured segments. The balloon is inflated with 30 cc of air or water and is kept in place 1 to 10 days.[6] The outer end of the catheter is taped to the patient's forehead. This method allows for the evacuation of the hematoma and for continuous irrigation and drainage of the antrum. The catheter is easily removed, after which the oroantral opening is repaired normally.

Conjunctival and Lower Lid Approaches

Approaches to the floor of the orbit include variations of conjunctival and eyelid incisions. Traction sutures are placed to evert the eyelid, and conjunctival incisions are placed midway between the fornix and the inferior aspect of the tarsal plate.

The dissection may take one of several routes to the rim or the floor of the orbit (Fig. 8–18). The conjunctival approaches may not adequately expose either extensive fractures of the rim or the floor of the orbit; in these instances, a cantothotomy extending to the lateral side may be employed. Similarly, the subciliary approach may not provide adequate access to associated extensive ZMC injuries.

In general, I have found the lower lid incision most desirable in terms of access and exposure of the fractured areas (Fig. 8–16). Various 2-cm curvilinear incisional lines are used, including one that is about midway between the infraorbital rim and the margin of

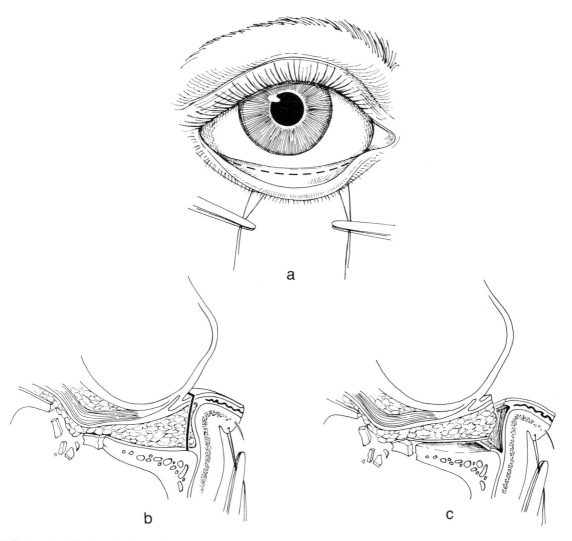

FIG. 8–18. Conjunctival surgical approaches to the infraorbital rim and the floor of the orbit. **a,** The eyelid is rolled anteriorly with traction sutures, and the incision line is made just through the conjunctiva. **b,** A dissection posterior to the orbital septum permits greater access to the area of a blow-out fracture. **c,** Elevation of the orbital contents to expose a blow-out fracture.

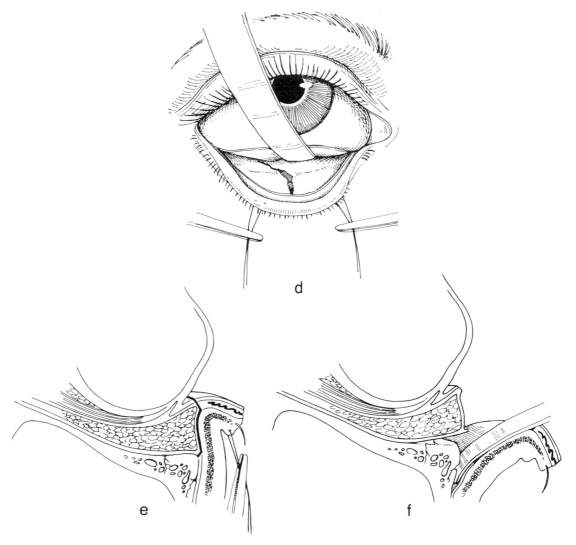

FIG. 8–18 (continued).   d, A dissection anterior to the orbital septum leads directly to a fracture of the infraorbital rim. **e** and **f,** Traction sutures and retractors expose a fracture of the infraorbital rim.

the lower eyelid: a landmark for placing this incision line is the lower border of the eyelashes of the inferior lid (Fig. 8–19). The subcutaneous soft tissues are bluntly dissected, the musculus orbicularis oculi fibers are separated, and the septum orbitale is followed down to the infraorbital rim. The soft tissues can be moved medially or laterally so that the entire infraorbital rim and floor can be inspected. The periosteum is incised along the periorbital rim for a distance equal to or greater than the length of the skin incision.

Following exposure of the rim or floor via any of the approaches (conjunctival, subciliary, or eyelid), the periorbita is then elevated.

The globe is atraumatically elevated and retracted by the curved end of brain spatula so that the periorbita, the bony orbital floor, and the contents of the infraorbital canal can be inspected. If a blow-out fracture exists, herniation of the periorbital tissues through the bony defect in the floor will be apparent. The herniation is elevated and an implant of any of various materials is placed. Freeze-dried bone or autogenous bone grafted from the anterior of the sinus or the coronoid process may be placed (Chapter 13). Most often, an alloplastic material, such as polytet (Teflon) or silicon rubber (Silastic) is used (Fig. 8–20).

The material is cut to match the contour of

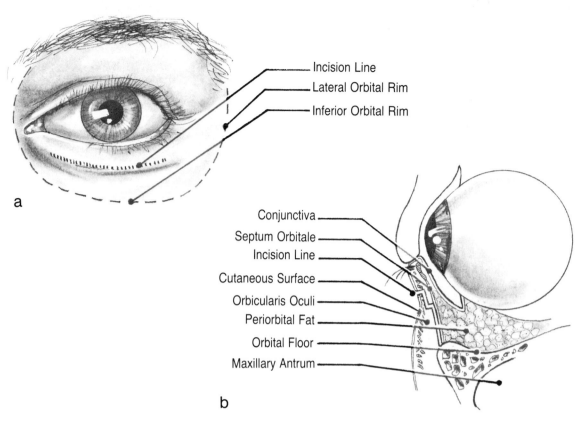

a

Incision Line
Lateral Orbital Rim
Inferior Orbital Rim

Conjunctiva
Septum Orbitale
Incision Line
Cutaneous Surface
Orbicularis Oculi
Periorbital Fat
Orbital Floor
Maxillary Antrum

b

FIG. 8–19. **a,** Lower lid approach to the infraorbital rim of the orbit. **b,** Lower lid approach to the floor of the orbit. (note Fig. 8–17)

the orbital floor and to be the proper size to include the defect. It should be notched to avoid pressure on the neurovascular bundle in the infraorbital canal. The implant is perforated with several small holes to allow for fixation of the implant by subsequent fibrosing through openings; the perforations in the implant also permit exchanges of fluids, thus avoiding accumulations of nonmetabolizing tissue fluid pockets that may produce an abscess.

Before the surgical site is closed, a traction test of the globe is conducted to help rule out extraocular muscle entrapment. The periorbita helps to hold the implant in position, and the implant is sutured to the periosteum along the infraorbital rim with interrupted stiches of 3-0 catgut suture. The fibers of the musculus orbiculars oculi need not be reapproximated, although reapproximation may be done, if desired, provided that care is taken not to include the septum orbitale. Suturing

the septum orbitale to the muscle fibers may produce ectropion of the lower lid, which is unaesthetic, impairs function of the lacrimal apparatus, and will require plastic surgical revision at a later date. The skin edges are coapted with interrupted stitches of 5–0 monofilament nylon or polyethylene suture.

The success of the treatment of blow-out fractures depends on early identification and management of the problem by either orbital floor reconstruction or intrasinal support. Usually not more than 14 days should be permitted to pass between injury and treatment to avoid diplopia and enophthalmos; however, some surgeons prefer to wait 2 to 6 weeks before correcting blow-out fractures.[5] Continuing consultation with an ophthalmologist is necessary. Postoperatively, treatment probably will be directed toward preserving balanced binocular vision and, if necessary, repairing extraocular muscles. Accurate diagnosis using CT studies, appropri-

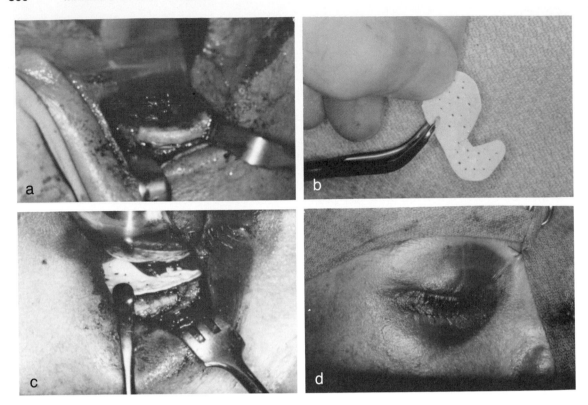

FIG. 8–20.   Placement of an alloplastic material via a lower lid approach for a blow-out fracture. **a,** Blow-out fracture in the floor of the orbit. **b,** Contouring an alloplastic material and placing holes to aid in tissue fluid transfers and in the stability of the implant. **c,** Placement of the alloplastic material. **d,** Soft-tissue closure.

ate surgical procedures, and effective post-operative care are necessary to avoid diplopia and enophthalmos.

Other Techniques

As an addendum to treatment techniques for ZMC fractures, screws and pins may be placed into the main body of the zygoma to achieve traction or fixation of the zygoma (Fig. 8–21). In general, however, the various transoral, extraoral, and intrasinal techniques provide a wide range of capabilities with more accurate results.

COMPLICATIONS

The postoperative results following reduction of ZMC fractures, including the modified blow-out type, are gratifying to both the patient and the surgical team. With the cosmetic defect eliminated and with normal function

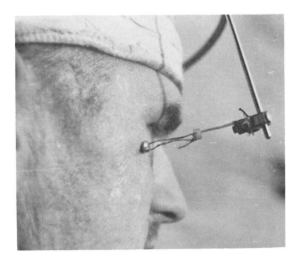

FIG. 8–21.   Use of a screw into the zygoma and traction to a headcap to support a depressed and unstable ZMC fracture.

restored after approximately 30 days, the patient is usually entirely asymptomatic. Certain complications are possible, however. For example, there may be bony nonunion, dacryocystitis, a hypo- or hypertropic state of the globe, edema, or ectropion of the lower lid, diplopia, unaesthetic cicatrix, persistent subacute or acute maxillary sinusitis, dysfunction of the maxillary division of the trigeminal nerve, and periorbital infection. If the ZMC fracture was relatively simple and displaced so minimally that the reduction was done extra-antrally, these complications are unlikely. The possibility of a complication increases if the zygomatic fracture was extensively comminuted and displaced and involved the orbital cavity or the maxillary antrum.

The fact that the natural thin bony floor of the orbit withstands less force than the globe and literally will blow out before the globe will rupture provides a "safety valve" when the eye sustains acute and direct trauma. When rigid implant material is used to restore the bony floor of the orbit, subsequent acute, direct trauma to the eye may result in a damaging injury with rupture of the globe.

The loss of vision following ZMC fracture was reviewed by Buckley and associates.[8] The literature revealed that loss of vision could occur from direct injury to the optic nerve by an implant, from increased intraorbital pressure producing retinal ischemia, and from direct interference with the optic nerve blood supply. Ord and El Attar discussed how the pressures of intraorbital hemorrhage are usually dissipated through fractures in the orbital floor and are manifested as epistaxis;[9] however, blockage of the fractures in the orbital floor of a sinus filled with a coagulum may prevent the spontaneous relief from hemorrhage pressures and thus fill the orbit with blood, causing proptosis. A rapidly occurring proptosis thus produced could collapse the thin-walled venous and lymphatic channels, which would further increase the intravascular pressure challenges to the central retinal artery. Under these conditions, the retina will appear pale, the vessels to the fundus will be in spasm or are constricted, and the retina's survival will be in jeopardy.

Buckley and associates described three categories of blindness that may accompany ZMC fractures; blindness immediately after trauma, blindness beginning hours or days following trauma, and blindness developing postoperatively.[8] Immediate blindness involves an immediate loss of vision that may gradually improve during the first few days; the improvement is short-lived, and optic atrophy occurs during the first 3 weeks. Intraocular pressures will produce the clinical sign of proptosis, and optic tears may be seen by CT. Contusion or concussion of the optic nerve followed by necrosis or hemorrhage is possible.[8] The causes of blindness beginning a few days after injury were described by Cullen and associates as edema of the optic nerve, necrosis of the optic nerve secondary to circulatory failure, or infarction secondary to vascular obstruction.[10] Postoperative blindness is usually associated with intraorbital pressure from edema, hemorrhage, an implant, and even a pressure bandage. Blindness is the most serious complication of a ZMC fracture, but it is rare. The status of the orbit must be evaluated continuously pre-, intra-, and postoperatively.

Bradycardia associated with ZMC or zygomatic arch surgery may be the result of oculocardiac reflex that is noted during ophthalmologic surgery and other surgical manipulations involving midfacial bones. This reflex is a function of afferent proprioception impulses to the mesencephalic nucleus from the trigeminal area of innervation and the efferent stimulation of the vagus from the nucleus. The vagus increases parasympathetic tone, producing bradycardia.[11] The reflex may be controlled by the administration of 0.4 mg atropine intravenously during the induction phase of anesthesia.

ACKNOWLEDGEMENT

Dr. Alston Callahan and the staff of the Eye Foundation Hospital, Birmingham, Alabama have extended, over the past several decades, a deeply appreciated collegial relationship, based on mutual respect, to the nation's oral and maxillofacial surgeons in the management of patients with injuries and deformities involving the bony orbit.

REFERENCES

1. Kwapis, B.: Treatment of malar bone fractures. J Oral Surg 27: 538–543, 1969.
2. Gillies, H.D., Kilner, J.P., and Stone, D.: Fractures of the malar-zygomatic compound with a description of a new x-ray position. Br J Surg 14:651, 1927.
3. Ellis, E., El-Attar, A., and Moos, K.F.: An analysis of 2,067 cases of zygomatico-orbital fracture. J Oral Maxillofac Surg 42:417–428, 1985.
4. Smith, B., and Regan, W.F., Jr.: Blow-out fracture of the orbits: mechanism and correction of internal fracture. Am J Ophthalmol 44:733–739, 1957.
5. Gilbard, S.M., Mafee, M.F., Lagouros, P.A. and Langer, B.G.: Orbital blowout fractures. Ophthalmology 92:1523–1528, 1985.
6. Lane, S.: The blow-out fracture. J Oral Surg 27:544–547, 1969.
7. Wilkins, R.B., and Havens, W.E.: Current treatment of blow-out fractures. Ophthalmology 89:464–466, 1982.
8. Buckley, S.B., McAnear, J.T., Dolwick, M.F., Aragon, S.B.: Monocular blindness developing 7 days after repair of zygomaticomaxillary complex fracture. Oral Surg Oral Med Oral Pathol 60:25, 1985.
9. Ord, R.A., and El Attar, A.: Acute retrobulbal hemorrhage complicating a malar fracture. J Oral Maxillofac Surg 40:234, 1982.
10. Cullen, G.C.R., Lvic, C.M., Shannon, G.M.: Blindness following blowout orbital fractures. Ophthalmic Surg 8:60, 1977.
11. Robideaux, V.: Oculocardia reflex caused by midface disimpaction. Anesthesiology 49:433, 1978.

9

NASAL-ORBITAL-ETHMOID FRACTURES

DAVID W. SHELTON

Trauma is the leading cause of death in the U.S. in people between the ages of 1 and 38.[1] Approximately 50,000 fatalities resulting from motor vehicle accidents were reported in 1983, and studies published by the National Safety Council indicate that for each person killed, 39 required hospitalization.[2] Of those hospitalized, an estimated 625,000 were treated for facial injuries.[3]

Nasal-orbital-ethmoid injury, although not frequently encountered, is difficult to treat and is often accompanied by significant functional and cosmetic complications.

Traumatic disarticulations and disruptions in the region of the nasal skeleton, interorbital area, medial orbital walls, and medial canthal ligaments have been identified by several names, such as naso-orbital fracture,[4] nasoethmoid fracture,[5] and nasoethmoid-orbital fracture.[6] In this discussion, the injury will be referred to as the nasal-orbital-ethmoid fracture, or NOE fracture.

This chapter will review the incidence and pathophysiology of injuries ot the structures in the nasal bridge–medial orbital region. The pertinent anatomic relationships, the goals of treatment, and the advantages of open exploration in severe and comminuted NOE fractures will be emphasized. Definitive management of this particular injury frequently requires a team approach and appropriate consultation. Complications that are most often encountered revolve around residual aesthetic and functional defects. On occasion and depending on the initial presentation of the injury, some of the complications can be difficult to avoid, even with the most meticulous of techniques.[7]

ETIOLOGY

The classic NOE fracture is not usually produced by low-velocity trauma. A light to moderate blow delivered to the nasal region may produce fracturing and dislocation of the nasal bones with varying degrees of septal involvement. With more severe trauma, such as that incurred during a violent motor vehicle collision in which the face is thrown against the steering wheel or dashboard, the resulting injury is frequently much more extensive.

NOE fracture consists of a disarticulation of the nasal skeleton from the curved nasal border of the frontal bone. The nasal bones, not infrequently comminuted, are driven posteriorly into the interorbital area, involving the ethmoid cells, and the medial walls of the orbits become crushed or splayed laterally.

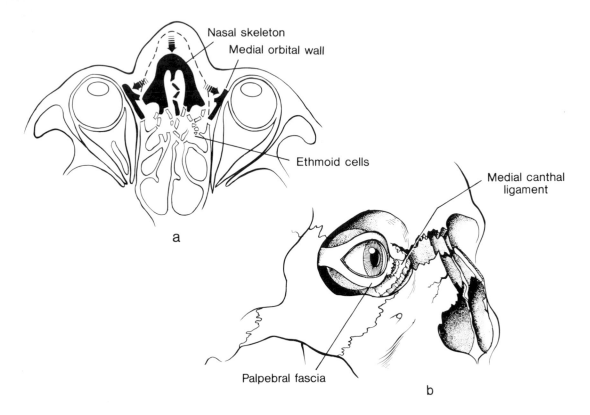

FIG. 9–1. **a,** Axial plane drawing through the orbit, nasal cavity, and ethmoid cells representing displacement of the nasal skeleton into the interorbital region, fracturing the nasal septum, and lateral splaying of the medial orbital walls. **b,** Mechanism of injury at the medial wall of the orbit involving detachment and tearing of the medial canthal ligament.

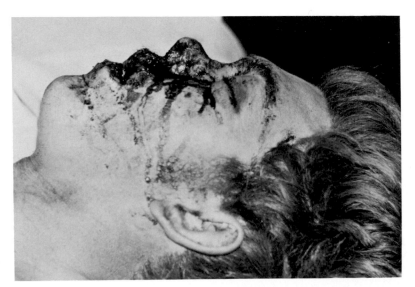

FIG. 9–2. Appearance of loss of the nasal bridge associated with multiple facial fractures and nasal-orbital-ethmoidal comminution.

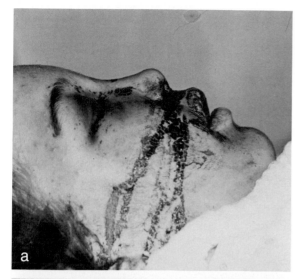

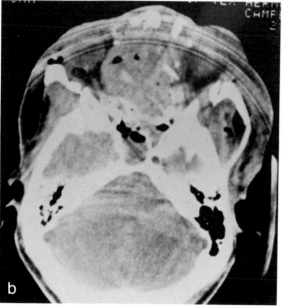

FIG. 9–3. **a,** Clinical appearance of edema-masked severe nasal-orbital-ethmoid fracture. **b,** CT scan radiograph demonstrating extensive comminution and displacement of underlying nasal-orbital-ethmoid structures.

The medial canthal ligaments become displaced laterally (Fig. 9–1).

DIAGNOSIS

These displacements cause many functional and cosmetic defects. In profile, the patient may appear to have lost the prominence of the nasal bridge (Fig. 9–2), although in some cases this defect may not be evident even though extensive displacement of the NOE structures has occurred (Fig. 9–3). Viewed from the front, the pertinent findings consist of widening and rounding of the medial palpebral canthi (Fig. 9–4). The rounded appearance of the medial canthal angle may be somewhat obscured if edema is present. A more subtle but very significant finding is loss of the natural depression between the prominence of the upper lid covering the globe and the medial aspect of the nose, an area that has been termed the "nasoorbital valley." This deformation indicates that the medial canthal ligament has lost its medial attachment and is no longer capable of holding the medial canthus against the globe. Marked periorbital ecchymosis and edema is characteristic; cerebrospinal rhinorrhea is a frequent finding, and on palpation the underlying bony structures are crepitant.

Other findings that may be associated with NOE injury are subconjunctival hemorrhage, nasal obstruction, subcutaneous emphysema, anosmia, regional cutaneous anesthesia, and neurologic symptoms.

ASSOCIATED INJURIES

OCULAR INJURY

One of the eye injuries most frequently associated with the NOE fracture is hyphema, which may predispose to secondary glaucoma. Vitreous hemorrhage, lens dislocation, rupture of the choroid or of the globe itself, retinal edema or detachment, commotio retinae, and traumatic mydriasis are among the eye lesions that may attend this type of fracture. Ophthalmologic consultation is mandatory early in the management of the patient.

CEREBROSPINAL RHINORRHEA

The diagnosis of cerebrospinal rhinorrhea is difficult to make unequivocally without special studies involving entry into the subarachnoid space, but absolute verification is seldom essential for the treatment of the frac-

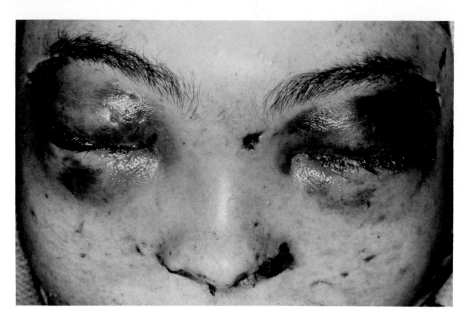

FIG. 9–4.   Traumatic hypertelorism caused by detachment of the medial canthal ligament in a nasal-orbital-ethmoid injury that accompanied other multiple facial fractures. Blunting of the medial palpebral angle, particularly on the right, is evident.

ture. Indeed, there would seem to be little advantage to waiting for the cerebrospinal rhinorrhea to cease before reducing the fracture, because manipulating the fracture might reopen the seal. In a series of 240 patients with major middle-third facial fractures, Steidler et al. reported cessation of cerebrospinal rhinorrhea in 60% of cases within 3 days after reduction and fixation of the fractures.[9] This finding is consistent with my experience and has been supported by the majority of consulting neurosurgeons. If cerebrospinal rhinorrhea is chronic, i.e., if it persists beyond 2 weeks after the inciting incident,[10] the appropriate consultant should then consider intervening.

FRONTAL SINUS INVOLVEMENT

Fractures that involve the frontal sinus can result in cosmetic defects, and, if only the anterior wall is involved, may require only simple elevation. More importantly, they can predispose the patient to a variety of serious sequelae. Obstruction of the frontonasal osteum as a result of the fracture will limit or prevent drainage of mucus, which may lead to the formation of a mucocele or pyocele several months to several years after the fracture;

fractures of the frontonasal osteum can require extirpation of the sinus mucosa and obliteration with an appropriate material. A direct communication into the anterior cranial fossa results from a fracture of the posterior wall of the frontal sinus and increases the risk of meningitis, brain abscess, and other intracranial complications. Fractures involving the posterior wall with depression and tearing of the dura might require craniotomy.

EPISTAXIS

Severe epistaxis associated with facial fractures generally is encountered infrequently; it is more often encountered with maxillary and midface fractures. Buchanan and Holtman reported incidence of epistaxis in 2 to 4% of their series of 312 patients with facial fractures but an incidence of 10-11% in patients with fractures of the midface.[11] Of the 312 patients in this report, 108 had sustained fractures of the maxilla or NOE complex and 12 experienced significant epistaxis, i.e., epistaxis that lasted more than 1 hr and required intervention. Six (50%) required nasal packing, transfusion, or both. Failure to recognize the gravity of epistaxis, especially in the patient who has suffered multiple body organ systems injuries, may play a major role in morbidity and mortality.[17]

When the bleeding is sustained and profuse, the source is apt to be the posterior region of the nose. As with virtually all bleeding, the initial method for control is pressure. A Foley catheter can be passed through the nose into the nasopharynx and inflated. An anterior nasal pack can then be placed. If these methods are not satisfactory, the catheter and nasal pack should be removed and replaced with a combination posterior and anterior nasal pack. Should bleeding occur through a well-placed anterior and posterior nasal pack, repacking often proves to be futile and other alternatives should be considered.

Anterosuperior nasal hemorrhaging most likely originates from the anterior ethmoidal artery, and, in keeping with the axiom that bleeding should be controlled as near to its source as possible and considering the extensive collateral vasculature of the area, exposing and clipping that vessel is the procedure of choice.[11,12] In fact, it is prudent to expose and clip the vessel at the time of operation if nasal bleeding is brisk and bright red and does not respond to packing. Transantral ligation or packing to occlude the internal maxillary artery is the procedure of choice for controlling severe posterior nasal hemorrhaging.[11,14] Other techniques involving radiographic contrast studies and embolization are available in selected situations.[15]

The benefit of ligating the external carotid artery to control epistaxis associated with NOE fractures is open to question. The artery is removed from the source of bleeding in an area well known for its collateral vascularity, and the ethmoidal arteries do not arise from the external carotid system.

Additional measures such as pharmacologic sedation and elevation of the head may be beneficial if not contraindicated.

SUPERIOR ORBITAL FISSURE SYNDROME

Although this syndrome is generally uncommon in facial trauma, because it is seen more frequently with the NOE fracture than with other fractures no discussion of NOE fractures should omit it. The clinical findings associated with the superior orbital fissure

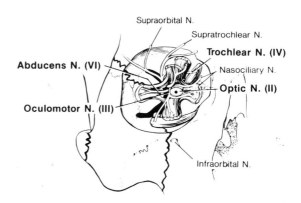

FIG. 9–5. Diagrammatic representation of cranial nerves involved in the superior orbital fissure syndrome.

syndrome consist of ptosis of the upper eyelid, fixed and dilated pupils with normal visual acuity unless other ocular injury is present, inability to adduct the eye, which may be fixed in a lateral gaze, absent corneal reflex with a normal fundoscopic examination, and regional cutaneous hypoesthesia or anesthesia.[16] The oculomotor, trochlear, and abducens cranial nerves are involved (Fig. 9–5). The syndrome has been noted with skull fractures, mandibular and zygomatic arch fractures, and fractures of the zygoma.[17-20] Gradual, complete or partial recovery is usually possible without surgical intervention in traumatic cases not involving severance of nerves.[21-23] Involvement of the optic nerve, in addition to those mentioned, is called the orbital apex syndrome.

TREATMENT

As with other traditional descriptions of midfacial fractures, such as the Le Fort classification, fractures described as NOE seldom conform conveniently to a set pattern. In addition, fracture-dislocations of the NOE variety do not commonly occur as isolated injuries, but rather as a component of the overall problem. In a series of 33 patients with NOE fractures reported by Cruse and co-workers, all of the patients had other facial injuries and fractures.[61] Hence, the surgeon must be intellectually flexible in his approach to treatment. Despite these considerations, the surgeon must be aware that the trauma has driven the nasal skeleton posteriorly into the interorbital region, the medial orbital walls are splayed laterally, and the medial canthal ligaments are displaced laterally.

CLOSED VERSUS OPEN REDUCTION

The surgeon's approach will be dictated by the nature and severity of the lesion in the patient. It may be possible to reduce and adequately fix some of these fractures using a conservative closed technique of intranasal elevation and cross-nasal splinting. However, in most significant NOE fractures, and in particular those in which the integrity of the medial canthal ligament is in doubt, without open exploration it is virtually impossible to ascertain the status of or adequately repair the medial canthal ligament and other anatomic parts involved in the injury.

The surgeon's decision to either open the area to permit direct repair or manage using a closed technique depends on his evaluation of the individual case and his experience in dealing with such injuries (Figs. 9–6, 9–7, and 9–8). Whatever methods are used, the goals are disimpaction, repositioning, and stabilization of the nasal bones to the frontal bone; centralization of the nasal skeleton and realignment of the nasal septum; repositioning of the medial orbital walls and reattachment of the medial canthal ligament; and re-establishment of alignment of the lacrimal apparatus.

Surgical exposure of the fracture site may be achieved through existing lacerations or by judiciously extended lacerations. When no such injuries exist or when they are inappropriate, the approach described by Converse and Hogan, or some variation of it, provides excellent exposure of the nasal skeleton and both medial canthal attachment areas.[24]

OTHER CONSIDERATIONS

The medial canthal ligament and the lacrimal collecting system are of particular interest and significance in the repair of this fracture.

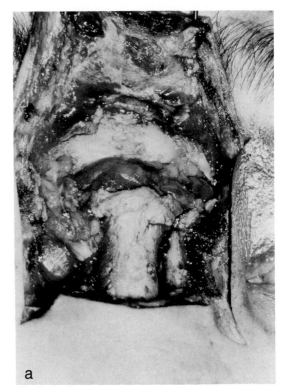

a

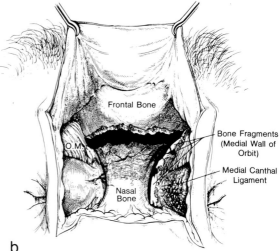

b

FIG. 9–6. **a** and **b,** Surgical exposure of typical NOE fracture. Note separation of the nasal skeleton from the curved nasal border of the fronal bone and posterior displacement into the interorbital ethmoidal region with lateral splaying of the medial orbital walls carrying the medial canthal ligaments.

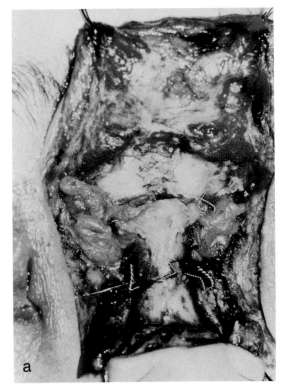

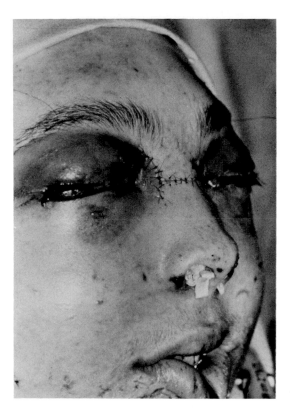

FIG. 9–8.   Closure of incision. Compare position of the medial palpebral angle to Figure 9–4.

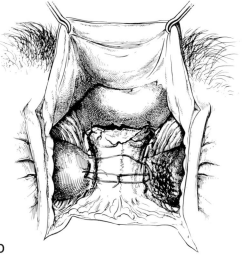

b

FIG. 9–7.   **a** and **b,** Reduction and internal fixation of the nasal skeleton to the frontal bone and the medial orbital walls, and replacement of the medial canthal ligaments.

Medial Canthal Ligament

The medial canthal ligament is inserted on the medial wall of the orbit and functions as the tendon for the musculus orbicularis oculi.[25] It is a strong, fibrous band and is a direct continuation of the two tarsal plates of the eyelids (Fig. 9–9a and b). Close to the tarsi it divides into a posterior limb and a strong, well-developed anterior limb that attaches to the anterior lacrimal crest on the frontal process of the maxilla.[26] The posterior limb is poorly developed and, along with some thin fibers of the musculus orbicularis oculi muscle (Horner's muscle), is weakly attached to the posterior lacrimal crest of the lacrimal bone.[25]

The precise role and importance of the posterior limb of the medial canthal ligament and Horner's muscle has been debated in the literature. In a study based on 14 surgical explorations and 6 cadaveric preparations, Robinson and Stranc found the posterior limb to consist of thin lacrimal fascia associated with areolar tissue and, invariably, of a few muscle fibers.[25] The posterior limb is attached to the very fine posterior lacrimal crest on the paper-thin lacrimal bone; the area of attachment was too small to measure. These authors concluded that the lack of bulk of muscle tissue associated with the posterior limb argues

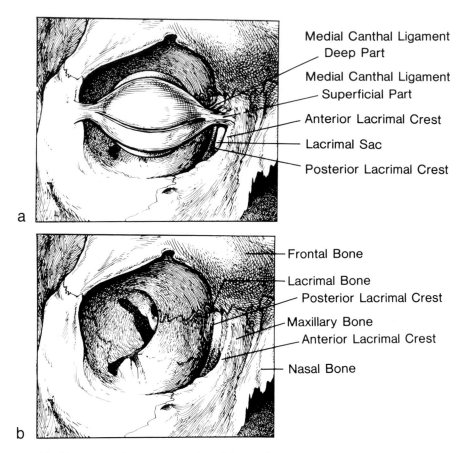

Medial Canthal Ligament
Deep Part

Medial Canthal Ligament
Superficial Part

Anterior Lacrimal Crest

Lacrimal Sac

Posterior Lacrimal Crest

Frontal Bone

Lacrimal Bone
Posterior Lacrimal Crest

Maxillary Bone
Anterior Lacrimal Crest

Nasal Bone

FIG. 9–9. **a** and **b,** Diagrammatic representation of the medial canthal ligament with its origin and insertion, the posterior limb attaching on the posterior lacrimal crest of the lacrimal bone, and the anterior limb attaching on the anterior lacrimal crest of the frontal process of the maxilla. Note the lacrimal sac intervening between the two limbs of the ligament at their insertions and continuing inferiorly as the nasolacrimal duct.

against the muscle's having any influence on tensing the tarsus and, that the primary anchorage of the medial canthus is the anterior limb. Robinson and Stranc postulated that the posterior limb and Horner's muscle structures are related to emptying the lacrimal sac and facilitating tear drainage either by expansion of the sac in a manner analogous to the action of the diaphragm on inspiration, or by direct compression of the sac.

In view of these relationships, it is clear that the most important part of the medial canthal ligament to be secured at the time of repair is the anterior limb. When the anterior limb is correctly and securely repositioned, fixed, and splinted, the complications of dacryocystitis, post-traumatic hypertelorism, epiphora, and widening of the nasal bridge are uncommon.

As in other situations in which detached muscle insertions seek out their own reattachments, the posterior limb of the medial canthal ligament reattaches itself; the accurate reattachment of the anterior limb is the key to the functional reattachment of the posterior limb and Horner's muscle structures.

Lacrimal Collecting System

The tear-draining apparatus begins at the lacrimal puncta, which are adjacent to the globe at the medial aspect of the upper and lower eyelids.[27] Failure to restore this relationship at the time of repair can result in improper or inadequate tear collection and drainage. The canaliculi are located within the anterior limb of the medial canthal ligament for most of their course and can enter the lacrimal sac separately or merge to form a common canaliculus before reaching the sac.[25] Injuries to the canaliculi must be addressed at the time of primary repair by passing a suture through the punctum, across the defect, into the severed end of the canaliculus, and into the lacrimal sac. The free end of the suture is brought out through the skin and tied.

The lacriminal sac is positioned within the lacrimal fossa between the anterior and posterior lacrimal crests. The sac is continuous with the nasolacrimal duct, which opens under cover of the inferior nasal concha. Anteriorly, its upper portion is protected by the anterior limb of the medial canthal ligament. It is free to be displaced laterally when so carried by the medial canthal ligament. The danger zones therefore are at the entrance into the nasolacrimal duct and within the nasolacrimal canal.[28] The risk of damaging the lacrimal sac and nasolacrimal duct in comminuted injuries by blindly and forcibly compressing and manipulating the underlying fracture fragments should be recognized.[25,28]

REFERENCES

1. Trunkey, D.D.: Trauma. Sci Am 249:28, 1983.
2. Dingman, R.O., and Converse, J.M.: The clinical management of facial injuries and fractures of the facial bones. In Reconstructive plastic surgery, Vol. 2. Edited by J.M. Converse. Philadelphia, W.B. Saunders, 1977, p.599.
3. Karlson, T.A.: The incidence of hospital treated facial injuries from vehicles. J Trauma 22:303, 1982.
4. Converse, J.M., and Smith, B.: Naso-orbital fractures. Trans Am Acad Ophthal 67:622, 1963.
5. Stranc, M.F.: Primary treatment of naso-ethmoid injuries with increased intercanthal distance. Br J Plast Surg 23:8, 1970.
6. Cruse, C.W., Blevins, P.K., and Luce, E.A.: Naso-ethmoid-orbital fractures. J Trauma 20:551, 1980.
7. Duvall, A.J., and Banovets, J.D.: Nasoethmoid fractures. Otol Clin N Am 9:507, 1976.
8. Blair, V.P., Brown, J.B., and Hamm, W.G.: Surgery of the inner canthus and related structures. Am J Ophthalmol 15:498, 1932.
9. Steidler, N.E., Cook, R.M., and Reade, P.C.: Residual complications in patients with major middle third facial fractures. Int J Oral Surg 9:59, 1980.
10. Chandler, J.R.: Traumatic cerebrospinal fluid leakage. Otolaryngol Clin North Am 16:623, 1983.
11. Buchanan, R.T., and Holtman, B.: Severe epistaxis in facial fractures. Plast Reconstr Surg 71:768, 1983.
12. Murakami, W.T., Davidson, T.M., and Marshall, L.F.: Fatal epistaxis in craniofacial trauma. J Trauma 23:57, 1983.
13. Weddell, G., Macbeth, R.G., Sharp, H.S., and Calvert, C.A.: The surgical treatment of severe epistaxis in relation to the ethmoidal arteries. Br J Surg 33:387, 1946.
14. Durisch, L.L., Jr., and Frable, M.A.: A surgical solution for posterior epistaxis. Surg Gynecol Obstet 133:669, 1971.
15. Kirchner, J.A.: Epistaxis: current concepts in otolaryngology. N Engl J Med 309:1,126–1,128, 1982.
16. Kruzer, A., and Patel, M.P.: Superior orbital fissure syndrome associated with fractures of the zygoma and orbit. Plast Reconstr Surg 64:715, 1979.
17. Banks, P.: The superior orbital fissure syndrome. Oral Surg 24:455, 1968.
18. Murakami, I.: Decompression of the superior orbital fissure syndrome. Am J Ophth 59:803, 1965.
19. Robinson, B.G.: Superior orbital fissure syndrome with Bell's palsy: report of a case. J. Oral Surg 31:203, 1973.
20. Bowerman, J.E.: The superior orbital fissue syndrome complicating fractures of the facial skeleton. Br J Oral Surg 7:1, 1969.
21. Watson, P.G.: The traumatic orbital apex syndrome. Its differential diagnosis and treatment. Trans Ophthalmol Soc UK 88:361, 1969.
22. Rowe, N.H., and Killey, H.C. (eds): Fractures of the Facial Skeleton. 2nd Ed. 251–275. Edinburgh, E. and S. Livingstone, Ltd., 1968, pp. 251–275.
23. Stallard, H.B.: Eye Surgery. Bristol, John Wright and Sons, Ltd., 1973, p. 848.
24. Converse, J.M., and Hogan, V.M.: Open sky approach for reduction of naso-orbital fractures. Plast Reconstr Surg 46:396, 1970.
25. Robinson, T.J., and Stranc, M.F.: The anatomy of the medial canthal ligament. Br J Plast Surg 23:1, 1970.
26. Morris' Human Anatomy, 11th Ed. Edited by J.P. Schaeffer. New York, The Blakiston Press, 1953.
27. Stranc, M.F.: Dacrocystography in midface fractures. Br J Plast Surg 25:269, 1972.
28. Stranc, M.F.: The pattern of lacrimal injuries in nasoethmoid fractures. Br J Plas Surg 23:339, 1970.

10

NASAL FRACTURES AND INJURIES

CHARLES C. ALLING III

The superior rim of the midface is composed of the zygomatic arches, the malar (zygomatic) bones, and the prominent nasal complex of bones and cartilages. The nasal complex, like other superior rim skeletal structures, may be fractured as the single injury or may be part of multiple associated injuries.

ETIOLOGY

Fisticuffs, assaults, sporting accidents, and falls are the most frequent causes of fractures limited to the nasal complex. Vehicular accidents, high-velocity missiles, and explosives may produce nasal injuries as one component of facial skeletal fractures. Nasal fractures may be either simple depressions and displacements or compound injuries with varying degrees of complexities. Compound fractures range from minor lacerations of the respiratory or olfactory mucous membranes associated with fractures of the anterior nasal bone and cartilaginous complex, to extensions into the ethmoidal or frontal sinuses, the cribriform plate, and the anterior cranial fossa. Any of the nasal fractures, from the simplest to the most complicated, may in-

volve wrinkling or displacement of the bony and cartilaginous nasal septum.

Injuries to the nasal hard tissues may involve one or all of the bones and cartilages that form and support the nose. The bones that may be involved include the paired nasal bones, the frontal (or nasal) processes of the maxillae, the nasal process of the frontal bone, the lacrimal and ethmoidal bones, and the anterior nasal spine of the maxillae.

ANATOMIC CONSIDERATIONS

The septal and paired lateral nasal and alar cartilages provide a flexible scaffolding for the anterior and inferior nasal structures (Fig. 10-1). All of the bones and cartilages are covered by relatively thin layers of mucous membranes or cutaneous tissues, richly endowed with a generous vascular network that aids in rapid repair.

Bilaterally, near the anterior aspect of the inferior meattus, formed by the inferior curvature of the inferior turbinate bones, are the orifices of the nasolacrimal ducts. The middle turbinates of the maxillae are positioned posteriorly with reference to the anterior aspect of the sinuses and the anterior portions of the ethmoidal sinal air cells. Positioned high in

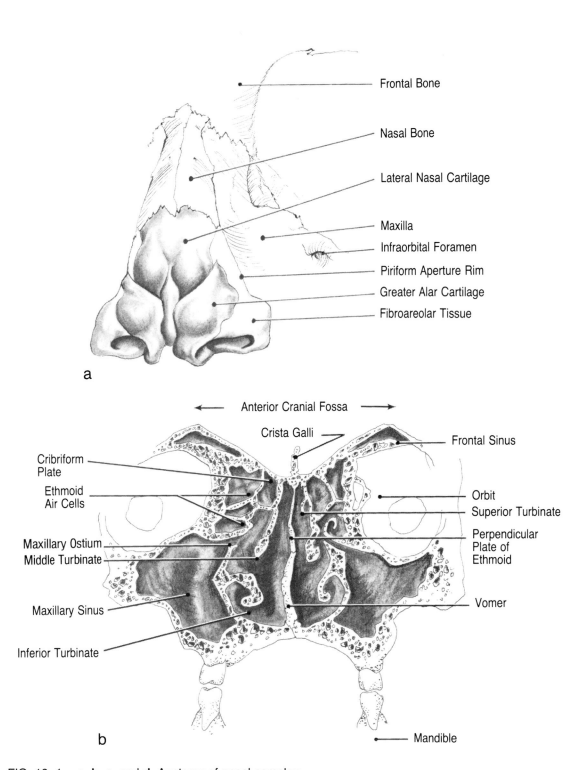

FIG. 10–1.   **a, b, c,** and **d,** Anatomy of nasal complex.

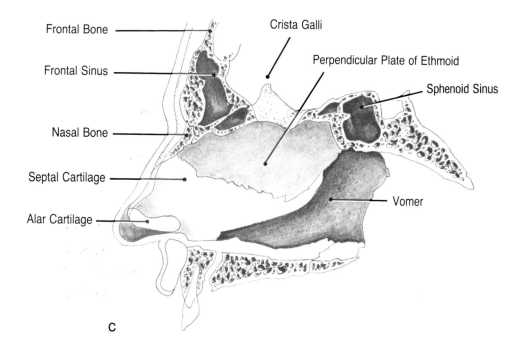

C

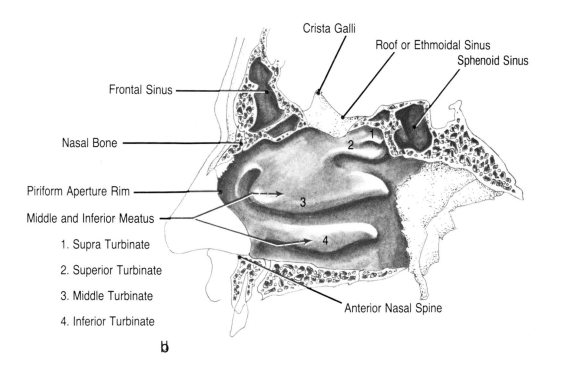

Crista Galli

Roof or Ethmoidal Sinus

Sphenoid Sinus

Frontal Sinus

Nasal Bone

Piriform Aperture Rim

Middle and Inferior Meatus

1. Supra Turbinate

2. Superior Turbinate

3. Middle Turbinate

4. Inferior Turbinate

Anterior Nasal Spine

B

FIG. 10–1 (continued).

the nasal cavity are the superior turbinates, which have small meattus, compared with the meattus of the middle and inferior turbinate bones and processes, through which drain the posterior ethmoidal sinal air cells. The sphenoidal sinuses drain into the superior posterior wall of the nasal cavity. The eustachian tubes open into the lateral nasopharyngeal walls posterior to the inferior turbinate bones. Respiratory mucous membrane covers all of the lower structures and blends into the olfactory mucosa above the superior turbinate processes.

The type, extent, and severity of nasal fractures resulting from different types of trauma vary with the mass and velocity of the moving body and the site of impact; the amount of damage also depends on the direction and intensity of the force (Fig. 10–2). The trauma may be directed from a frontal, inferior, or lateral direction. Frontal trauma usually results in comminution and displacement of the nasal complex including the nasal septum. Trauma from the inferior often results in fractures limited to the anterior nasal spine. However, more severe trauma from this direction can damage the nasal septum and the alar cartilages, and can produce lacerations of the nasal mucosa and the skin of the nose and cause fracture of the turbinate bones and possibly of the maxillary nasal processes and na-

sal bones. Fractures from lateral forces can vary from unilateral medial displacement of the bony fragment to lateral displacement of the entire nasal complex. When nasal fractures are a component of Le Fort II or III midfacial fractures extending across the bridge of the nose, the nasal complex may be moved posteriorly, inferiorly, and laterally as part of the midface skeleton and without significant additional injury to the nose.

Injuries to the soft tissues can produce airway occlusion from fibrosis secondary to hematomas and from synechia between lacerated tissues on the medial and lateral nasal walls. Injuries may produce loss of the sense of smell, thinned membranes that are easily injured by subsequent trauma, and damage to the orifices of the nasolacrimal ducts, the eustachian tubes, or the several paranasal sinuses.

DIAGNOSIS

The physical examination of nasal complex fractures should best be performed very soon after the trauma because edema will rapidly obscure the relatively fine bones and cartilages and the delicate soft-tissue membranes that constitute the structure.

Nasal fractures limited to the anterior nasal

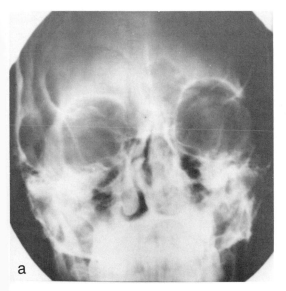
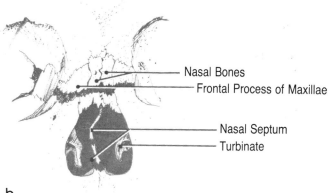

Nasal Bones
Frontal Process of Maxillae

Nasal Septum
Turbinate

a

b

FIG. 10–2. **a,** Radiograph of facial fractures, including nasal complex. **b,** Diagram of intra- and extranasal fractures.

spine produce pain to the upper lip, edema (usually without ecchymosis), and acute tenderness to the base of the columella. Fractures of the nose involving the nasal bones and frontal processes of the maxillae usually produce edema of the cheeks and periorbital tissues with ecchymosis of the eyelids. Nasal fractures extending into the frontal sinuses produce periorbital ecchymosis as well as edema over the frontal sinuses. Often, the midfacial injuries obscure the displacement of the nose, and the fractured nasal complex will not be clinically evident by inspection and palpation (Fig. 10–3).

It is important to obtain a history regarding the time of injury, the nature of the trauma, previous operations, and pre-existing deformities.

A gentle, systematic, and thorough inspection and palpation of the nasal structures will aid in the diagnosis and planning of treatment, especially if the patient is examined shortly after the trauma and before hematomas and edema obscure the physical findings. Intranasal inspection and extranasal palpation may require local and regional or general anesthesia for children and for many adults. If the lateral nasal bones are fractured, gentle manual pressure may produce crepitus. Hypermobility of the nasal bony complex may not be present in cases of either posteriorly displaced or superiorly impacted Le Fort II and III fractures until disimpaction and reduction of the midfacial fractures have been performed.

The examination of the intranasal structures may reveal nasal obstructions resulting from large blood clots or active hemorrhage from torn mucosae, which must be controlled to allow evaluation of the extent of the injury. Blockage of the airway may result from edema of the mucosa, displacement of the nasal septum, and fracturing and displacement of the cartilaginous structures. Although hypermobility and crepitus are signs of fractures, palpation should be performed carefully to prevent additional soft-tissue damage, further bony displacement, and possible involvement of the anterior cranial fossa.

Radiographic examination of the nose may include paranasal sinus views, projections of lateral facial bones, a submentovertex view, and CT scans (Fig. 10–4). An occlusal radiograph of the maxilla will be helpful in evaluating the status of the nasal septum and the anterior nasal spine.

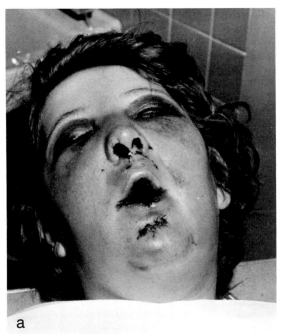
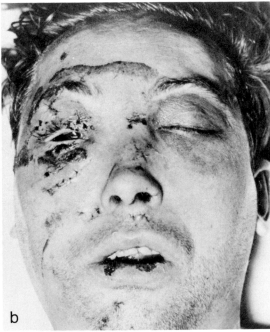

FIG. 10–3. **a** and **b,** Multiple facial skeletal fractures, including the nasal complex.

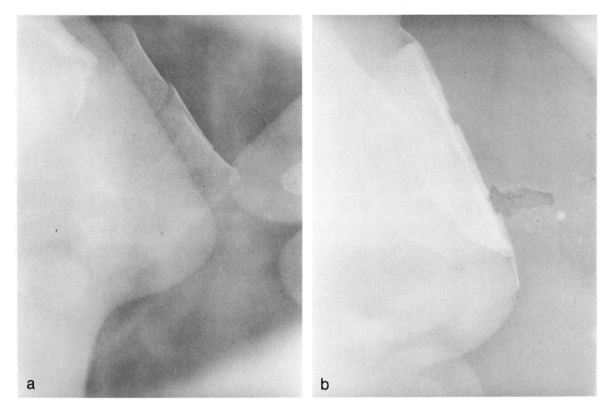

FIG. 10–4.   **a,** Detailed lateral radiographic view of preoperative nasal complex fractures. **b,** Postoperative view.

TREATMENT

Every effort should be made to reduce and treat isolated nasal fractures within the first few hours after injury and prior to the development of an obscuring edema. The majority of nasal complex fractures involve structures in the anterior portion of the nasal cavity and may be managed by manipulation and contouring. Children and many adults will be managed most easily under topical and local anesthesia supplemented by general anesthesia or intravenous deep sedation.

UNCOMPLICATED NASAL FRACTURES

Depressed fractures of the nasal complex are elevated using an elevator or a nasal complex disimpaction forceps intranasally while concurrently contouring using digital pressure extranasally (Fig. 10–5). A wrinkled or displaced nasal septum is straightened and repositioned in the maxillary groove with a nasal complex disimpaction forceps, such as an Asche forceps, whose beaks are placed on both sides of the septum. The surgeon may prefer to cover the elevator and the beaks of the forceps with rubber or plastic tubing. Care is taken during this maneuver to avoid applying crushing trauma to the columella (Fig. 10–6). A large-curved hemostat may be substituted for these devices, its beaks covered with plastic or rubber tubing to avoid injury to the soft tissue; obviously, the beaks should not be closed over the columella. The surgeon can use the disimpaction forceps or the hemostat to manipulate and reduce displaced nasal fractures by placing one beak inside the nose and the other beak outside. Careful placement of the instrument is important to avoid damage to the intranasal mucosa that could result in a fibrotic mass or a synechia between the septum and the turbinates.

When the entire nasal complex is shifted off of the midline, with moderated displacement but minimal comminution, the maneuvers summarized above provide a means of moving the nasal bony and cartilaginous pyramid to its proper position in the midline.

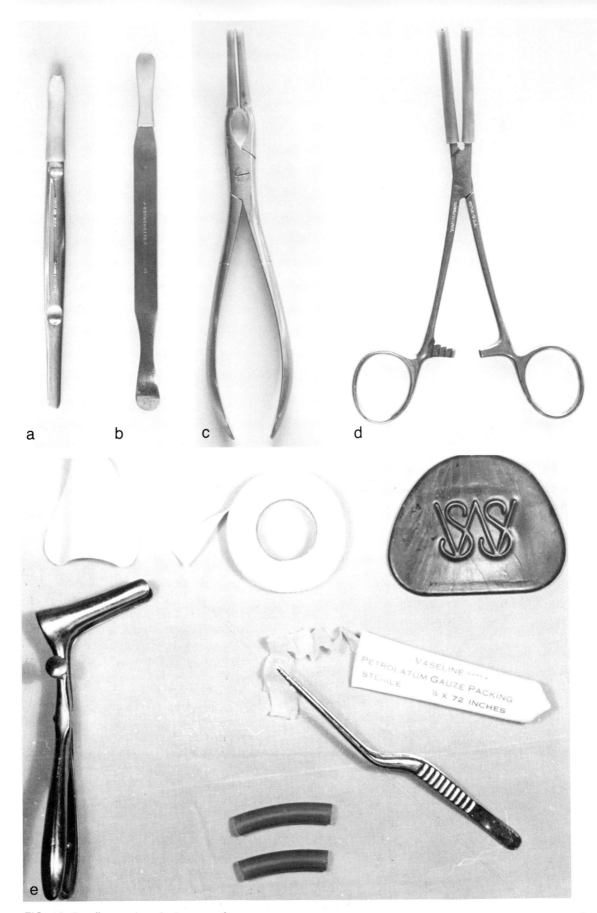

a   b   c   d

e

FIG. 10–5. (Legend on facing page.)   ⟶

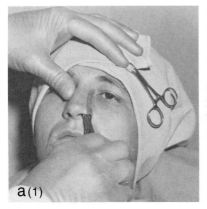
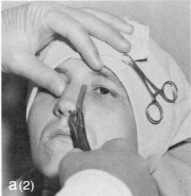
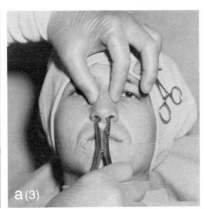

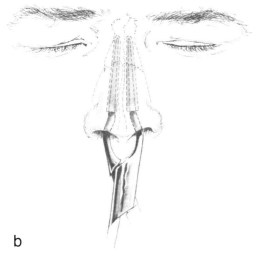

FIG. 10–6. **a** (**1, 2,** and **3**) and **b,** Reduction of nasal complex fractures.

A submucosal dissection, usually very limited, may be necessary to reposition the vomer. The reduction of fractures of the vomer and the lateral nasal cartilages and bones usually involves closed reduction and manipulation. Open reduction with direct wiring or placement of miniplates is rarely indicated except in association with frontal and nasoethmoid extensions of the fractures.

MULTIPLE NASAL FRACTURES

If the nasal fractures are apparently displaced and are a part of multiple facial fractures, their reduction should be delayed until all the other fractures, including the orbital and ethmoidal fractures, are disimpacted, reduced, and immobilized. This delay is advisable because stabilization of the midfacial fractures will provide bony landmarks for manipulation of the nasal complex.

SPLINTS AND PACKING

Following reduction of most nasal fractures, the nose should be packed for hemostasis and support. The packing, which is sat-

FIG. 10–5. Instruments for managing the usual nasal complex fractures. **a,** Sayre submucous elevator. **b,** Seldin elevator. **c,** Asche forceps. **d,** Kelly hemostatic forceps. **e,** Nasal packing, rubber tubing, compound and padded splints, and speculum.

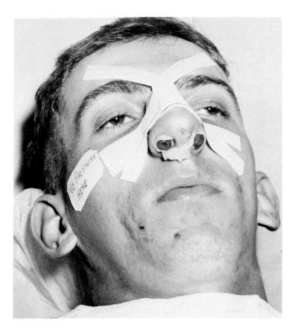

FIG. 10–7. Postreduction of nasal complex and ZMC fractures, including stabilization with a metal extranasal stent and intranasal airway tubing and packing.

urated with bacitracin or another ointment, is placed after elevation and reduction of the fractures. In patients with immobilized mandibles who have a full complement of teeth and do not have a tracheotomy, placing tubing for an airway in both nostrils may be necessary prior to packing the nasal cavity. The external surface of the nose is splinted by a commercial padded plate, a stent of malleable metal, dental compound, or plaster of Paris and taped securely in place. Pressure ulcerations of the skin in the area of the external splints is avoided by eliminating sharp, irritating edges and lining the inner surface of the metal with moleskin fabric, aerated plastic, or another cushioning material. The packing is removed in 5 to 7 days and the splint in 7 to 10 days (Fig. 10–7).

Extensive compound, comminuted nasal complex fractures may require packing as described above and application of extranasal metallic splints that are secured to the nasal complex by stainless steel wires passing through the splints and through the nasal structure (the nasal processes of the maxillae and the vomer). The wires usually are placed in the horizontal suture configuration using straight surgical needles to pass through the nasal structures. This technique provides for firm immobilization of the metal splints over the fractured bones that are supported by the intranasal packing, and it allows more rigid fixation than that achieved by external surface splints, which are secured to only the cutaneous tissues.

If avulsive losses of the nasal structures have occurred, early consultation by the team member who will be responsible for the reconstruction is in order.

COMPLICATIONS

Epistaxis, septal abscess and hematoma, and massive facial edema are early complications that are seldom serious. Hemorrhage from the nose is usually of short duration and is controlled by the tamponading effect of intranasal packing. A septal hematoma should be evacuated by aspiration or should be incised and drained to avoid complications of septic pyemia, airway occlusion, septal abscess, or necrosis. Septic pyemia resulting from an infected septal hematoma is managed by incision and drainage of the abscess and general systemic metabolic supports, as indicated.

HEMORRHAGE

In acute trauma to the nasal complex, as with many other conditions, the hemorrhage is usually from Kiesselbach's plexus located on the anterior aspect of the nasal septum. Pinching the nostrils with finger pressure for 50 to 10 min may arrest the hemorrhage. For more aggressive hemorrhages, the bleeding site should be identified with direct vision using a speculum and aspiration. A vasoconstricting agent, 1:1,000 epinephrine on a cotton application wooden stick or crystalline silver nitrate supplied on a stick, should be applied. A small gauze pad containing an antibiotic ointment or plain petroleum jelly can be placed over the area for 8 to 12 hrs with a tuft of microfibrillar collagen hemostatic material between the bleeding site and the gauze. Hemorrhage from the deeper structures that may accompany a fracturing process may require placement of anterior and posterior nasal packs (Fig. 10–8). The flow may be slowed by a trigeminal second-division anesthetic block via one of several routes—through the pterygopalatine canal, posterior to the tuberosity, or laterally through the mandibular (sigmoid) notch area. Regardless of the route of the needle, a solution of 2% lidocaine with 1:100,000 epinephrine will produce a vasoconstriction of the palatine and nasal vessels as well as anesthesia at the area of the manipulations.

EMPHYSEMA

Subcutaneous emphysema may develop from nasal complex fractures when air dissects through torn subcutaneous tissue or the mucoperiosteum and spreads into the contiguous tissues following surgery, sneezing, or efforts to blow the nose. Subcutaneous emphysema resolves without specific treatment, although prophylaxis by antibiotics is warranted.

CEREBROSPINAL RHINORRHEA

Cerebrospinal fluid rhinorrhea may occur with nasal fractures. It is not always necessary for the cerebrospinal flow to cease before definitive treatment of the nasal or midfacial fractures is performed (Fig. 10–9). In the presence of nasal, ethmoidal, and midfacial fractures, cerebrospinal rhinorrhea can continue for days or weeks. With appropriate antibiotic and metabolic therapy and clearance by the neurosurgeon, however, the nasal, ethmoidal, and the midfacial fractures can be reduced, and the cerebrospinal rhinorrhea usually will cease in a matter of hours after the bones are repositioned and stabilized.

INTRANASAL OBSTRUCTIONS

Abnormal healing of lacerations may produce unusual unions of the mucosal tissues overlying the turbinate processes, the bones, and the septum. These unions may obstruct the osteums of the sinuses, the nasolacrimal ducts, and the nasal airway. The surgeon should consider direct surgical contouring with soft-tissue flaps, as indicated, followed by 10 days of packing as a dressing.

Problems that may develop in the months following trauma to the nose include partial or complete obstruction of the nose resulting from organization of fibrotic masses on the nasal septum, as mentioned above. The masses, which can be quite dense and large

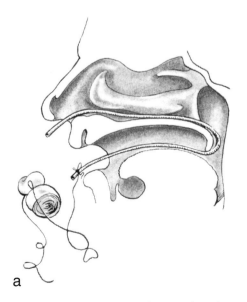

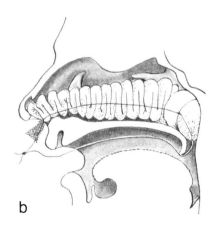

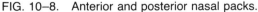

FIG. 10–8.   Anterior and posterior nasal packs.

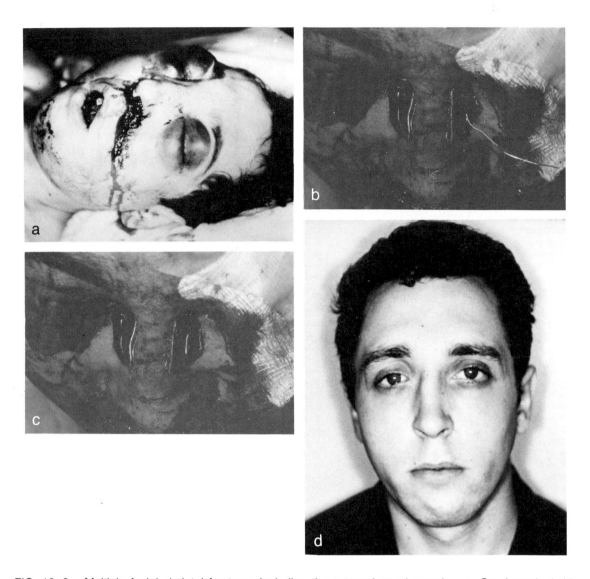

FIG. 10–9. Multiple facial skeletal fractures including the external nasal complex. **a,** Cerebrospinal rhi-norrhea from a patient with mandibular, maxillary, and nasal fractures. Nasal fractures were managed by intranasal packing and lateral nasal splints. **b** and **c,** Placement of splints. **d,** Postoperative appearance.

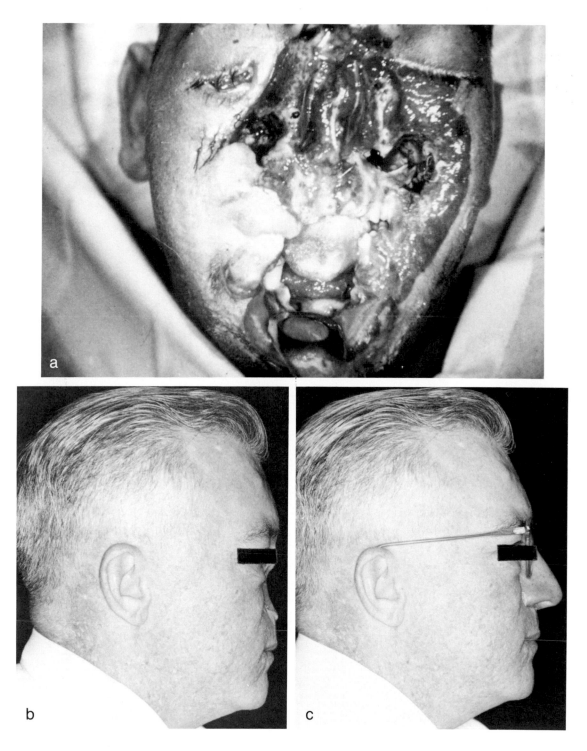

FIG. 10–10.   **a,** Avulsive loss of nasal structures caused by gunshot injury. **b** and **c,** Restoration of loss of nasal structures by a maxillofacial prosthesis. (Courtesy of Colonel Peter Margetis, D.C., U.S. Army.)

and can contain bony elements, result from perichondromal and subperiosteal hematomas that were either not evacuated or not absorbed. In some cases, instead of developing into an occluding fibrotic mass, these hematomas can become infected, resulting in necrotic loss of nasal structures and functional and aesthetic deformities that will require reconstructive surgery.

NASAL PROSTHESES

Maxillofacial prostheses might be indicated as the treatment when loss of tissue from the primary injury or from an infection is extensive (Fig. 10–10).

11

DENTITION AND ALVEOLAR PROCESS INJURIES

ROBERT A. J. OLSON

Traumatic injuries to the teeth and supporting structures occur frequently and, compared with other types of injuries, may not be considered serious. However, because teeth have the lowest potential of any tissue for returning to a normal, healthy state following injury, most injuries to the teeth and supporting structures require immediate evaluation and treatment.[1]

Most dental injuries sustained by children between the ags of 1½ and 2½ are caused by falls.[2] Subluxated and displaced teeth are the most common injuries in these children, followed by fractured crowns.[3] School-age children are injured in playground or bicycle accidents and most commonly have fractured crowns or teeth with subluxation and displacement. Young teenagers' injuries are usually associated with automobile accidents.[4] Adults sustain dental injuries primarily in automobile accidents and altercations. In adolescents and adults the most common injuries are fracture of the teeth, followed in order first by subluxation and then by displacement or avulsion.

If adequately and promptly treated, retention of fractured or avulsed teeth is possible. The sequelae of injuries to the primary dentition can include failure to continue eruption, discoloration, infection and abscess, ankylosis, injury to the developing permanent teeth, abnormal exfoliation, and loss of space within the dental arch. Sequelae of injuries to the permanent dentition can include discoloration, infection and abscess, loss of space in the arch, loss of alveolar bone support, ankylosis, resorption of root structure, abnormal root structures, and abnormal root development. Often the full extent and significance of traumatic injuries to dentition may not be manifest for months or possibly years after the original trauma.[5] Close followup of these injuries is essential.

When triage directs the multiply injured patient toward definitive care, because of the extent and severity of the associated injuries the dentoalveolar problems sometimes are overlooked or postponed to a much later time, beyond the optimum treatment phase. However, considering the cosmetic and functional impact on the patient and the scientific acumen and technical skill necessary to manage these injuries, these relatively peripheral injuries become major factors in the appropriate total management of the patient. Early care of dentition injuries is urgent because survival of the odontogenic-osseous complex requires very early stabilization.

ANATOMIC CONSIDERATIONS

The periodontal ligament buffers blows to the teeth somewhat. The ligament itself may be damaged, however, with or without an associated bony fracture. Additionally, the apical neurovascular bundle could be severely torqued by traumatizing lateral movements of the teeth. The alveolar processes have areas of obvious weakness; these are a concavity in the anterior mandibular area at the junction of the alveolar process and the base of the mandible; a similar area in the anterior maxillary region; the nasal cavity; and the maxillary sinuses, especially when an alveolar extension of the sinuses is present. Fractures of the alveolar processes in response to accidental or iatrogenic trauma may occur in any of these areas.

Areas of potential fracture in the dentition are associated with alignment of enamel rods and dentinal tubules, constrictions in the cervical area, and the presence of radicular trifurcations and bifurcations. Though fractures can occur at any point along the length of the tooth, the areas of fractures are usually described according to "thirds of coronal" or "thirds of the radicular portion" and in terms of the damaging exposure of the pulp chamber.

DIAGNOSIS

Thorough evaluation of the injured area is important to ensure proper diagnosis and treatment of the traumatized teeth and the supporting structures. Factors to be evaluated include the patient's ability to cooperate, the type of dentition involved, the location and type of injury, the condition of the remaining teeth and the patient's oral health, and concomitant injuries.

The soft tissues of the area must be inspected and palpated to determine the extent of trauma and contamination. Often associated with dentoalveolar injuries are soft-tissue injuries to the lips or the mucosal structures of the oral cavity. These injuries include contusions, abrasions, lacerations, and punctures.

If a tooth has been avulsed, either totally or partially, the lamina dura of the alveolus may be undisturbed although the tooth is moved from its normal position. A tooth that has been luxated or loosened within its socket will have an intact lamina dura, but the width of the periodontal ligament space will be uniformly increased.

Fracture of alveolar bone may be manifest by a radiolucent line. When present, this line extends over a large area of two or more teeth and appears to run between the teeth or beyond the apex of the teeth rather than through them and, depending on where the alveolar bone is fractured, it may be superimposed over the tooth. Fracture of the alveolar process is found more often in older patients then younger patients.

The clinical signs of fracture of the alveolar bone may include displacement of the teeth; mobility of the entire fractured portion of bone (i.e., when checking mobility of a single tooth all the teeth in the segment move; hemorrhage or ecchymosis in the area of fracture; and malocclusion.[6] Displacement of a single tooth, particularly an anterior tooth, often results in fracture of the alveolar socket wall, which is manifest by mobility and crepitus on palpation. The degree of trauma involved and the presenting signs and symptoms can indicate the possibility of a fracture of the alveolar process of the body of the mandible, or of the maxilla.

A tooth or the supporting structures may be damaged without early clinical or radiographic evidence. The periodontal ligament may be damaged even if the teeth are not injured. The apical neuromuscular bundle can be damaged by the trauma and can cause disruption of the neurovascular supply to the teeth.[7]

Radiographs are essential in the evaluation of traumatic injuries, although damage to a tooth or the supporting structures can occur without radiographic evidence. The panoramic film offers an overall view for evaluation of the full extent of the trauma, while occlusal and periapical views of smaller areas provide better definition of suspected sites of injury, which are inconclusive on the panoramic radiograph. Radiographs are used to verify the presence, number, and sites of fractures; the direction and types of fractures; displacement or deformity of teeth; and complicating factors. Following treatment, radiographs reveal the adequacy of treatment and the progress of healing. A fracture in a tooth appears in a radiograph as a radiolucent line within the tooth structure extending to the edge of the tooth but not beyond.[8] Fractures of the teeth may not be evident radiographically if the x rays cannot pass through a line of cleavage; hence taking radiographs from several directions may be necessary to confirm the diagnosis of tooth fracture.

The condition of a patient who has sustained trauma to teeth or the supporting structures should be followed so that possible complications can be managed. Pulp testing performed immediately after injury is very unreliable and hence is of no value in the initial evaluation.[3,6,9] After 4 to 6 weeks, the tooth will begin to show response to electrical stimulation and will respond to pulp testing fairly predictably, and based on the results the surgeon can decide whether endodontic treatment is required. Follow-up radiographs are a part of the post-traumatic routine to evaluate for possible complications.

Pulpal responses to electrical and thermal tests which measure the pulp's vitality, give information on the ability of the pulp to respond to sensory and nociceptor perceptions; the tests are most useful when they indicate pulpal vitality. When the pulp is not fully vital, other evaluations are necessary to provide diagnostic and prognostic data; these include the color of the tooth, its mobility, signs and symptoms of inflammation, and information revealed in radiographs.

CLASSIFICATION AND TREATMENT

For many patients who experience traumatic insult to the teeth, the only clinical evidence is a local edema or an abrasion. The clinical and radiographic findings do not suggest any problem. These patients require no immediate treatment but do need periodic follow-up examination. Although teeth may not respond to pulp testing immediately, by 8 to 12 weeks they should respond in the normal range. A progressive discoloration in a permanent tooth indicates that it is probably nonvital and may require endodontic therapy. A deciduous tooth showing discoloration can be left in place without treatment until it exfoliates; no damage will be done to the unerupted and developing permanent teeth unless a periapical inflammation develops, in which case the damaged deciduous tooth should be removed and the space held by a space maintainer, because periapical inflammation may cause enamel hypoplasia of the permanent dentition.[2]

CORONAL FRACTURES

Fracture of the tooth crown occurs quite frequently (Fig. 11–1). Andreasen[9] in 1972 described four categories of fracture of the crowns of teeth.

The Class I category involves those teeth that have a fracture of only the enamel portion of the tooth. These can be treated quite easily by smoothing the rough edge with a sandpaper disc or stone or by a simple restoration.

The Class II fracture of the crown involves both enamel and dentin and requires a protective restoration and limited use for 10 to 14 days; because the tooth has received significant trauma, long-term evaluation after restoration is necessary to determine its continuing vitality. An acid-etched enamel restoration causes minimal further trauma to the tooth[10] (Fig. 11–2). The tooth is first cleaned with pumice and then isolated with cotton rolls. Any loose or unsupported enamel is removed and the fractured enamel surface is beveled approximately 45° which increases the surface area of bonding, strengthens the restoration, and avoids a butt joint. Calcium hydroxide is placed over the exposed dentin.

The acid-etch liquid (phosphoric acid solution) is applied to the prepared enamel surface of the fractured tooth to cover at least 2 mm beyond the margin for 90 sec. The tooth is then rinsed thoroughly with water and air dried, leaving the prepared enamel with a chalky appearance. If the chalky appearance is not present, the acid etch is repeated.

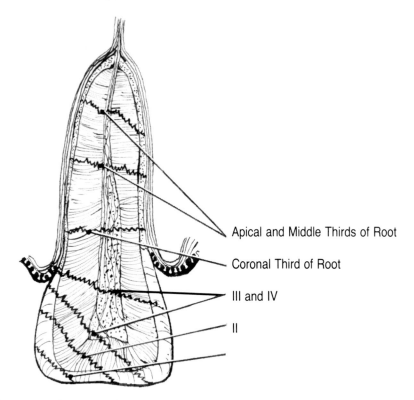

Apical and Middle Thirds of Root

Coronal Third of Root

III and IV

II

FIG. 11–1.   Diagram of fractures of the crown and root.

The resin is prepared by mixing a drop of catalyst with a drop of base resin, and the mixture is applied to the treated enamel surface with a small sponge. One of three types of composite resin can then be placed: self-polymerizing, ultraviolet light–cured, and visible light–cured. I presently prefer the ultraviolet light–cured resin because of the rapidity of the polymerizing. After the material has set, the excess is removed with burs and stones and the restoration is polished with fine discs and polishing strips.

These restorations are useful in children in whom a crown preparation is not yet feasible or when pulpal stability is not certain. They may be used as a temporary restoration as an alternative to a crown, or when damage is slight and aesthetics is a prime concern.

Class III fractures have a slight degree of involvement of the pulp in addition to dentin and enamel. These teeth require pulp capping with calcium hydroxide, restoration, and close follow-up with both pulp testing and radiographs to evaluate viability. When a substantial coronal fragment is fractured and is recovered intact, a one-step endodontic procedure combining dentinal bonding and acid-etch techniques may be used.[11]

The Class IV fractures of the crown have irreversible open trauma to the pulpal chamber. At the initial treatment, an attempt is made to maintain the vitality of deciduous teeth or permanent teeth with wide apices by performing coronal pulpotomies. On fully developed permanent teeth the entire pulp should be extirpated and root canal treatment initiated.

Any traumatized tooth should be checked to ensure that it is not in occlusion, particularly in lateral excursions. The teeth often are not loose but may be sensitive and should have only limited use (the patient should be on a soft diet for approximately 14 days) to ensure survival.

ROOT FRACTURES

The prognosis for the survival of nondisplaced fractures of the apical third of the root that have not received endodontic care increases as the level of the fracture moves toward the apex; that is, an apical tip fracture

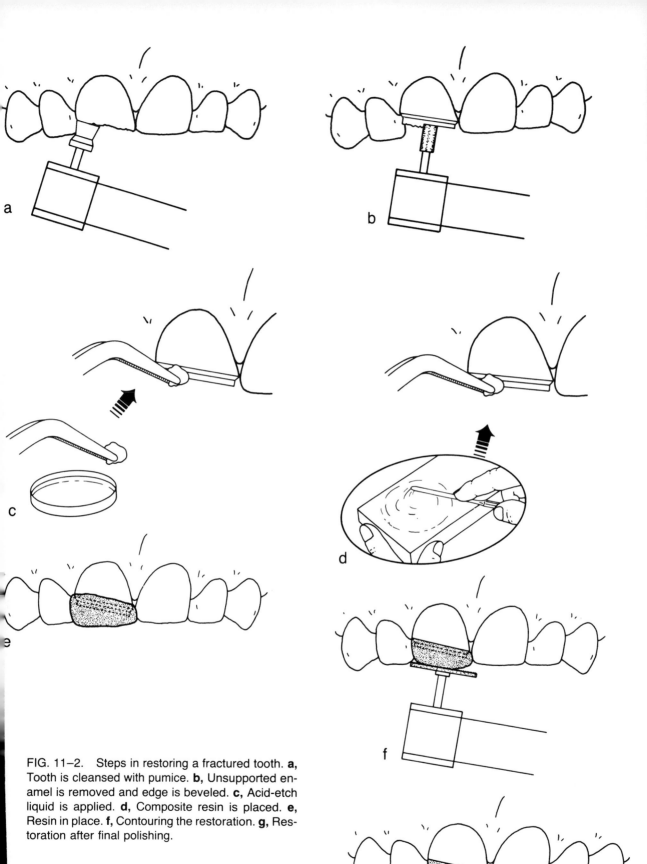

FIG. 11–2. Steps in restoring a fractured tooth. **a,** Tooth is cleansed with pumice. **b,** Unsupported enamel is removed and edge is beveled. **c,** Acid-etch liquid is applied. **d,** Composite resin is placed. **e,** Resin in place. **f,** Contouring the restoration. **g,** Restoration after final polishing.

has a better prognosis than a fracture at the level of the apical third of the root (Fig. 11–1). Fractures in the middle third of the root have a poor prognosis for retention of the entire tooth with or without stabilization and endodontics; however, some teeth with middle-third radicular fractures have been saved with stablization, with and without endodontic treatment. Following endodontic treatment, loss of the crown by fracture at the cervical neck can provide a stable, retained root that can be used to support a fixed prosthesis.

Root fractures can heal by several routes. In some instances, the fragments are united by a solid, bony type of union. The uniting substance has various compositions, from tubular or atubular dentin to bone or cementum. In some cases, healing produces a fibrous tissue union that does not become calcified and displays a radiographic fracture line of the root; with the passage of years, considerable rounding at the edges of the fractured root segments can occur. These teeth can function well provided that the root structure on the coronal segment is long enough to give the necessary stability.

Trauma may produce fracture of the roots of teeth. Early considerations depend on the level of the root fracture. Vitality of the tooth must be considered. More often than trauma primarily to the crown, injury causing root fractures can result in ankylosis.

When the root fracture is in the apical third the tooth can be moved more than 2 mm in any direction, and the apex has not fully formed, the tooth will require immobilization for 4 to 6 weeks, which by reducing subsequent trauma at the apex can maintain the tooth's vitality. If the tooth becomes nonvital or if the root has a closed apex, root canal therapy with apicoectomy to remove the apical fragment and seal the apex is indicated.

If a fracture occurs in the middle third of the root and is not displaced, the tooth might maintain its vitality and should be stabilized for 4 to 6 weeks to allow callus or cementum to form and stabilize the tooth; however, the tooth will probably become nonvital and require endodontic therapy.

The fracture that occurs in the cervical third of the root or the fracture and that travels through the crown and past the root can be treated by immediate endodontic therapy, by removing the root, or by retaining the root if it is stable and the patient understands the possibility of eventual infection and loss of a retained, burried root. If the root is removed, immediate or early placement of implants may be considered. If endodontic therapy is successful, the retained root may be an excellent base for a postcrown restoration.

LUXATED AND DISPLACED TEETH (Fig. 11–3)

The entire tooth may remain intact following trauma, and its displacement with relation to the alveolus can be defined as intrusion, medial or lateral displacement, extrusion, or avulsion; an alveolar process fracture is usually associated with a displaced tooth. Regardless of the type and location of injury, whether on the tooth or in the alveolar bone, the periodontal ligament must be protected because it provides a vital life support to a tooth. Therefore, if a tooth is completely avulsed, the patient is instructed to protect the periodontal ligament that still may be attached to the tooth. The prognosis for the pulp depends on the age of the patient, the size of the apical opening, the level of the fracture, and the amount of displacement of the fractured segments. If the apical opening is still immature, uncalcified, and bell shaped, the prognosis for retaining the tooth without endodontic therapy is excellent.

Luxated Teeth

Luxated teeth, those loosened within the alveolar socket but not displaced, present with varying degrees of mobility. If no mobility or only slight mobility (movement of 0 to 2 mm in any direction) is present, stabilization is not generally required.[12] These teeth must not be in traumatic or heavy occlusion, and only light function should be permitted. Should vitality, confirmed by clinical and radiographic findings, not return within 8 to 12 weeks, endodontic treatment should be carried out. If mobility is excessive, greater than 2 mm, the tooth should be immobilized 8 to 12 weeks and then tested for stability and evidence of vitality, to be followed by appro-

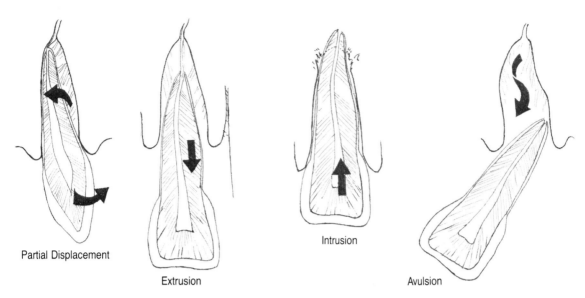

Partial Displacement

Extrusion

Intrusion

Avulsion

FIG. 11–3.   Diagram of intra-alveolar displacements and avulson of an anterior tooth (arrows).

priate therapy. If the buccal or lingual plates of bone are fractured so that the tooth is unstable in more than one direction, if periodontal disease has destroyed the surrounding bone so that stability cannot be achieved, or if periapical pathosis was present previously, the teeth should be removed.

Displacement or avulsion of teeth may be partial or total. The partial displacement may be intrusion or extrusion.

The intruded tooth is of particular importance when the deciduous dentition is involved. Intrusion of the primary teeth into the proximity of the permanent teeth may cause injury to the permanent teeth.[13,14] Injuries to the permanent dentition can include discoloration, malformation, hypocalcification, and ectopic eruption; the most common injuries are enamel hypoplasia and dilaceration of roots. Fewer abnormalities are found in the permanent teeth when the deeply intruded deciduous tooth is extracted than when it is left to exfoliate by itself.[13] If the tooth is expected to exfoliate within 6 months, efforts to retain it are not worthwhile and the tooth should be removed. If the deciduous tooth is not affecting the permanent tooth, the deciduous tooth can be allowed to re-erupt. If it does not move in 12 weeks, orthodontic assistance could help to bring the tooth into position; otherwise, the tooth will have to be removed.

The first consideration in evaluating an intruded permanent tooth for possible retention is its stage of development. In the young patient with an intruded permanent tooth with an open apex, the tooth should be allowed to re-erupt on its own or with orthodontic help if it has not begun to reposition itself within 6 months. When the permanent tooth is intruded and the apex of the tooth is fully formed and closed, the tooth should be surgically repositioned and stabilized for 6 to 8 weeks. Root canal therapy will probably be required.

The partially avulsed tooth in the deciduous dentition must be evaluated from the standpoint of future use. If the tooth would exfoliate within 6 months, attempts at retention are not very successful and the tooth should be removed. Sufficient root structure must remain for retention to be feasible. If the tooth is not suitable for retention or cannot be retained, a space maintainer should be considered if more than 4 months will elapse before the eruption of the permanent tooth. Deciduous teeth that have been partially displaced will require repositioning and stabilization for approximately 3 weeks to prevent ankylosis. Occlusion should allow light function but should prevent any traumatic occlusion.

Every attempt should be made to retain a partially displaced permanent tooth, even if comminuted fracture of the bone wall had oc-cured. Permanent teeth with wide-open api-ces often will retain their vitality and have the best chance for survival. Those with closed apices will normally require endodontic ther-apy but have an excellent chance for long-term survival if comminution of the alveolus is minimal or not present. These permanent teeth must be returned to their normal posi-tions, have their functional load reduced, and be stabilized. Permanent teeth should be sta-bilized for a longer period then deciduous teeth because ankylosis is less likely. The sta-bilization period is 8 weeks.

The partially displaced tooth can be stabi-lized with bonding splints, or wiring tech-niques (Fig. 11–4). The advent of the acid-etch bonding technique has greatly facilitated stabilization. The tooth is repositioned and the area is isolated with cotton rolls to keep the teeth dry (Fig. 11–5). The facial and lin-gual surface of the displaced and adjacent teeth are cleaned with pumice and the prox-imal surfaces are lightly roughened with a diamond bur disc. These surfaces are acid-etched for approximately 90 sec and the area rinsed and dried thoroughly. The binding ma-terial is then mixed and applied directly to the etched surfaces, and the displaced tooth is held firmly in the desired position for 3 to 5 min. The excess is then removed with a disc or a bur. The occlusion is checked in all ex-cursions to prevent excessive trauma, and en-dodontic treatment can be instituted when-ever indicated.

Avulsed Teeth

A completely avulsed deciduous tooth has a very poor chance of survival if reimplanted and should not be replaced. If necessary, the space can be held with a space maintainer until the permanent tooth erupts.

The surgeon must be selective in choosing the avulsed permanent teeth to be replaced. If the tooth were nonfunctional, or overe-rupted, its replacement would be illogical. If the dentition was severely over-crowded, the loss of the tooth might be helpful to the total arch length. Advanced cariously diseased teeth can have pulpal decay and can be poor candidates for retention, and the general den-tal condition of the patient may be such that retention of the tooth is not a high priority. The patient's periodontal condition must be satisfactory to allow retention of the tooth; severe periodontal conditions militate against the success of reimplantation. Other situa-tions in which reimplantation is undesirable are fracture of middle or cervical third of the crown and a fractured alveolar socket not suf-ficiently intact to support the tooth.

Reimplantation is optimal for a tooth that has an open apex in a healthy patient with an intact dentition and an alveolus that is not fractured. Two other factors of primary im-portance when considering reimplantation of a tooth are the time interval between the in-jury and treatment[3,15] and the conditions un-der which the tooth has been preserved.[7] Pa-tients in whom the tooth has been avulsed 30 min or less prior to seeking treatment have a 90% chance of successful retention. Resorp-tion of the root occurs in approximately 95% of patients in whom the tooth has been out for more than 2 hrs. The outside limit for suc-cessful reimplantation is 48 hrs, although in-juries treated within 1 or 2 hrs have the best chance for survival. To maximize the chances of success, the tooth can be stored in the al-

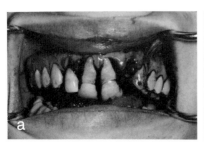
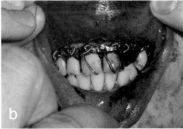
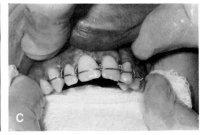

FIG. 11–4. Wiring techniques for replanting teeth. **a** and **b,** Arch bar supporting hammock-type wiring. **c,** Wiring to stabilize replantation of both central incisors. (Courtesy of Dr. Hugh P. Brindley.)

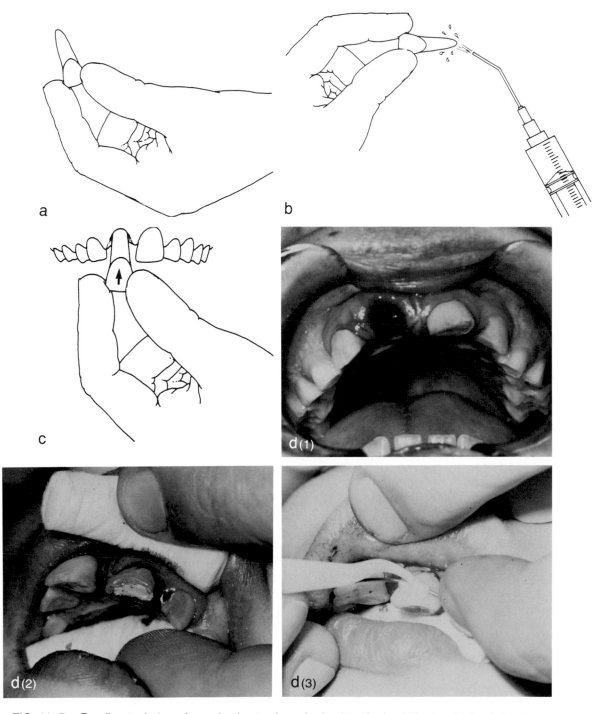

FIG. 11–5.   Bonding technique for replanting teeth. **a,** Avulsed tooth should be handled only by the crown. **b,** Foreign debris is rinsed, not scrubbed, away. **c,** Tooth is replanted in the alveolus. **d,** Clinical steps in replacing and stabilizing an avulsed tooth. (Courtesy of Dr. Nolan Downs.) **(1),** Right central incisor (no. 8) was avulsed; left central incisor (no. 9) has a class II coronal fracture. **(2),** no. 8 replanted; no. 9 treated with calcium hydroxide. **(3),** no. 9 restored with composite resin; passive labial arch bar is being placed.

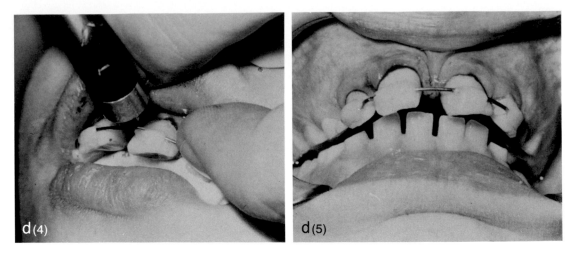

FIG. 11–5 (continued). **(4),** Polymerization with ultraviolet light. **(5),** no. 8 replanted and stabilized; no. 9 restored.

veolus from which it was avulsed, under the tongue, or in the vestibule of the mouth. Other alternatives are to store the tooth in milk, saline, saliva, or a wet handkerchief. The tooth should be handled as little as possible, and then only by the crown.

With the patient under local anesthesia and usually sedation, the socket area should be inspected and gently irrigated to remove debris. The tooth is inspected for fractures and to determine its stage of development and the degree of contamination, and a radiograph of the socket area is made to rule out fracture of the adjacent teeth or the cortical plate of bone. The root should not be handled and should not be scrubbed or dried. Foreign material present on the root should be merely rinsed away by irrigation with normal saline in order to leave the periodontal tissue attached to the root surface.

If the apex of the permanent tooth is closed, a bevel of approximately 1 to 2 mm may be cut to allow better seating in the socket. At this point, an access opening into the tooth pulp can be made and the pulp extirpated, and the access opening can be sealed with cotton and a temporary filling. The tooth is then inserted into the cleansed socket and seated to place. A radiograph may be taken to ensure proper seating. The tooth is stabilized with acid etching, splint, or wire treatment for approximately 8 weeks. Conventional endodontic treatment can be started

about 1 week after the stabilization. The canal should be filled with calcium hydroxide to prevent resorption and ankylosis.[16]

The avulsed tooth with a wide-open apex will be treated in a similar manner except that the pulp is not removed. Because maintaining the vitality of this tooth is possible, after the tooth is gently cleansed it is repositioned into the socket, stabilized, and observed for an indefinite period. Endodontic treatment can be instituted whenever indicated.

The possible results of reimplantation are diverse. The tooth with open apex may survive as if no trauma occured. If it becomes nonvital, internal resorption, manifest by a radiolucent increase in the area of the canal, may occur. Resorption can be treated with root canal therapy and has a fair prognosis. If external resorption occurs, as manifested by erosion of the external root surface, the prognosis is poor, and the tooth will probably not survive. External resorption is usually related to trauma to the periodontal membrane associated with the root. Other results seen with reimplanted teeth are ankylosis and hypercementosis, which do not affect tooth survival but can make possible removal of the teeth more difficult.

ALVEOLAR PROCESS INJURIES

The severity of alveolar process fractures may vary from a simple linear fracture line along an alveolus to complete fracture of the alveolar process with displacement into adjacent structures. The presence of teeth in the alveolus may complicate the bony repair of the alveolar fracture line, as would any tooth in a line of fracture. The treatment of alveolar process injuries is directed toward preserving the alveolar process and retaining dentition by repositioning and stabilization. If the teeth cannot be salvaged, as much alveolar bone should be preserved as possible to provide the best base for a subsequent rehabilitation of the mouth as well as to preserve normal intra- and extraoral facial features and contours.

When the teeth are so severely injured or displaced that their removal is necessary, the procedure should be carried out with the utmost care. Separating these teeth or their roots from the loosened alveolar segment without completely detaching the entire segment from the mucoperiosteum is frequently a very difficult procedure. Sometimes the loose segment can be stabilized with finger pressure while the tooth to be removed is separated from its alveolar attachments. The thin blade of a light elevator or curette can be inserted into the periodontal space to gently dislodge the tooth. If this procedure is unsuccessful, the tooth can be stabilized more firmly with a forceps while an attempt is made to dislodge the tooth with the elevator. The teeth should be removed without reflecting the mucoperiosteum, if possible, in order to maintain the maximum blood supply to the loose alveolar segment. Relatively large bone fragments with a minimal amount of attached mucoperiosteum will often survive when repositioned and covered with the detached mucoperiosteum. Sharp edges should be trimmed with a bone rongeur or a machine-driven bur prior to closure of the soft tissues.

Alveolar process injuries of the maxilla can include a portion of the palatal process. When the alveolar process is displaced laterally or distally to any great degree, the palatal tissues will usually be torn, exposing the palatal fracture line.

Maxillary Sinus

Displacement of one or more of the teeth into the maxillary antrum with distal displacement of the maxillary tuberosity is seen occasionally as a result of a high-speed motor vehicle accident, usually in the driver of the automobile rather than the passengers. It probably occurs when the head is forced forward at the moment of impact and the opened mouth contacts the rim of the steering wheel, which fractures and displaces the teeth, usually the bicuspids and first molar, into the maxillary sinus. The remaining molar teeth and the maxillary tuberosity may be fractured and displaced distally or inferiorly in such an injury. Teeth, fragments of teeth, and other foreign bodies displaced into the maxillary antrum should be removed and primary closure of the oroantral opening should be accomplished. Palatal soft-tissue injuries should also be sutured early in treatment. When teeth are present in the fractured tuberosity, reduction and immobilization can often be accomplished by intermaxillary fixation. The use of a palatal splint will be useful in stabilizing the loose fragment.

Maxillary Tuberosity Fractures

Fractures of the maxillary tuberosity can also occur from the complex vectoring of forces in trauma or during the process of extracting a maxillary molar, especially in extraction of teeth with long, divergent, and sometimes ankylosed roots. Another common anatomic feature that predisposes to fracturing during extraction is an alveolar extension of the maxillary sinus (Fig. 11–6). Fractures can occur without the application of an excessive amount of extraction force in many instances if the alveolar process is in a weakened condition. The doctor will note a sudden cracking noise, after which mobility of the tooth and the maxillary tuberosity as a single unit will be evident. This weakened condition of the alveolar process is usually related to an excessively enlarged maxillary antrum with extensions into the interseptal and trifurcation areas that are normally occupied by cancellous bone. Additional weakening of the alveolar process will be present when the tooth anterior to the one being extracted has been missing for a year or more.

Maxillary tuberosity fractures resulting from extractions may be treated by removing

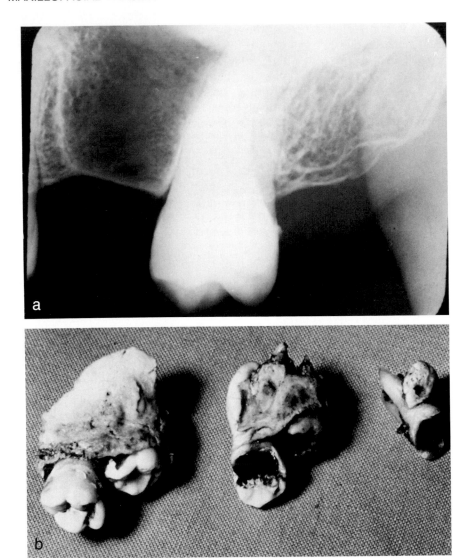

FIG. 11–6. **a,** Radiographic view of a tuberosity weakened by an alveolar extension of the maxillary sinus. **b,** Examples of tuberosities avulsed during exodontia procedures.

the tooth from the fractured tuberosity, stabilizing the tuberosity until it heals and then removing the tooth, or immediately removing the tuberosity.

When the roots are not too divergent, an attempt may be made to remove the tooth from the alveolar bone with a thin elevator. The procedure usually involves reflecting the mucoperiosteum sufficiently to expose a portion of the alveolar bone over the buccal roots. A fissured bur is used to remove part of the alveolar bone. The roots are then sectioned with the bur, and the crown and palatal root are removed as a single unit. The bur should

be used to extend a groove around the roots to aid in their removal with a thin elevator. The roots should be removed while the tuberosity is stabilized with forceps or finger pressure. After removal of the tooth or teeth, the mucoperiosteum is sutured back into position.

To stabilize the tuberosity and then surgically remove the tooth, the fractured tuberosity is immobilized with a palatal splint for 6 to 8 weeks to allow the fracture to heal. After the splint has been wired into place, the cusps and occlusal surfaces of the teeth in the fractured fragment should be reduced by occlusal adjustment sufficiently to free them from any occlusal interferences. When the fracture has repaired, the tooth is sectioned and removed.

In immediate removal of the tuberosity, the greatest disadvantage is the permanent loss of the alveolar process and maxillary tuberosity that are so necessary for denture stability. The palatal and buccal mucoperiosteum is reflected to completely free the loose segment of the tuberosity. Following the removal of the tuberosity, the buccal and palatal mucoperiosteal flaps are sutured together.

The selection of an appropriate method of stabilization will depend on numerous factors—the patient's occlusion, the condition of adjacent teeth, the type of alveolar process injury, and the extent of injury to the dentition.

Stabilization Techniques

Various wiring techniques provide versatile approaches to stabilization of dentition. Eyelet wiring, Essig wiring, Stout wiring, and other methods will stabilize injured dentition to adjacent noninjured teeth; it is helpful, in many cases, to apply either self-curing acrylic material into the wire splints or to use composite restorative materials to help with the stabilization and retention of fractured dentition. Dental floss or suture material may be applied in a continuous figure-of-8 technique to stabilize fractured teeth and overlying composite restorative material, and allowing aesthetic maintenance.

Labial arch bars are used in many instances. It is important to adapt the arch bar to the expected contour of the dental arch and to ligate it to a sufficient number of adjacent teeth for long-term stability of the dentition.

Palatal and lingual splints may be constructed on reassembled stone casts. The casts are made from impressions of the dental arches and are sectioned with the displaced segments realigned and placed in correct relationships. Either acrylic or metal may be used for the construction of the splint.

SUPPORTING CARE

A soft diet is essential following trauma to the dentition, particularly when displacement of the tooth has occurred. Postoperative pain medication such as nonsteroidal anti-inflammatory agents are also beneficial in reducing discomfort and inflammation. Antibiotic coverage with penicillin or a substitute, if the patient is allergic to penicillin, for a 7- to 10-day period is advisable to prevent infection.

REFERENCES

1. Calaldi, C.R.: Injuries to the teeth. *In* Sports Injuries: The Unauthorized Epidemic. Edited by F.F. Vinger and E.F. Hoerner. Littleton, Mass., PSG Publishing Co., Inc., 1981.
2. Josell, S.D., and Abrams. R.G.: Traumatic injuries to the dentition and its supporting structures. Pediatr Clin North Am 22:717, 1982.
3. Sowray, J.H.: Localized injuries of the teeth and alveolar process. *In* Maxillofacial Injuries. Edited by N.L. Rowe and J.L. Williams. New York, Churchill Livingstone, 1985.
4. Johnson, R.: Traumatic injuries to the teeth and supporting structures. *In* Pediatric Dentistry: Scientific Foundation and Clinical Practice. Edited by R.E. Stewart, et al. St. Louis, C. V. Mosby Co., 1982.
5. Torneck, C.D.: Effects and clinical significance of trauma to the developing permanent dentition. Dent Clin North Am 26:481, 1982.
6. Andreasen, J.O.: Traumatic Injuries of the Teeth. 2nd Ed. Philadelphia, W.B. Saunders Co., 1981.
7. Alling, C.C.: Personal communication.
8. Stoneman, D.W.: Radiology of trauma to the teeth and jaws. Dent Clin North Am 26:591, 1982.
9. Andreasen, J.O.: Traumatic Injuries of the Teeth. St. Louis, C.V. Mosby Co., 1972.
10. Sebor, R.J.: Restoration of Class IV lesions and fractures with acid-etch composite. Compend Contin Educ 4:510, 1983.
11. Ludlow, J.B., and LaTurno, S.A.L.: Traumatic fracture—one visit endodontic treatment and dentinal bonding reattachment of coronal fragment: report of a case. Dent Assoc 110:341, 1985.
12. Levine, N.: Injury to the primary dentition. Dent Clin North Am 26:461, 1982.
13. Selliseth, N.E.: The significance of traumatized primary incisors on the development and eruption of permanent teeth. Report of Congress, European Orthodontic Society, 443, 1970.
14. Van Gool, A.V.: Injuries to permanent teeth germs after trauma to the deciduous predecessor. Oral Sur Oral Med Oral Pathol 35:2, 1973.
15. Kozen, B.H.: Endodontic treatment of traumatized teeth. Dent Clin North Am 26:505, 1982.
16. Pulver, F.: Treatment of trauma to the young permanent dentition. Dent Clin North Am 26:525, 1982.

12

FACIAL SKELETAL RECONSTRUCTIVE SURGERY

CHARLES C. ALLING III
ROCKLIN D. ALLING
DONALD B. OSBON

Injuries of the maxillofacial region include complex avulsions of portions of both the soft tissue and the underlying bony structures. Avulsive injuries of the maxilla and mandible often result in continuity defects with subsequent loss of function of the facial area. Whereas many maxillary injuries can be restored successfully by prosthetic means, continuity defects of the mandible usually require bony reconstruction. In a survey of 9439 patients with maxillofacial injuries in the Vietnam War, 9.4% exhibited avulsion of a significant portion of the mandible, and long-term reconstructive therapy was required to return the patients to acceptable function and facial aesthetics.[1]

The management of maxillofacial injuries consists of three phases, early, intermediate, and late. Definitive reconstruction, such as use of bone grafts, is usually performed in the late phase; the foundation for successful intermediate and late-phase treatment, however, begins with the initial care in the early phase.

Reconstructive treatment must be predi-cated on thorough and continuing examinations and planning. Certain factors stand out as being significant influences in the success or failure of bone graft reconstruction. These include proper wound management in the early and intermediate phases of treatment to ensure a healthy recipient site; an adequate soft-tissue bed to permit coverage of the bone graft and closure of the surgical site without tension; watertight closure of the oral aspects of the injury; very conservative debridement of comminuted areas of bones; avoidance of open spaces in the soft tissue that invite formation of hematomas and infection; satisfactory general health of the patient; asepsis in all aspects of the direct surgical care, including control or suppression of oral microbes; deft, delicate, and accurate handling of the graft to avoid mechanical injury; absolute immobilization of the graft to the recipient site; and superior general supportive care of the total metabolism of the patient.

Attention must be paid to the the basic principles of bone grafting for consistently satisfactory results. Although continued development of techniques and materials is anticipated, success will continue to depend on adherence to the basic surgical principles and the special factors associated with bone grafting to the oral and maxillofacial tissues.

EARLY CARE

Patients with maxillofacial injuries can have in addition many other body injuries consisting of wounds of the head, chest, abdomen, and extremities. Obviously, priority must be given to performing triage for life-preservation procedures: the establishment and maintenance of a patient's airway; arrest of hemorrhage; and recognition and treatment of shock, associated head injuries, and severe trauma to the extremities, thorax, and abdomen. The initial triage involving a complete physical examination should establish the priority of treatment. Because maxillofacial injuries are not generally life-threatening, their treatment will usually be a lower priority.

MANAGEMENT OF WOUNDS

Wound Preparation

The majority of maxillofacial wounds are contaminated and require cleansing and preparation using vigorous irrigations. Irrigation is usually performed with several liters of isotonic saline or sterile water in conjunction with a surgical soap solution applied with a brush or sponge. The use of the water-jet lavage is helpful in the debridement of wounds containing particles of foreign matter that may be overlooked on inspection of the wound. Debris that is permitted to remain in the tissues will produce a permanent tatoo that is difficult to eradicate later or that may complicate reconstruction.

Intraoral Wounds

Injuries of the oral structures may vary in severity from lacerations of the oral mucosa and lips to avulsive wounds of the palate, alveolar process, and floor of the mouth. In extensive injuries involving oral cutaneous communications, a watertight mucosal closure is imperative. Prior to soft-tissue closure, all fractured teeth in the line of fracture that cannot be salvaged or used for immobilization should be considered for removal to reduce the incidence of infection and wound breakdown resulting in possible nonunion of a fracture.

In avulsive wounds of the palate, an effort should be made to close the defect by mobilizing the remaining palatal mucosa and suturing it to the buccal mucosa or the alveolar mucoperiosteum. If the remaining tissue is not sufficient to cover a palatal defect, a plastic or vinyl splint may be fabricated to cover the defect and permit as much granulation of the mucosa as possible. Definitive care should be planned at a later date and may consist of many procedures.

Soft-Tissue Wounds

Timing is extremely important in the management of soft-tissue wounds of the face. Primary closure is best performed within the first 24 hrs following the injury for best results and minimal scar formation, although the use of wet dressings may make possible a delay of a few days when necessary. Thorough conservative wet debridement, hemostasis, careful tissue handling, and meticulous closure of tissues in layers to as normal a position as possible will produce the best results. Conservative wound margin trimming, undermining, and plastic modification of lacerations lines, where indicated, are the bases for closure of cutaneous wound margins.

Using the concept "inside first, outside second," the surgeon should direct his attention first to intraoral wounds. Injuries of oral mucous membranes must be corrected by suturing techniques that permit primary closure of the oral mucosa and provide a watertight seal to the oral cavity. A monofilament suture material, usually placed in a running horizontal suturing technique, will help prevent penetration of the contaminated oral fluids into the submucosa. Prior to closure is an excellent time to make impressions of the dental arches for construction of splints and to place fixation devices, arch bars, eyelet wiring, and continuous loop wiring.

Avulsive wounds with tissue deficiencies in the perioral region should be managed by suturing the mucous membranes to the skin. This technique permits primary healing of the residual mucosal and cutaneous tissues and prevents the development of excessive scarring. Areas of avulsed cutaneous tissues should be covered by a medicated, moist dressing in preparation for future coverage by soft-tissue flaps or grafts.

Bone

Conservative management of fragments of bone is important in comminuted or avulsed injuries. Soft-tissue attachments to bony fragments must not be stripped away in an attempt to provide fixation by internal wiring or plating. Often, these fragments may be molded into position and maintained by soft-tissue closure and major fragment stabilization.

Extraskeletal pin fixation can be used to stabilize small fragments of bone by supporting the major segments in an anatomic alignment. Extraskeletal pin fixation devices are applicable in a variety of locations and situations, including stablization of comminuted fractures (Fig. 12–1). The small comminuted fragments may be considered as a "bag of bones" in an admixture of bony elements and periosteum; the fragments will unite if protected from infection and movement. The use of intraoral splints with wires that cradle the bag of bones will produce union with minimal sloughing of bony structures.

Drains

Many injuries about the face will require drainage to minimize hematoma formation. Wounds involving the relatively thin tissues of the cheeks, lips, and upper face should be closed in a manner that eliminates open spaces and requires no drains. Wounds involving the floor of the mouth, base of the tongue, retromandibular area, infratemporal fossa, and neck usually will have some open spaces and require drainage. Placement of a drain is most important with wounds involving the loss of mandibular bony structure and the oral cavity. After the oral mucosa is closed,

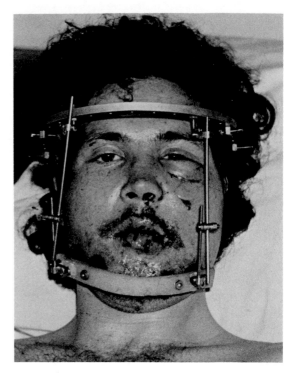

FIG. 12–1. Multiple facial fractures treated with a Morris headframe and biphasic system for extraskeletal reduction and fixation.

the periosteum should be closed into and over the space occupied by the mandible. A thin rubber or plastic tube drain should be placed superficial to the periosteal repair. A drain placed on bone tends to cause breakdown of the tissues with formation of an oro-cutaneous fistula.

INTERMEDIATE CARE

Intermediate care encompasses a variable time span; of the utmost importance during this phase is the status of the patient relative to future treatment. Treatment performed in the early phase is reviewed and evaluated, and major modifications are instituted only if the initial efforts were not successful. Additional diagnostic and planning procedures may be necessary at this time, including making impressions of the dental arches for the preparation of stabilizing devices, if these impressions were not obtained at the early phases. If reduction and immobilization of facial fractures was not performed during the early phase, it should be accomplished at this time.

Airway adequacy should be assessed continuously, and during the intermediate phases a decision may be necessary concerning the retention of a tracheostomy tube. Retention depends on the future surgical and anesthetic needs and the patient's ability to handle secretions and diet with the jaws fixated.

Proper wound care in the intermediate phase is extremely important and includes suture and drain removal, dressing changes, irrigations, oral hygiene maintenance, and observation of the wound status.

The antibiotic program is reviewed and revised on the basis of culture and sensitivity testing when drainage is present. Removing fractured or infected teeth, debriding necrotic bone or soft tissue, and incising, draining, and irrigating deep wounds that have become necrotic may be necessary. Antibiotic therapy cannot be relied on to alter the course of an infection in the absence of correct local wound care. Resistant organisms may develop at this stage and establish soft-and hard-tissue infections that are difficult to control.

The general supportive care of the patient during this phase includes a well-balanced, high-calorie diet, perhaps administered through a nasogastric tube. Oral hygiene must be emphasized to both the patient and the nursing personnel.

LATE OR RECONSTRUCTIVE PHASE

The late or reconstructive phase of treatment will involve those patients who have residual defects and those who have developed complications. If a continuity defect of bone exists, bone grafting should be planned at the earliest practical time. Sufficient soft tissue is fundamental to provide coverage of bony grafts. Remaining dentition must be maintained, as it may be used as an additional, if not the primary, source of stabilization during reconstruction and used to support a prosthesis.

BONE GRAFTING

Theories of Bone Regeneration

Many theories have explained the process of bone regeneration as it applies to bone grafting. A composite theory combines the osteoblastic theory and the induction theory that was defined and refined by Urist.[2,3] The osteoblastic theory proposed that bone marrow and periosteum survive transplantation and produce bone. Urist contended that transplanted bone undergoes aseptic necrosis and is replaced with bone produced by the connective tissue fibroblasts of the recipient bed and host bone. The composite concept postulates two phases of bone regeneration: the first is the cellular phase, and the second is the induction phase. Urist further subdivied these two phases.[4]

The first and physiologically most important phase, the bone induction phase, originates in the pre-existing osteoblasts and begins soon after grafting. The endosteal osteoblasts proliferate and lay down new bone on the surface of necrotic bone that has not survived transplantation. In addition to endosteal osteoblasts, mesenchymal fibroblasts of the marrow spaces and hematopoietic cells of the marrow survive transplantation. The amount of cellular survival during this phase will influence the quality of bone produced by transplantation.

The second phase associated with the bone induction principle of Urist, is stimulated by the necrosis of bone.[5] During the second phase, mesenchymal cells proliferating from phase one differentiate to produce bone. The bone is produced in a random fashion by endosteal osteoblasts and differentiated mesenchymal cells. In addition, host mesenchymal fibroblasts and vessels invade the graft. During this phase, the disorganized bone becomes organized in relation to soft-tissue volume and function. Urist described this process as a system of inducing cells and responding cells; Urist has isolated the inducing substance, bone morphogenic protein (BMP), from human bone as well as from bovine bone.[6,7] BMP is part of the organic matrix of bone and is concentrated primarily in the cortical bone. Apparently BMP has the ability to stimulate committed cells to produce bone and to genetically influence uncommitted mesenchymal fibroblasts to produce bone collagen.

This process of bone regeneration is further influenced by the rate of revascularization of the graft. During transplantation, the viability of the osteocytes is jeopardized by the loss of the vascular supply. It has been demonstrated, however, that some surface cells in the deep layers of the periosteum, the endosteum, and the cells on the surface of the trabeculae are able to survive even in the absence of blood supply.[8] These cells appear to be nourished by circulating plasma derived from the surrounding soft tissue.[9] Nevertheless, the rate of revascularization becomes important because even these cells, which survive and are nourished by tissue fluids, must re-establish a blood supply if they are to survive long term. Dying osteocytes appear to influence the cells lining the capillary sinusoid system, causing proliferation of osteogenic vessels.[10] Autogenous grafts are rapidly revascularized and return to a normal vascular pattern in approximately 3 weeks; homogenous grafts have a normal vascular pattern in 7 weeks.

Early vascularization depends on not only the viability and type of graft, but also the physical characteristics of the graft.[11] Cancellous bone provides a network for easy penetration by vascular ingrowth with less need for osteoclastic resorption.[12] A definitive correlation exists between the rate of revascularization and the ultimate incorporation of the graft. Remodeling and maturation of the graft depend on the vascular ingrowth's bringing circulating monocytes to form local osteoclasts. In addition, fibroblasts provide cells for induction of bone formation that replace and remodel early phase-one bone, and they may even form a type of functional periosteum.

In summary, phase two of bone regeneration involves bone production, maturation, and remodeling.

Functions of a Bone Graft

A successful bone graft to the mandible should restore continuity and function, restore normal facies, form a framework for im-

mobilization of the donor tissue to the recipient site, and furnish a source of viable osteogenic cells, which act as a precursor for bone induction.

Principles of Bone Grafting

Regardless of the type of bone graft system or procedure selected, required in all cases are satisfactory general health, asepsis, a healthy graft recipient site, an uninjured graft, immobilization of the graft, and proper closure of the surgical site.

The patient should be in the best possible health, and unacceptable nutritional or systemic debilities should be corrected before surgery. Improved healing with fewer postsurgical complications are benefits of adequate nutrition during the pre-and postoperative periods. Dietary regimens are complicated in bone graft cases because often long periods of maxillomandibular fixation are required.

To maintain the sterility of the graft bed, indirect stabilization devices, arch bars, splints, eyelet wiring, and continuous loop wiring can be placed as part of the immediate preoperative preparation of the patient. Ideally, the devices could be placed under regional anesthesia 1 or 2 days preoperatively to save time and prevent possible contamination of the surgical site in the operating room.

Every effort must be made to provide aseptic conditions during the grafting of a mandibular continuity defect. In the days prior to surgery, oral prophylaxis can be performed, especially when a graft is being placed through a transoral or an extraoral approach. For both approaches, in addition to the usual cutaneous surface scrubbing and preparation at the time of surgery, a throat pack should be placed and the intraoral tissues dried and then scrubbed with an antiseptic solution (a toothbrush is useful when dealing with dentition and intraoral stabilizing devices). If the surgical approach is extraoral, the intraoral preparation is performed before the extraoral preparation. If the approach is transoral, the cutaneous scrub and preparation is performed before the intraoral preparation. Usually the throat pack need not be left in place when the approach is extraoral.

Systemic antibiotics are used for all bone graft operations. Pencillin and cephalosporins are very effective first choices. Intravenous antibiosis is initiated on the morning of surgery with 4,000,000 units every 4 hrs for 7 days. Another antibiotic regimen consists of 1 g of cefazolin given IV 1 hr preoperatively and then continued at the rate of 500 mg to 1 g IV or 1M four times per day for 7 days.

Prior to surgically opening the graft site, whenever possible the major segments of the mandible should be stabilized against the maxilla by intermaxillary rubber bands. This stabilization will orient the surgical site anatomically and facilitate placement of the graft.

The recipient tissue bed must consist of healthy soft tissue free of infection and having an adequate supply of blood. Scar tissue should be excised whenever possible to improve the recipient tissues. Obviously, in many cases placement of the graft must await soft-tissue plastic procedures.

For an extraoral approach, the submandibular incision should be placed as low as practical in the neck, because the increased facial bulk resulting from the graft will cause the incision to move superiorly. The incision should be extensively undermined in the subcutaneous layer and on the surface of the platysma muscle, and the dissection is carried to the level of the fascia over the digastric muscles. The dissection should then expose the ends of the proximal and distal mandibular segments. The tissue between the segments is carefully prepared to receive the graft, with due regard for prevention of an oral perforation.

The extraoral entry to the placement of a graft may use the principles of Z-plasties to provide a more relaxed soft-tissue coverage of the surgical site. A series of Zs, accompanied by a generous undermining, will make additional tissues available to the injured site and will change a linear scar, which might contract into a deforming fibrous band, into a more acceptable, multidirectional incisional line (Fig. 12–2).

The graft is handled carefully to prevent contamination and mechanical injury. Every effort should be made to place the graft into the recipient tissue as soon as possible after harvest. The harvested bone should immediately be placed in saline solution,[13] or it can be wrapped in a saline-soaked cotton gauze sponge. If the donor bone is cancellous bone marrow, it is placed in a stainless steel cup and covered with a saline-moistened gauze. Although antibiotic solutions can be used with allogeneic bone, because the solutions may be cytotoxic they should not be used for autogenous bone.

The major reason for bone graft failure in the mandible is improper or inadequate immobilization of the graft and the recipient site. Maxillomandibular fixation should be used if the patient has remaining teeth, and the major segments can be approximated by intermaxillary fixation or elastic traction. The elastic traction permits modest movement of the recipient sites while the graft is being placed.

After the graft has been placed, firm intermaxillary wire fixation can be used. If no teeth are proximal to the canine area on the side of the graft, a lingual splint may be fabricated with an extension arm engaging the maxillary teeth above the defect. This technique prevents torquing of the mandible that distorts the graft-host interfaces. Additional tension can be relieved by removing the coronoid process to eliminate the influence of the temporal muscle on the proximal fragment.

In edentulous patients, splints are used instead of the appliances worn on teeth. Extraskeletal pin fixation may be used in both dentulous and edentulous patients to supplement the intraoral and the graft site immobilization. In nearly every case, rigid fixation of the grafted area is provided by a bone plate, by a metallic crib, or by the bone graft itself. As a general rule, if possible at least two forms of fixation are used in addition to that provided by the graft. For example, the surgeon should use combinations of two or more of maxillomandibular, bone plate, extraskeletal, and splint fixation techniques.

When the quality and quantity of the recipient sites and the graft will permit, and assuming a cooperative, well-motivated patient, rigid osteosynthesis can be employed; due regard must be given to the use of long-span plates to nullify the adverse torquing at the two graft and recipient site interfaces.

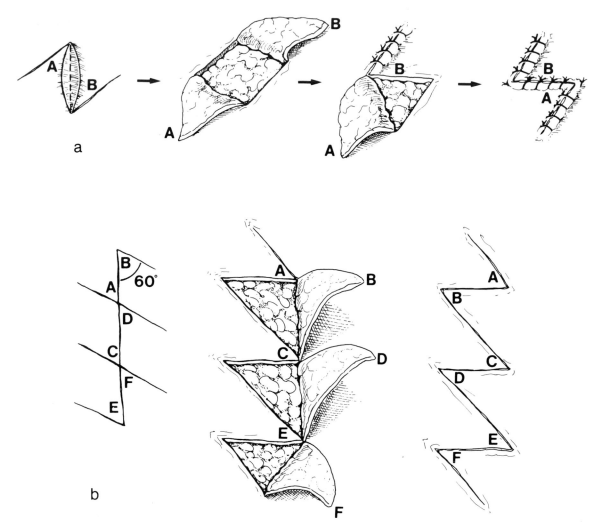

FIG. 12–2. **a,** A Z-plasty produces additional length by transferring the triangular flaps. **b,** Multiple Z-plasties are combined to release tension and provide a linear lengthening of available soft tissue. This procedure may be applicable in managing scar tissue overlying a surgical site.

The surgical site should be closed in layers without tension on the soft tissues. Any open space should be eliminated to prevent hematoma formation around the graft. If the deep tissues are inadequate to cover the graft, they should be sutured to the graft or to a crib supporting the graft. The layers of tissue that were established during the initial dissection should be reapproximated. If necessary, additional undermining is performed to eliminate all tension.

Bone Grafting Systems

Autogenous hematopoietic marrow and autogenous cancellous bone containing marrow appear to be the only types of bone graft material that are capable of actively inducing osteogenesis. Sources for mandibular bone grafting include solid corticocancellous grafts using iliac crest, rib, particulate cancellous marrow bone, and the mandible. Freeze-dried allogeneic bone is used both to carry autogenous bone and to provide structural support within the graft site.[1,14–17] Other graft systems include alloplastic devices and materials, osteomyocutaneous grafts, and microvascular bone–periosteal grafts.

Iliac Solid Corticocancellous Graft System. The iliac solid corticocancellous graft system is extremely dependable. The graft is taken from either the lateral or the medial aspect of the ilium, avoiding creation of a total-thickness iliac crest defect. Generally, grafting from the medial aspect of the ilium is less traumatic to the patient and reduces the postoperative morbidity. The graft is usually placed on the medial aspect of the mandible with an overlap of approximately 1.5 to 2 cm at the host recipient site to allow for mortising of the graft to the proximal and distal segments (Fig. 12–3). The medial surfaces of the host segments should be contoured to permit close opposition at the interface and to provide a viable bleeding surface. The graft

is immobilized with mattress wires to firmly seat the graft to the recipient site. Usually a bone plate is contoured and placed on the lateral surface. After the graft is secured, additional particulate cancellous bone and marrow are generously packed over the lateral aspect of the graft, particularly at the interface areas. This procedure may be critical to the success of the graft, because the particulate bone contains additional endosteal osteoblasts and marrow mesenchymal cells for the first phase of regeneration. Wound closure is completed as described above.

The graft obtained from the inner surface

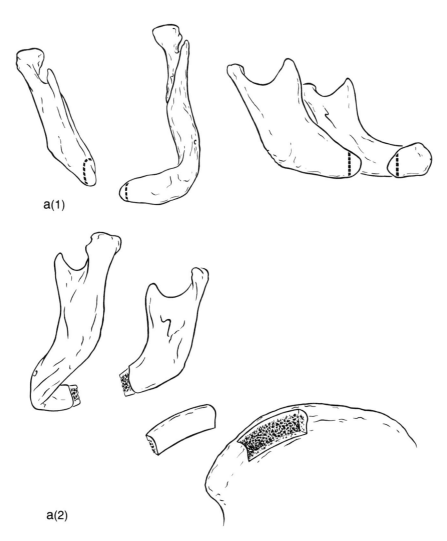

a(1)

a(2)

FIG. 12–3.   Iliac grafts to the medial aspect of the mandible. **a (1, 2, 3, and 4),** Greater structural stability, a shorter graft, and abundant soft-tissue coverage are achieved when the donor bone is placed on the mandibular medial surface instead of on the lateral surface.

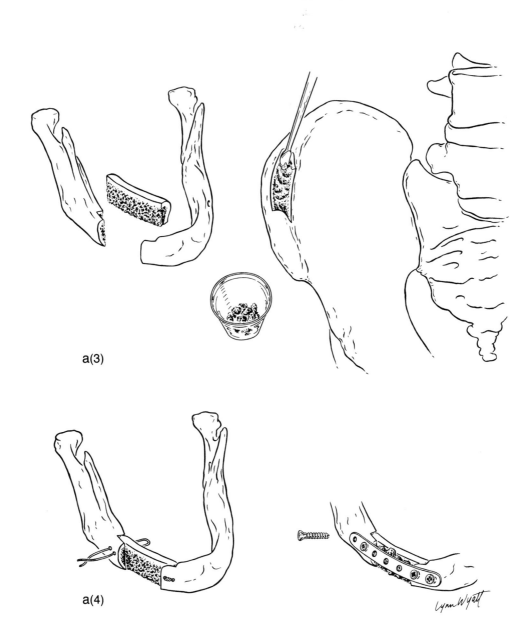

a(3)

a(4)

FIG. 12–3 (continued).

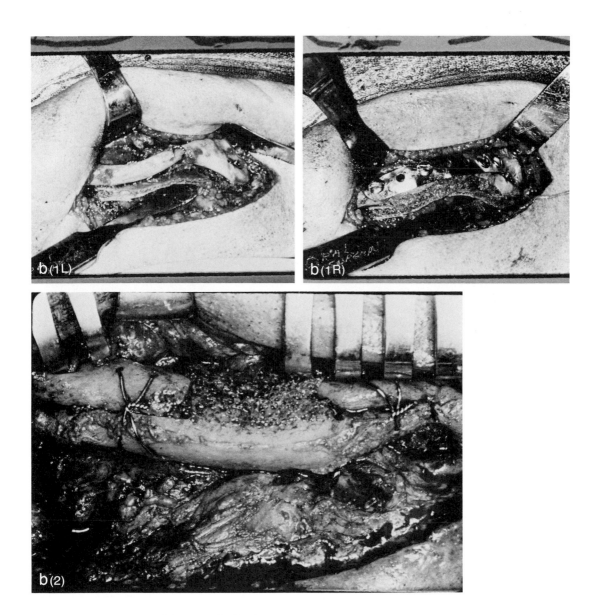

FIG. 12–3 (continued).   **b (1) L** and **R,** Medially placed iliac corticocancellous and particulate cancellous graft supported by transosseous wiring, bone plate, and intermaxillary fixation. **(2),** Reconstruction of the left angle of the mandible with a medially placed iliac corticocancellous and particulate cancellous graft supported by transosseous wiring and a compression bone plate.

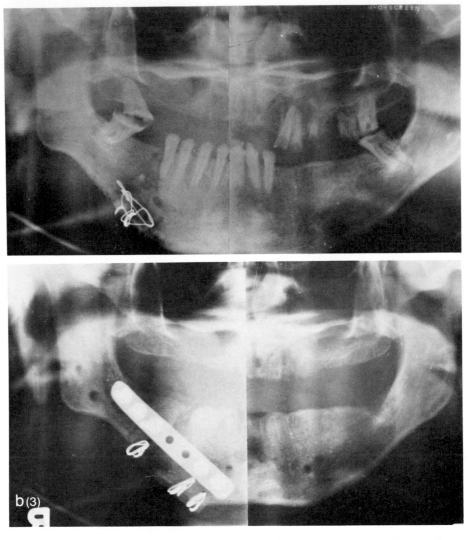

FIG. 12–3 (continued). **(3) L** and **R,** Attempt by others at fracture management by a collection of wires and no other fixation resulted in a nonunion. The patient was then managed by removal of the nonrestorable teeth, followed by use of a medially placed iliac bone graft, compression double transosseous wiring, and a compression bone plate.

of the ilium usually has a curvature comparable to the body of the mandible on the same side of the patient. The graft may be placed on the medial side of mandible with the iliac cortical border extending superiorly, thus producing an alveolar ridge. If indicated, the cortical margin can be placed inferiorly.

Compared to the crib and particulate cancellous bone technique, the corticocancellous grafting system offers several advantages. The width of the graft is not limited; also, when the surgeon is reconstructing the body of the mandible, the rounded cortical margin can be placed either superiorly as an alveolar ridge or inferiorly as a base of the mandible. In addition, the surgical instruments required are basic with the possible addition of a small orthopedic bone plate for rigid osteosynthesis.

Autogenous Rib Grafts. Autogenous rib grafts are used in cases that require a graft with a particular shape or additional length. The use of solid rib grafts is limited, however, because the graft may resorb rapidly with very little satisfactory bone replacement (Fig. 12–4). If using the rib, the surgeon should

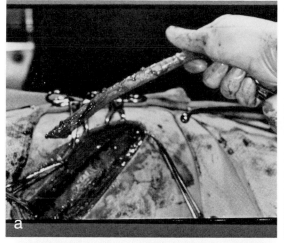
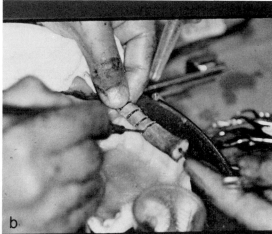
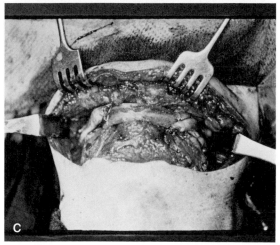

FIG. 12–4. Rib grafts. **a,** The ninth rib is harvested. **b,** The donor rib is contoured for specific size requirements. **c,** The graft is secured to the anterior mandibular area.

consider splitting and combining the sections with cancellous bone and marrow from the ilium. Costochrondral rib grafts are used to replace the condyle and varying lengths of the mandibular ramus and body of the mandible.[18] The cartilage is trimmed to fit the glenoid fossa, leaving a 3- to 5-mm gap superior to the cap of cartilage to prevent bony union and the formation of pseudoarthritis. Freeze-dried bone, additional sections of ribs, and bone from the ilium may be placed to reinforce the costochrondral graft.

Reconstruction of a hemimandibular loss, after the soft-tissue bed is established, may be a phased operation. First, a segment of cancellous cortical bone from the medial crest of the ilium is grafted to the remaining anterior segment of the mandible and held with a bone plate in the cantilever fashion as it extends posteriorly to the ramus area. After

the union of the anterior mandible and graft has been achieved, the posterior reconstruction is performed with, for example, a costochrondral graft.

Crib and Cancellous Bone Marrow Technique. Boyne was instrumental in developing the crib and cancellous bone marrow technique for reconstruction of the mandible.[19,20] The crib can be lined with a nylon-reinforced cellulose ester filter of 0.45-μm pore size. The filter permits tissue fluid passage and prevents fibrous tissue ingrowth, and the metallic crib establishes the desired structure. This technique is not always necessary and is undesirable if local infection is present or if oral fluids could seep into the graft site (Fig. 12–5 and 12–6).

Particulate cancellous bone and marrow grafts within alloplastic cribs are very adaptable and provide an excellent method for re-

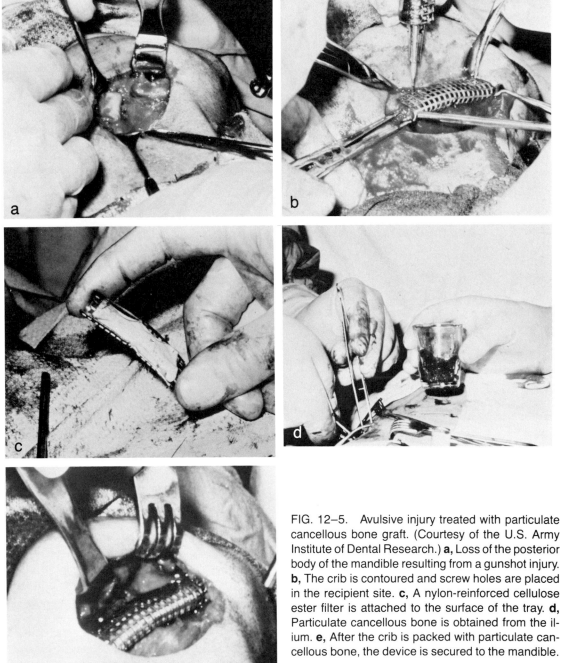

FIG. 12–5.   Avulsive injury treated with particulate cancellous bone graft. (Courtesy of the U.S. Army Institute of Dental Research.) **a,** Loss of the posterior body of the mandible resulting from a gunshot injury. **b,** The crib is contoured and screw holes are placed in the recipient site. **c,** A nylon-reinforced cellulose ester filter is attached to the surface of the tray. **d,** Particulate cancellous bone is obtained from the ilium. **e,** After the crib is packed with particulate cancellous bone, the device is secured to the mandible.

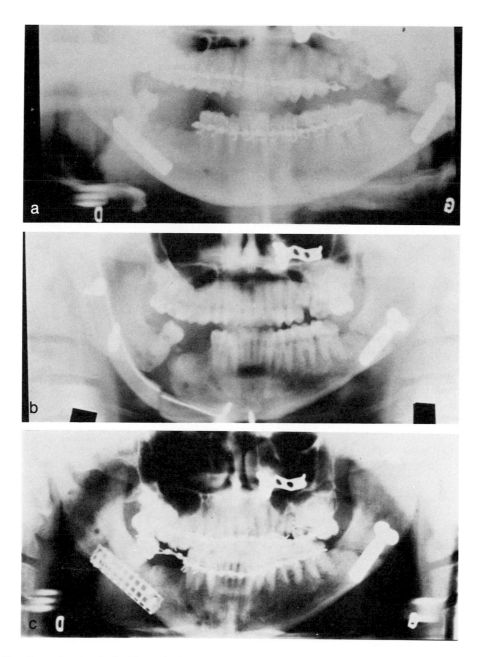

FIG. 12–6.   Nonunion treated with particulate cancellous bone graft. **a,** Displaced mandibular fractures and depressed left ZMC fracture were initially treated with rigid osteosynthesis fixation. **b,** One month postoperatively, an infection developed in the right mandibular area. The bone plate was removed and the mandible was stabilized with the Morris extraskeletal fixation device. A nonunion ensued in the infected area, however, evident by the eburnated proximal and distal segments 6 months following the initial reduction and fixation with bone plates. **c,** Successful treatment concluded with placement of particulate cancellous bone harvested from the ilium. The graft was placed in a tray without a filter 9 months following the original injury.

construction of traumatic defects of the mandible. Because the graft consists only of particulate bone and cancellous marrow, many osteoblasts and mesenchymal cells survive transplantation and revascularization takes place rapidly. The alloplastic crib holds and supports the particulate cancellous bone and marrow. Various types of cribs and trays have been used, including titanium trays [21] and chromium cobalt alloy cribs; the latter may be designed with adaptable wrought segments at each end for attachment to the host fragments.[15] The cribs adapt well to various contours of the mandible and can be fabricated to any length (Fig. 12–7).

A disadvantage of the crib, as with the fracture plate placed over the graft site for rigid fixation, is the need to remove the crib or plate if it interferes with the prosthetic rehabilitation. Removal of the devices may be recommended to avoid stress shielding. However, in our experience with over 400 bone graft reconstructions of the mandible, we have observed no instances of stress shielding as manifested by atrophy or by fracturing after the removal of the bone plate or wire mesh. Unlike the bones of the leg, which bear heavy loading stresses, the mandible is subjected to torquing tensions. Because the body of the mandible is a flat bone that is curved, metallic devices on one surface do not completely shield the mandible from stresses; such shielding may occur in other, straight bones.

A Dacron and urethane tray has been developed that is semirigid, lightweight, porous, and radiolucent and can be shaped with scissors at the time of surgery. The trays are biocompatible and can be autoclaved for sterilization.[22]

Mandibular Grafts. The mandible of the patient is another source of bone graft material (Fig. 12–8). Several areas that are easily accessible and provide a versatile autogeneic supply of grafting material include the outer cortical plate of the mandibular angle and the coronoid process. The angle region is structurally similar to the anatomic floor of the orbit. After harvesting of this region, a customized bony platform can be fashioned and used in the reconstruction of an orbital floor blowout fracture. The coronoid process can be used in a similar fashion or can be pulverized

to provide a dense cortical mix for other grafting needs.

A decade-old technique has been to obtain a graft, with its periosteal attachments often intact, from the adjacent base of the mandible. Material from other donor areas in the mandible, such as the parasymphyseal and retromolar regions, may be obtained using, for example, trephine techniques. The parasymphyseal bony anatomy can provide wafers of bone through the surgical approach used for genioplasty procedures.

Freeze-Dried Bone. Cribs and plates of freeze-dried allogeneic bone are biocompatible and provide support for particulate cancellous bone and marrow. The function of the allogeneic bone is purely passive in the osteogenic process. No active osteogenic stimulation occurs, but new bone from the host grows over the absorbable surfaces of the freeeze-dried bone. The active regenerative phase of the bone grafting is stimulated by particulate cancellous bone and marrow contained in the allogeneic crib. Because this freeze-dried bone is resorbed and replaced over an extended period of time, a second operation may not be needed to remove the allogeneic plate or crib. Freeze-dried bone is adaptable and can be used in a number of different forms.[23,24]

Freeze-dried bone from the iliac crest can be contoured, thinned, shaped, and secured to the segments of the mandible and can then be packed with particulate cancellous bone and marrow (Fig. 12–9). Although allogeneic ribs are thin and friable and not very flexible, the ribs can be used, usually split, to form a box between the recipient site segments that will contain the bone.

When available, allogeneic mandibles may be hollowed and packed with cancellous bone and marrow, making ideal grafting systems.

Alloplastic Materials. Alloplastic materials for reconstruction of the mandible include hydroxyapatite and similar materials, temporomandibular joint prostheses, and ramal-condylar metallic devices.[25–27] Hydroxyapatite and similar materials do not add to the structural integrity of the mandible unless used in conjunction with an admixture of cancellous bone; rather the materials are used to add to the contours of the facial skeleton and alveo-

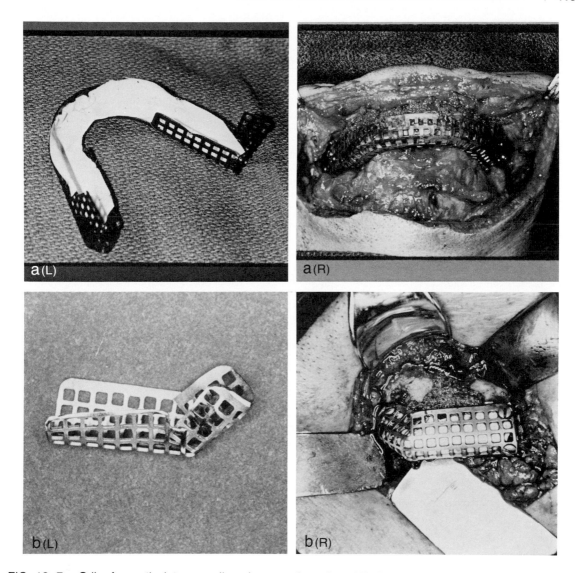

FIG. 12–7. Cribs for particulate cancellous bone grafts. **a** L and **R,** Restoration of the entire body of the mandible. **b** L and **R,** Reconstruction of the angle of the mandible.

lar processes. The condylar joint prostheses are especially indicated to correct the rare post-traumatic problems of temporomandibbular joint degeneration and ankylosis. Ramal-condylar metallic devices have been used since the 1920s (Fig. 12–10).

Osteomyocutaneous Grafts. Osteomyocutaneous grafts consist of bone and associated soft tissues on a vascular pedicle[28,29] This technique transplants viable osteocytes and maintains the blood supply to the segment of bone. One graft that has been advocated consists of a segment of rib with associated greater pectoral muscle and overlying skin.[30] Another type uses the me-

dial third of the clavicle with a pedicle consisting of the sternocleidomastoid muscle arising from the origin of the muscle at the mastoid process of the temporal bone.[31] Disadvantages include morbidity associated with the operations and a limited amount of available bone. The development of surgical techniques can make osteomyocutaneous grafts practical for restoration of mandibular defects secondary to trauma.

Microvascular Bone–Periosteal Grafting Techniques. Microvascular bone–periosteal grafting techniques permit the transfer of vascularized bone segments into areas with poor blood supply, heavily scarred tissue beds,

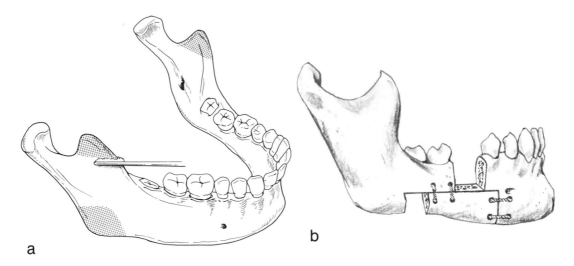

a

b

FIG. 12–8. Mandibular donor sites. **a,** The shaded areas represent potential donor sites in the gonial angle areas and the coronoid processes. **b,** Diagram of an osteoperiosteal sliding bone graft.

and irradiated areas. Donoff reported success in re-establishing periosteal blood flow in dogs and humans using vascularized rib grafts.[32] The operation requires an intrathoracic harvest of the anterior and middle third of a rib with the anterior intercostal artery and draining vein. Recipient vessels are located in the neck, and the anastomosis in completed under the microscope, with the vessels accompanying the rib graft. The bone is positioned and immobilized in the usual manner. The risks and complications of this technique include failure of the anastomosis, resulting in the possible loss of the graft. Because the rib harvest requires closed chest drainage,

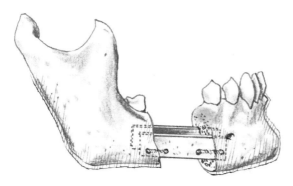

FIG. 12–9. An application for freeze-dried bone. Allogeneic bone (also, autogenous ribs and cortical plates) can be fashioned into boxes to hold particulate cancellous bone.

pleural effusions and pneumonias are possible risks. The expected evolution of technical procedures will make this a reliable and commonplace reconstructive technique.

RECONSTRUCTION OF THE MAXILLA

Most defects in the middle facial skeleton are restored successfully with a maxillofacial prosthesis. Avulsive wounds may produce extensive scars or oronasosinal communications. Soft-tissue repair of the intraoral areas can usually decrease and often eliminate the communications. Preprosthodontic surgical techniques, including implants for stabilizing prosthodontic devices, are an important part of the final restoration of function to the oral cavity.[33] Obturators may be indicated for extensive palatal losses of bony structures.

Bone graft reconstruction of periorbital injuries, including blow-out fractures, uses grafts with autogenous bone, allogeneic bone, and alloplastic materials. Augmentation of facial prominences, the malar eminence and the nasolabial area, may be indicated, and hydroxyapatite and similar materials are usually used. Bicoronal and hemicoronal flaps are useful for the placement of the augmentation materials in the zygomatic and frontal areas, because the coronal approach assures little to no tension on the surgical site, and scalp incisional lines are hidden in the hair.

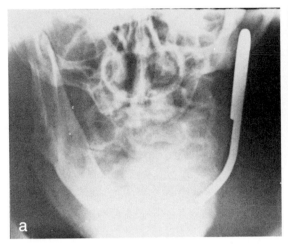
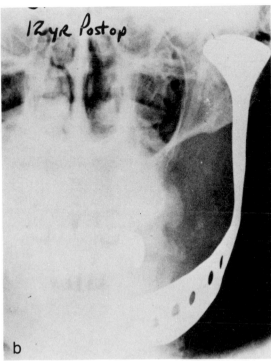

FIG. 12–10.   Alloplastc ramus-condylar prostheses. **a** and **b,** Metallic condylar prostheses restoring form and function. (Courtesy of Colonels William B. Irby and Jack B. Caldwell, D.C., U.S. Army, Ret.)

COMPLICATIONS OF BONE GRAFT RECONSTRUCTION

When undertaking reconstructive procedures of the maxillofacial area, one should keep in mind the potential complications at the donor and recipient sites.

Donor Site

The most common complication following harvest of a graft from the iliac crest is pain on ambulation. The degree of discomfort is associated with the trauma of the surgery, the amount of the soft tissue reflected, and the amount and area of bone harvested. When removing only particulate cancellous bone and marrow, the reflection of a bony flap, with periosteum and musculature attached, will minimize postoperative discomfort. Corticocancellous grafts are usually taken from only the medial or lateral surface of the ilium and produce very little postoperative pain when compared to a full-thickness graft that involves both cortices.

A postoperative hematoma may develop but in most cases is prevented by control of bleeding at the donor site with absorbable microfibrillar collagen or bone wax and, for full-thickness graft that included both cortices, by the placement of a drain or an automatic suction device (Hemovac). Infection occurs very rarely and should be managed by antibiotic therapy, drainage, and frequent irrigation. A postoperative ileus may occur secondary to a retroperitoneal hematoma. A temporary ileus may occur as a normal postoperative sequela.

Postoperative morbidity in the form of pain, particularly with deep breathing, may be associated with the harvesting of a rib graft. Additionally, lung expansion could be restricted. A complication of rib resection is pneumothorax.

Recipient Site

Infection at the recipient site is a major concern in the reconstruction of facial skeleton. When the wound infection develops in the graft site of a patient with a mandibular continuity defect, the graft might fail.[13] Every effort must be made to eliminate those factors

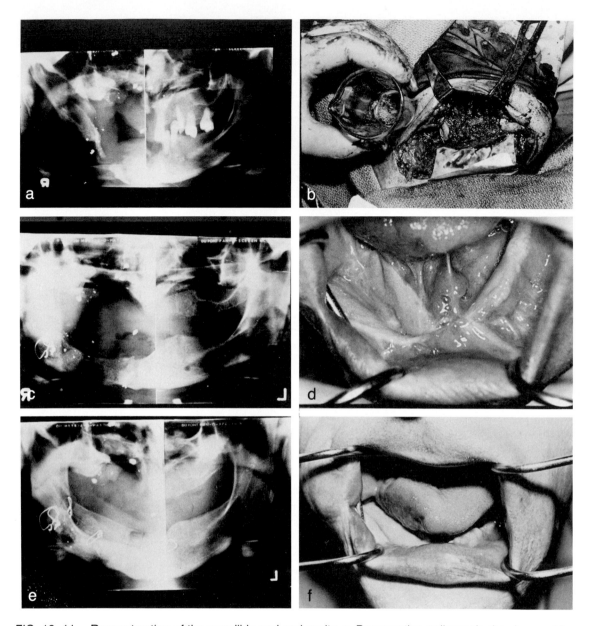

FIG. 12–11.   Reconstruction of the mandible and oral cavity. **a,** Preoperative radiograph showing avulsion of the right body of the mandible resulting from a gunshot injury. **b,** Medial placement of the usual inner superior rim of the iliac crest and particulate cancellous bone were stabilized by the double wire compression technique and an extraskeletal facial fixation device. A Millipore filter was wrapped around the graft to protect it from possible oral contamination. **c,** Postoperative view of the successful bone graft. **d,** Intraoral skin graft. **e,** Postoperative view of the transoral placement of a graft to create an alveolar ridge to support either a conventional denture or implants. **f,** Intraoral view of the mandibular ridge form.

that contribute to the development of infections. The bone segments and the recipient soft-tissue bed should be adequately debrided before a graft is placed; debridement includes the removal of nonvital teeth and foreign bodies close to the graft site. Every effort should

be made to prevent hematoma formation in and around the graft, because hematoma is a potential culture medium for bacteria, and its presence interferes with the early nutrition of the graft. The best method to prevent hematoma is to close the wound carefully and eliminate open spaces. If infection occurs, early and aggressive management is necessary.

Experience gained during the Korean War, which coincided with the widespread availability and use of antibiotics, suggested that the deferring of bone grafting procedures be reduced from the usual 3-month period between the last signs of infection and placement of the graft. With technical advances, improved antibiotics, and continuing improvement in supportive pre- and postoperative care, the length of deferral of bone graft placement should be reduced. At present, grafts are placed almost immediately or after a delay of just weeks.

Perforation of the oral mucosa that is not corrected creates a significant complication, because the contaminated wound markedly increases the possibility of infection at the surgical site. A perforation that occurs at the time of surgery should be repaired with a watertight closure. If the perforation occurs in the presence of a particulate cancellous bone and marrow graft with a metallic crib, prognosis for survival of the graft is poor.

In cases in which adequate soft-tissue flaps are not established and the tissues are under tension because of the closure over the bone plate or crib, dehiscence may occur. Treatment may consist of daily irrigations with no attempt to close the soft tissues surgically.

Another complication is aseptic necrosis, which may arise without clinical signs of infection and usually is associated with instability of the graft-host interface.

INTRAORAL RECONSTRUCTION

Watertight closure of the oral mucosa is a primary consideration in all of the surgical phases, from the initial treatment through the reconstructive phases. The closure may result in distortion of the oral structures that will inhibit normal function and interfere with the construction and wearing of a prosthesis or will lead to periodontal maladies. Nevetheless, the objective of a watertight closure should not be compromised. During the late reconstructive phases of treatment, the surgeon can perform procedures usually associated with preprosthodontic surgery, such as

vestibuloplasties and modification of the floor of the mouth using mucosal or skin grafting procedures (Fig. 12–11).

REFERENCES

1. Jones, J.C., et al.: Mandibular bone grafts with surface decalcified bone. J Oral Surg 30:269, 1972.
2. Urist, M.R., et al.: The bone induction principle. Clin Orthop 53:243, 1967.
3. Urist, M.R.: Bone formation by autoinduction. Science 150:893, 1965.
4. Urist, M.R.: Fundamental and Clinical Bone Physiology. Philadelphia, J. B. Lippincott Co., 1980, p. 331.
5. Breine, U., and Branemark, P.I.: Reconstruction of alveolar jaw bone. An experimental and clinical study of immediate and preformed autologous bone grafts in combination with osseointegrated implants. Scan J Plast Reconstr Surg 14:23, 1980.
6. Urist, M.R., Mikulski, A.J., and Boyd, S.D.: A chemosterilized antigen extracted bone morphogenetic alloimplant. Arch Surg 110:416, 1975.
7. Urist, M.R., Mikulski, A.J., and Lietze, A.: Solubilized and unsolubilized bone morphogenetic protein. Proc Natl Acad Sci 76:1828, 1979.
8. Sabet, T.Y.: Bone grafts: cellular survival versus induction. J Bone Joint Surg 45A:337, 1963.
9. Hurley, L.A., Stinchfield, F.E., Bassett, C.A.L., and Lyon, W.H.: The role of soft tissues in osteogenesis. J Bone Joint Surg 41A:1243, 1959.
10. Truetta, J.: The role of vessels in osteogenesis. J Bone Joint Surg 45B:402, 1963.
11. Stringa, G.: Studies of the vascularization of bone grafts. J Bone Joint Surg 39:395, 1957.
12. Emeking, W.F., and Morris, J.L.: Human autologous cortical bone transplants. Clin Orthop 87:28, 1972.
13. Marx, R.E., Snyder, R.M., and Kline, S.N.: Cellular survival of human marrow during placement of marrow-cancellous bone grafts. J Oral Surg 37:712, 1979.
14. Osbon, D.B., Lilly, G.E., Thompson, C.W., and Jost, T.: Bone grafts with surface decalcified allogeneic and particulate autologous bone: report of cases. J Oral Surg 35:276, 1977.
15. Osbon, D.B.: Intermediate and reconstructive care of maxillofacial missile wounds. J Oral Surg 31:429, 1973.
16. Pike, R.L., and Boyne, P.J.: Use of surface-decalcified allogeneic bone and autogenous marrow in extensive mandibular defects. J Oral Surg 32:177, 1974.
17. DeChamplain, R.W.: Mandibular reconstruction. J Oral Surg 31:448, 1973.
18. MacIntosh, B.R.B., and Henny, F.A.: A spectrum of application of autogenous costochondral grafts. J Maxillofac Sur 5:257, 1977.
19. Boyne, P.J.: Restoration of osseous defects in maxillofacial casualities. J Am Dent Assoc 78:767, 1969.
20. Boyne, P.J.: Autogenous cancellous bone and marrow transplants. Clin Orthop 73:199, 1979.
21. Boyne, P.J.: Tissue transplantation *In* Textbook of

Oral Surgery. 5th Ed. Edited by G.O. Kruger., St. Louis, C. V. Mosby Co., 1979, p. 286.

22. Leake, D., and Habal, M.B.: Mandibular reconstruction and craniofacial fairing. Br J Oral Surg 16:198, 1979.

23. Marx, R.E., et al.: The use of freeze-dried allogenic bone in oral and maxillofacial surgery. J Oral Surg 39:265, 1981.

24. Kline, S.N., and Rimer, S.R.: Reconstruction of osseous defects with freeze-dried allogeneic and autogenic bone. Am J Surg 146:471, 1983.

25. Alling, C.C.: Hydroxylapatite augmentation of edentulous ridges. J Prosthet Dent 52:828, 1984.

26. Kent, J.N., et al.: Temporomandibular condylar prosthesis: a ten year report. J Oral Maxillofac Surg 41:245, 1983.

27. Kent, J.N., et al.: Experience with a polymer glenoid fossa prosthesis for partial or total temporomandibular joint reconstruction. J Oral Maxillofac Surg 44:520, 1986.

28. Panje, W., and Cutting C.: Trapezius osteomyocutaneous island flap for reconstruction of the anterior floor of the mouth and the mandible. Head Neck Surg 3:66, 1980.

29. Green, M.F., Gibson, J.R., Bryson, J.R., and Thomson, E.: A one-stage correction of mandibular defects using a split sterum pectoralis major osteo-musculocutaneous transfer. Br J Plast Surg 34:11, 1981.

30. Bell, M.S., and Barron, P.T.: The rib-pectoralis major osteomyocutaneous flap. Ann Plast Surg 6:347, 1981.

31. Barnes, D.R., Ossoff, R.H., Pecaro, B., and Sisson, G.A.: Immediate reconstruction of mandibular defects with a composite sternocleidomastoid musculoclavicular graft. Arch Otolaryngol 107:722, 1981.

32. Donoff, R.B., and May, J.W.: Microvascular mandibular reconstruction. J Oral Maxillofac Surg 40:122, 1982.

33. Fonseca, R., and Davis, W.H.: Reconstructive Preprosthetic Oral and Maxillofacial Surgery. Philadelphia, W. B. Saunders Co., 1986.

13

COMPLEX MAXILLOFACIAL INJURIES

GUY A. CATONE

This chapter will describe the sequencing of care in complex maxillofacial fractures and will include examples of management of complicated fractures of the midfacial skeleton.

Usually, the maxillofacial surgeon manages facial skeletal fractures from the inferior structures to the superior structures by establishing a stable mandible and then reducing midfacial fractures from the occlusal plane in a cephalad direction toward a stable cranial base. Elective orthognathic and craniofacial surgical techniques often use a superior to inferior sequencing of surgery; this order can also be used in panfacial trauma, especially if the mandibular injuries include bilateral dislocated condylar process fractures or avulsive losses of sections of the mandible.

Advances in imaging technologies have featured computed tomography (CT), which permits the development of three-dimensional programs and hence the generation of models of the facial skeleton. The models assist surgeons in assessing damage and calculating quantitative injury and guide reconstruction in the operating room. Also, the recent acceptance of bone plates for skeletal rigid fixation has opened new options for treatment of facial skeletal fractures.

Though new technologies abound, the historical orthopedic principles of the 4 Rs of fracture management, recognition, reduction, retention, and rehabilitation, are still fundamental in managing facial fractures.

THE IMPACT OF TRAUMA

Complex maxillofacial injuries usually co-exist with multiple-system trauma and rarely exist in isolation (Fig. 13–1). Trauma is the leading cause of death and disability in patients between the ages of 1 and 38[1,2] and ranks as the fourth leading cause of death in the U.S. overall, superseded only by heart

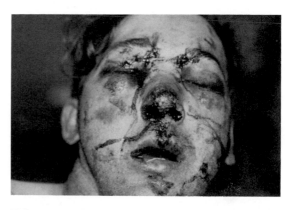

FIG. 13–1. Typical multiple complex maxillofacial injury after a highway vehicular accident. Note asymmetry and elongation of the face.

disease, cancer, and cerebrovascular disease. Because trauma victims are disproportionately younger, the cost of unnecessary loss of productive life is incalculable.

Statistics compiled by the Department of Health and Human Services showed that, for Americans between the ages of 15 and 24, the combined death rates from motor vehicle accidents, homicides, and suicides has risen 50% since 1976. The contribution to this mortality rate of motor vehicle accidents has risen steadily throughout this century, now exceeding 45%. Multiple-system trauma results in more than 50% of all deaths in the pediatric population from ages 1 through 14.[3] In both age groups, motor vehicle accidents are the major source of traumatic events. By far, the greatest lethality is seen in young male drivers associated with drug and alcohol abuse (Fig. 13–2).

Trunkey described a trimodal distribution curve representing the pattern of death from trauma. The death rate is plotted as a function of time after injury, producing three peaks in the graph (Fig. 13–3). The first peak represents immediate deaths, patients who die very soon after an injury. These deaths can be attributed to lacerations of the brain, the brain stem, the spinal cord, the aorta, or the heart. In the best of conditions, only a very small proportion of patients with these injuries can be salvaged. The second peak on the graph represents early deaths. These people die within the first few hours after a traumatic event, usually with major internal hemorrhage involving the intracranial region (epidural or subdural hematomas), hemopneumothorax, abdominal injuries, pelvic fractures, and major long-bone fractures. Many smaller simultaneous injuries that result in extensive blood loss also contribute to this peak. This second peak represents injuries that are treatable with current medical technology. If the interval between the traumatic event and resuscitation can be decreased, the statistical probability of recovery

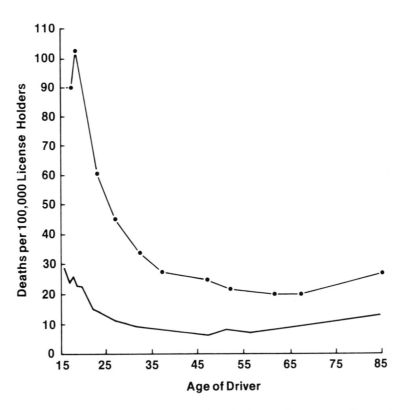

FIG. 13–2.   Graph indicating sex and age with regard to death rate from traumatic events involving motor vehicles. Peak indicates high percentages of young male drivers, usually alcohol abusers. (Solid line = females; dotted line = males)

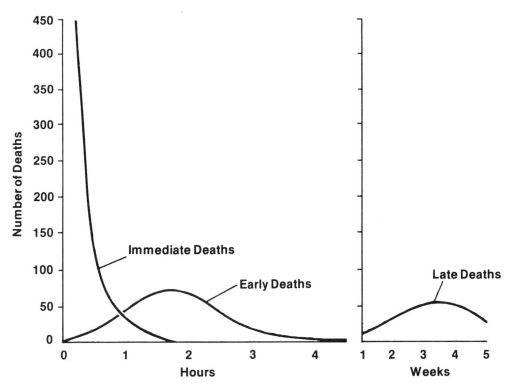

FIG. 13–3.   Trunkey's trimodal wave.[4]

is enhanced, and coexisting maxillofacial in-juries can be addressed. The last peak in Trunkey's trimodal curve is described by Trunkey as late deaths. These patients die days or weeks after an injury, in 80% of cases from multiple organ failure or sepsis.

Patients in the first peak of the trimodal curve represent 50% of all trauma deaths. A small number of patients in this category could have been saved by emergency trans-portation systems and trauma centers com-mitted to providing 24-hour coverage by general surgeons or traumatologists, neuro-surgeons, anesthesiologists and supporting surgical specialties. Trunkey noted that, of patients showing signs of life at the scene of an accident or in transit to the hospital who are described as dead on arrival, 20% can be resuscitated in the emergency room and will eventually leave the hospital without per-manent neurologic damage.

Approximately 30% of the deaths from trauma occur in the second peak. Patients who survive early death in Trunkey's trimo-dal curve have treatable maxillofacial injuries. Survivors in this category can be classified as

having one of two major pathologic condi-tions, neurologic injuries and various hem-orrhagic phenomena. About 22% of all hos-pital admissions in the U.S. are for head and spinal cord injuries, representing 34,000 cases of intracranial bleeds treated annually. If sur-gical intervention for intracranial bleeding is delayed for more than 4 hr after an injury, the most probable outcome is death or per-manent disability. Definitive surgical care within the first 4 hr improves outcome sig-nificantly. Prompt attention to injuries result-ing in hemorrhage can affect outcome posi-tively. Hemorrhage is assigned various grades; in severe hemorrhage, the rate of blood loss exceeds 150 ml/min, resulting in at least 1500 ml of blood loss in the first 10 min (or one third of the blood volume) and one half of the blood volume in 20 min after the injury. In moderate hemorrhage, with bleed-ing rates between 30 and 150 ml/min, life-threatening blood loss will occur within 1 hr after the injury. In minor hemorrhage, with rates of less than 30 ml/min, 1 hour can elapse before surgical intervention is necessary. Prompt intervention with intravenous lines started before arrival at the hospital keeps up with the bleeding.

In recent years, the character of treated maxillofacial injuries in multiple-trauma victims has changed somewhat because of advances in medical and surgical technology, improved coordination of emergency medical services, development of regional trauma centers, and rapid evacuation of injured patients to such treatment centers. Of critical importance is the interval between injury and surgical intervention (Fig. 13–4). During World War I, the interval between injury and surgery averaged between 12 and 18 hr, and the overall mortality rate was 8.5%. This time was reduced in World War II to between 6 and 12 hr, with the mortality rate falling to 5.8%. During the Korean War, MASH units decreased the average time lag to within 2 and 4 hr and reduced the mortality rate to 2.4%. In the Vietnam War, the average interval between injury and definitive surgical management was reduced to 65 min and mortality rates fell to 1.7%.[4] During all phases of the Vietnam War, fully trained surgical specialists, including oral and maxillofacial surgeons, were located throughout the combat zones. The saving of lives, and the salvaging of destroyed faces, was without parallel in the history of land warfare.

While these results seem dramatically significant, they had very little impact on civilian attitudes toward the care of trauma victims, and legislation and implementation of regional trauma units was slow in Western countries.

THE TRAUMA CENTER

In the mid-1960s, a regional trauma center was established at the Cooke County Medical Center in Chicago.[5] This center led to improvements in evacuation and transportation of patients injured in traffic accidents or industrial traumatic events. It also established an experimental milieu in which to study the effects on civilian casualties of rapid evacuation to and communication with regional center staffed by general surgeons who had basic interests in trauma. Later, as the concept of regional trauma centers began to be accepted, the trauma team evolved to encompass more than general and orthopedic surgeons, and included neurosurgeons and the surgical specialties. The organization of regional trauma centers led to legislation that integrated a system of standardized quality control and pro-

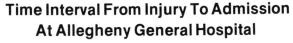

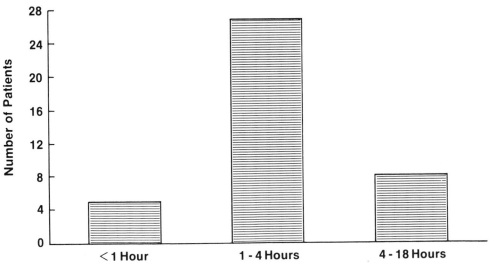

FIG. 13–4.   A study of actual intervals of treating consecutive trauma patients admitted to the Trauma Unit at Allegheny General Hospital, Pittsburgh, Pennsylvania.

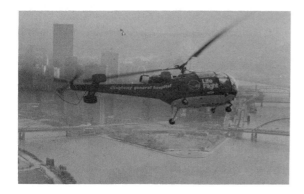

FIG. 13–5. Typical helicopter used as part of a rapid evacuation system for trauma patients coordinated through a Level 1 trauma center in a civilian setting in Pittsburgh, Pennsylvania.

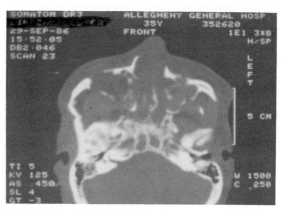

FIG. 13–6. Axial CT scan of high-impact force directed over a broad surface of the facial skeleton, resulting in extensive comminution and fragmentation.

vided economic incentives for the establishment of such centers.

A Level I trauma center is a center where comprehensive care will be delivered to a patient immediately on arrival. Head injuries sustained in traffic accidents are usually seen by a neurosurgeon immediately, along with the traumatologist who initially cares for the patient. In Level I trauma centers, 24-hr availability of CT scanning, intracranial pressure monitoring, early operative decompression, and intensive care nursing have had a profound effect on the multiply injured patient with a life-threatening head injury. The rapid initial treatment by general surgery of injuries of the thorax and abdomen has enabled the maxillofacial surgeon to manage patients who in the past would have succumbed to their multiple-system traumata.

As a tertiary care institution, Allegheny General Hospital (AGH) in Pittsburgh, Pennsylvania, committed its resources to becoming a regional Level I trauma center in western Pennsylvania, serving regions of Pennsylvania, Maryland, Ohio, West Virginia, and New York. Under the name "Life Flight," the regional emergency medical air transport service was instituted in 1978. Since that time, the program has expanded from one helicopter to a service of three jet-assisted helicopters combined with a fixed wing aircraft capability (Fig. 13–5). Life Flight serves public safety and emergency medical service agencies, hospitals, and other health care facilities, recreational areas, businesses, and industries

within a 130–air mile radius of Pittsburgh. Life Flight works with approximately 200 health care facilities in its service area as well as major specialty centers in eastern United States. Since its inception, Life Flight has logged more than 10,000 flights. The monthly flight average has risen from 33 in 1978 to 165 flights as of December 1986.

The AGH Life Flight staff includes 20 flight nurses, 5 dispatchers, 6 pilots, 3 mechanics, a medical director, a program manager, an outreach coordinator, and secretarial staff. The Life Flight nurses are all registered nurses who are certified in advanced cardiac life support, have audited advanced trauma life support training sponsored by the American College of Surgeons, and have completed a special 160-hour training program before being assigned to the helicopters. The entire trauma support staff is managed by a traumatologist–general surgeon who directs activities of other surgical specialists, trauma fellows, residents, and educational and research programs arising from the trauma center.

PATTERNS OF MAXILLOFACIAL INJURIES

The high-impact force that is characteristic of road accidents is responsible for the extensive comminution and fragmentation of the maxillofacial skeleton seen in those with multiple-system injuries who survive early death (Fig. 13–6). Dolan and Jacoby[6] showed that

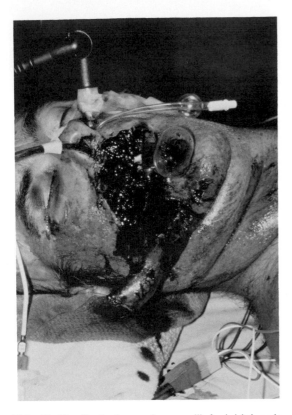

FIG. 13–7. Typical complex maxillofacial injury in which at least two of the facial thirds are involved in severe bony comminution and avulsion of hard and soft tissues.

high impact distributed over a broad area of the facial skeleton produces extensive comminution and atypical patterns of maxillofacial bony disruptions. Thus, the historical classifications of facial skeletal dislocations in many instances do not apply to the high-velocity, high-impact facial injury.

A casual review of the literature and an examination of the AGH trauma registry reveals an increasing number of maxillofacial trauma patients with complex maxillofacial injuries and associated general injuries. Complex maxillofacial injuries can be defined as those injuries involving two thirds or more of the facial skeleton in patterns that do not coincide with historical classifications or are characterized by significant loss of hard or soft tissue (Fig. 13–7). Midfacial fractures and composite injuries consisting of disruptions involving combinations of upper, middle, and lower facial structures has increased. Some European centers have reported that midfacial trauma

has increased as much as 554% since World War II.[7] In addition, the ratio of midfacial fractures to mandibular fractures has steadily increased. In addition to a quantitative increase in the number of orbital floor fractures, we at AGH have noted an associated increase in severity, as in loss or avulsion of the orbital floor into the maxillary antrum, necessitating primary or delayed reconstruction by bone grafting (Fig. 13–8). The severity and complexity of the maxillofacial injuries, combined with loss of substance and the need to manage the systemic complications of multiple-organ system involvement in multiple-trauma patients, has led to a reassessment of the classic management of facial trauma. Specifically, surgeons have applied craniofacial technologies designed to treat developmental orthognathic and congenital facial skeletal anomalies and rigid orthopedic fixation techniques to the problems associated with repair of unusual fragmentation of the maxillofacial complex.

The historical classification of midfacial fractures into three categories by Le Fort[8] has been used by surgeons in this century to diagnose, classify, and design treatment plans to manage such injuries (Fig. 13–9). This classification, while still useful, is not always applicable to the high-velocity, high-impact complex maxillofacial skeletal injury when fracture lines overlap and extensive comminution or avulsion of tissue is present. Most complex maxillofacial injuries do not easily fit into the Le Fort classification. Instead, the classification of complex maxillofacial injuries is based on the major craniofacial skeletal regions involved and cephalad-caudad combinations including transverse and coronal planes.

In addition to complex injuries of the maxillofacial skeleton, disruption of the superior aspects of the facial skeleton with the frontal bone can occur, allowing coexistence of frontobasilar skull fractures and nasal-ethmoidal-orbital injuries (Fig. 13–10). Nasoethmoidal injuries can exist with complex orbital injuries in which loss of substance is characteristic. All of these midfacial injuries can coexist with unusually comminuted or dislocated fractures of the mandible. Complex maxillofacial injuries can be categorized by using the above

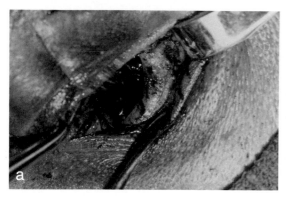 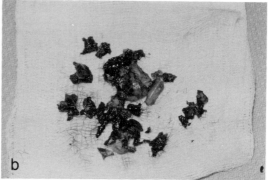

FIG. 13–8.   Orbital floor fracture. **a,** Total disruption of the orbital floor in severe maxillofacial injury. **b,** Multiple bony fragments of the fractured orbital floor retrieved from the maxillary sinus.

Le Fort classification, in which injuries would involve two or more thirds of the face, as in frontobasilar, nasoethmoidal, or complex orbital trauma; mixed Le Fort fractures involving right and left sides with different Le Fort classifications; and combinations of the Le Fort classification in which two or more Le Forts coexist. Lastly, the entire midfacial skeletal fracture complex could occur with a severely fractured mandible.

All other factors being equal or stable, the earliest possible care of facial injuries is essential to avoid irreparable deformity or dysfunction. The major objectives in complex maxillofacial trauma are to preserve life, restore function, decrease deformity, and allow reconstruction of any residual deformity. Hence, complex craniomaxillofacial trauma is managed by a team usually combining many specialties, especially neurosurgery and maxillofacial surgery. With comminution of the cranial vault, it may be necessary to consider first providing rigid interosseous fixation of the cranial vault, followed by fixation of the maxillofacial skeleton to the cranium. With avulsion of cranial bony elements it may be prudent to repair the maxillofacial skeleton and fixate the reconstructed face to the remaining cranial vault, followed immediately by primary bone grafting using split or intact ribs. These surgical approaches to direct repair will require access through the primary

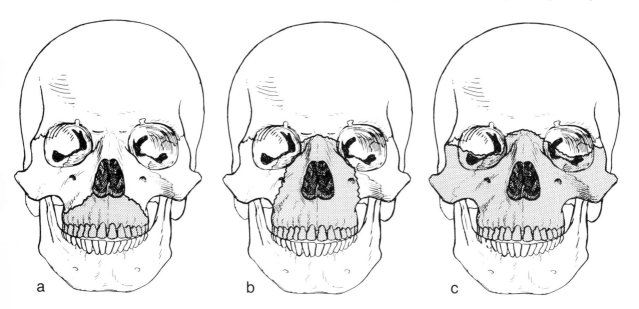

FIG. 13–9.   Le Fort fracture lines. **a,** Le Fort I. **b,** Le Fort II. **c,** Le Fort III.

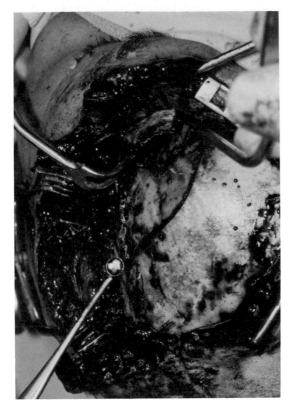

FIG. 13–10. Typical frontobasilar skull fracture co-existing with a midfacial component.

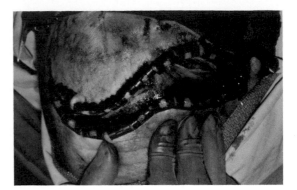

FIG. 13–11. Coronal flap, as usually used during the elective-in-time treatment of craniofacial anomalies, is applied to the management of complex maxillofacial injuries.

laceration or an extension thereof or the use of designed craniofacial flaps. Therefore, the usual application of closed reduction techniques and internal suspension with the focus on the mandible as the initial bone to be reconstructed can, in selected instances be replaced by craniofacial techniques that advocate multiple open procedures with variations of coronal flaps (Fig. 13–11) and direct bony apposition using rigid osteosynthesis and primary or delayed bone grafting (Fig. 13–12). Other new technologies applied to complex maxillofacial injuries include the early use of CT scanning and three-dimensional imaging and modeling (Fig. 13–13) to enhance the surgical planning and probability of a favorable surgical outcome.

GENERAL PRINCIPLES IN THE SEQUENCING OF CARE IN PATIENTS WITH COMPLEX MAXILLOFACIAL INJURIES

Traditional methods of sequencing and surgical management of maxillofacial injuries

that follow conventional classic fracture lines are no less important in the management of complex maxillofacial trauma. However, some modifications must be considered when dealing with complex multiple-region fractures of the facial skeleton. These modifications have their origin in orthognathic and other craniofacial surgical procedures and in the use of rigid skeletal fixation. If the patient has a severely comminuted mandible and midfacial fractures, the usual method of first treating the mandibular fractures to establish a mandibular occlusal plane, followed by inferior to superior skeletal reconstruction, is not possible when there is no reproducible mandibular plane from which to reconstruct the midface. In these cases, the principles of orthognathic and craniofacial surgical technology are used so that each fractured bone is repaired in sequence from superior intact structures. The bones of the upper and midface are repaired directly by rigid fixation followed by reconstruction of the mandibular plane. A corollary to this technique is seen in orthognathic surgery in which the maxilla is first repositioned relative to the cranial base via an interim splint, followed by osteotomy and repositioning of the mandible to the established maxillary occlusal plane.

AIRWAY

Complex maxillofacial injuries often involve the nasal complex and comminution of the mandible. These conditions pose a serious threat to survival because of partial or com-

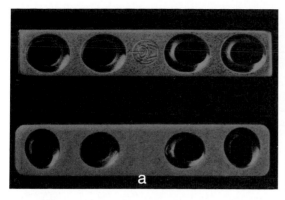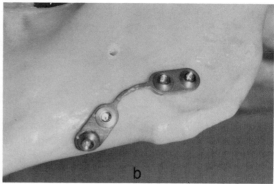

FIG. 13–12.   Rigid osteosynthesis. **a,** Rigid fixation bone plate commonly used in mandibular fracture management. **b,** Hall Reconstructive Systems bone plate designed for ease in contouring and using splined screwheads.

plete airway obstruction. In most major road accidents in which a high-velocity, high-impact event has occurred, an endotracheal tube has already been placed before the patient is brought to the hospital. If the patient is arriving from a primary or secondary care hospital, he may already have had a tracheostomy. However, if an airway is not provided, the first objective of care is to provide a patent airway.

In addition to factors such as foreign bodies, secretions, and hemorrhage into the oral cavity, oral pharynx, and upper airway, comminution of the mandible will result in posterior displacement of the tongue. The impact of forces will rapidly cause edema of the epiglottis, lateral pharynx, retropharynx, larynx, or laryngeal-hypopharyngeal region and will cause air emphysema when the upper airway passages have ruptured. High-velocity anteriorly directed forces, e.g., a steering wheel that directs the larynx posteriorly against the unyielding cervical spine, also result in blunt and penetrating trauma to the larynx and hypopharynx. This impact vector of force will produce occult disruptions of the cartilage mucosa of the endolarynx or will perforate or rend the hypopharynx. Unfortunately, such occult injuries are not seen by the tertiary care clinician. In the multiple-trauma patient, hoarseness, dysphonia, dysphagia, and stridorous respirations may suggest the diagnosis. In most cases, superficial abrasions in the anterior cervical region and a noticeable loss of the prominence of the thyroid cartilage occur. There may also be crepitus from subcutaneous emphysema.

In such blunt and penetrating trauma to the larynx, immediate tracheostomy can be life-saving. Significantly, CT scanning of the patient's intracranial status, which is performed after many laryngeal-hypopharyngeal injuries, can be extended to the cervical region so that a laryngeal fracture can be diagnosed definitively. At the AGH Trauma Center, oral or nasal intubation is contraindicated in controlling the airway in a suspected laryngeal fracture; triple endoscopy can be performed to determine whether open repair is needed. Attempted endotracheal intubation might cause pseudopassage formation, hemorrhage, and edema, and the significantly compromised airway can be completely obstructed, necessitating emergency surgical intervention. Usually, a tracheotomy is established low, at the level of the third or fourth tracheal ring. Higher entrances into the trachea would not establish a patent airway. The indications for tracheostomy include thyrohyoid separation, thyroid or cricoid cartilage fractures, vocal cord injury, mucosal rents with underlying cartilage, and perforation of the hypopharynx.

Complex fractures of the midface or crush injuries traversing the nasal airways are also factors resulting in loss of normal airway patency. Moreover, severe comminution of the midface results in retroposition and loss of airway. Attempting to open the airway with a nasopharyngeal or oral airway is not usually feasible and many times is contraindicated because severe comminution in these regions and the placement of airways may stimulate

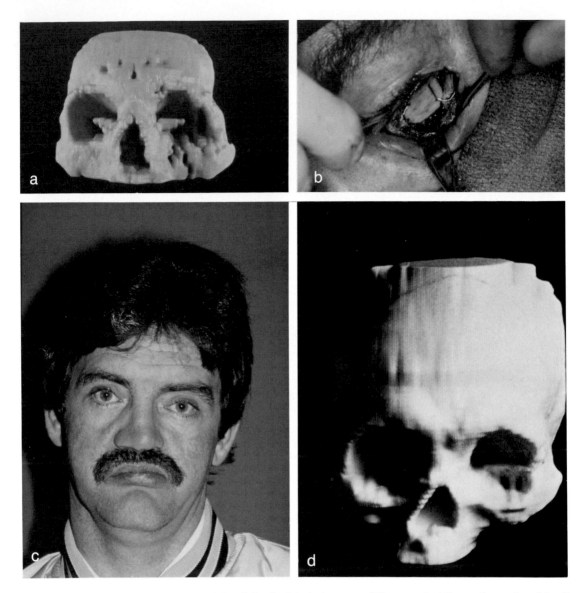

FIG. 13–13.   Three-dimensional models of the facial skeleton. **a,** CT-generated three-dimensional Lucite model of complex orbitozygomaticomaxillary injury with destruction of the orbital floor. **b,** Rib bone graft to the left orbital floor. The planning and operative phases were facilitated by the model of the patient's facial bones. **c,** Facies, and **d,** CT-generated three-dimensional Lucite model of a patient with untreated malunited midfacial fractures. The patient was subsequently treated with osteotomies to reposition the ZMCs and augmentation with Proplast malar implants.

emesis and possible aspiration. Most patients with comminution of the facial skeleton will arrive at the hospital with an endotracheal tube or an emergency cricothyrotomy or tracheotomy.

When obvious blunt trauma to the upper airway involving the larynx and/or superior tracheobronchial tree has occurred, a tracheostomy is performed. Complex maxillofacial trauma usually coexists with multiple system injuries, and while immediate tracheostomy is not required, a limited surgical entrance into the airway using a cricothyrotomy has been used at the AGH Trauma Center with success and low morbidity. A tracheostomy or cricothyrotomy enables the surgical management of many traumatically involved body systems and the use of general anesthetics.

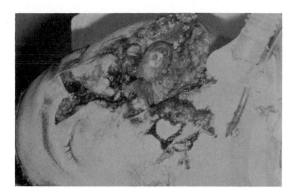

FIG. 13–14.   Typical close-range maxillofacial gunshot wound with immediate threat to the airway, necessitating tracheostomy.

Table 13–1.   Problems of Prolonged Endotracheal Intubation

1. Loss of airway from significant edema or hemorrhage after inappropriate early removal
2. Irritation and laceration of the mucosa of the upper airway
3. Entrance into the intracranial fossa during intubation (nasal) when significant traumatic disruption of the cribriform plate is present
4. Contamination of the superior nasal cavity and the development of subsequent retrograde meningitis
5. Occlusion of the distal lumen by blood clot and/or mucus plugs
6. Pulmonary complications resulting from lack of capability to provide aggressive pulmonary toilet

While tracheostomy may have complications, it is used in those maxillofacial injuries involving crush trauma to the midface that destroy the nasal airway, such as are caused by high-velocity motor vehicle accidents; close-range gunshot wounds (Fig. 13–14); gunshot wounds to the tongue and oropharynx; closed and open head injuries causing significant cortical and lower center obtundation such that the patient is unable to maintain a patent airway; when significant disruption of the cribriform plate has occurred with concomitant cerebrospinal fluid leakage; and when maxillomandibular fixation and edema further compromise the airway.

The use of tracheostomy in isolated maxillofacial trauma has declined since the introduction of endotracheal tubes fabricated from soft, flexible polyethylene that create significantly less trauma to the mucosal lining of the larynx and trachea; these tubes can be left in place for days or weeks provided that appropriate care and surveillance is maintained. On the other hand, the use of the short-term cricothyrotomy to gain access to the airway has improved the management of severe complex maxillofacial injuries and provides total access to the facial bones for improved reconstruction without the encumberances and complications associated with prolonged endotracheal intubation. The complications of prolonged endotracheal intubation are well known to the maxillofacial surgeon (Table 13–1). While the use of a cuffed endotracheal tube prevents further aspiration of blood and other fluids, it also seals off the peripheral

space between the trachea and the endotracheal tube, so that in the event of distal occlusion of the lumen of the endotracheal tube, there is no possibility of any exchange of air or the entry of oxygen.

HEMORRHAGE

Massive hemorrhage in isolated maxillofacial injuries is uncommon and hypovolemic shock from maxillofacial hemorrhage is rare. However, hemorrhages in the airway and from the scalp and massive hemorrhages in the nasal-ethmoidal-orbital regions can be life threatening.

Nasopharyngeal and Scalp Hemorrhages

Aspiration of blood from persistent hemorrhage from the nasopharyngeal region can complicate surgical management and can result in significant morbidity and mortality. Persistent undetected hemorrhage from apparent and occult scalp lacerations can result in significant blood loss, even to levels producing shock (Fig. 13–15). Such insidious scalp hemorrhage results from the maintenance of scalp vessel patency by contiguous elastic fibers of the galea aponeurotica.

Nasal-Ethmoidal-Orbital Hemorrhages

Midfacial hemorrhage usually occurs in nasal-ethmoidal-orbital injuries and Le Fort II and III fractures. In nasal-ethmoidal-orbital injuries, bleeding usually occurs from the angular or infraorbital arteries, and retrobulbar

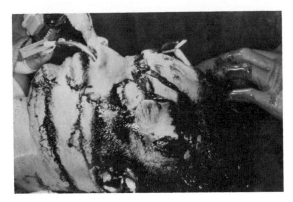

FIG. 13–15.   Multiple scalp lacerations resulting in a large blood loss that could cause hypotension.

hemorrhage can accompany nasoethmoidal and Le Fort II and III fractures (Fig. 13–16) (Table 13–2). Retrobulbar hemorrhage and the development of hematomas are rare because the blood will flow by gravity into the adjacent paranasal sinuses (Fig. 13–17). However, as the complexity and severity of the injury increase, the incidence of retrobulbar hemorrhage is more likely, and a hematoma is a sign of fracture of the base of the skull. In midfacial injuries such as fracture of the zygomatic complex, retrobulbar hemorrhage has been observed in 0.3% of cases.[9] When retrobulbar hemorrhage is suspected, the management must be immediate and effective if vision is to be preserved.[10]

It is assumed that such a hemorrhage occurs within the muscle cone and leads to pressure on the short posterior ciliary arteries.[11] This pressure causes a significant alteration of the perfusion pressure of the globe. As a consequence, intraocular pressure rises, causing an anterior displacement of the iris and occlusion of the aqueous drainage system of the anterior chamber resulting in a traumatic glaucoma. There is eventual ischemia, then collapse of the central retinal arteries associated with edema and venous congestion surrounding the optic nerve head.

The management of retrobulbar hemorrhage focuses on reducing edema, the inflammatory reaction, and vascular spasm and on surgical operations designed to decompress the intraconal space. The survival time of the optic nerve and retinal cells, which are anatomically part of the central nervous system, after total loss of blood supply is not much better than that of brain tissue, and hence treatment must be prompt. Rowe advocates the medical management of retrobulbar hemorrhage based on the intravenous use of mannitol 200 ml of a 20% solution and 50 mg of acetazolamide, which have been used to reduce the hydration of the vitreous and the rate of formation of aqueous humor. Intravenous administration of papaverine causes a relaxation of vascular spasm of the retinal arterioles. The use of high-dose steroid regimens such as dexamethasone sodium phosphate intravenously at a dose rate of 4 mg/kg of body weight as a loading dose, reduced to 1 mg/kg at 6-hour intervals for 48 hours, has also been used. Surgery designed to decompress the orbit and the intraconal space is approached above and below the lateral palpebral ligament through the septum orbitale. For a lateral canthotomy, the approach should be through the lateral canthus to allow the globe to move farther forward. The problem of retrobulbar hemorrhage and blindness must be addressed by the ophthalmologist

Table 13–2.   Retrobulbar Hemorrhage (Orbital Apex Syndrome)

Observations	Etiology
Pain	Retrobulbar neuritis
Tense, hard globe	Increased intraocular pressure
Proptosis	Physical presence of retrobulbar blood
Pupillary dilatation	Interference with parasympathetics of oculomotor nerve
Ophthalmoplegia	Extraocular muscle involvement secondary to cranial nerves III, IV, VI
Decreased visual acuity, diplopia	Possible optic nerve ischemia Possible anterior displacement of globe

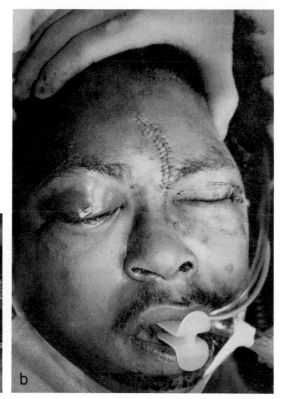

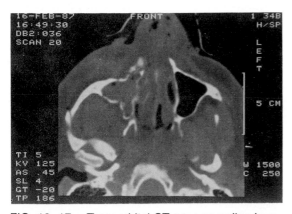

FIG. 13–16.   Proptosis. **a,** Severe proptosis secondary to retrobulbar hemorrhage. Patient was struck by a pipe in the right ZMC region. **b,** The patient was treated with enucleation of the right eye, temporary globe prosthesis, and tarsorrhaphy.

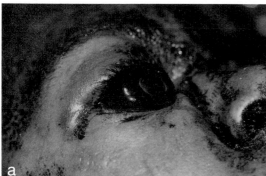

FIG. 13–17.   Transorbital CT scan revealing hemorrhage into the sphenoidal, ethmoidal, and maxillary sinuses. These repositories for bleeding allow decompression of the orbit and reduce the potentially morbid retrobulbar bleeding.

during this critical phase following trauma. The most important factor in dealing with retrobulbar hemorrhage is early diagnosis, and CT scanning has enabled early detection of the site and nature of displacement of bone on the soft tissues (see Chapter 3, Part II). Manfredi et al.[12] noted that if CT showed hemorrhage in the ethmoidal air sinuses and sphenoidal sinuses, optic nerve impairment or compression was likely (Fig. 13–17).

Further injury to the eye should be assessed by the ophthalmologist as part of the protocol in the initial assessment of the multiple-trauma patient with coexisting maxillofacial trauma. Patients with periorbital ecchymosis and edema or lid lacerations associated with chemosis and proptosis should be suspected of having occult injuries involving the globe. In a group of over 700 maxillofacial injury patients who had ophthalmologic evaluation, 67% sustained some form of ocular injury. This percentage increased to 76% in a group of patients with midfacial injuries.[13] Major injury to the globe such as rupture and laceration with loss of sight has varied widely. However, Luce reported an incidence of 2.5%.[14] Of course, the incidence of ophthalmologic injuries increases in patients with orbital trauma; this has been reported in 29% of such patients.[15]

More obvious injuries such as hyphema, soft globe, loss of light perception, scleral laceration, and herniation of the vitreous can all be detected on the initial examination by the trauma surgeon or oral and maxillofacial surgeon. Though curious injuries such as superior orbital fissure syndrome have dramatic clinical presentation, ophthalmologic signs usually resolve (Fig. 13–18) (Table 13–3). All patients with injuries to the midface and upper face such as the frontobasilar skull region, the nasal-ethmoidal-orbital and zygomatic area, and the maxillary complex should be seen by the ophthalmologist either initially or soon after stabilization.

Hemostasis

Hemostasis is usually obtained by immobilizing the maxillofacial skeleton using an appropriate Barton's bandage. Persistent bleeding from the palatal suture or inferior alveolar arteries can be controlled by temporary maxillary fixation or simple bridging wires across the fracture sites using the teeth for stability. Using an external bandage and maxillomandibular fixation, the maxilla is stabilized against the base of the skull, resulting in tamponade of vessels in this region. The decrease in maxillary and mandibular movement provided by immobilization allows effective co-agulation of blood and the arrest of hemorrhage in most cases.

In the emergent phase, most hemorrhage is controlled by direct pressure over the persistently bleeding site. Unless there is a clear indication of a lumen, direct clamping and ligation of arteries is not performed. Nonspecific clamping and attempted ligation often results in injury to proximal and distal segments of important nerves such as the facial nerve. Digital pressure over proximal arterial trunks in an attempt to control distal hemorrhage especially over the carotid artery should not be performed; digital pressure over the carotid artery, especially in older patients, can result in severe intracranial circulatory compromise, especially during the hypotension of the acute post-traumatic phase. The maxillofacial surgeon should also be aware of the possibility of injury to the carotid artery, if there is blunt cervical trauma from a mandibular fracture as part of the total maxillofacial injury. Blunt trauma to the carotid artery can result in a delayed hemiparesis because of dislodgement or fragmentation of an intraluminal thrombus and is associated with a 50 to 60% mortality rate[16] (Fig. 13–19).

Persistent nasopharyngeal hemorrhage is usually controlled and a patent airway provided using a small nasal inflatable device or balloon inserted into the nasal passage and nasopharynx and gently inflated (Fig. 13–20). The use of a nasal balloon device should be weighed against the possibility of meningitis if the device is left in place in excess of 48 hours.

Massive Hemorrhage

After resuscitation, the maxillofacial complex can undergo massive hemorrhage after

Table 13–3. Superior Orbital Fissure Syndrome

Observations	Etiology
Exophthalmos	Paresis of extraocular muscles Retrobulbar hemorrhage
Retrobulbar pain	Injury to first division of trigeminal nerve
Ophthalmoplegia	Paresis of extraocular muscles secondary to cranial nerves III, IV, VI
Fixed, dilated pupil	Injury to parasympathetics of iris (cranial nerve III)
Anesthesia (skin, cornea)	Injury to branches of maxillary division of trigeminal (V2)
Loss of corneal reflex arc	Injury to branches of V2

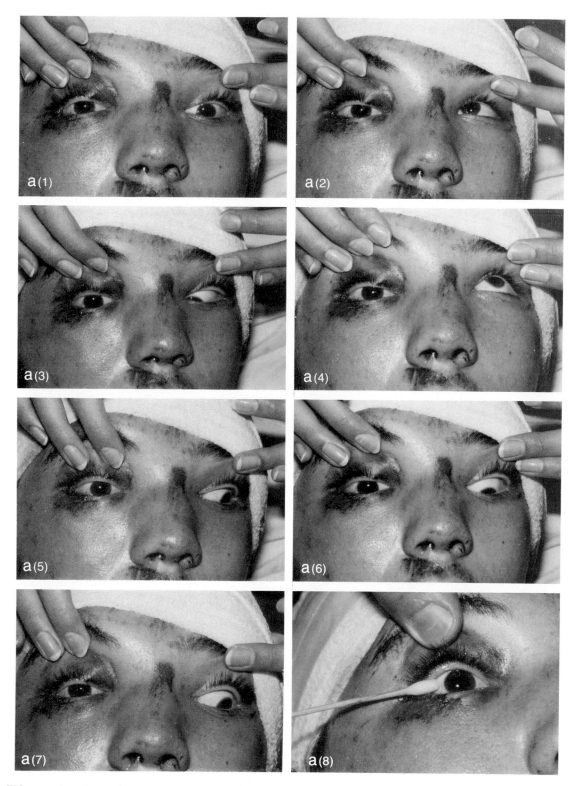

FIG. 13–18.   Superior orbital fissure syndrome. **a,** Complete ophthalmoplegia of the right eye through all cardinal movements of the eyes. **1,** Superior orbital fissure syndrome. **2,** Intorsion, adduction of the upward gaze, left eye. **3,** Intorsion, adduction of the downward gaze, left eye. **4,** Upward gaze. **5,** Extorsion, abduction of the lateral gaze, left eye. **6,** Downward gaze, **7,** Extorsion, abduction of the downward lateral gaze, left eye. **8,** Anesthesia of the cornea.

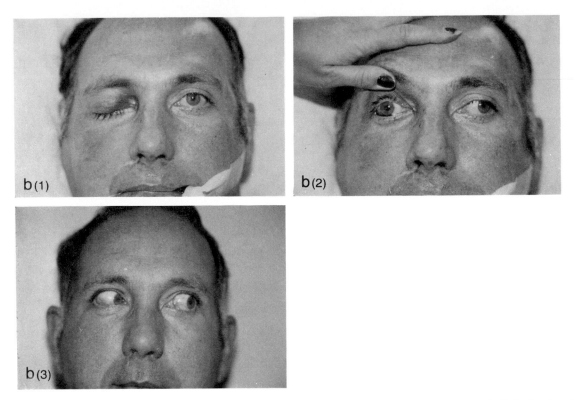

FIG. 13–18 (continued). **b,** Resolution of signs during the intermediate postoperative period. **1,** Ptosis of right eyelid. **2,** Ptosis of right eyelid, ophthalmoplegia, right eye. **3,** Patient at 4 months post-trauma demonstrates resolution of disturbed extraocular muscle.

successful therapy for shock increases blood pressure; hemorrhage usually indicates the presence of wide fracture sites within the midfacial skeleton. These fractures allow blood to flow unencumbered into the nasal cavity and then into the pharyngeal and oral cavities. The origin of bleeding may be the pterygopalatine segment of the internal maxillary artery, lacerated at a fracture site between the posterior wall of the maxillary sinus and the pterygoid process. If the venous plexus circumscribing the artery is lacerated, the bleeding will be even more severe.

If hemorrhage from the nasopharyngeal region is not responsive to tamponade, direct ligation of the internal maxillary artery must be planned. The internal maxillary artery can be approached through an entrance into the maxillary sinus by a Caldwell-Luc maneuver and from there through the medial posterior wall of the sinus, followed by application of arterial clips on the bleeding vessels. The presence of adipose and loose connective tis-

sue in this region can complicate this approach. The transantral approach to the internal maxillary artery is facilitated by comminution of the walls of the maxillary sinus, which can occur in severe complex maxillofacial injuries. This approach may not be successful, however, especially in massive facial trauma in which persistent hemorrhage fills the maxillary sinus.[17]

An alternative to the transantral approach to the peripheral branches of the internal maxillary artery is intraoral ligation of the internal maxillary artery, proposed by Macri and Makielski.[18] In this procedure, the internal maxillary artery is identified through an incision made in the mucogingival fold just posterior to the maxillary tuberosity and lateral to the first and second molars. The dissection is carried down to the temporalis muscle through which the artery is identified; vascular clips are applied on the artery, two on the proximal side and one on the distal side. While this maneuver does not address

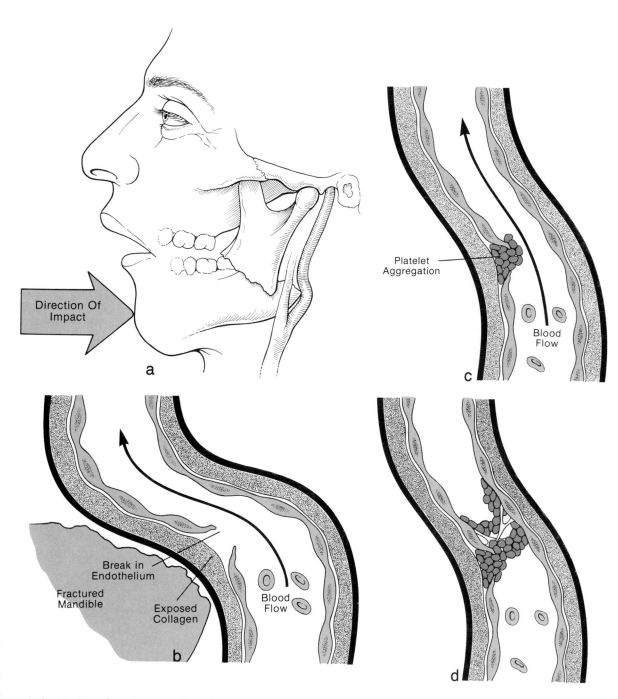

FIG. 13–19.   Carotid artery thrombosis. **a,** Fracture displacement of the mandible resulting in blunt injury to the carotid arterial system. **b,** The blunt trauma can result in a rent in the intima. **c,** A rent in the intima results in platelet aggregation and eventual thrombus formation. **d,** The intraluminal thrombus almost complete, with resultant arterial occlusion.

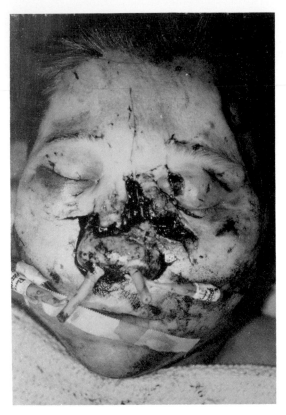

FIG. 13–20. Nasal balloons for control of naso-pharyngeal hemorrhage.

the most distal branches of the artery, it is enough to decrease the pressure gradient at the nasal capillary bed without rendering the nose avascular.

Posterior epistaxis can also be controlled by ligating the anterior and posterior ethmoidal arteries, which are branches of the internal carotid system. The anterior and posterior ethmoidal artery is approached through a curvilinear vertical incision at the medial canthal region of the orbit. The dissection is carried bluntly along the medial wall of the orbit and the lamina papyracea of the ethmoidal bone. The anterior and posterior arteries are then identified along the medial wall of the orbit and clipped with small vascular clips. External carotid artery embolization or ligation has been used to treat persistent epistaxis but may not be completely effective because of collateral vessels.

The external carotid artery has numerous collateral vessels and affects the blood supply of the superficial temporal, posterior auricu-

lar, and internal maxillary arteries. Ligation of the external carotid artery at the mandibular angle may not be effective because the artery is proximal to the bleeding sites of midfacial injuries. Nonetheless, ligation of this vessel has been used to control or to decrease hemorrhage from the maxillofacial complex. The usual justification for ligation of the carotid artery is massive bleeding from the nasopharyngeal or maxillary region of the oral cavity uncontrollable by nasal tamponade. After an incision in the skin at the angle of the mandible, the platysma muscle is exposed and divided. The dissection is carried deep between the angle of the mandible and lower pole of the parotid gland to expose the upper margin of the stylohyoid muscle and posterior belly of the digastric muscle. The external carotid artery is immediately below these structures.

During the treatment of soft-tissue injuries, the bleeding branches of the facial artery and vein or other distal arteries of the midface are identified, clamped, ligated, or electrocoagulated. Rarely is ligation of the lingual artery necessary in maxillofacial trauma. Ligation of the lingual artery is undertaken only when closure of injuries involving the floor of the mouth and tongue does not result in hemostasis and when persistent bleeding into the neck originates from the wounds of the tongue and the mouth floor. Ligation of the lingual artery is carried out through a submandibular incision. After the submandibular gland is identified and retracted superiorly, the hyoglossus muscle is identified just posterior to the proximal edge of the mylohyoid muscle. An incision through the hyoglossus muscle will locate the lingual artery and its posterior branches supplying the posterior tongue and floor of the mouth. After adequate exposure, the artery can be occluded with vascular clips.

NEUROLOGIC CONSIDERATIONS

Closed and open head injuries often coexist with maxillofacial injuries. It is important that the neurosurgeon and maxillofacial surgeon coordinate their efforts relating to the timing of operative intervention so that unnecessary use of anesthetics or duplication of surgical operative sites will not follow.

Concurrent Neurosurgical and Maxillofacial Injuries

At the AGH Trauma Center, significant head injuries are monitored and managed by the neurosurgical department. The maxillofacial injuries are addressed in most cases when the patient's neurologic status has stabilized and he has a high Glasgow Coma Score. In the majority of severe head injuries, a ventriculostomy is performed to monitor intracranial pressure (ICP). When the ICP is stabilized within the normal range or has reached a reasonable equilibrium, maxillofacial surgery is scheduled. The ICP can be controlled to some extent by drawing off cerebrospinal fluid (CSF) when pressures become dangerous.

Adjacent maxillofacial injuries and neurosurgical injuries can be treated simultaneously. Extension of the scalp lacerations and utilization of appropriate craniofacial flaps combined with selected maxillofacial surgical incisions will allow excellent exposure and visualization for repair of neurosurgical, craniofacial, orbital, and midfacial injuries. The neurosurgical procedure is performed first, because guaranteeing vitality of the brain has priority and because operations involving maxillofacial reconstruction usually take longer.

Cervical Spine Injuries

Of primary importance in the sequence of care in maxillofacial trauma is the early diagnosis of cervical spine injuries (Fig. 13–21), the only diagnosis that must be made prior to any intervention or manipulation of the patient. Most patients arriving at the hospital have been intubated using traction on the cervical spine so that the intubation is performed "in line," minimizing injury to the cervical cord. Most trauma patients will also have a Philadelphia collar that is removed only after radiographic studies ensure that there is no fracture dislocation of the cervical spine. When the results are uncertain, the lateral cross table cervical spine radiograph can be supplemented by the swimmer's view or the use of pluridirectional tomography or CT scanning of the cervical spine region. Determining the status of the cervical spine is especially critical when there is a question involving the area of C7 and T1 (see Chapter 3, Part II).

At autopsy, the frequency of cervical spine fractures in motor vehicle accidents is 25%.[19] Incidence of cervical spine injuries in patients with concomitant maxillofacial skeletal injuries has been recorded as 2 to 4%.[20] There is a biomechanical relationship between injuries of the cervical spine and soft tissue and maxillofacial skeletal injuries.[21] Lewis, et al. studied the relationship between maxillofacial trauma and cervical spine injury in two major trauma centers. Similar to the study by Trunkey,[4] the population examined was young adult males associated with a high frequency of alcohol abuse injured in motor vehicle accidents. Of 982 patients with spinal cord injury examined by Lewis and co-workers, 190 (19.3%) had associated soft-tissue and skeletal injuries. The majority of these spinal injuries involved the lower cervical spine, with smaller percentages in the middle and upper regions. Significantly, the most frequent spinal injury was a fracture dislocation with subgroups of hangman's fracture and high cervical fracture. The hangman's fracture is a bilateral avulsion fracture of the arch of C2 combined with an anterior fracture dislocation of the axis through the interspace of C2-C3.[22] This location is of special importance to the maxillofacial surgeon because at the levels of the hangman's fracture, the spinal canal is wide relative to the cord, so that the chances of permanent neurologic injury are less. Lewis and others found that among the facial and skeletal injuries there were 138 soft-tissue injuries (in 14% of patients) and 84 fractures (in 8.6% of patients). In the majority of instances, these fractures involved the mandible and were related to injuries of the upper cervical spine. The facial soft-tissue lacerations, affecting mostly the upper face and skull, occurred with greatest frequency in injuries of the lower cervical spine.

Lacerations of the scalp and face associated with cervical cord injury are treated after management of the cervical injury, usually in

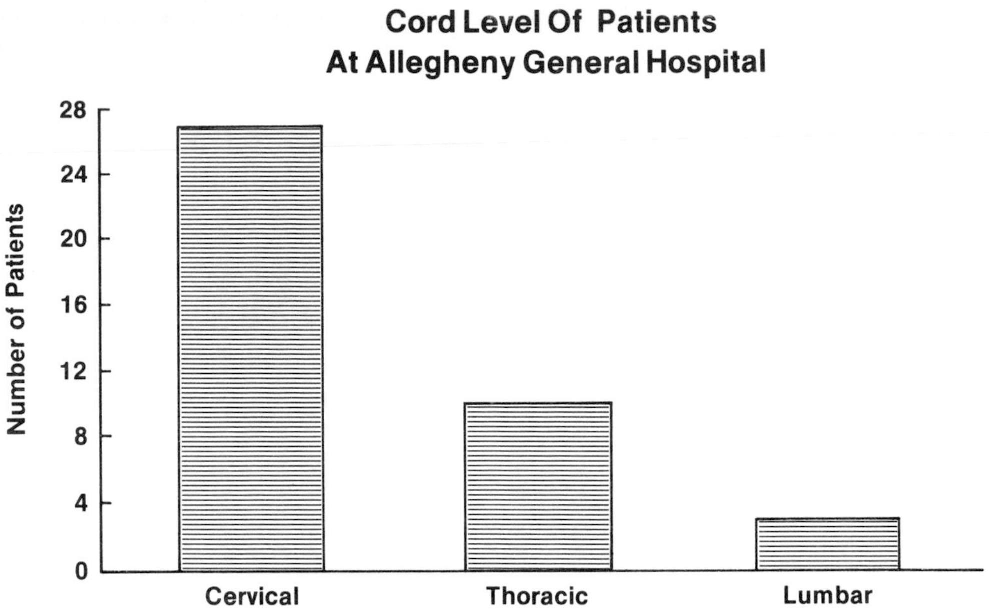

Cord Level Of Patients
At Allegheny General Hospital

FIG. 13–21.   A study of the level of spinal cord injuries in consecutive trauma patients admitted to Allegheny General Hospital, Pittsburgh, Pennsylvania.

the trauma unit, where appropriate soft-tissue instrumentation is provided. Unusual wounds that involve extensive avulsion or necessitate extensive debridement are managed in the operating room after halo frame stabilization of the cervical spine. Maxillofacial injuries can be addressed after the patient is fixed on the operating table and the table is rotated along its long axis to the appropriate position to gain access to the injury. In the AGH Trauma Center, reconstructive procedures are deferred until the patient is stabilized or is brought to the operating room for associated procedures. After cervical injuries are stabilized with halo frames, external skeletal fixation using Morris appliances can be useful to overcome the difficulty of obtaining access for open reduction. When open mandibular procedures are indicated, however, it may be necessary to operate despite the vertical rods extending from the halo to the thoracic shell. The patient's table can be rotated as long as the halo frame remains fixed to enhance access to the mandible.

Cerebrospinal Fluid Leakages

Patients with midfacial/frontobasilar fractures may have leakage of CSF (Fig. 13–22).

Though CSF leakage may present as rhinorrhea or otorrhea, CSF can leak from any site, such as from a frontal laceration. Definitive localization of the site of leakage can be determined by contrast studies involving appropriate CT scanning (see Chapter 3, Part II). The patient's bed is elevated in a semi-Fowler's position to approximately 40 to 60°. This position allows soft tissue superior to the intracranial communications to plug or bridge the rents in the dura at the base of the skull. A ventriculostomy (ICP monitor) will assess CSF pressure, and CSF can be drawn off at the ventriculostomy site to decrease the loss of CSF externally and to control rising CSF pressure. Valsalva maneuvers are avoided, and nose blowing, sneezing, and coughing are monitored and controlled by the nursing staff. Antibiotics are selected based on culture of the nasal secretion and ability to cross the blood-brain barrier in the maxillofacial trauma setting.

Early reduction and fixation of midfacial fractures will reduce the CSF leakage; CSF discharge should cease in 5 to 14 days. If the CSF discharge persists longer than 2 weeks or is intermittent, or if a delayed leak persists for 2 weeks or an expanding pneumocephalus occurs, craniotomy with dural repair may be

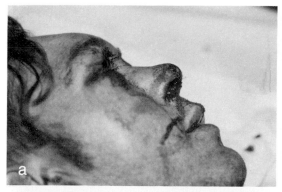

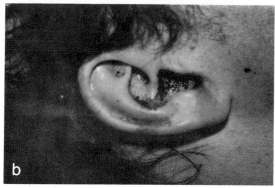

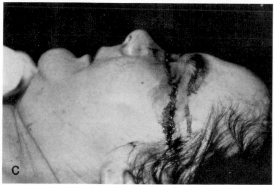

FIG. 13–22.   Cerebrospinal fluid leaks. **a,** Spinal rhinorrhea in a patient with Le Fort III fracture. **b,** Clear fluid otorrhea collecting in the ear concha. This fluid was confirmed as spinal fluid, an indication of a basilar skull fracture. **c,** Patient with a fracture of the posterior wall of the frontal sinus with CSF discharge directly through the open laceration.

imperative. Because the CSF discharge causes decompression and can mask the occult presence of an expanding intracranial mass of vascular origin, patients with CSF discharge should be monitored continuously via ventriculostomy.

MANAGEMENT OF COMPLEX MAXILLOFACIAL INJURIES

The surgical management of complex maxillofacial soft-tissue injuries is based on general surgical principles and sequencing dictated by the nature of the injury. In most complex maxillofacial injuries involving many sites, a tracheostomy is performed soon after wounding using either local anesthesia or, if an endotracheal tube is being placed, general anesthesia.

SOFT-TISSUE INJURIES

After securing the airway, controlling hemorrhage, and managing shock, neurosurgical injuries, and other systems injuries, the surgeon treats soft-tissue wounds of the facial region. Road accidents and industrial acci-

dents usually produce wounds contaminated with dirt, road tar, and other foreign bodies. By using a nitrogen-driven intermittent irrigation jet (Sympulse), the amount of contamination and the presence of foreign matter in the wound can be significantly reduced (Fig. 13–23). After irrigation and debridement, the underlying facial skeletal fractures are eval-

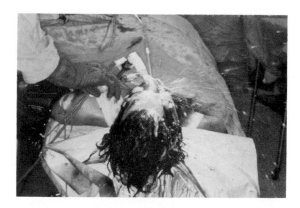

FIG. 13–23.   Nitrogen gas–powered irrigation device (Sympulse) in use to irrigate severe facial laceration caused by ejection through a windshield of an automobile in a highway accident. The operating team should wear protective eyeshields when using the device.

uated, and open reduction of obvious fractures can be performed through soft-tissue lacerations.

Injuries involving the parotid duct are treated using a small polyethylene catheter to bridge the rupture in the lumen of this structure. The duct can then be sutured directly under 2.5-power loupes. During debridement, distal and proximal stumps of severed branches of the facial nerve can be tagged with colored sutures and later repaired under the microscope using an epineural approximation. In the midface, the medial and lateral canthal ligaments can be resutured either to themselves or to contiguous bone using non-resorbable sutures of fine braided stainless steel wire. Injured lacrimal structures are usually not repaired immediately. Their repair can be delayed by enlarging the lacrimal fossa with a trephine and placing within the nasal cavity a catheter that exits in the lacrimal fossa; a soft silicone rubber cannula is placed through the inferior aspect of the lacrimal duct and then through the lumen of the catheter (Fig. 13–24) and is left in place at least 3 months. In frontobasilar nasoethmoidal injuries in which significant damage to the nasofrontal duct has occurred, the neurosurgical department may elect to re-establish the patency of the duct by placing a catheter from

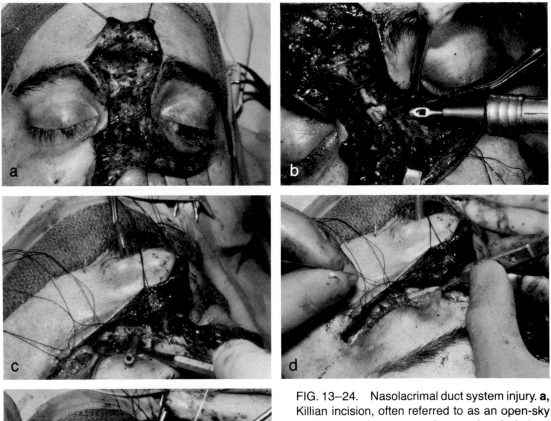

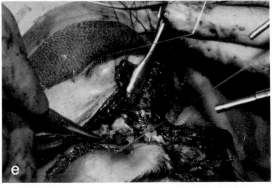

FIG. 13–24. Nasolacrimal duct system injury. **a,** Killian incision, often referred to as an open-sky incision, used to approach associated skeletal injuries and provide access to the nasolacrimal duct system. **b,** Trephine bur used to enlarge the region of the bony entrance into the nasal cavity from the lacrimal sac. **c,** Foley catheter threaded into the nostril and brought into the wound via the trephination entry hole. **d,** Silicone rubber tube placed into the canaliculus and threaded through the Foley catheter. **e,** Silicone rubber catheter (Gabor catheter) in place. The ends of the catheter will be brought together and will remain in place for 3 months.

the opening of the nasofrontal duct in the floor of the frontal sinus and from there into the superior nasal cavity to exit the nares. The frontal sinus can be obliterated by many means, depending on the character of the injury and the preference of the surgeon.

INFERIOR TO SUPERIOR RECONSTRUCTION (Caudad to Cephalad)

The management of maxillofacial skeletal fractures centers on establishing a stable and functional occlusal relationship. Usually the sequence of surgical care of facial fractures depends on establishing an intact mandible and then building on the occlusal plane superiorly to the next stable bone in a cephalad direction.

Managing the Mandible

If the mandible is not fractured or if its fractures can be reduced, management of facial fractures is directed to the establishment of the occlusal plane. The mandible can be reestablished by using closed and open reduction modalities including double wire compression fixation and by using rigid fixation by eccentric dynamic compression bone plates. Bilateral condylar fractures are treated by managing at least one side with an open reduction (Chapter 6). If a burst fracture of the condyloid process or vertical ramus complex exists, a costochondral rib graft (Fig. 13–25) is used to represent the lateral aspect of the vertical ramus; if a portion of the prox-

imal horizontal ramus is intact, it is placed against that bone. The need for early mobility may dictate the use of lag screws in strategic locations to fixate the costochondral graft.

Application of a maxillary arch bar usually results in the reduction and stabilization of a midline palatal fracture. Unless this fracture is severely displaced, open reduction is usually not indicated, as has been shown in numerous orthognathic surgical procedures in which the palate is sectioned and maxillomandibular fixation holds the palatal bones passively until bony union. In addition, as part of this phase, soft-tissue lacerations involving the tongue, soft palate, midline of the hard palate, buccal mucosa, and floor of the mouth can be closed using a resorbable gut suture or a longer-lasting polyglycolic acid suture.

A stable mandible, or an intact mandible in the presence of midfacial injuries after application of arch bars, can be brought against the maxillary occlusal plane to determine the anteroposterior position of the maxilla, and maxillomandibular fixation wire can be applied. This maneuver does not assure the vertical dimension of the face which is achieved by direct reduction and fixation of the midfacial bony structure by intrasinal packing and support procedures (Chapter 7).

The bony fragments of the maxilla that may be partially impacted must be mobilized, as is performed in orthognathic surgical procedures of the midfacial skeleton. If the maxilla is impacted posteriorly, disimpaction and reduction can be accomplished using the ap-

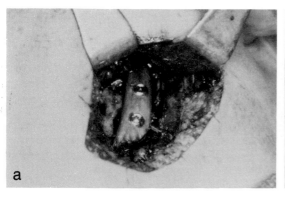 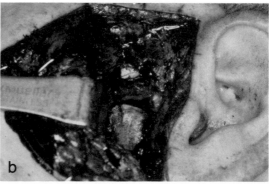

FIG. 13–25.   Costochondral rib graft. **a,** Two lag screws hold a costochondral rib graft in place on the lateral aspect of the mandibular vertical ramus. **b,** View of the superior aspect of a costochondral graft as it abuts the glenoid fossa.

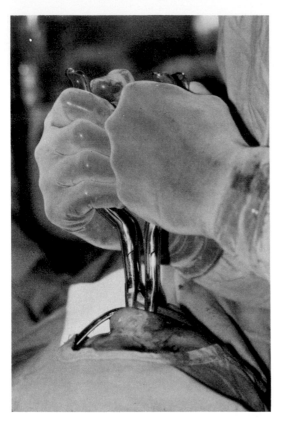

FIG. 13–26. The use of the Rowe disimpaction forceps to re-establish an antatomic alignment of the facial skeleton. The fractured segments must be completely mobilized to allow subsequent maxillomandibular fixation to be passive.

Table 13–4. Steps in the Surgical Management of Complex Maxillofacial Injuries

1. Tracheostomy (or limited cricothyrotomy), if indicated
2. Debridement (use of pulsatile irrigation) and management of injuries to soft tissues
3. Repair of intraoral lacerations, and removal or salvage of avulsed and partially avulsed bone and tooth structure
4. Application of arch bars or other indicated fracture devices
5. Reduction and fixation of dentoalveolar components and palatal fracture
6. Disimpaction of the maxilla or midface
7. Maxillomandibular fixation
8. Establishment of integrity of mandible, if indicated, with open reduction and transosseous fixation
9. Final confirmation of AP dimension of face with special attention to the condyloid process of the mandible
10. Reduction and fixation of midfacial components
11. Reassessment of need for external skeletal fixation

propriate disimpaction forceps (Fig. 13–26). The disimpaction forceps will allow anterior repositioning of the maxilla to meet a stable mandibular occlusal plane. The maxilla and mandible should rest passively against one another prior to the application of rigid skeletal fixation, which is usually performed from a cephalad direction. If bilateral condyloid process fractures of the mandible are present, the surgeon should avoid attempting to re-establish the anteroposterior relationship of the maxilla to the mandible. At least a unilateral open reduction of a condyloid process fracture should be performed to establish the position of the face in the anteroposterior dimension. Usually the open reduction of the condyloid process is carried out on either the most severely dislocated side or the side with the longest proximal segment. In unusual cases such as bilateral burst fracture of the condyloid processes in the presence of an intact glenoid fossa, an anatomic position of the maxilla relative to the cranial base is established. Maxillomandibular fixation and open reduction of the condyloid process, removal of the stump or fragments, and placement of costochondral rib grafts bilaterally follow to establish AP relationships. With bilateral fractured condyloid processes without fragmentation, in order to begin to establish AP and vertical relationships, the surgeon might need to apply external skeletal fixation using a light-weight Morris headframe with struts extending to the angles of the mandible. A pin can be placed at the angle or at the midbody region of the mandible and be fixated to the vertical strut to establish a vertical position and to assist in establishing the AP dimension of the face (Table 13–4).

After the anteroposterior facial dimension is established and the vertical dimension is first confirmed, with special attention to the condyloid processes of the mandible, fractures of the midfacial complex can then be addressed. The first phase of the biphasic device can be secured to the angle of the mandible and can be finally tightened when open reduction is performed on midfacial fractures. Open reduction is usually employed in those complex injuries in which a headframe has been placed. If using suspensory techniques, the surgeon prevents a telescoping of the midface by intrasinal supports, bone plates, or both.

Le Fort Fractures

Most classic Le Fort fractures can be stabilized either by performing direct transosseous internal reduction through an open approach or by suspending the midfacial fractures between the mandible and cranial base using several suspending wires. The suspending wires arise from the zygomatic arches, lateral infraorbital rims, piriform aperture, anterior nasal spine, and zygomatic processes of the frontal bone. Usually, intraspinal supporting packing or balloons are necessary for vertical stability. Whether external skeletal fixation will be used should be decided on early in the intermediate phases of treatment, as it is usually the first maneuver that is performed during the surgical reduction and fixation of maxillofacial injuries. A Morris or Irby headframe or halo-type apparatus is applied to the calvarium. These halo-type headframes can be used even if portions of the skull are fractured. In these cases, the fracture sites must be well known by the surgeon, and intact calvarial bone must be chosen to support the frame. Vertical rods can be attached to the lateral aspect of the headframe and thus provide support and fixation for the mandible, or ZMC. A vertical wire in the midline of the face can support a severely depressed nasal bridge after wires have been passed through the lateral nasal bones and attached through suspensory wires to the vertical midline outrigger of the headframe.

Headframes secure the midface against the cranial base and enable an early release of maxillomandibular fixation. In some cases, maxillomandibular fixation can be eliminated through the use of rigid bone plate support of mandibular fractures. Headframes are especially indicated when mobile midfacial fracture components coexist with bilateral fractures of the condyloid process of the mandible and in fractures of the midface to maintain vertical dimensions where extensive comminution or avulsion of the bone has occurred.

In edentulous patients, the patient's dentures or a Gunning splint can be used to establish anteroposterior and vertical dimension of the face. The mandibular splint is fastened using circummandibular wire ligatures of 24 or 25-gauge wire placed in the midline and at each parasymphysis or body of the mandible. Maxillary splints are stabilized to the maxilla by various methods, such as passing perialveolar wires through the alveolus of the maxilla, into the palate, and around the maxillary splint through a hole in the palatal aspect of the splint. Splints can be fastened to the alveolus of the maxilla by passing threaded or nonthreaded Kirschner wires through the acrylic flanges of the maxillary denture or splint directly through the alveolar bone across the palate and into the body of the zygomas. Direct wiring of a maxillary splint to the anterior nasal spine and the buttresses of the zygomas bilaterally will secure the apparatus to the maxilla. The procedure can be varied by suspending the prosthesis from the upper face, depending on the level of the midfacial fracture. One can place suspension wires from the zygomatic arch or the lateral orbital rim to the posterior aspect of the maxillary prosthesis in Le Fort II fractures. In Le Fort III fractures, suspension wires from the zygomatic process of the frontal bone to the posterior maxillary prosthesis can be used. In those instances, the apparatus is ligated to the anterior nasal spine.

When external skeletal fixation is used on the mandible and severe midfacial injuries are present, a biphasic device used to stabilize the mandibular fractures can be attached to vertical struts from a headframe.

Usually, isolated Le Fort I fractures of the maxilla are managed by maxillomandibular fixation and suspension from the zygomatic buttresses. The surgeon can use intraoral incisions to gain access to the entire anterior and lateral wall of the maxilla. In cases of combined Le Fort I and II fractures, direct open reduction of the maxilla can be performed with transosseous wire sutures or small bone plates at the piriform aperture and on the zygoma where the buttress makes its inferior-medial bend toward the lateral wall of the maxilla. Exploration can be directed superiorly to the infraorbital rims. Le Fort II frac-

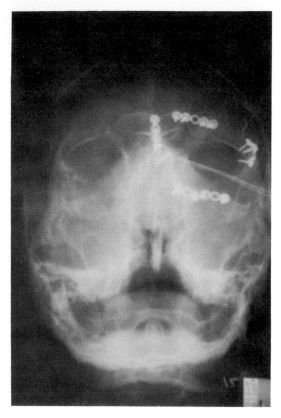

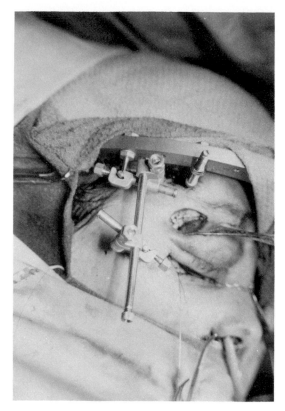

FIG. 13–27. Radiograph displaying osteosynthesis bone plates used to reconstruct the periorbital bony rim. Adaptation-type plates are seen at the supra- and infraorbital margins. A rigid bone plate at the frontozygomatic suture may be used to treat many ZMC fractures.

FIG. 13–28. Immobilization of a severely dislocated, unstable fractured zygoma by an intramedullary pin placed into the body of the zygoma and attached to a headframe.

tures can be reduced and fixed by placing an orbital rim wire or minibone plate lateral to the infraorbital neurovascular bundle.

In cases of severe impaction of the maxilla in which retropositioning and fragmentation has occurred in the region of the pterygoid plates, the surgeon can place autogenous or allogeneic bone blocks in the regions of the pterygoid plates to assist in securing an anterior repositioning of the maxilla.

Access to the body of the zygoma can be gained through intraoral incisions, and ZMC fractures can be reduced with an elevating instrument and can be fixed with bone plates or transosseous wire to the infraorbital rim, in addition to being fixated at the frontozygomatic suture (Fig. 13–27). In cases of very mobile, apparently irreducible zygomas, a Morris pin can be placed into the body of the

zygoma and the zygoma fixated to a strut dropped from a headframe (Fig. 13–28).

In Le Fort III fractures, a craniofacial dysfunction, many methods to secure stabilization, in addition to reduction and fixation at the frontozygomatic suture line, must be performed. In most cases, an incision is made directly over the frontozygomatic suture into the hair of the lateral portion of the eyebrow, and the bones of the frontal process of the zygoma and the zygomatic process of the frontal bone are identified. Holes are drilled from anterior to posterior into the temporal fossa through the superior and inferior bony segments. A horizontal mattress suture of 24- or 25-gauge stainless steel is passed from anterior to posterior through each hole and the wire-twisted stump is buried in the posterior aspect of the zygomatic process of the frontal bone.

Bone Grafts for Avulsive Midfacial Defects

In large avulsive defects of the midface, one can place bone grafts through a transoral incision. The integrity of the bone graft can be better assured by closing in layers when surgery is completed.

To succeed, bone grafts require firm contact with the recipient sites, soft-tissue coverage, freedom from infection, and immobilization. If these factors cannot be provided in treatment of a midfacial skeleton shattered by trauma, the surgeon must rely on time-proven techniques of reduction and fixation of the fractures by molding and manipulating bony fragments and providing intrasinal support by packing or balloons. In most cases, of course, the surgeon can use a variety of techniques, including approaches to the skeleton through lacerations, intraoral incisions, facial incisions, and coronal incisions; placement in intrasinal supports of packing or balloons; and transosseous wires or small plates, as indicated.

The bone grafts of the midface can be placed in strategic areas, at once bridging the bony defect and providing additional internal support for the facial complex. A frequently observed avulsive injury is one in which the anterior wall of the maxilla and infraorbital rims have been lost and the entire floor of the orbit might be missing (Fig. 13–8). Split-rib grafts are placed on the anterior wall of the maxilla and bridge gaps in the bone from the body of the zygoma to the piriform and dentoalveolar region of the maxilla. The bone grafts can be secured using Kirschner wires (Fig. 13–29). After the graft is fastened into position, the threaded Kirschner wire is cut off with a small fissure bur. In the region of the lost orbital floor, a full-thickness rib graft can be cantilevered by driving a small unthreaded Kirschner wire through the body of an intact zygoma and skewering the rib graft (Fig. 13–30). The Kirschner wire is cut off approximately 1 cm from the stab incision in the skin overlying the zygoma and covered by a sterile rubber stopper or cork. The Kirschner wire is left in place 6 weeks and removed under local anesthesia. Thus, the architecture of the midface can be preserved using the struts of split ribs as an additional fixation device to not only establish aesthetics and contour but also assure healing.

Orbital Floor and Wall Fractures

If the surgeon suspects that the orbital floor will need support inferiorly, an antrostomy can be performed by direct vision, and a balloon or packing can be placed into the antrum to reduce and support the orbital floor. Exploring the orbital floor through the maxillary antrum using a Caldwell-Luc approach and attempting to reduce a significant fracture of the orbital floor usually is not adequate. If significant comminution of the lateral wall of the antrum exists and many entrances have been made into the midface through the mouth, it is preferable to perform an antrostomy and to support the lateral wall and floor of the orbit and any potential bone graft with antral packing, brought out through the antrostomy site. After fixation of the midfacial bones has been assured, the antral packing can be removed in 48 hours, unless it is the principal means of support.

In complex maxillofacial injuries, the surgeon usually must explore the orbital floors through a subciliary incision in the lower eyelid (Fig. 13–31). Therefore, it may not be necessary, even in the presence of severe comminution, to enter the lateral wall of the maxilla to explore the maxillary antrum, unless one suspects the need for primary bone grafting in this region or unless a supporting pack on balloon must be placed.

To repair Le Fort II fractures and other midfacial fragmentation, direct transosseous wire fixation and bone plates can be used through a buccal vestibular incision. The midfacial bones of the Le Fort II or pyramidal fracture are stabilized bilaterally at the zygomatic buttresses and at the lateral aspects of the infraorbital rims. The surgeon can observe the status of the infraorbital rims and get an idea of the integrity of the orbital floors through this incision. Classic Le Fort II fractures can be reduced and fixated by bilateral circumzygomatic suspensory wires with secondary wires to the mandible, zygomatic buttress wires, and lateral orbital rim wires. If Le Fort II fractures coexist with unstable infraorbital rims or blowout fractures of the orbital floors,

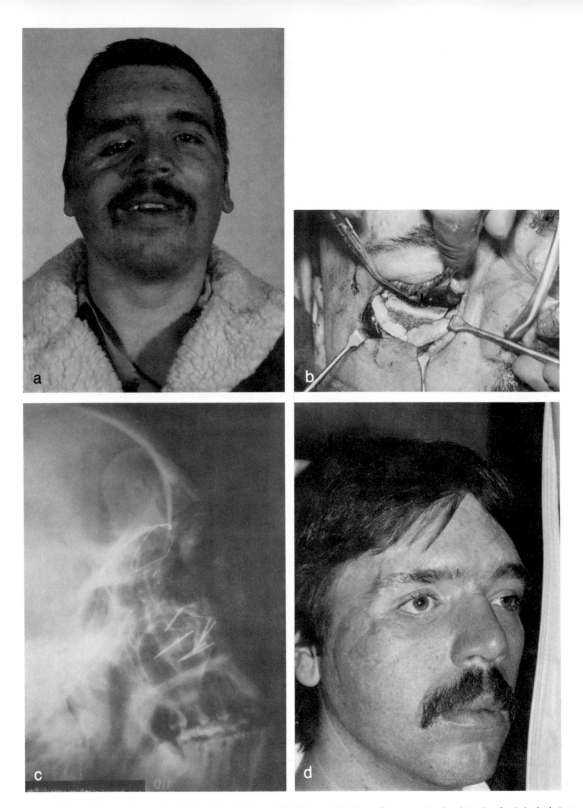

FIG. 13–29.   Rib grafts to the midfacial skeleton. Multiple split-rib grafts are attached to the facial skeleton by threaded Kirschner wires. After the grafted bone has been adapted and fixed it can be contoured using machine-driven rotary burs operating under a lavage of saline and suctioning. **a,** Preoperative view of a 26-year-old male with a malunited ZMC following a motorcycle accident. Earlier treatment of the ZMC was precluded by a cranial injury. **b,** Multiple split-rib grafts were used to rebuild the right zygoma and maxilla. **c,** Postoperative radiograph. **d,** Postoperative view. Note partial restitution of the vertical position of the right globe and recontouring of the right ZMC and maxilla.

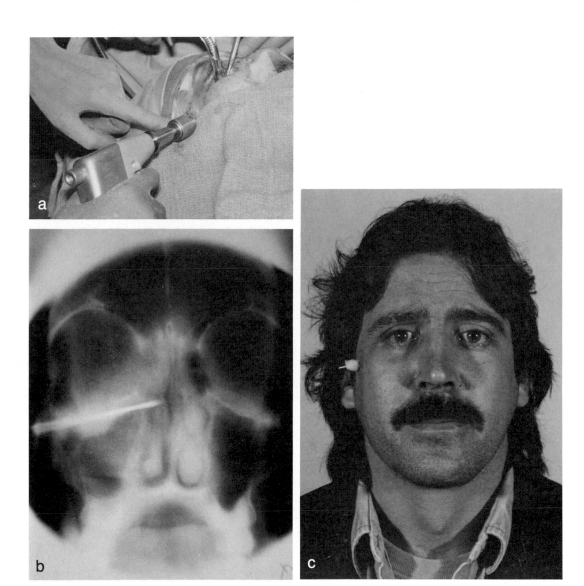

FIG. 13–30.   Kirschner wire used to skewer a bone graft to the orbital floor. The Kirschner wire is removed in 6 months in an outpatient procedure. **a,** Skewering the Kirschner wire through the body of the zygoma. Direct visualization of the progress of the Kirschner wire through the zygoma and bone graft must be maintained at all times to avoid injury to the globe or other normal structures. **b,** Tomogram displaying Kirschner wires through the body of the zygoma and the bone graft of the orbital floor. **c,** Postoperative clinical photograph displaying normal binocular vision and extraocular muscle integrity.

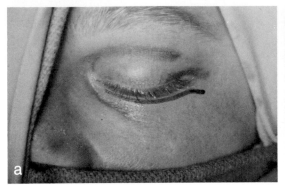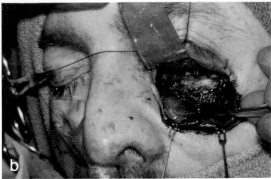

FIG. 13–31.   Subciliary incision. **a,** Subciliary incision that is often used for access to the infraorbital rim and floor. **b,** The wide exposure provided by the subciliary incision is useful for bone grafting procedures.

the floor of the orbits and infraorbital rims can be approached through a subciliary incision into the lower eyelid. The integrity of the infraorbital rim can be re-established using transosseous wire, a bone plate, or staple fixation. If the lateral aspect of the infraorbital rim is comminuted, it can be repaired but cannot be used for suspensory purposes in reducing the Le Fort II fracture.

The periorbita is reflected superiorly with special orbital retractors (Donovan) and the orbital floor completely explored for fracture. Fractures may occur with simple stepping off, nondisplacement, or a significant trapdoor effect that tethers the periorbital extraocular muscles and viscera and the infraorbital neurovascular bundle. In a large percentage of cases in which significant damage has occurred to the orbital floor, there is also involvement of the medial orbital wall. Significant rupture of the floor of the orbit with herniation of orbital contents into the maxillary antrum can be reduced from above and an antrostomy performed, followed by insertion of a Foley catheter balloon or sinal packing into the maxillary antrum directly beneath the herniated soft tissue and bony portions of the orbital floor. The orbital viscera and bony segments of the floor are elevated from the antrum using fine tonsil clamps and the bones of the floor are manipulated into alignment. The balloon is then inflated or packing is placed, thus repositioning the bones superiorly into a reduced state. If the medial and lateral shelves of bone constituting remnants of the orbital floor are adequate, a rayon-reinforced silicone rubber implant can be placed

over the defect (Fig. 13–32). This implant ensures that the periorbita will not create a cicatrix with the schneiderian membrane and periosteum of the maxillary sinus; it will also provide support for the globe and eliminate the tethering effect at the fracture site involving the inferior oblique and inferior rectus muscles.

Complex maxillofacial injuries can be associated with total loss or avulsion of the floor of the orbit with complete inferior herniation of small fragments of bone previously constituting the medial and lateral walls of the orbit. Even when medial and lateral canthal ligaments and Lockwood's suspensory ligament are intact, an aggressive approach to repair of this defect is necessary. With large avulsive defects of the orbital floor, a small

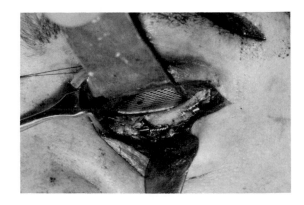

FIG. 13–32.   Silicone rubber sheeting cut to appropriate size and shape to provide a bridge across the defect of the orbital floor. I have noted no morbidity in 15 years' of experience with this implant.

segment of rib in either split or full thickness can be used to bridge the defect. The segment can also be used to support the midfacial structures when medial comminution is present. The full-thickness rib graft is rotated 180° from its original anatomic position because its radius of curvature is approximately the same as the inferior wall of the orbit. It is then cantilevered from the body of the zygoma, as discussed above. Smaller defects of the orbital floor without major midfacial fragmentation associated with enough damage of the floor to preclude the use of silastic sheeting, such as loss of medial and lateral bony shelves, can be repaired by using a simple split-rib graft locked into position by grooves produced on the medial and lateral margins of the bone graft. At AGH, we have found this procedure to be useful in reconstructing the midface because a large portion of rib can be used to repair other defects of the midfacial skeleton.

The amount of rib to be harvested from the donor site can be determined by measuring tomograms, CT scans, or models of the patient's maxillofacial complex produced by CT scan. When either a bone graft or silastic implant is used to repair a damaged orbital floor, the surgeon must preserve the periorbita. The periorbita can then be used to support the graft or implant using an accurate suturing technique.

Nasal-Ethmoidal-Orbital Wall Fractures

In the classic Le Fort II fracture, disimpaction of the midface followed by maxillomandibular fixation with or without suspension by the zygomatic buttresses or use of circumzygomatic wires will reduce the nasofrontal fracture region. Complex maxillofacial injuries are usually associated with involvement of several facial regions, and the nasal-ethmoidal-orbital region is often severely damaged in cases of severe Le Fort II and III fractures. This damage results in a new constellation of injuries in which the nasal bones are comminuted and in which the medial canthal ligaments may be free-floating, either still attached to bony fragments or lacerated and pulled laterally by the orbicularis oculi. Lateral pulling results in a characteristic clinical picture of telecanthus, hypertelorism, dysto-

pia, rounding of the lacrimal lake, and pronounced anatomic impaction and distortion with widening of the nasal bridge.

In treating simple nasoethmoidal fractures in which comminution is limited, we at AGH have found the following method of closed reduction useful. A modification of an accepted technique is used to create lateral support to the nasal bones that would ultimately repair the defect in the nasal bridge and pull the medial canthal ligaments toward the midline. A spinal needle, with the hub cut off by a bur, can be used as a drill with the trochar of the spinal needle placed within its lumen. This modified spinal needle and enclosed trocar are mounted in an air- or gas-powered drill and driven through the nasal bones while the medial canthal ligaments are held. Two such drillings are performed, producing two holes within the lateral nasal bones on each side. The original spinal needle is left in place while a second set of holes is drilled with a new needle. On removal of the trocars, stainless steel wire segments are placed within the lumens of each spinal needle. The spinal needles are then removed while the wires are held firm, leaving the wires in place within the bone and soft tissue. Commercially available padded plates can be used to support the nasal bridge on each side. These must be trimmed with wire-cutting forceps to coincide with the anatomy of the patient. Holes are drilled into the plates and the wires are passed through them. When the plates are next to the skin of the lateral surface of the nose, the operator can hold the lateral nasal bones in position while the assistant twists the wires on each side down to the padded plate while applying gentle pressure (Fig. 13–33). It may be of value when support for the nasal complex is desired in an anterosuperior vector from a locus on a headframe (Fig. 13–34). Premature removal of the plates can lead to collapse of the nasal bridge.

In multiple complicated midfacial fractures that include nasoethmoidal injuries, placement of the globes in their proper position requires reducing nasofrontal fractures and re-establishing the anatomic positions of the medial canthal ligaments; the preferred technique is open reduction, which may be referred to as the open-sky technique. For ex-

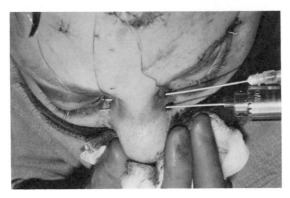

FIG. 13–33.   Technique of drilling through the gracile nasal bone structures using a spinal needle as a step in placing nasal plates. (This is adapted from a method proposed by Dr. Lee Chewning, Division of Oral and Maxillofacial Surgery, Allegheny General Hospital.)

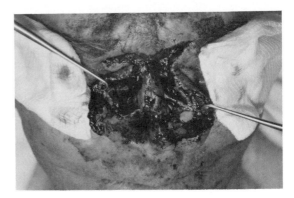

FIG. 13–35.   Access to the medial canthal region and ligaments provided by compound fractures.

ample, a frontal laceration can be extended with an incision to provide access to the frontal bone and the medial canthal ligaments (Fig. 13–35). If there is no frontal laceration that can be used for access, we use Killian incisions at the medial aspect of the nose or modified Killian incisions across the midline in a ''W'' fashion to reduce later visibility of the repaired incision line (Fig. 13–36).

When a craniotomy is being performed for a concomitant intracranial injury such as an anterior dural laceration or for an approach to the posterior wall of the frontal sinus, the nasofrontal and medial orbital region can be approached through a bicornal flap combined with subciliary incisions (Fig. 13–37). The gracile nature of the bones in the nasoethmoidal region dictates that very fine gauge stainless wire sutures be placed in a chain-link fashion. Larger bones superior to the nasoethmoidal region involving the glabellar region of the frontal bone can be linked together with adaptation bone plates (Fig. 13–38) or smaller osteosynthesis bone plates. Avulsion defects in the region of the midline with loss of portions of the frontal and nasal bones can be reconstructed by split-rib grafts across the bony defect in the frontal bone, and costochondral rib grafts can be cantilevered from the frontal bone with the cartilaginous portion of the rib directed against the alar cartilages.

SUPERIOR TO INFERIOR RECONSTRUCTION
(Cephalad to Caudad)

High velocity, high-impact trauma to the craniomaxillofacial region can result in frac-

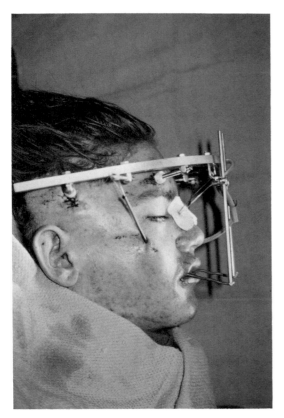

FIG. 13–34.   Gentle anterosuperior traction applied by using a transnasal wire attached to a strut from a Morris headframe.

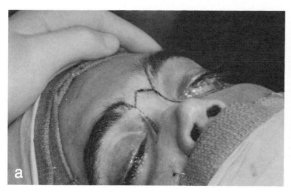 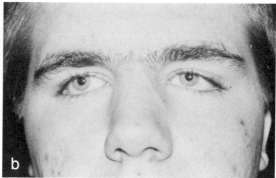

FIG. 13–36.   Modified Killian incisions to provide surgical visibility and access to the nasoethmoidal region. **a,** Killian incision. **b,** Postoperative results after Killian incisions with eyebrow extensions.

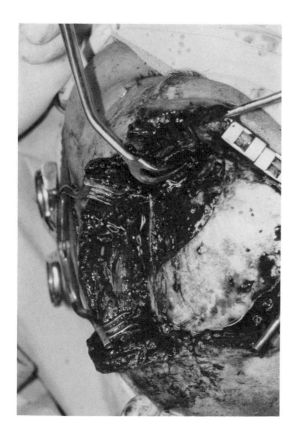

FIG. 13–37.   Frontal craniotomy provides concomitant access to superior aspects of the facial skeleton. Simultaneous use of subciliary incisions provides excellent surgical access to the midfacial skeleton.

tures of both the maxillofacial complex and the cranium. In isolated fractures of the craniofacial complex, the supraorbital, glabellar, or cranial vault can be involved. Cranial injuries can also be associated with Le Fort II or III fractures and regions of the nasal-ethmoidal-orbital complex. Finally lateral orbitozygomatic fractures can have intracranial involvement and could coexist with fractures of the supraorbital region and cranial vault. Extension into the parietal and temporal bones can occur in these kinds of injuries, as can intracranial complications. Craniomaxillofacial injuries with complete avulsion of bone through large skin lacerations and/or deep soft-tissue avulsions are also seen. This avulsion of bone may be so extensive as to prohibit adequate stabilization of bone.

Complex maxillofacial injuries many times

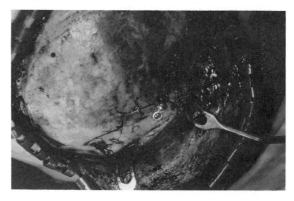

FIG. 13–38.   Bone plates are used to give stability to fractures of the frontal bone. These plates give outstanding stability to the maxillofacial skeleton when the fractures are approached from a superior to an inferior direction.

result in severe comminution of the mandibular arch form, and the establishment of a useful occlusal plane to reconstruct the midface when concomitant midfacial injuries exist is not possible. Therefore, it is necessary to use techniques that will allow direct access to the fracture sites in the upper face and midface, thus establishing an accurate alignment of these fractured bone sites and enabling one to relate the maxilla to the cranial base. At the AGH Trauma Center, while we usually use the inferior to superior methods, for severe midfacial craniofacial skeletal fractures we occasionally will use a superior to inferior sequencing, especially with comminution of the mandible and coexisting intracranial injuries or dural lacerations.

In complex craniomaxillofacial injuries, it is often necessary to begin with neurosurgical procedures in the frontal region and follow inferiorly with reduction and fixation of midfacial fractures until the inferior portion of the maxilla and mandible can be relocated to the re-established cranial base. The maxilla is reduced against the cranial base by direct approximation of the maxillary bone against stable zygomatic and nasal (piriform) buttresses, if present. The mandible can then be related to the maxilla, as in orthognathic surgical procedures. Superior to inferior sequencing might be necessary with avulsive losses of sections of the mandible and in some instances of inoperable bilateral fracture dislocations of the mandibular condylar processes.

The need for frontal sinus exploration or dural repair may necessitate a bicoronal flap. This flap, combined with Killian incisions or incisions across the midline and subciliary incisions, can expose the entire midface for total reconstruction. It is common to reduce and fixate fractures of the orbital rims and then relate the fractured maxilla to a re-established cranial base. Appropriate bone grafts can then be placed for midfacial contour, and avulsive injuries of the mandible are repaired with bone grafting and costochondral rib grafting. Rigid fixation using compression bone plates can be used in all phases of the facial skeletal repair and reconstruction. Complete immobilization of the midface, if necessary, can be secured by a headframe.

Extent of Injuries

Craniomaxillofacial trauma can be differentiated from conventional complex maxillofacial injuries by several parameters: direct involvement of the cranium; usually, many fractured bones of the maxillofacial skeleton; unusual instability and mobility of the fractures; fragmentation of individual bones; avulsion of segments of the facial skeleton; marked asymmetry of the overlying tissues, including the face and cranium; and importantly, usually an inadequate mandibular occlusal plane from which to rebuild the maxillofacial complex. Extension of the cranial injury to the midface often involves fracture of the nasal-ethmoidal-orbital region with all its signs and symptoms. The methods used to address craniomaxillofacial injuries vary considerably. In general, the surgical approach will involve open reduction using techniques derived from craniofacial reconstructive surgery and, in the majority of instances, a superior to inferior sequencing of the surgical steps.

Assessing the Fracture Patterns

The clinical diagnosis of craniomaxillofacial trauma is obscured by edema, ecchymosis, hemorrhage, and gross deformity. The earliest possible elucidation of the underlying bony problem is imperative because reconstructive planning can be initiated immediately and surgical intervention accomplished as soon as traumatic edema has subsided.

A major advance in the diagnosis of craniomaxillofacial trauma has been the early imaging of the craniofacial region with CT scanning (see Chapter 3, Part II). CT scanning offers many advantages over conventional radiography and pluridirectional tomography because of the versatility permitted by its improved high resolution, its range of soft-tissue and bone windows, its capability for image reformatting, image reversal, creation of mirror images, image manipulation, magnified mode capability, selected direct image generation (in the absence of cervical spine injury), data storage, and three-dimensional soft- and hard-tissue presentation; and importantly, the immediate ability of the traumatologist to determine both the intracranial and craniomaxillofacial status. Intracranial contents and craniomaxillofacial trauma from injury to the vault and frontal sinus can be assessed by transaxial views. Transaxial CT scans can be used to explore the superior to inferior expanse of the orbits and nasoethmoidal region, thus enabling the surgeon to assess injury to the inter- and intraorbital anatomy including the extraocular muscles, globe, optic nerve, and ethmoidal complex. All walls of the orbit can be assessed for rupture, and either extrusive or intrusive (encephalocele) injuries can be detected. Direct impingement on the optic nerve by bone fragments can be located definitively, thus assisting in the surgical decompression of the nerve. The CT scan does not merely confirm the clinical impression, but indeed establishes the diagnosis; we have found that CT scanning has discovered facial fractures or soft-tissue disruptions not detected by clinical examination or conventional radiography.

A joint surgical effort by the neurosurgical and maxillofacial teams is planned in severe craniomaxillofacial trauma when intracranial extension is suspected or demonstrated by clinical or CT evidence. Prior to repair of the maxillofacial complex, the neurosurgical team explores and repairs lacerations or avulsions of the dura. In caring for craniomaxillofacial traumatic injuries, the sequencing of the care can be reversed. While "conventional" injuries can be repaired from the inferior or mandibular fracture sites to the midfacial or superior injuries, craniomaxillofacial fractures with severe comminution of the cranial vault might require stabilization of the vault with rigid interosseous fixation followed by maxillofacial surgical repair against the surgically repaired intact cranial vault. When cranial tissue or bone is lost, maxillofacial skeletal injuries are repaired first. The maxillofacial complex is then stabilized to the remaining cranial vault. This stabilization is followed by assessment of the quantity of missing bone or measurement of the size of the existing defect(s). Bony defects will be replaced by primary rib bone grafting; full-thickness rib grafts are used to provide the lost supraorbital margin.

Surgical Approaches

To surgically expose the multiple fractures constituting a severe craniomaxillofacial injury, the surgeon uses many of the incisions used for complex conventional facial trauma. In obtaining the necessary access to the supraorbital, orbital, and naso-orbital regions, we have used a unicoronal or bicoronal flap (Fig. 13–39). This incision is commonly used by the neurosurgeon in performing a frontal craniotomy when direct access to the dura or intracranial contents is required. After neurosurgical repair, the versatile coronal flap can be extended to provide access to the midface. Other local incisions can be designed with the coronal flap to repair regional maxillofacial trauma not accessible by the coronal flap.

The standard periorbital incisions used to further visualize the midface include the subciliary, conjunctival, Killian, lateral brow, and buccal vestibular approaches (Fig. 13–40). The subciliary incision, mentioned earlier with reference to conventional complex injuries, is our preferred approach to the infraorbital rim and floor. Its extension provides excellent access to the floor of the orbit, zygoma, and superior maxilla. This incision can be combined with a coronal incision to provide a direct approach to the medial and lateral orbital walls. The subciliary incision is designed to avoid the ectropion and subsequent epiphora observed from more inferior incisions near the infraorbital rim. If placed too high, the incision can disturb the normal lid-conjunctival seal, resulting in cicatrization of the superior lid margin, inadequate tear discharge into the lacrimal punctum, and an unaesthetic result. A characteristic thickening of the superior margin of the lower eyelid persisting for months has been observed.

Use of a convenient skin crease present in almost all individuals on the superior aspect of the lower eyelid approximately 3 to 4 mm from the upper margin provides good cosmetic result. Lateral extensions of this curvilinear incision can be made to enhance access, especially when dealing with lateral orbital rim fractures or disruptions of the corpus of the zygoma or to facilitate bone grafting. The lateral arm of the subciliary incision is usually curved inferiorly to be placed in the "crow's

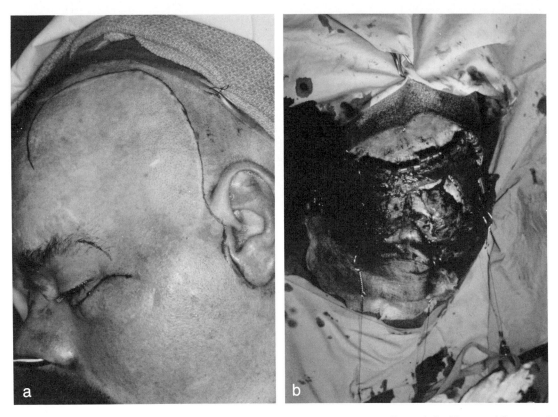

FIG. 13–39.   Coronal flaps. **a,** Unicoronal flap used when the injury is unilateral. **b,** Bicoronal flap used to provide bilateral access to the frontal bone and superior facial bones.

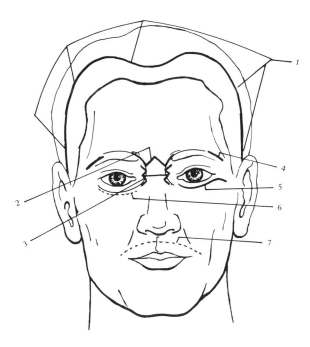

FIG. 13–40.   Possible incisions for surgical access to the upper and middle facial fractures. Bicoronal (1). Killian (2). Direct open-sky approach (3). Lateral eyebrow (4). Subciliary (5). Conjunctival (6). Buccal vestibule (7).

feet" or "laugh line" of the lateral canthal region. After the skin is divided with no undermining of the subcutaneous layers, the incision is carried down to the orbicularis oculi. The surgeon enters this muscle at the midpoint of the incision paralleling the muscle's transverse curving fibers using sharp tenotomy scissors. The dissection is then carried through the muscle layer to the glistening white septum orbitale. The remaining lateral muscle bundles are divided in the transverse plane, thus completely exposing the underlying septum from the medial to the lateral margin of the wound. Dissection is then carried inferiorly along the anterior surface of the septum to its attachment to and confluence with the periosteum of the infraorbital rim. Just lateral to the dissection and lying variably along the lateral inferior margin of the orbital rim is a fat pad, the presence of which might be incorrectly interpreted as the result of an inadvertent rent into the septum behind which the periorbital fat is located. By "stepping" the incision in this fashion, the surgeon quickly reaches the infraorbital rim. A sharp incision can be made along the infraorbital rim to expose the subjacent bone. From the anterior margin of the rim, blunt dissection can be used to expose the region of the orbital floor. A layered suturing technique is not used after surgery using the subciliary incision because of the possibility of binding the septum orbitale/orbital periosteum to the orbicularis oculi, which would cause vertical shortening of the lower eyelid and thus dysfunction of normal approximation of the palpebral fissure. The use of the conjunctival incision is limited to isolated orbital trauma when wide exposure is not required. This incision must be combined with other incisions to visualize the lateral orbit.

The "open sky" is a direct approach to the nasoethmoidal region. In this incision, the base of the letter "W" lies against each lateral aspect of the base of the nasal bridge in the medial canthal region. The midportions of the Ws are connected by a horizontal incision across the bridge of the nose in the midline. Direct access to the nasoethmoidal region can also be provided by modified Killian incisions, curvilinear incisions at the medial aspect of the bridge of the nose, which can be

connected across the midline with a zigzag type of incision to decrease its unaesthetic consequences. The coronal incision does not provide the amount of access necessary to manage nasoethmoidal trauma completely, especially when bone grafting and more complex procedures involving the medial wall and floor of the orbit are anticipated. The lateral brow incision is used to provide access to the frontozygomatic suture region and has been mentioned with reference to the management of Le Fort III fractures. This incision has obvious limitations in craniomaxillofacial trauma when greater visibility is needed. An eyebrow incision extending from the medial to the lateral aspect of the eyebrow has been useful in dealing with supraorbital injuries. Such an incision is acceptable cosmetically and can be used in combination with the superior arm of the Killian incision to create wide access to frontoethmoidal injuries.

Finally, direct access to the maxilla is provided through buccal vestibular incisions. These incisions can expose the entire anterior and lateral wall of the maxilla. Concomitant use of vestibular and subciliary incisions assures wide access to the orbit and zygomaticomaxillary complex. It is useful when dealing with a transoral approach to attempt to obtain a double layer closure to produce a water-tight wound seal, especially when grafting bone or using rigid fixation with bone plates. The vestibular incision can be made inferolaterally to the depth of the vestibule so that the final wound will not lie in the sulcus or buccal gutter itself. A mucosal flap is raised, dissection is carried down to the musculature overlying the maxilla, and another incision is made into the muscles and periosteum. The muscle layer is closed first, followed by the mucosa. By employing the above incisions and combinations, access to the entire maxillofacial complex can be gained.

Reduction and Fixation

In severe craniofacial injuries it may be necessary first to perform open reduction on the fractured bones of the upper face. The midface is then placed into maxillomandibular fixation, after which the midfacial fractures are fixated and then stabilized to a stable cranial base or the upper face. Small, fine-gauge wire is used to fixate tiny fragments of bone of the midface. The small fragments of craniofacial membranous bone that have been completely stripped of periosteum usually often survive if adequate internal fixation and stabilization is performed. The fragments are chain-linked together using multiple wires in one transosseous hole, thus preventing excessive weakening of the bone. The maxillofacial surgeon will expose all fracture sites and compare the injury with the radiographs. When all fracture sites are exposed and the "global" pattern of the injury is identified, the surgeon can begin to perform fragment-by-fragment reduction and fixation, either by interosseous wiring using a chain-link method or by rigid compression bone plates. By their very nature, craniomaxillofacial injuries include a statistically high incidence of comminuted or avulsed bone mass that ideally should be supported or reconstituted with primary bone grafts consisting of split ribs. Such bone grafts, if not placed immediately, should be considered as early as possible after wounding. Their purpose is to replace lost or fragmented bony substance and to provide internal fixation, re-establish "normal" bony stress buttresses, and effectively restore the topographic architecture of the maxillofacial complex. The surgeon may find, when treating craniofacial injuries by direct visualization of the multiple fracture sites and placement of a network of transosseous wires, bone plates, or bone grafts, that cephalad internal and external suspensory techniques might not be necessary.

Bone Grafts to the Midface

As noted, severe craniofacial trauma is often associated with severely damaged or lost bone. This is replaced and contour defects are re-established by primary bone grafting. At AGH, we have attempted to provide bone grafting as early as possible, depending on the systemic status of the patient. We also have used several donor sites, including rib and the split inner and outer table of the skull, which is particularly useful when a neurosurgical flap has been raised. We prefer rib grafts because they are membranous bone, have a natural curvature, and can be easily split and bent to the contour of the defect. They can be useful as full-thickness grafts at the supraorbital margin or as costochondral grafts for nasal reconstruction. In my experience, rib grafts have survived despite communication to the oral cavity as occurs in oroantral openings and bone grafting to the orbital floor of orbital defects. While the iliac crest has been useful in specific situations, such grafts are better suited for mandibular replacement and are less useful in large craniofacial avulsion defects. Primary bone grafts can be used to reconstruct avulsed bone or contour deficits in any region of the craniomaxillofacial skeleton. We have used primary full-thickness and split-thickness rib grafts to reconstruct defects of the skull, nasal region, walls of the orbits, maxilla, and mandible. We have also found that alloplastic materials such as Proplast (Vitek Corporation, Houston, Texas) can be used to re-establish facial contour, especially in the zygomatic region when there is actual loss of substance, in addition to treating malunited fractures of the maxilla that have healed in retroposition. It is difficult to perform Le Fort II osteotomies on these latter patients because of the extensive scarring and morbidity involved.

FRONTAL-NASAL-ETHMOIDAL-ORBITAL INJURIES AND RECONSTRUCTION

Most patients have a characteristic appearance after a frontal nasoethmoidal fracturing injury. The impact causes fractures and posterior dislocation of small bony fragments underneath the frontal bone, with comminution of the body of the ethmoidal and lacrimal bones. Approximately 35 to 50 gravity units of force in the nasoethmoidal region produces fractures that have characteristic indentation of the supraorbital and glabellar region and nasal bones. The indentation causes a superior repositioning of the nasal tip, and inspection can imply incorrectly that the nasal bones have shortened. There is an increased acuteness of the nasoglabellar angle.

The actual traumatic event on the soft tissues of the face will cause hematoma, lacerations, and edema, which may mask the above findings. Such soft-tissue injuries can obscure the presence of a significant depression of the frontal bone. A subgaleal hematoma can give the appearance of a frontal depression.

Frontoethmoidal fractures can also be associated with comminuted midfacial Le Fort II and III fractures. In these cases the face has a characteristic "dished out" or concave appearance. Frontoethmoidal fractures frequently involve the medial canthal ligaments, either by laceration by the injuring object or by severe comminution of the supporting bones of the midface. The patient thus exhibits pseudohypertelorism. If there is comminution of the medial aspect of the orbit, especially in the region of the attachment of a trochlea of the superior oblique muscle, the superior gaze would be impaired. However, because of the strength of the attachment of the ligament and the thickness of the bone involved, this impairment occurs rarely.

Most patients present after injury with periorbital ecchymosis and edema and usually there are lacerations over the eyebrow or upper eyelids and skin of the forehead. Often, traumatic ptosis with severe lid edema occurs. Crepitation or subcutaneous emphysema is palpable in the tissues of this region because of underlying air.

Associated Ophthalmologic Injuries

A high incidence of related ophthalmologic injuries makes ophthalmologic consultation mandatory, although the trauma surgeon and maxillofacial surgeon can rule out the more obvious ocular injuries that would need immediate attention. Injury is suspected especially in the presence of a Marcus Gunn or amaurotic pupil. The diagnosis of these defects must be corroborated by CT scanning in at least two planes to rule out direct injury to the optic nerve which can occur by several means. Direct extension of bone fragments can impinge or lacerate the optic nerve; neural injury can occur from stretching, torquing, or ischemia within the canal. Intracanalicular ischemia from loss of direct blood supply is one of the more common post-traumatic events resulting in blindness. The CT scan can provide some insight into the diagnosis if fracture

or an air-fluid level is present in the sphenoidal, ethmoidal and maxillary sinuses. When all three sinuses are involved, it is likely that the ocular apparatus is damaged even when radiographs do not display this directly. In many instances, edema or patient combativeness or conscious state can make definitive ophthalmologic evaluation difficult. CT scanning can show indirect neural injury, displacement of the nerve, or, in some instances, subdural hematoma involving the optic nerve sheath. Most patients will also present with neuropathy and neuropraxia involving the distribution of the supraorbital nerve.

Neurosurgical Considerations

Significantly, CSF rhinorrhea is a common sequela of frontoethmoidal injuries. Therefore, one of the objectives of neurosurgical treatment is to eliminate such discharges. The neurosurgical procedure should be performed first, either by directly extending the lacerations involving the forehead and frontal scalp, or by creating appropriate coronal or bicoronal flaps to gain access to the frontal bone. Usually, the patient is operated on before the CSF leak ceases because, depending on the volume of leakage, it may be impractical to wait for a spontaneous resolution of the discharge.

Following formal craniotomy or direct extension into the lacerations, the surgeon elevates any depression of the frontal bone. The frontal bone can be stabilized after repair of the intracranial injury by interosseous wire fixation or minibone plates. The neurosurgeon removes bone fragments and necrotic bone within the brain and, depending on a favorable neurologic outcome in the frontal brain, debrides the injured site. Depending on its size, the dural laceration can be closed by pericranium, fascia lata, or lyophilized or freeze-dried dura. Next, the frontal sinus is explored surgically; if the posterior wall is involved, the neurosurgeon can use one of several approaches. If the posteromedial wall is fractured, the neurosurgeon can elect to obliterate the frontal sinus using either muscle or fat and thus occlude the entrance to the nasofrontal ducts. In severe comminution of the posterior wall of the sinus, the wall can be removed and the frontal sinus cranialized. In relatively benign lesions of the sinus, we have elected to re-establish drainage through the nasofrontal duct.

Imaging

CT scanning has revolutionized the care of injuries to the frontoethmoidal region. CT in the transaxial reconstructed coronal plane, overcoming the inability to manipulate the multiple-trauma patient, helps ascertain the presence or absence of fracture of the anterior and posterior walls of the frontal sinus, rupture of the cribriform plate, or rupture of medial orbital walls. The viscera of the orbit, including the extraocular muscles and optic nerve, can also be viewed using appropriate soft-tissue windows. CT can display the distribution of fracture, the dislocation of the nasal bones, the ethmoids including the perpendicular plate, and the relationship of these structures to the frontal bone. Air-fluid levels within the sinuses can point to involvement of the optic nerve and CSF leakage.

We have found that the clinician can be misled about the presence of subjacent injuries by the clinical and radiographic examination. To be sure, the radiographic evaluation involving CT scanning has been invaluable and has, indeed, been the basis of diagnosis. However, despite accurate CT evaluation and clinical evaluation, which can be limited by the presence of profound edema, hemorrhage, lacerations, and tissue contusion, often diagnosis is possible only by surgical exploration. If significant disruption of the frontoethmoid complex exists, surgical intervention will be necessary anyway. At issue is the extent of neurosurgical intervention and whether primary bone grafting will be necessary.

CSF fluid leaks into the nose and nasopharynx usually by way of intracranial fossa either through the frontal sinus and into the middle meatus of the nose, or directly through the cribriform plate. CSF leakage can also occur from the middle cranial fossa through the sphenoid sinus and from the middle and posterior cranial fossa through the middle ear and eustachian tube. The pa-

tient usually will sense a salty taste when supine; CSF drainage usually increases in a prone position, in a hanging head position, or with compression of the internal jugular vein. The classic test of CSF discharge onto a handkerchief or paper tissue is useful in general for screening patients: CSF fluid dried on a handkerchief or paper tissue leaves the material with the same consistency that was present prior to wetting, whereas nasal secretions, containing mucin, will cause stiffening of the handkerchief or tissue. Alternatively, because normal nasal secretions, unlike CSF, do not contain reducing sugars, one can differentiate between nasal secretions and CSF by a Dextro-Stix test. When the patient has significant nasal hemorrhage or a persistent ooze, blood will give a false positive test. Importantly, because lacrimal secretions also contain reducing substances, if they are present significantly they may give a false positive diagnosis.

Radiographic analysis of the presence and location of the leak may be helpful, although it is also fraught with interpretative controversy. CT of the roof of the intraorbital space will show a pneumocephalus and hence locate the region of the entrance of air, which is also the exit of CSF discharge. However, CT can easily show a diffuse pneumocephalus and not specifically the focus of discharge. Finally, one can use methods such as intrathecal dyes (see Chapter 3). Repositioning the patient in the prone position for intrathecal injections is not often practical in the acute trauma patient. The use of 0.5 ml of 5% fluoresceine dye diluted in 3 to 4 ml of spinal fluid can be used, but the patient must be placed in a prone position and examined within 30 minutes. Placement of intranasal pledgets of cotton into the cribriform area, in the middle meatus, and in the sphenoid recess is helpful in localizing small leaks.

Pseudohypertelorism, Telecanthus, and Nasolacrimal Apparatus

Pseudohypertelorism and telecanthus must be addressed in repairing frontoethmoidal injuries. Frontoethmoidal injuries are associated with lateral displacement of the medial palpebral ligament resulting from pseudohypertelorism and telecanthus of the nasal

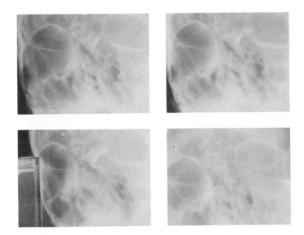

FIG. 13–41. Dacrocystogram performed by cannulating the nasolacrimal duct canaliculus through puncta and injecting a radiopaque medium. Note the lack of flow into the nasal portion of the duct.

bone, lacrimal bone, and lamina papyracea. Action of the orbicularis oculi on the medial palpebral ligament is unopposed because of disintegration of medial or midline attachments. Thus, there is an increase in distance between the right and left medial canthi, flattening in the region, rounding of the medial canthus, and disappearance of the medial prominence. The posterior filaments of the medial ligament associated with Horner's muscle, which has been displaced by the similar displacement of the medial attachment of the ligaments to the muscle, produce sagging of the lacrimal puncta. This sagging causes epiphora, which can be mistaken for obstruction of the nasolacrimal apparatus. Injury to the nasolacrimal apparatus can be identified in several ways, one of which is simple injection of radiopaque material into the puncta and subsequent radiographic examination (Fig. 13–41). In addition, one can place fluorescine dye into the fornix of the eye and cotton pledgets beneath the inferior turbinate. Yellow staining of the cotton shows the integrity of the nasolacrimal apparatus. In our experience in dealing with frontoethmoidal and nasoethmoidal injuries, we have not been impressed with the acute repair of nasolacrimal injuries because the edema of the trauma and of the subsequent surgery will falsely obstruct the duct. Therefore, a one-step dacrocystorhinostomy should be done several

weeks to a month after the injury to re-establish patency of the nasolacrimal apparatus.

Case Report One

A 46-year-old man was transferred via the Life Flight helicopter to the AGH following an accident in which his tractor trailer plunged approximately 33 m down an embankment. On arrival at the emergency room the patient had vital signs within normal limits, and he was amnesic to the event. The trauma team evaluation listed his Glascow coma score (GCS) as 15 and his trauma score (TS) as 16. The patient's injury complex (Fig. 13–42) included a right open frontal skull fracture, a nasal-ethmoidal-orbital complex injury, multiple facial lacerations, an L-1 compression fracture, and a possible renal contusion. The patient was stabilized in the emergency room for transfer to the trauma intensive care unit.

Initial laboratory data including chest radiograph, ECG and cervical-spine radiographic series were negative. In the operating room, preliminary exploration and uneventful primary closure of multiple facial lacerations was accomplished. Maxillofacial imaging included orbital tomograms and facial CT (Fig. 13–43). One day post-trauma the patient showed a Le Fort II maxillary midface fracture with severe nasal-ethmoidal, orbital, and frontal sinus involvement. Because of the severe nasal comminution and possible avulsion of bone, it was decided to harvest a costochondral graft for repair of the comminuted nasal-ethmoidal-orbital injury. The technical plans for surgery was coordinated by the oral and maxillofacial surgery team and neurosurgical team.

The patient was returned to the operating room 8 days post-trauma for right frontal craniotomy and elevation of the frontal fracture (Fig. 13–44), exenteration of the frontal sinus and internal fixation of the frontal bone, open reduction and internal fixation of the nasal-ethmoidal-orbital fracture, costochondral grafting to the nasoethmoidal region, and rigid fixation of the displaced right zygomaticomaxillary complex fracture. A costochondral graft consisting of the right seventh rib was performed. A right frontal craniotomy

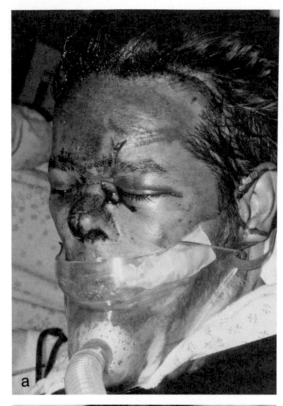

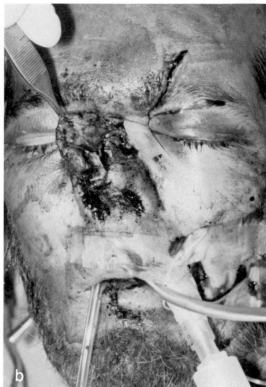

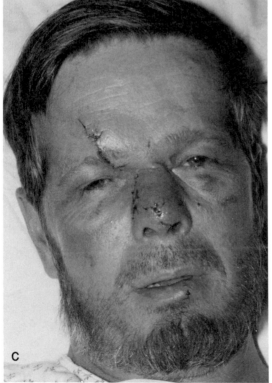

FIG. 13–42.   Case Report One. An adult male was involved in a motor vehicle accident. His injuries were confined to the upper and midfacial skeleton. **a** and **b,** Immediately post-trauma. **c,** After resolution of edema.

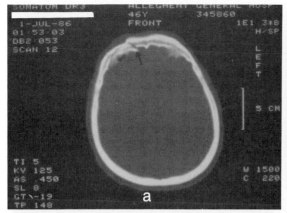
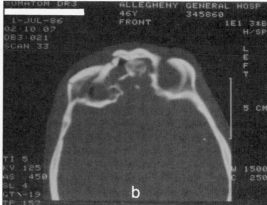
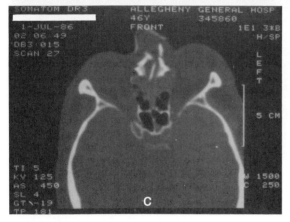

FIG. 13–43.   Case Report One. Facial CT scans of frontal bone and nasoethmoidal fractures. **a** and **b**, CT scans of frontal sinuses. **c**, CT of midface including the nasoethmoidal fractures.

was accomplished with a right frontal incision. The patient had multiple comminuted fragments in the right frontal region and a slightly depressed area immediately over the frontal sinus. Multiple small fragments of bone of the outer table of the frontal sinus were removed. The frontal fracture was mobilized and elevated until the right frontal sinus could be entered. The mucosa in the right frontal sinus was completely exenterated, and the sinus was obliterated with muscle taken from the right temporalis region and placed into the sinus and nasofrontal duct. The remaining small confines of the sinus were filled with antibiotic ointment. Bone fragments of the frontal bone were reduced and fixated with bony wire fixation. Normal right frontal contour was re-established by placing the pieces of outer table together and wiring them in place with interosseous fixation.

To gain access to the nasal-ethmoidal-orbital region, a bilateral Killian incision was established along with a "W" upper eyebrow

incision and right subciliary incision. After appropriate incisions were made, the fracture sites were identified; the patient had fractures specifically in the right supraorbital region, one extending in a lateral direction and one extending into the superior frontal region at the medial aspect of the supraorbital ridge. The right infraorbital rim was fractured in two segments, the fracture sites extending down to the anterior wall of the maxilla to the region of the piriform aperture. The right nasal bony complex was severely comminuted and displaced, and some very small fragments had to be removed. The nasal bone was completely distracted in a posterior superior position at its attachment to the frontal bone.

These segments were reduced and stabilized using reconstruction bone plates. Initially a five-hole reconstruction plate was placed over the medial supraorbital ridge fracture in a horizontal direction and stabilized with 6-mm screws; then, the lateral right supraorbital fracture was stabilized with a four-hole reconstruction plate. The nasal bone was

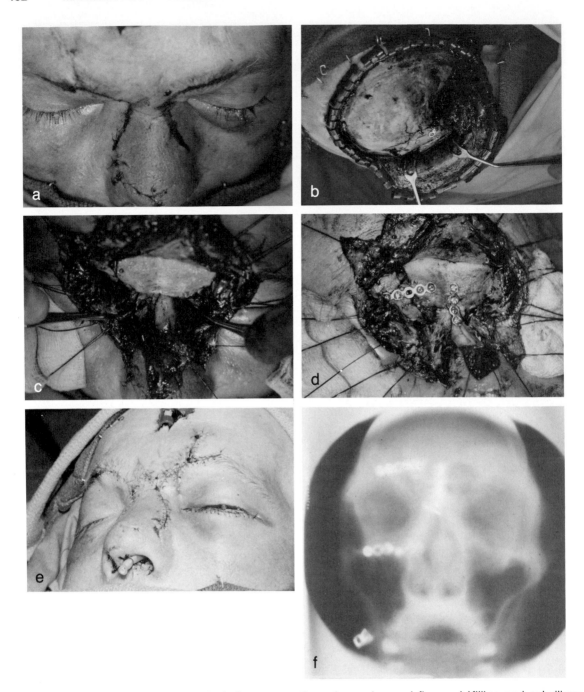

FIG. 13–44. Surgical procedures including access through a unicoronal flap and Killian and subciliary incisions. **a,** Brilliant green dye indicating the flap design. **b,** Unicoronal flap. **c,** Access to fractures. **d,** Adaptation of bone plates at the nasofrontal suture region. **e,** Soft-tissue closure. **f,** Postoperative radiograph.

elevated with Asch forceps, and another four-hour reconstruction plate, meticulously contoured to fit the region of the frontonasal suture area, was placed. The bone was then stabilized to the frontal bone with a four-hole reconstruction plate and 6-mm screws.

The right infraorbital injuries were treated by placement of a three-hole reconstruction plate over the midaspect of the right infraorbital rim, spanning the fracture with approximately 2 mm between the fracture site because of the loss of fractured segments.

Another three-hole construction plate was used to span a diagonal area from the initial infraorbital plate to stabilize the other segment to the anterior wall of the maxilla.

The left nasal bone was intact but laterally displaced. This bone was returned to its anatomic position by use of elevators and finger pressure, and the right nasal bone was found to be avulsed. A costochondral graft was then contoured to overlie the nasal bone and part of the nasofrontal suture, with the cartilage aspect extending toward the tip of the nose. After adequately contouring this piece of bone the surgeon placed a lag screw in a cantilevered fashion to the nasal process of the frontal bone. Placement of the right and left lateral nasal bones in their correct anatomic position reconstructed the nasal bridge. In addition, the medial canthal ligament on the left was brought into proper alignment into the right orbital floor, and the medial wall was explored. The comminuted ethmoidal bones in the midline were meticulously realigned, and overcontouring was established by anterior repositioning of the nasal bridge. A .020 silicone rubber sheet was placed in the right orbital floor region. It was then necessary to place an antral balloon via an antrostomy into the right maxillary sinus.

Postoperative progression was uneventful. A postoperative ophthalmology consultation indicated that the extraocular muscles were intact with no visual field defect. There was some ptosis of the right eyelid presumably secondary to edema from the unicoronal flap. The patient was discharged 8 days postoperatively with no diplopia, good visual acuity, and good wound healing. The patient was seen 10 days after surgery and the antral balloon was removed. Subsequently, he was seen weekly for 2 weeks and then monthly (Fig. 13–45).

Discussion

While the patient had severe deformity of the nasal bridge and comminution of the medial wall of the orbits, the entire nasoethmoidal complex was rigidly fixed without movement postoperatively, and reconstruction, basically of the ethmoidal complex including the canthal ligaments that were not

lacerated but simply moved out of position, was completed. The diagnosis of frontoethmoidal orbital injuries and the possible need for a combined neurosurgical maxillofacial approach is dictated by the nature of the injury.

In this patient the following signs of nasoethmoidal complex injury were noted: traumatic telecanthus, depressed and disrupted bony architecture of the nasal complex, orbital involvement with enophthalmos, and a rounding out of the medial canthal region. This patient also had a mobile displaced right zygomaticomaxillary complex with a blowout fracture of the right orbital floor. Because of retrotelescoping of the ethmoidal complex, the medial orbital wall was explored. In this case, the medial walls were explored via the Killian incisions bilaterally, with more exposure on the right side. The small pieces of bone making up the medial wall were placed into position; more importantly, reconstruction of the nasal bridge to correct deformity enhanced the position of the medial canthal ligament definitively. Exploration of the nasolacrimal duct system at the close of the operation revealed no obstruction. However, because the edema from trauma and surgery can mimic signs of obstruction, we wait for the symptoms of naso-lacrimal duct occlusion to develop postoperatively before reconstructing the nasal lacrimal system with a dacrocystorhinostomy.

Primary reconstruction of the medial orbital wall is important when indicated by volumetric changes in the orbit. A severely telescoped and retropositioned medial orbital wall cannot be repositioned adequately by simple manipulative measures. The bone graft serves to decrease orbital volume and provide a partition between the ethmoidal sinuses, nasal cavity, and orbital cavity. Neurosurgical repair of CSF discharge by dural grafting, for example, does not interfere with the manipulative procedures in the region of the ethmoid, orbital area, or midface. Addressing the neurosurgical aspects first seems practical because of the amount of time that it takes to repair facial injuries.

Our experience also shows that re-establishing the integrity of the orbital rims is important to protect the globe as well as provide an appropriate aesthetic result. Re-establish-

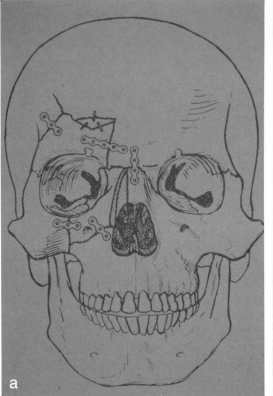

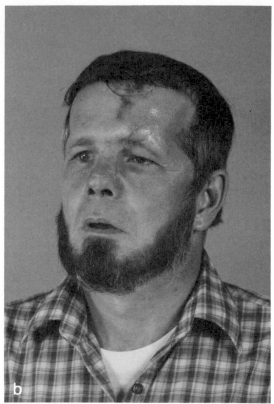

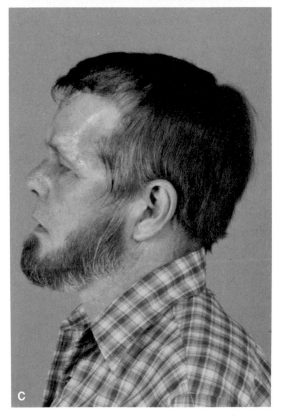

FIG. 13–45.   Case Report One. **a,** Diagram representing treatment of the patient's injuries. **b** and **c,** Postoperative photographs.

ment of the walls of the orbit to their original integrity is therapeutic in addressing volumetric changes in the orbit, and indeed, primary bone grafting of the floor of the orbit is useful in cases of total loss of this structure with persistent diplopia.

Despite such careful reconstruction of the orbital bony architecture, ocular problems can persist into the postoperative phase, despite normal horizontal position of the globe and re-establishment of both medial and lateral orbital walls and despite the re-establishment of the medial and lateral suspensory ligaments. The rationale for reconstruction of the bony orbit, including exploration of all walls in severe frontoethmoidal injuries, is based on that fact that persistent ocular injuries would be much more severe if exploration is not carried out. Traumatic enophthalmos and diplopia are very difficult to treat, and surgical intervention to enhance aesthetics and function more than justifies the results.

We have noted in the treatment of frontal nasoethmodial-orbital injuries that 1) treatment of nasofrontal and frontobasal ethmoidal injuries should involve maxillofacial surgery, neurosurgery, and other specialties such as ophthalmology; 2) serious injuries involving the frontal sinus should dictate ablation of this structure; 3) neurosurgical procedures can be assisted greatly by maxillofacial attention to rigid fixation of frontal bone fragments after elevation by the neurosurgeon; and 4) reduction of very severely comminuted nasal skeletal injuries produces poor postoperative aesthetic results and primary reconstruction with bone grafts is much more practical.

Case Report Two

A 14-year-old male was involved in an accident while riding a dirt bike. In addition to a CSF leak, he incurred the following injuries on the right side of his craniofacial skeleton: depressed frontal bone fracture, orbital roof fracture, nasoethmoidal complex fracture, scleral rupture of the eye, and lacerated superior and inferior canaliculi. He was treated initially by enucleation of the right eye and repair of a laceration of the nasolacrimal canal. His intermediate surgery included a bifrontal craniotomy and repair of dural lacerations, obliteration of the frontal sinuses, and a frontalis fascia oversew of the frontal sinus. Approximately 10 months following the accident, a three dimensional CT scan was used in the fabrication of a three-dimensional Lucite model (Cemax, Mountain View, California). The model was used in the operating room to assist in replacement of the defect with split-rib bone grafts. The right supraorbital region was reconstructed with a full-thickness rib graft. The postoperative ptosis was subsequently repaired with a brow lift plastic procedure along with reconstructions of the supratarsal folds (Fig. 13–46).

Case Report Three

A 25-year-old male was involved in a motor vehicle accident. CT scan revealed a depressed fracture of the right frontal region with an underlying contusion and pneumocephalus. Also present were an extension of the skull fracture through the frontal sinus, a displaced right ZMC fracture, and posterior orbital wall fractures.

He was treated initially by a right frontal craniotomy, cranioplasty, and obliteration of the frontal sinus. The upper facial skull was stabilized by bone plates. Open reduction of the right ZMC fractures was performed with suspension and fixation of the body of the zgyoma from a headframe. Postoperative ptosis, which is often characteristic of a coronal flap procedure occurred (Fig. 13–47).

COMPLEX NASAL-ETHMOIDAL-ORBITAL FRACTURES

Complex nasal-ethmoidal-orbital fractures are those injuries that do not involve the cranial vault but involve significant orbital volumetric changes, fractures of other facial bones, or severe avulsion of soft tissue or bony components requiring primary or secondary bone grafting. These fractures are distinguished from the isolated nasal-ethmoidal-orbital injury, in which a closed operative procedure may be satisfactory.

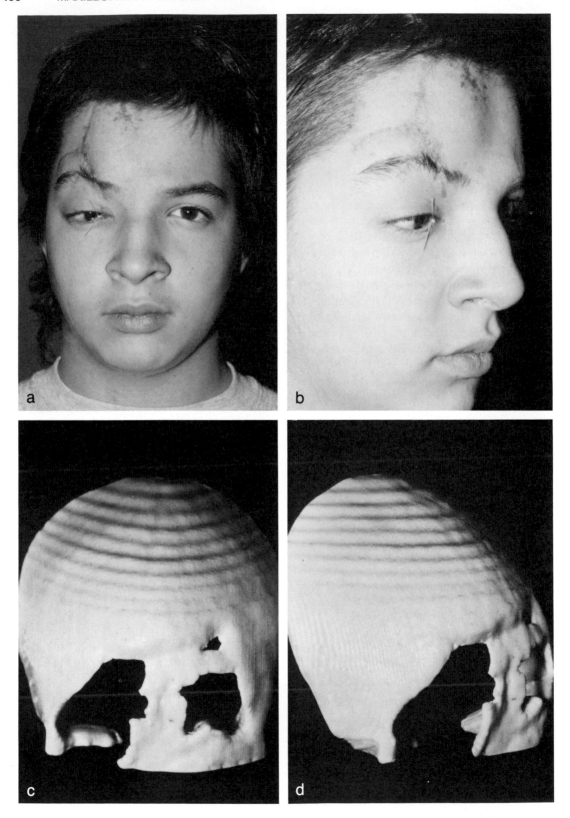

FIG. 13–46. Case Report Two. A 14-year-old boy was injured in a motorcycle accident. **a** and **b,** Extensive defect in the right frontal bone and an avulsive defect of the right supraorbital rim. **c** and **d,** Lucite model of frontal and supraorbital regions as generated by three-dimensional CT program.

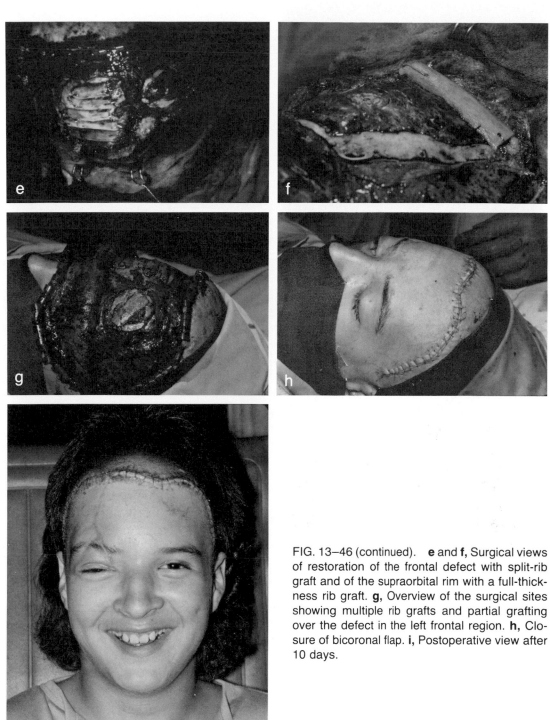

FIG. 13–46 (continued).   **e** and **f,** Surgical views of restoration of the frontal defect with split-rib graft and of the supraorbital rim with a full-thickness rib graft. **g,** Overview of the surgical sites showing multiple rib grafts and partial grafting over the defect in the left frontal region. **h,** Closure of bicoronal flap. **i,** Postoperative view after 10 days.

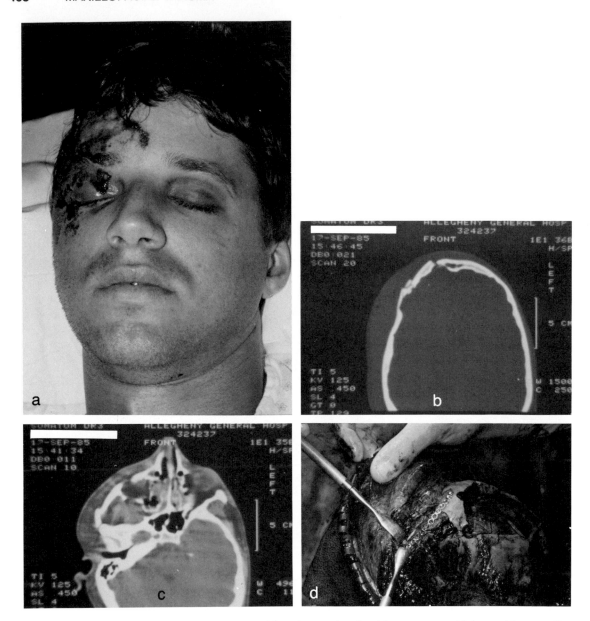

FIG. 13–47.   Case Report Three. A 25-year-old male was involved in a motor vehicle accident. **a,** Post-trauma view. **b,** CT scan of the patient showing a fractured skull. **c,** CT scan demonstrating the fractured right ZMC. **d,** Surgical view of the use of bone plates to stabilize fractures of the frontal bone and supraorbital ridge and demonstrating the use of freeze-dried dura.

Clinical Considerations

The characteristic clinical presentation of nasal-ethmoidal-orbital injuries makes the diagnosis of such lesions straightforward. Some of the clinical signs and symptoms were discussed with frontal nasoethmoidal injuries. An abbreviated case report follows, illustrating the significance of support of the nasal bridge and the problems associated with ex-

ternal support using metal or other plating devices. It also points out the difficulties in delayed or secondary bone grafting of such injuries.

We have been impressed by primary bone grafting of nasal-ethmoidal-orbital injuries, especially when the CT scans show severe comminution in the region of the nasal-ethmoidal-orbital complex. This region is relatively intolerant to impact force; the existence

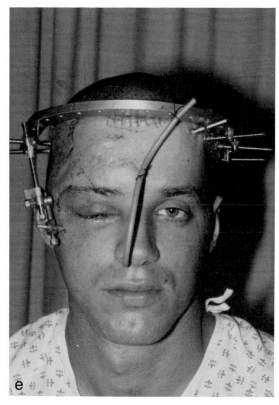

FIG. 13–47 (continued). **e,** Immediate postoperative photographs. Note the suspension of the right zygoma from the headframe.

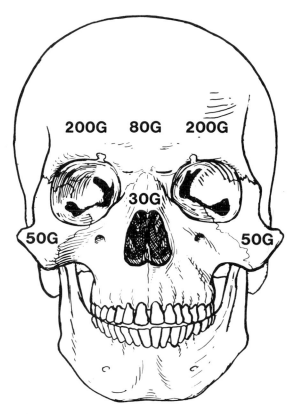

FIG. 13–48. Diagram representing the lower gravity units (G forces) necessary to produce fracturing. (After Swearingen, J.J.: Tolerances of the human face to crash impact. Reprint #65–20, Federal Aviation Agency, Oklahoma City, Oklahoma, 1964.)

of such injuries in isolation implies that the impact force was localized (Fig. 13–48). Large-impact forces delivered over a broader aspect of the face will cause fracture of the frontal bone and of the nasoethmoidal complex. A very localized force will cause an isolated injury to the anatomy in the nasoethmoidal complex.

The complex anatomy of the interorbital area was described previously in relation to treatment of isolated nasal-ethmoidal-orbital injuries (Fig. 13–49). Complex isolated nasoethmoidal injuries can be differentiated from isolated injuries by the fact that whereas the isolated nasal-ethmoidal-orbital injury can be reduced by a closed or open reduction with interosseous wiring chain-link techniques, the complex nasal-ethmoidal-orbital injury usually requires immediate or delayed bone grafting and is associated with fractures of the central maxilla. Thus, a severe, localized force to the nasoethmoidal region may

produce extensive comminution or avulsion of the perpendicular plate of the ethmoid, the maxillary crest, the vomerine bone, and the region of the nasomaxillary buttresses, with a concomitant crushing of the cartilaginous nasal septum (Fig. 13–50). This results in loss of cartilaginous and bony nasal support. A classic sign of this type of injury is seen by putting pressure on the nasal tip and producing a prolapse of the distal nose into the piriform aperture. Thus, a difference between isolated nasal-ethmoidal-orbital injuries that are relatively straightforward and those that are complex is in the loss of distal nasal support and the subsequent need for primary or secondary bone grafting. It must be stated, however, that secondary bone grafting is difficult after scarring has occurred because of the loss of resiliency of the soft tissue.

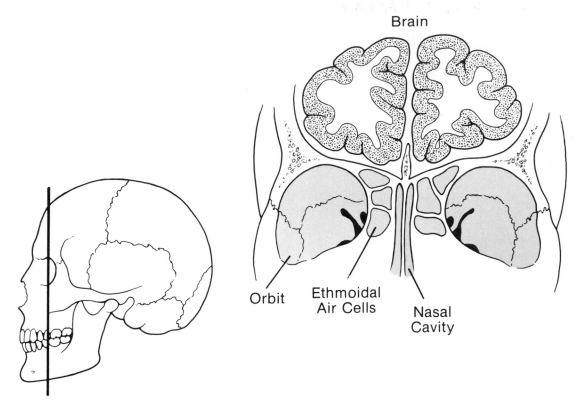

FIG. 13–49.   Interorbital anatomy. Note the proximity of the frontal lobes of the brain to underlying ethmoidal and orbital complexes.

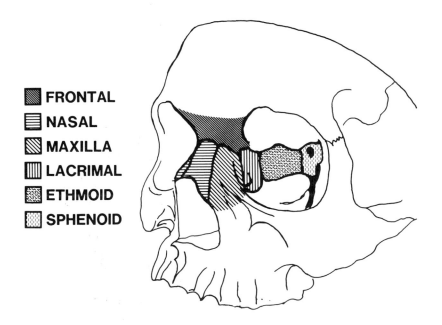

FIG. 13–50.   Bones of the nasoethmoidal region.

TECHNICAL CONSIDERATIONS

Fractures isolated to the bony nasal-ethmoidal-orbital region are often repaired by open reduction through pre-existing lacerations, a coronal incision, a Killian incision, or an open-sky approach and by direct interosseous wiring at the frontonasal and medial orbital region. In isolated injuries that are relatively simple, cartilaginous or distal nasal support is always maintained. The medial canthal ligament and its attachment to the anterior lacrimal crest become laterally displaced, producing traumatic telecanthus. In more complex nasal-ethmoidal-orbital injuries, loss of distal cartilaginous nasal support occurs, often with crushing of the cartilaginous nasal septum. When extensively comminuted and combined with dislocation of bony components posteriorly, laterally, and inferiorly the medial orbital rim and wall are located inferior and posterior to the intact portion of the inferior orbital rim. Because the nasal bones are inaccessible, the surgeon cannot successfully employ a method that uses a blind transnasal approach to attempt to skewer the fragmented nasal bones. An open exploration is indicated so that all fragments can be disimpacted. If this method is unsuccessful, appropriate bone grafting can be used to re-establish normal medial wall contour to support the nasal dorsum, and to restitute medial canthal ligament attachments. Interfragmentary wiring can be used to establish continuity and contour and stabilize the region of the frontal process of the maxilla and bony nasal dorsum. If distal cartilaginous support is lost, however, bone grafts must be used to re-establish stability and contour. The nasal dorsum can be reconstructed using a costochondral rib graft with the bony portion cantilevered against the nasal process of the frontal bone and with the distal cartilaginous portion of the graft in the alar cartilaginous tip (Fig. 13–51).

Some of the dangers inherent in the use of laterally applied lead plates against the nose (Fig. 13–52) are inability of the surgeon to accurately place the wires through the comminuted bones; inability to adequately correct medial canthal laceration, or lateral migration of bones to which the ligament is inserted;

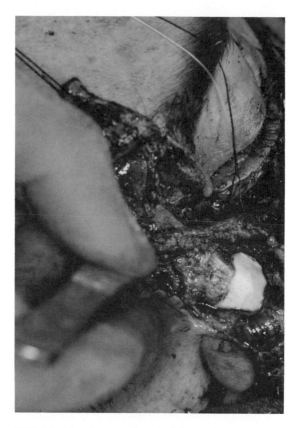

FIG. 13–51.   A costochondral rib graft cantilevered from the nasofrontal region.

often, unaesthetic results because of overcorrection during wire tightening; inadvertent early removal of the plates with collapse of bony support; iatrogenic obstruction of the nasolacrimal duct caused by scarring or displacement of bone fragments as a result of plate pressure; and possible postoperative infection of the portal of entry of the transnasal wires.

Primary Bone Grafting

Certain nasal-ethmoidal-orbital injuries often require both primary correction and numerous secondary procedures to correct posttreatment deformities; comminution of the medial orbital wall and orbital floor, which frequently lead to enophthalmos and diplopia, can be corrected only by primary bone graft replacement. Central maxillary crush injuries associated with loss of distal nasal support can be corrected only by primary nasal bone grafting. Severe comminution or bone

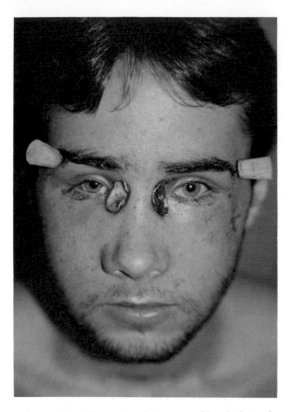

FIG. 13–52. Example of the use of lead plates for support of lateral nasal bones in nasoethmoidal fracture. Their use is fraught with many complications and is usually contraindicated when there is a loss of distal cartilaginous support.

loss in the frontozygomatic or maxillary regions is best stabilized by immediate grafting of the missing or destroyed bone. A patient described by Merville and Real[23] required secondary nasal bone grafts to correct the nasal deformity. As seen in the following case report, a secondary bone graft was needed to repair the nasal bridge collapse following premature removal of the transnasal support plates.

The use of primary bone grafting in the care of severe nasal-ethmoidal-orbital injuries has resulted in a decline in secondary septorhinoplasty for nasal airway obstruction. Use of costochondral grafting improves the appearance of the nasal tip and lessens the risk of its resorption. We have found that split-thickness rib grafts over the body of the zygoma seem not to do as well as full-thickness grafts. In multiple-trauma patients who have had many surgical procedures and are not good

surgical candidates, we use alloplastic material such as Proplast (Vitek Corporation, Houston, Texas) in these regions to rebuild the facial contour.

An unexplained enophthalmos after adequate repair of the orbital floor might result from a medial wall loss. This kind of delayed complication can be prevented by exploring and repairing medial wall damage with appropriate bone grafting at the time of injury. One can suture the medial canthal ligament through a bone graft when the ligamentous attachment is lacerated from the medial orbital bone (Fig. 13–53). Severe nasal-ethmoidal-orbital injuries often result in delayed nasolacrimal duct system problems, especially when many lacerations are present and when many procedures have been done to correct deformity.

Case Report Four

A 30-year-old man was involved in a motor vehicle accident in which his automobile struck a concrete bridge abutment. He suffered loss of consciousness but no hypotension. The patient was transferred from a secondary care hospital to the Allegheny General Hospital Trauma Center with a GCS of 15 and a TS of 16.

His vital signs were stable on arrival. Head and neck examination revealed loss of midfacial contour, gross muscle entrapment of the left globe, periorbital ecchymosis and edema, and scleral hemorrhage (Fig. 13–54). The remaining physical examination was within normal limits with the exception of a chest contusion and a suspicious right hemidiaphragm. Rupture of the diaphragm was ruled out by a laparotomy. CT scan of the head and abdomen revealed no abnormality; facial CT revealed a comminuted, displaced nasal-ethmoidal-orbital fracture including a left ZMC fracture and a fracture of the left orbital floor at the medial surface. Asymptomatic impingement of fragments of bone on the optic nerve was also noted.

On the fifth day post-trauma, open reduction was performed on the left ZMC fracture by exposure of the inferior orbital rim fracture and the fracture at the frontozygomatic suture. At both sites, the fractures were fixated

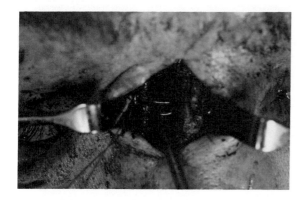

FIG. 13–53.   Reconstruction applying bone grafts to the medial orbital wall and direct insertion into the bone graft of the medial canthal ligament.

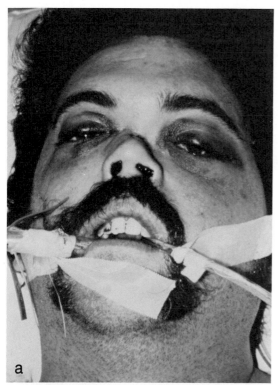

FIG. 13–54.   Case Report Four. Post-trauma photographs of a patient with the usual signs of injury to the nasoethmoidal complex: superior positioning of the nasal tip, telecanthus, concave deformity of the nasofrontal angle, periorbital ecchymosis, and edema. **a** and **b,** Post-trauma photographs. **c,** Post-trauma photograph after resolution of edema; note the deformity of the nasal dorsum.

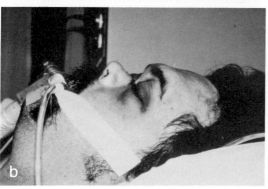

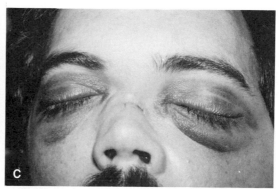

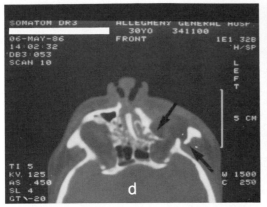
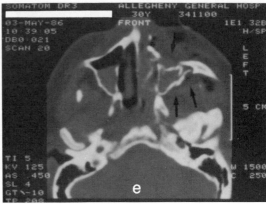
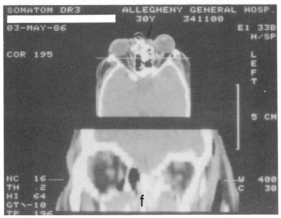

FIG. 13–54 (continued). **d, e,** and **f,** CT scans displaying multiple disruptions of the nasoethmoidal region. Note CT reconstruction of the blow-out fracture of the left orbit.

with 26-gauge stainless steel wire sutures. The fracture of the medial surface of the orbital floor was repaired by placing on it a segment of silastic sheeting.

Attention was then directed to the nasoethmoidal region, where bilateral Killian incisions were made on the anterior lateral aspect of each side of the nose. The superior arms of these incisions were connected by an inverted "V" across the midline (Fig. 13–55). The dissection was carried down through skin and through the overlying musculature and periosteum of the nasal bones, frontal bone, maxilla, and ethmoidal region to the depths of the medial orbital walls. The surgeons found comminuted fracture of the nasal bones, of the nasal process of the frontal bone, of the perpendicular plate of the ethmoidal bone, and of the inferior aspect of the frontal bone just superior to the nasal process. There was also comminution of the lacrimal bone and the nasal process of the maxillary bone. After being reduced with Asche forceps, these bony segments were wired into

position by interfragmentary chain-link wiring. After the nasal bony architecture was reestablished, the surgeons decided to reinforce the lateral nasal bones by use of nasal plates. These plates were secured using a modification of the spinal needle technique.

The patient's postoperative recovery was uneventful. However, on postoperative day 10, the nasal plates were removed prematurely, causing collapse of the nasal dorsum because of lack of distal cartilaginous support (Fig. 13–56). Two months later, the patient developed a left periorbital cellulitis and was admitted to the hospital several days later. Though ophthalmology consultants thought the cellulitis was an infectious process, infectious disease consultants found no incidence of infection in the patient's systemic response. Nonetheless, the left inferior orbital rim wire and silastic implant were removed and a drain inserted. The drain was removed in 24 hr after dramatic improvement, and the patient was discharged 2 days after surgery on oral penicillin and metronidazole. Recur-

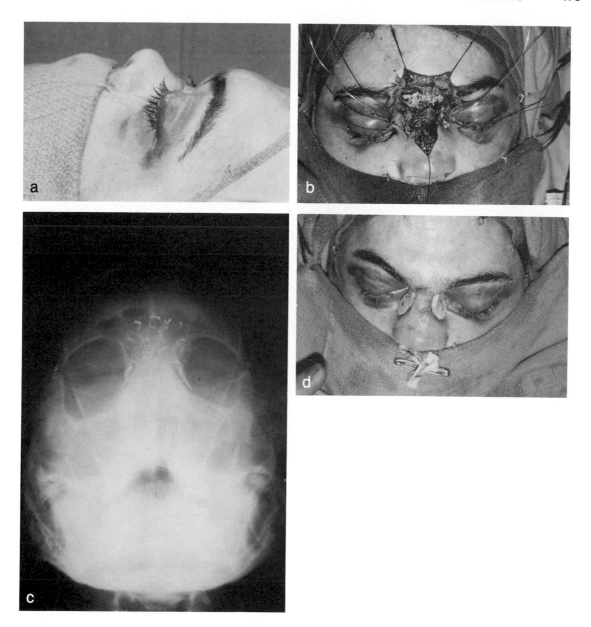

FIG. 13–55.   Case Report Four. Modified Killian incisions used to obtain access to the nasoethmoidal region. **a,** Preoperative photograph. **b,** Killian incision with wide exposure and interfragmentary wiring. **c,** Radiograph showing multiple interfragmentary wires. **d,** Use and premature removal of nasal plates that could have contributed to the collapse of the nasal dorsum.

rent swellings of the left lower eyelid were treated by antibiotics and two attempts at obtaining drainage. A dacryocystogram revealed obstruction of the left nasolacrimal duct system. The patient was subsequently admitted to the hospital for dacryocystorhinostomy and reconstruction of the nasal dorsum and left infraorbital rim using a costochondral graft (Fig. 13–57). The patient was

discharged 3 days later on gentamicin ophthalmic drops, penicillin, and metronidazole. To treat the ectropion that had developed over time as a result of the presence of lacrimal fluid within the tissues and subsequent multiple surgeries of the lower eyelid, a transpositional temporal flap was used to increase the vertical height of the left lower eyelid (Fig. 13–58).

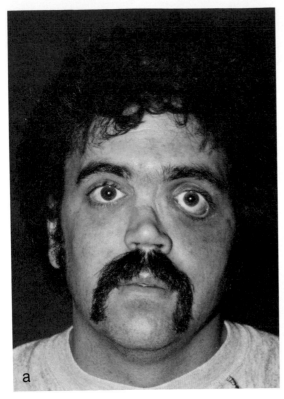 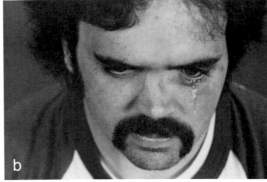

FIG. 13–56. Case Report Four. **a,** View 10 days postoperatively demonstrating collapse of the nasal dorsum and developing ectropion. **b,** View 2 months postoperatively showing dacrocystitis and obstruction, presumably related to the use of plates. Note ectropion caused by numerous surgeries and the ectopic presence of lacrimal secretions.

Discussion

This case illustrates the problems inherent in managing complex nasal-ethmoidal-orbital injuries. With loss of distal cartilaginous support, the patient should have had a primary bone graft to support the central bones of the nasal complex. Although use of the nasal plates for postoperative nasal support indicates that the interfragmentary wiring was adequate, the entire complex lacked total support following surgery. The nasal plates did not provide the needed support, and their premature removal further aggravated the collapse of the bony nasal dorsum. The nasal bones on the left side were telescoped posterior and inferior to the left infraorbital rim, which was itself proximal to its original anatomic position. This positioning created a need for delayed bone grafting of not only the nasal dorsum, but also the left infraorbital rim and maxilla. Moreover, the use of the nasal plates could have caused the obstruction of

the left nasolacrimal drainage system. The nasal cosmetic defect, the inferior/proximal malposition of the orbital rim and maxilla, the occluded nasolacrimal duct system, and ectropion are all sequelae that might have been avoided by open reduction, interfragmentary wiring, and primary bone grafting at the first operation, when lack of distal cartilaginous support was noted.

COMPLEX ORBITOZYGOMATICOMAXILLARY INJURIES

Complex orbitozygomaticomaxillary fractures involve extensive soft-tissue and bony damage to the orbit and its associated ZMC. Isolated ZMC fractures are differentiated from complex injuries by several features. Complex injuries to the orbitozygomaticomaxillary region transcend the more common varieties of zygomatic bone fractures when they involve loss of bony substance and in-

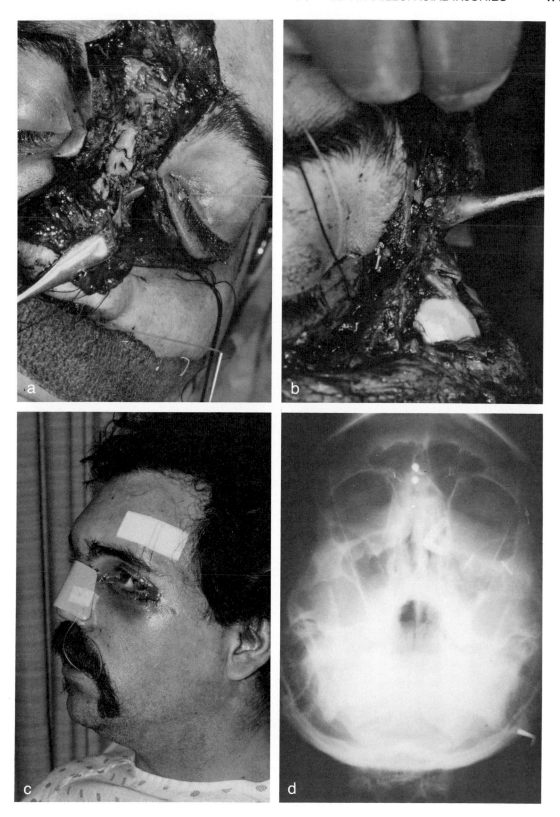

FIG. 13–57.   Case Report Four. **a,** Steps in performing a dacryocystorhinostomy. **b,** Bone graft to the nasal dorsum and left infraorbital rim. **c,** Immediately after DCR, with Frost suture elevating the lateral canthus. **d,** Radiograph of postoperative nasal reconstruction and dacryocystorhinostomy.

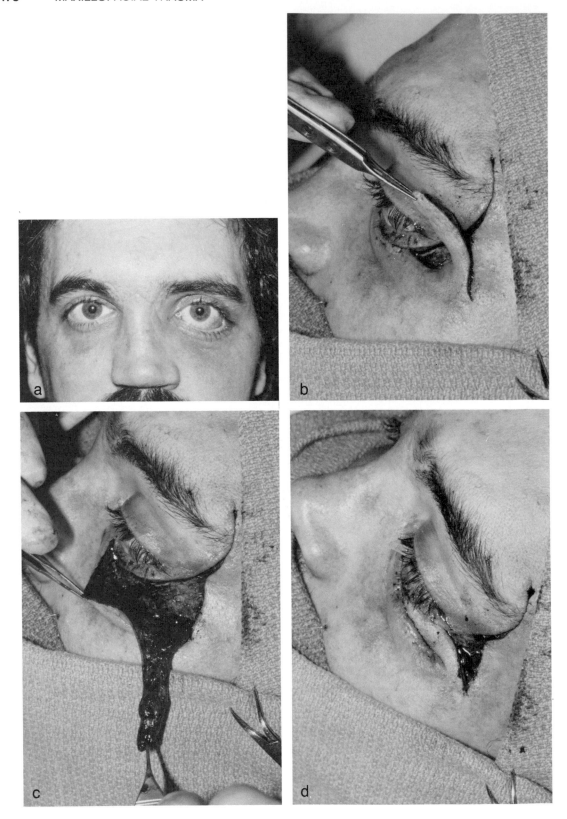

FIG. 13–58.   Case Report Four. Postoperative management of ectropion. **a,** Following repair of nasal dorsum and left infraorbital rim. Ectropion is improved but is still present. **b, c, d,** and **e,** Steps in creating a transpositional temporal soft-tissue flap to increase the vertical height of the lower eyelid.

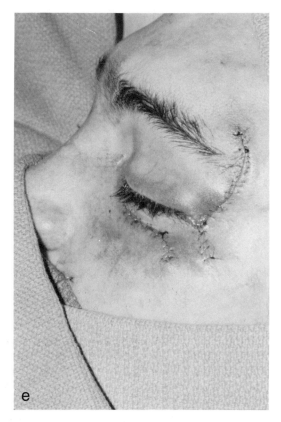

e

FIG. 13–58 (continued).

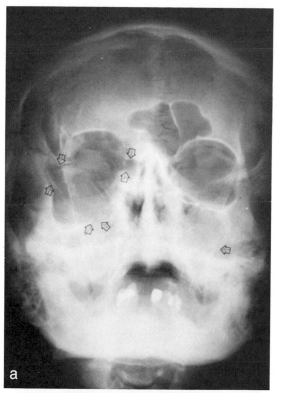

a

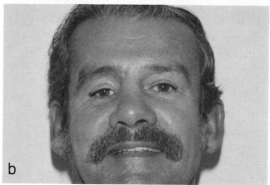

b

stability in bony fractures. A case report will describe a so-called isolated injury that was actually complex because it involved loss of substance, instability, and the need for bone grafting. In addition, this particular case required delayed alloplastic implantation.

Clinical Considerations

In complex severe injuries involving the ZMC with orbital involvement, changes in the volume of the orbit produce extensive displacement or dystopia of the globe (Fig. 13–59). In addition, substance of the floor of the orbit and/or body of the zygoma is lost. In these severely displaced and dislocated fractures, the support of the zygomatic region is unstable, and interosseous wiring many times is not effective in re-establishing the stability of the bone to support the lateral orbital rim. Indeed, the loss of substance of the orbital process of the zygoma causes volumetric changes of the orbit that must be addressed

FIG. 13–59. A 46-year-old male was injured in a motorcycle accident in which the right side of his face bore the brunt of the trauma, demonstrating severe orbital dystopia and an increase in volumetric changes in the right orbit. **a,** Waters radiograph displaying the large change in orbital volume. Complete interfragmentary wiring was performed without bone grafting to decrease the orbital volume. **b,** One year postoperatively the patient had residual traumatic enophthalmos with loss of the supratarsal fold and persistent diplopia in the vertical lateral gaze. Bone grafting in the immediate post-trauma phase may have prevented or lessened the patient's subsequent symptoms.

if traumatic enophthalmos and diplopia are to be avoided.

Loss of the orbital floor or inferior displacement of the orbital floor due to loss of bone from the zygoma causes various degrees of disorganization of the orbital viscera and disrupts the function of the globe. Associated frequently, neuropraxia involving the infraorbital nerve can be addressed immediately or after a delay. Assuming that the medial canthal region is intact, restoration of the separation of the frontozygomatic suture will re-establish the continuity and suspensory function of Lockwood's ligament. However, if comminution is present at the insertion of Whitnall's tubercle, fastening the lateral aspect of the lateral canthal ligament into a bone graft in this region might be necessary. Major lacerations or disruptions of the soft tissue overlying the region of the zygoma provide direct access to the bones; however, the standard subciliary incision and the incision at the lateral aspect of the eyebrow are adequate to gain access to the critical areas to manipulate the fractures. Extension in a lateral inferior direction of the lateral aspect of the subciliary incision can enable the surgeon to place bone grafts in cases of ZMC-orbital injuries that are not associated with extensive soft-tissue lacerations.

The maxillofacial surgeon must be aware that manipulation of impacted or laterally displaced ZMCs can be fraught with severe complications because of possible retrobulbar hemorrhage, blindness, and cardiac arrest. The major objectives in treatment of dislocated fractures of the ZMC are to restore orbital volume, establish horizontal global symmetry, provide support for the ocular globe, and prevent traumatic enophthalmos and diplopia. Re-establishment of facial contour and periorbital bone integrity are other objectives.

In ZMC-orbital injuries that involve loss of substance, the orbital floor, anterior maxilla, body of the zygoma, or zygomatic arch can be replaced by full- or split-thickness rib grafts. In addition, the stability of such fractures can be enhanced by application of bone plates. In some cases, when other fractures of the facial skeleton coexist, it may be advantageous to apply a headframe external skeletal cranial device to support the body of

the zygoma. A vertical strut to an intramedullary pin can be driven into the body of the zygoma (Fig. 13–47). Bone grafts can be placed in an undercut around the remaining shelves of bone that represent the fractured medial and lateral orbital floor or the bone graft can be secured by driving a Kirschner wire through the body of the zygoma and into the bone graft under direct vision (Fig. 13–60). High-velocity impact injuries are associated with atrophy of the periorbital fat, which leads to a persistent traumatic enophthalmos.

Surgical Approaches

To approach the comminuted zygomatic arch, a preauricular incision is made along the temporal skin at a 45° angle anteriorly, relative to the body of the zygomatic arch. The incision can be modified as a rhytidectomy incision (Fig. 13–61) and carried through skin and subcutaneous tissue to the temporal fascia; dissection follows down to the fascia's attachment along the previously intact zygomatic arch. Direct incision of the fascia exposes the fragments of the zygomatic arch. If the arch is comminuted, a rib graft is placed in the region extending from its most distal fragmentation to the temporal process of the zygomatic arch near the bony auditory meatus.

To approach the infraorbital rim and floor of the orbit, a modified subciliary incision is used; the modification is a small "crow's foot" that is extended laterally and inferiorly to gain further access to the floor of the orbit and to facilitate bone grafting procedures. A large bony defect or comminution in this region after severe injuries requires careful approach to the medial and lateral infraorbital rims. Many times it is necessary to bluntly dissect the void between the medial and lateral bony segments with a fine forceps. The periorbita can then be followed inferiorly, and the separation between the maxillary antrum and the orbital cavity be identified. Donovan retractors can be used to maintain a separation between the infraorbital nerve and the maxillary antrum. The maxillary antrum is then irrigated thoroughly through the large void at the floor of the orbit and the residual hema-

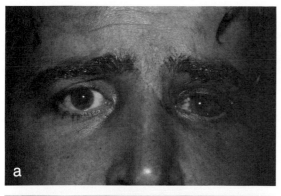

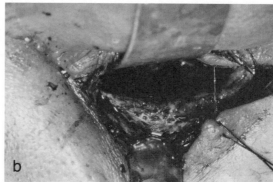

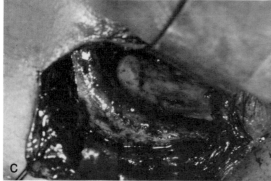

FIG. 13–60.   A 26-year-old male involved in a motorcycle accident. **a,** Preoperative view. **b,** Total loss of the orbital floor. **c,** Treatment consisted of rib grafts to replace the orbital floor.

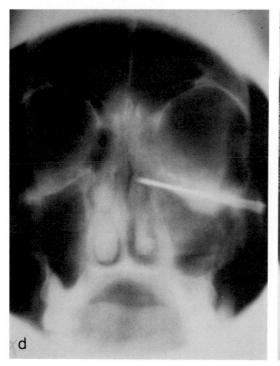

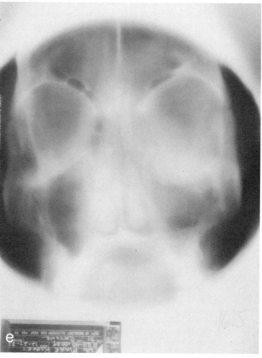

FIG. 13–60 (continued).   **d,** Radiograph shows the graft skewered onto Kirschner wires, which are inserted into the body of the zygoma and then, under direct vision, into the bone graft. **e,** Postoperative radiograph displays stable graft.

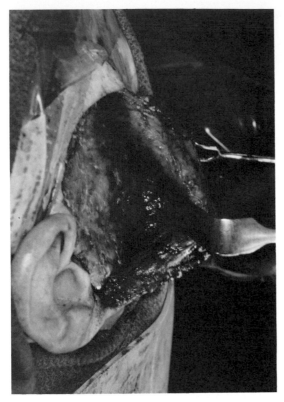

FIG. 13–61.   Modified rhytidectomy incision to provide surgical access to the posterior zygomatic body and arch.

toma and bone fragmentation is debrided (Fig. 13–62).

If there is a significant rent or amputation of the infraorbital nerve, a primary microsurgical epineural repair can be performed at this time. This procedure is facilitated by the access to the infraorbital nerve obtained by the separation of the fragments when the segments are disimpacted by the surgeon or by the laterally displaced condition of the segments. The fragility of this nerve repair must be recognized during subsequent manipulations of the ZMC. The wound is then assessed for the amount of bone lost from the orbital floor, rim, and zygoma.

The frontozygomatic suture region fracture is repaired with transosseous wire ligature. Attention is then directed to the infraorbital incision, and the mobility of the zygoma is tested. If the zygoma is quite mobile and substance has been lost between the medial and lateral segments of the infraorbital rim, it may be necessary to bridge the gap using bone grafting techniques or a specially fashioned staple constructed from a Kirschner wire.[24] This staple can be used subsequently to hold the fragments of infraorbital rim or a bone graft placed in this region (Fig. 13–63). To enhance stability at the frontozygomatic suture region by securing the infraorbital rim, it may be necessary to place a minibone plate and a staple. With a stable frontozygomatic area and infraorbital rim, the surgeon can drive a Kirschner wire through the body of the zygoma into the bone graft of the orbital floor under direct vision.

In the patient in Case Report Five, surgeons performed secondary bone grafting because primary bone grafting appeared to be contraindicated by the amount of wound contamination by many fragments from an exploded

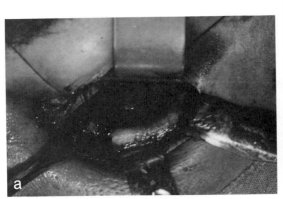

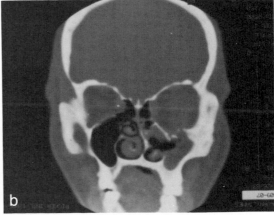

FIG. 13–62.   An example of fragmentation of the orbital floor. In such cases, it is prudent to reconstruct the orbital floor with a bone graft. **a,** Clinical, and **b,** CT scan views of the destruction of the orbital floor.

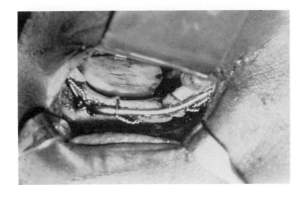

FIG. 13–63. An example of a bent Kirschner wire used as a staple to hold an unstable zygoma laterally when stable bone is present at the naso-orbital buttress and medial infraorbital rim. Note that the bone graft is further stabilized by the collapsing zygoma.

grinding wheel. In any case, elevation of the body of the zygoma in the anterior and lateral position or return of the zygoma to its original anatomic location are usually carried out through the frontozygomatic suture region.

Delayed Treatment

Delayed treatment of an old ZMC fracture is usually carried out with an osteotomy of the frontozygomatic region and the infraorbital area just lateral to the zygomaticomaxillary suture and with an osteotomy of the anterior aspect of the zygomatic arch. This procedure mobilizes the zygoma, which can be placed into proper alignment with the rest of its anatomy. This delayed osteotomy is difficult, especially if there is an associated large defect of the orbital floor that cannot be treated conservatively. If ZMC fracture and this defect coexist, it is often necessary to graft the orbital floor. If several weeks to months elapse after injury, atrophy of the periorbital fat and enophthalmos will be present.

Often associated with injuries to the ZMC are injuries to the infraorbital nerve, as described. In persistent neuropraxia, which in some patients becomes quite significant, especially in cases of anesthesia dolorosa, it may be necessary to take a small segment of the infraorbital rim, remove the segment above the infraorbital nerve, and perform an epineurectomy using either loupes or a microscope (Fig. 13–64). The fragment of bone can

be replaced over the nerve after surgery or simply eliminated. We have found that the use of a machine-driven drill with diamond bur tips will essentially remove bone and not destroy the nerve, whereas steel burs that have flutes may catch and injure soft tissue. The nerve is then held in position with vascular loops, and an epineurectomy is carried out involving approximately 4 mm of the infraorbital nerve. When the nerve is found bound to the membrane of the sinus, it must be released.

Case Report Five

A 54-year-old man sustained multiple injuries in an industrial accident in which a large grinding wheel rotating at 1750 rmp exploded in his face, throwing him backward into another grinder. The patient was amnesic for the event but suffered no loss of consciousness. He was intubated and evacuated by air. On arrival at the trauma center he was awake, alert, and moving all extremities. He was also hypotensive to 90 over palpable and hypoxemic with a PO_2 of 65. His GCS was 15, and his TS, 14. Peritoneal lavage, performed on his arrival, was negative.

Physical examination revealed a large, open avulsion injury over the left zygomatic region extending into the maxillary sinus, as well as a large frontal laceration extending down to the galea aponeurotica. Many smaller lacerations of the midface were noted, with associated blast effect, or tatooing of the facial skin. There was massive periorbital ecchymosis and edema (Fig. 13–65). The pupils were equal and reactive. The left ocular globe was significantly displaced in an inferior direction, although extraocular muscle function was intact. The left half of the maxilla was very mobile, with many associated fractured teeth of the maxillary left quadrant.

Examination of the thorax revealed massive contusions to the left anterior chest. There was tenderness of the ribs to palpation bilaterally with crepitation noted in the left lateral region. Numerous small puncture wounds were present over the chest wall bilaterally. Breath sounds were present throughout and equal bilaterally. Chest radiography revealed numerous rib fractures bilaterally but no flail component.

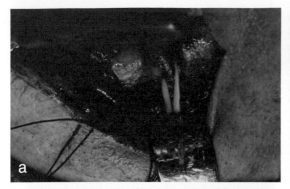

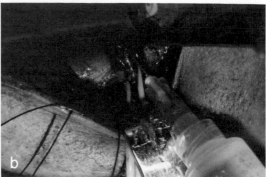

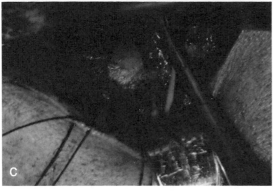

FIG. 13–64.   Microsurgical neurorrhaphy managed by epineurectomy of the infraorbital nerve. The nerve is dissected free from the infraorbital canal and outlined with vascular loops. Bone overlying the nerve is removed with a diamond bur mounted on a handpiece. An epineurectomy is performed with microscissors after saline is injected beneath the nerve sheath. **a,** Identification of the nerve. **b,** Proximal and distal vascular loops and injection of saline. **c,** Epineurectomy with microscissors.

The patient was taken to the operating room after initial fluid resuscitation and after appropriate review of head and face with CT and cervical-spine films. This first operation involved extensive debridement of the face and excision of many fragments of grinding wheel material from the facial wounds. The nitrogen-driven (Sympulse) irrigation device was used extensively to enhance the debridement procedure. After the wound was thoroughly debrided, wound assessment at surgery revealed an extensively comminuted left orbital-ZMC. The body, arch, and buttress of the left zygoma were fragmented into many bony segments that remained attached to the periosteum. Most of the left midface could be pedicled from its posterior base, the anterior margin of the wound lying along the lateral ridge of the nose and upper lip. Exploration of the orbital floor disclosed total disruption of the left orbital floor with many fragments lying in the maxillary antrum. The left globe was dystopic and the orbital viscera was herniated through the missing inferior wall. The anterior and lateral walls of the left maxilla were also comminuted, with free movement of the left maxilla at the palatine suture.

Surgeons decided to perform primary re-construction of the left zygomatic region using interfragmentary wiring to reconstitute the entire superior, lateral, and inferior orbital rim. Similar interosseous wiring was carried out on the remaining bones of the walls of the maxilla (Fig. 13–66). The massive facial pedicle flap was thoroughly undermined, and on selected sites the periosteum was sharply released to allow primary closure of the facial wound without tension. In view of the gross contamination and severity of the patient's rib fractures, it was decided not to perform primary bone grafting of the left face or orbital floor. Maxillomandibular fixation was used to reduce the occlusal disharmony caused by maxillary fracture. The wound was then closed in the usual fashion and drained. The patient progressed well postoperatively and was discharged on post-trauma day 12. Because his pulmonary status was still of concern, it was decided to defer further maxillofacial reconstruction until improvement was noted.

The patient was admitted again 18 days after the accident and the left fifth rib was harvested and used as a graft to the left orbital floor. The patient progressed well following the orbital floor reconstruction and reconsti-

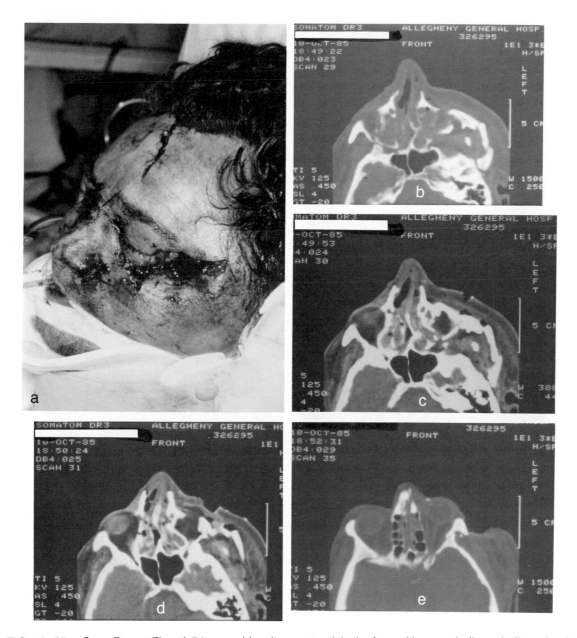

FIG. 13–65.   Case Report Five. A 54-year-old male was struck in the face with an exploding grinding wheel. **a,** Most of the facial injuries were confined to the left side. **b, c, d,** and **e,** Preoperative CT scans reveal the extensive damage to the bony architecture of the left ZMC and orbital areas.

tution of horizontal symmetry of the eyes. Over the ensuing postoperative months, the patient developed increasing ankylosis of the mandible. A left coronoidectomy was performed after tomograms revealed fusion of this process to the lateral wall of the maxilla.

Approximately 8 months after the injury, the patient's left zygoma was augmented with placement of a Proplast zygoma implant (Vitek Corporation, Houston, Texas). Later, sev-

eral smaller procedures such as dermabrasion of facial tatoos and facial scar revisions were done.

PANFACIAL TRAUMA

These patients' case histories emphasize that significant trauma can exist in separate sites of the maxillofacial complex or at overlapping sites, and while they may affect a spe-

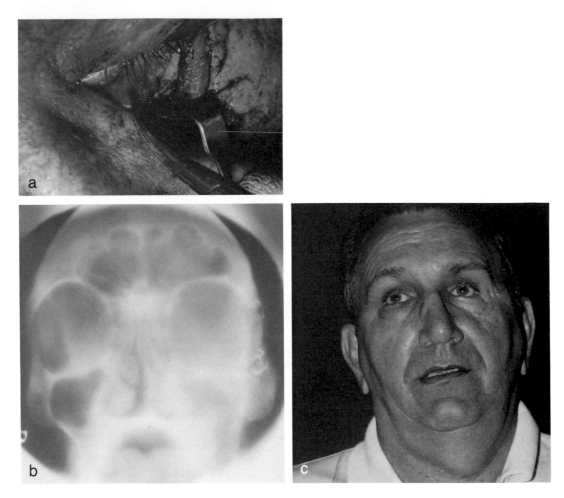

FIG. 13–66.   Case Report Five. Intraoperative and postoperative views. **a,** Intraoperative view of rib grafts to the left orbital area. **b,** Postoperative radiograph showing interfragmentary wiring. **c,** Postoperative view of patient.

cific anatomic area, some fractures (such as a distally unsupported nasoethmoidal injury) are of greater magnitude than a nondisplaced and distally supported nasoethmoidal injury. The panfacial or complex multiple-site maxillofacial skeletal injury is defined by those injuries that do not adhere to any specific classification, involve many sites, often each site being as complex as the cases described above, and involving avulsion or comminution of bone requiring primary and secondary bone grafting.

Sequencing of Treatments

It is important, not only to guarantee the overall physiologic well-being of the patient,

in whom coexisting multisystem trauma may contraindicate immediate maxillofacial intervention, but also to facilitate operative management of facial injuries, that the maxillofacial surgeon and the traumatologist coordinate their resources and philosophies so that the patient can be treated as soon as possible after trauma. Indeed, because of the development of trauma centers and the rapid resuscitation of severely injured patients, it is often possible to treat patients within 6 hr after the accident, before massive edema associated with these injuries develops. We have observed that once this massive panfacial edema occurs, at least 1 week must pass before the surgeon can operate with relative ease.

At the AGH Trauma Center, when panfacial injuries crossing many facial skeletal lines occur in addition to thoracoabdominal injuries, intracranial injuries, and extremity injuries, it is important that the traumatologist be involved with the initial facial treatment. While thoraco-abdominal injuries are being treated, initial early care of the maxillofacial injuries can be provided. When there are no significant intracranial injuries and the thoracoabdominal injuries are stabilized, care of the panfacial injury must be begun. Initial treatment involves a tracheostomy, so that the maxillofacial surgeon can complete his care in an unobstructed surgical field.

Preliminary maxillomandibular fixation prevents supraglottic airway obstruction, and the traumatologist and pulmonary specialist can assist in maintaining pulmonary function. In the early care of panfacial injuries, attention is then directed to immediate resuscitation, correction of dislocations within the thoracoabdominal complex, establishment of long-term airway access with tracheostomy and pulmonary toilet, nasogastric intubation and suction, and in the multisystem-injured patient, a feeding pharyngostomy. Debridement of all the soft-tissue lacerations, as discussed in a previous section of this chapter, follows. Next, intraoral lacerations are closed after application of arch bars on an intact dentition, or the taking of impressions for casts of the upper and lower jaws to later construct fracture appliances to ensure normal AP dimensions of the facial skeleton. The maxillary and mandibular teeth or arches are brought into fixation, if possible, with maxillomandibular fixation wires.

With the patient thus stabilized, the maxillofacial surgeon can begin to treat the multiple injuries based on a clinical and facial CT evaluation. If no cranial injuries complicating maxillofacial skeletal injuries are present, injuries can be addressed according to standard procedure. The sequencing thus becomes the re-establishment of a mandibular occlusal plane and the caudad to cephalad reduction and fixation of each fracture site separately. The mandibular fragments are realigned first with arch bars and then by open reduction and internal fixation using eccentric dynamic compression bone plates or bone plates with small self-tapping intramedullary screws. If several mandibular fracture sites are present, in order to establish the mandibular occlusal plane it may be necessary to open each fracture site individually and place appropriate bone plates. This procedure is done after the surgeon is assured that the occlusal interdigitation is appropriate. The re-established mandibular arch serves as a guide for reassembly of the midface.

Establishing Vertical and AP Facial Dimensions

In patients with bilateral fractured mandibular condyles, at least one condyle is opened to re-establish vertical dimension and attempt to re-establish normal AP dimension of the midface. If there is a severe burst fracture of the mandibular condyle ramus complex, applying a costochondral graft to the affected side might be necessary. The costochondral graft is placed against the existing glenoid fossa after debridement of hematoma and bone fragments from the region of the injury. Thus, the mandibular arch is re-established and attention is turned to the midface fractures.

An alternative to suspension of the midface from the intact cranial base and reconstructed mandibular arch is rigid fixation of the maxillary fragments. This fixation is done after disimpaction of the maxilla, maxillomandibular fixation, and checking of the dental occlusion. Rigid fixation can be used bilaterally in the anteromaxillary and posteromaxillary buttresses. To place the buttress plates at anterior and posterior maxilla, a vestibular incision is made through the buccal sulcus, and bone plates are applied directly. Subciliary incisions are used to expose the infraorbital rims, and the frontozygomatic suture area is approached through a lateral brow skin incision.

Following disimpaction of the midface, and establishment of normal AP dimension of the facial structures, the zygomas are suspended bilaterally using rigid fixation and minibone plates at the frontozygomatic sutures. To complete the rigid fixation structure, bilateral infraorbital rim plates can also be used. The amount of bone loss in the anterior wall of the maxilla, zygomas, and orbital floor is evaluated; split ribs can be placed in these regions to establish contour of the midface in addition to providing support for the globe in the region of the floor of the orbit.

In some cases, at the time of the initial debridement, closure of intraoral lacerations, and placement of arch bars after the initial tracheostomy, a headframe can be applied. Many times, with coexistence of a fractured skull, strategic calvarial pins can be placed at a distance from the skull fractures. Later, the bone grafting can be fixed with Kirschner wires driven into the bodies of the zygomas or secured simply by placing undercuts to lock the bone into position. The mandibular complex can then be fastened to the headframe with vertical struts. Collapse of the midface can be further prevented by placement of appropriate traction wires from the maxillary arch bar or, transcutaneously, to vertical struts arising from the headframe (Fig. 13–34). Additionally, bone grafts can be placed in the pterygomaxillary region to further assist in stabilizing the maxilla. This may prevent secondary recession of the maxilla after removal of the stabilizing devices.

Case Report Six

A 21-year-old female jumped out of a motor vehicle moving approximately 55 mph, landed on her face, and skidded on the pavement. The patient was flown to the trauma center by Life Flight from an outlying hospital. The patient arrived at the hospital already intubated with an endotracheal tube. There was a bloody drainage from the right ear, mouth, and nose. Her GCS was 15 and TS was 16. The presumptive diagnosis was Le Fort III fracture, basilar skull fracture, pelvic fracture, and bladder perforation. Tracheostomy, operation for a feeding pharyngostomy, and repair of multiple lip lacerations were performed. The patient was found at that time to have a symphyseal mandibular fracture and right burst fracture of the condyloid process and ramus (Fig. 13–67). Many teeth were extracted and intraoral soft-tissue lacerations were closed during the same operative procedure, and the orthopedic department placed an external fixation device (a pelvic Hoffman) at this time. A small tooth

fragment lodged in the lower right lung quadrant was removed via bronchoscopy. The bladder injury was confirmed by the urology department and a catheter was placed. On the fourth day post-trauma, the maxilla/midface was disimpacted to be freely mobile. Arch bars were placed and tentative maxillomandibular fixation was established. A right costochondral graft was placed, thus repairing the right ramus condyloid process complex. The mandible was completely repaired using a bone plating technique.

Following reconstruction of the mandibular occlusal plane and reconstruction of the right mandibular condyle and ramus with a costochondral graft, a bicoronal incision was developed and the flap was retracted inferiorly. The flap was then returned to its natural position and bilateral subciliary incisions were made. These incisions exposed the infraorbital rims.

Using a different set of instruments, the maxilla was approached through the oral cavity and a transverse incision was made through the alveolar mucosa. This buccal vestibule incision was carried to the bone, and reduction was performed after disimpaction of the maxilla using seven Luhr plates and two wires. A four-hole plate was placed across the left inferior orbital fracture, which surgeons considered adequately stabilized the left nasal orbital rim fracture; a four-hole plate was placed in the left anterior maxillary buttress, and another four-hole plate in the left posterior maxillary buttress. The right frontozygomatic suture was partially reduced using stainless steel wire passed through holes made in the bone. The globe was protected while all plates and wires were placed by using malleable retractors and Donovan retractors. Having partially reduced the frontozygomatic suture, the surgeons reduced the right inferior orbital rim with a four-hole plate, followed by performing a four-hole plate reduction of the right anteromaxillary buttress. Having achieved stability on the right frontozygomatic area, the right zygomaticofrontal area was reduced by tenting the wire and securing the bone with a five-hole Luhr bone plate.

When the nose and its surrounding structures were palpated, a step was felt along the right nasomaxillary junction. Because this

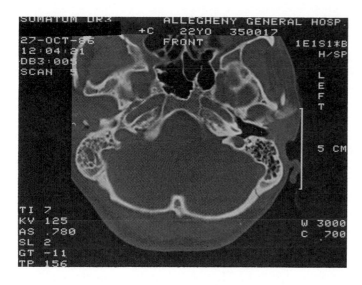

FIG. 13–67. Case Report Six. A 21-year-old female jumped from a moving vehicle and sustained multiple injuries to the upper, middle, and lower facial skeleton. CT scan of the injuries show absence of the right condyloid process.

step was extremely hard to visualize through the subciliary or coronal incisions, a W-shaped incision was made longitudinally along the medial aspect of the nasion and carried down to the fracture, which was found to be at the most medial portion of the right infraorbital rim. This was reduced and held in position with a small-gauge wire.

An additional rib was obtained using the chest incision, and then split with small osteotomes, cut into size with rongeurs, bent manually, and placed along the right orbital floor. The wounds were all closed in the usual manner and the patient was returned to the trauma intensive care unit. On post-trauma day 9, the patient was transferred to a regular hospital floor. Her major postoperation problems involved atelectasis and rhonchi.

RIGID INTERNAL FIXATION

In complex maxillofacial skeletal injuries, the treatment of mandibular fractures follows the same basic orthopedic principles as have been established for long bones: reduction of the fractured segments to anatomic position, establishment of the pretrauma dental occlusion, immobilization of the fracture to facilitate healing, establishment of early physiological function, and prevention of sepsis or gross movement that would lead to malunion or nonunion. Since the beginning of the Civil War, the treatment of fractured mandibles has involved maxillomandibular fixation applied

in an open or closed procedure with internal wire fixation.

Bone plating is a historical method of general orthopedic fracture fixation used in Europe and the British Isles since the latter part of the nineteenth century. The use of bone plates but not necessarily axial compression had been used in the recent past.[25-28] Static bone plating methods were not widely accepted because, in many cases, they frequently led to postoperative infection, osteomyelitis, and malunion or nonunion because of distraction at the fracture ends. Other fixation procedures were advocated in addition to static bone plates. More recently, an increase in interest and knowledge relating to the physiology of bone, as well as its biomechanics, paralleled the more sporadic use of static bone plates; as biotechnical knowledge developed, the operative techniques improved, as did the designs of the devices and the alloys used to construct the bone plates. Bone plates of diverse designs have been developed for the mandible and maxilla and have been reported by numerous authors.[29-34]

In recent years, the Association for the Study of Internal Fixation (ASIF) has provided fundamental improvements in design and clinical research that have enhanced maxillofacial surgeons' understanding and acceptance of the concept of rigid internal fixation in fracture management.[28]

INDICATIONS

Rigid internal fixation is indicated in patients who are edentulous or partially edentulous or who are elderly and for whom early function would enhance psychologic and social interaction and improve nutritional status; in complex maxillofacial injuries associated with discontinuity defects resulting from gunshot wounds, explosions of automobile or truck tires, or high-velocity motor vehicle accidents; in patients who are medically compromised and require special medical support, such as those with severe cardiac and pulmonary problems or those who have a problem with epilepsy or alcohol or drug abuse; and in psychologically disturbed patients who have a very difficult time in compliance. In multiple-trauma patients who will require anesthesia several times for various operative procedures, the use of rigid fixation greatly facilitates its administration.

Although rigid internal fixation is not a panacea and there are some specific problems with its use, for the selected patient it is a useful, successful, low-morbidity method of fracture management.

However, inappropriate use of rigid fixation must not be allowed to service the surgeons' natural intellectual interest in renewed and newer technology. With their appreciation for finely machined instrumentation, surgeons' use of rigid fixation devices might occasionally be a case of "a treatment seeking a malady." Rigid fixation devices involve expensive equipment; in the nasal-ethmoidal-orbital area and the orbital rims, the devices can be very bulky compared to transosseous wires; the surgical time required for their placement might be significantly longer than that for other techniques of reduction and fixation of maxillofacial fractures and might mandate inpatient care or longer hospitalizations; also, the placement of the devices is technique-sensitive and could result in rigid fixation of slight malunions.

SURGICAL TECHNIQUES FOR THE MANDIBLE

In the management of complex maxillofacial injuries with a mandibular fracture component, dynamic compression bone plates or eccentric dynamic compression bone plates can be applied through the full-thickness lacerations. Low morbidity is associated with placement of the bone plates through transoral incisions. However, when no pre-existing full-thickness lacerations expose the compound fractures of the mandible, extraoral approaches facilitate the placement of eccentric dynamic compression plates. The eccentric dynamic compression bone plates are placed in the basal portion of the mandible where the bone is thickest and the screws can be below the root structures and the inferior alveolar neurovascular canal of the mandible.

The first and fundamental consideration in rigid internal fixation when using eccentric dynamic compression bone plates or dynamic compression bone plates is establishment of the dental occlusion and maxillomandibular fixation. This is especially important in dynamic compression bone plating, in which only axial compression is exerted, rather than in eccentric dynamic compression bone plating, in which the bone is rotated clockwise in relation to the distal fragment and counterclockwise in relation to the proximal fragment, thus bringing the alveolus into compression at the superior margin toward the teeth. The supplemental application of an arch bar can maintain bone contact at the superior aspect of the fracture in the tooth-bearing portion of the mandible. In the presence of coexisting midfacial and other anatomic disruptions of the maxillofacial skeleton in complex maxillofacial injuries, maxillary and mandibular arch bars rather than eyelet loops are used. While certain isolated mandibular fractures can be treated with rigid fixation and without maxillomandibular fixation, we have found that severe complex maxillofacial disruptions are better handled by maxillomandibular fixation for 3 weeks.

After the establishment of the occlusal plane through maxillomandibular fixation, an extraoral incision is made at the fracture site, and the inferior border of the mandible and the fracture site are exposed. Even after maxillomandibular fixation there may be a transverse rotation and axial gapping at the fracture site. The maxillomandibular fixation and occlusal intercuspation allow reduction pliers to be used to develop a preload on the mandible because they ensure that the eccentrically applied force is transformed into axial compression (Fig. 13–68). Pressure rollers on

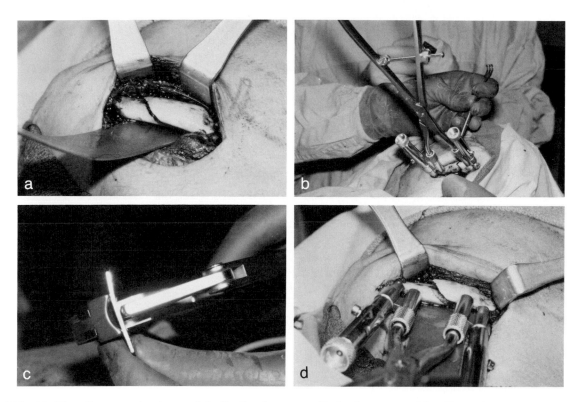

FIG. 13–68. Compression bone plate fixation for a mandibular fracture. **a,** Mandibular fracture exposed through a submandibular surgical approach. **b,** Use of reduction forceps at the inferior border of the mandible. **c,** Contouring the bone plate with bending forceps. **d,** Gradual tightening of the reduction forceps.

the reduction pliers ensure an increase in pressure. By adjusting the reduction forceps, the surgeon can use axial compression to provide complete stability and approximation of the fracture site. An eccentric dynamic compression bone plate based on the principle of spherical geometry is used—that is, if a sphere is theoretically rolled down an angular cylindrical tube, the vertical dropping of the sphere through the lumen of the cylinder will change into a horizontal movement of the sphere. The head of the intramedullary screw that is used in rigid internal fixation is a hemisphere (see Chapter 5). Also, a portion of a negative hemisphere is imprinted within the openings of the dynamic compression bone plate, making up the entire eccentric dynamic compression bone plate. When the reduction pliers are used to bring the fractured segments into actual compression, the eccentric dynamic compression bone plate is placed at the appropriate site on the mandible, bridging the fracture site. The plate is bent with the special instruments and forceps. A slight

overbending is necessary to enable the lingual portion of the mandible to be compressed. With reduction and compression assured by the reduction forceps and compression performed by tightening the rollers of the forceps with additional superior support by the maxillomandibular fixation, the surgeon can then place two vertical intramedullary screws adjacent to the fracture site.

The surgeon first places the distal screw through the bone plate and into the bone but not into a tightened position. The proximal screw is then inserted and tightened firmly. When the proximal screw is being tightened, its head moves on the gliding plane of the bone plate so that the plate moves proximally. As soon as the plate meets the distal screw head, the screw draws the fragment in the same direction. The distal screw is then tightened firmly and the plate is drawn distally and moves the proximal fragment toward the fracture site. The screw on the distal segment which is firmly anchored in the distal fragment, creates resistance producing compres-

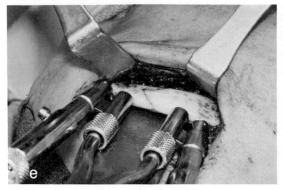

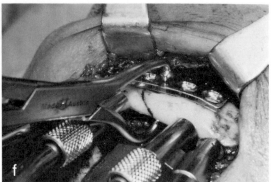

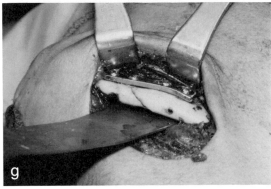

FIG. 13–68 (continued). **e,** Reduction of the fractured segments. **f,** Compression bone plate in place. **g,** Reduction forceps removed.

sion of the fracture line. If transverse holes are present on the outer aspect of these screws, placing intramedullary screws in the transverse holes will cause compression of the superior aspect of the mandibular fracture as well as axial compression. Multiple bone plates can be used throughout a multiply fractured mandible.

Small T-shaped phalangeal bone plates can be used to repair fractures at the neck of the mandibular condyle. Other mandibular fracture locations for transoral fixation using bone plates include the third molar region and the parasymphyseal area.

SURGICAL TECHNIQUES FOR THE MIDFACIAL SKELETON

Miniplates using compression, adaptation plates without compression, or lag screws are used to treat various fractures of the midfacial complex (Fig. 13–69). Minibone plates can be used in the regions of the frontozygomatic suture, the medial and lateral orbital rims, the zygomaticomaxillary buttress and the naso-maxillary buttress at the piriform aperture. In addition, in fractures overlying the frontal

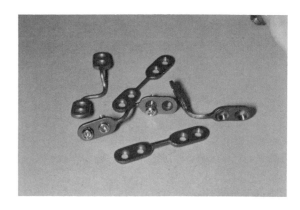

FIG. 13–69. Miniplates, especially those designed for ease of contouring, can be placed at various locations throughout the mid- and upper facial skeleton. They can be used in the mandible as a substitute for superior margin transosseous wiring in the mandibular third molar region and for unicortical direct wiring in the body of the mandible, especially in the parasymphyseal area. (Courtesy of Hall Reconstructive Systems, Santa Barbara, California.)

sinus and frontal bone and supraorbital ridge, compression osteosynthesis plates can be used. Adaptation bone plates have been used in the region of the nasal bone at the junction of the frontal and the nasal process of the frontal bone. Adaptation bone plates in the regions of the lateral wall of the maxilla may be employed where the bone is extremely thin; in these cases, the adaptation bone plates do not exert compressive forces.

Simple fracture of the zygomaticomaxillary complex without mobility and without significant displacement can be treated by a rigid fixation minibone plate placed at the frontozygomatic suture, which may obviate the need for a fixation wire at the infraorbital margin. Duker and associates[35] compared 26 cases of zygomaticomaxillary fractures treated with interosseous wiring with 24 cases treated with plate osteosynthesis. They noted that in at least half of the cases treated with interosseous wiring, the frontozygomatic suture ligature had to be supplemented with a ligature at the infraorbital margin, but with the plate osteosynthesis, all that was required was a frontozygomatic buttress plate. Very mobile ZMC fractures can be supported by a bone plate placed at the buttress of the zygoma, in addition to the two-point fixation mentioned above.

Miniplates will support Le Fort II fractures at the nasomaxillary and zygomatic buttresses and in some cases at the infraorbital rims. Le Fort III fractures can be secured at the frontozygomatic sutures bilaterally in the nasofrontal region, and in the midline. The surgeon can stabilize combination fractures at nasomaxillary, zygomaticomaxillary, nasofrontal, infraorbital rim, and frontozygomatic locations. It might be more appropriate to secure Le Fort II fractures at the lower orbital margins rather than at the zygomaticomaxillary buttresses. Palatal fractures that have splayed the maxilla laterally can be secured across the fracture line in the midline of the maxilla by an osteosynthesis plate at the lower margin of the piriform aperture. Maxillomandibular fixation should be removed at the conclusion of the operation in which bone plates and lag screws are placed if there is no skeletal fixation cephalad of the midfacial fracture sites to oppose the muscle forces that distract the midfacial fractures because the compression screws are weak relative to these muscle forces.

In the placement of rigid fixation to the midface, the drill bit 1.5 mm in diameter through a drill and tap sleeve is used to protect the soft tissue contiguous to the drill site. The hole must be drilled precisely, the drill bit not being allowed to wobble, to avoid producing an eccentric hole. A self-tapping screw is then placed, or a 2-mm tap is used to provide grooves for the screw.

In lag screw osteosynthesis of the midface, miniscrews with a diameter of 2.5 mm are used. For the gliding hole, a 1.5-mm twist drill bit is needed. The drill guide and tap have an outer diameter of 1.5 mm. The depth gauge is the same as for the 2-mm screws. The screwdriver is specially constructed for a 1.5-mm screw. In addition, an appropriate counter-sink is needed. Where there are thick bone lamellae, the 2-mm miniscrews can also be used, with corresponding equipment for lag screw osteosynthesis.

To explain application of osteosynthesis to midfacial fractures, it may be useful to discuss a fracture at the frontozygomatic suture region. The surgical approach to the fracture is usually through a lateral brow incision. A stainless steel wire of 24 or 25 gauge can be used to hold the frontozygomatic suture in place while the manipulation is carried out and an adequate reduction is achieved and stabilized. Attention is directed to the inferior or distal fracture segment or the frontal process of the zygoma. A screw hole is drilled into the bone with a 1.5-mm twist drill after the miniplate is adapted to the flat portion of the lateral aspect of the frontozygomatic suture region. This 1.5-mm drill size corresponds to the core diameter of the 2-mm miniscrew. The orbital viscera is protected with a malleable retractor. The screw length is then measured with a depth gauge and the thread is cut with a 2-mm tap. The adapted bone plate is applied and fixed in a loose manner with a 2-mm miniscrew. The superior hole on the proximal segment or the zygomatic process of the frontal bone is then placed in a similar way. The miniscrew is placed and tightened at the zygomatic process of the frontal bone, bringing the fracture site together. Those screws are tightened firmly and the outer screws are placed, after which the transosseous wire is removed.

Neutral osteosynthesis is undertaken in the regions of the piriform aperture and in the area of the zygomatic buttress. These fracture sites can be secured with four- or six-hole adaptation bone plates with round holes without compression. The bone fragments are then secured using 2-mm intermedullary screws.

LAG SCREWS

Lag screws can be used with excellent success in placing a cantilevered bone graft or onlaid bone graft of the nasal bridge and grafting in the region of the zygomatic buttress and infraorbital margin. Lag screws can be used in mandibular reconstruction after trauma, especially if there is an oblique fracture line; however, for most mandibular fractures we have not found it as useful as eccentric dynamic compression and bone plating. Lag screws are indicated for stabilizing and fixating costochondral grafts to the ramus of the mandible.

Bone grafts involving split ribs and full-thickness ribs can be adapted for contour and for stability using miniplates or lag screws. In adapting laterally positioned bone grafts to the facial skeleton, lag screws are used in the following manner. The initial hole is drilled through the onlaid bone graft with a drill bit 2.7 mm in diameter. When manual or tactile sensation indicates that the cortex of the underlying bone has been reached, a 2-mm drill bit is used to drill through the underlying bony tissue. A 2.7-mm tapper is dropped through the bone graft itself (the descent should be unimpeded because of the diameter of the screw hole drilled in the bone graft). The underlying bone hole, which is 2 mm in diameter, is then engaged. Tapping is then carried out, the tapper is removed, a depth gauge is used to determine the length of the screw, and appropriate miniscrews 2.7 mm in diameter are used to fasten the overlying bone graft to the underlying bone.

COMPLICATIONS

Complications of bone plating to the midfacial skeleton and the mandible are consist-ent with the use of any interosseous fixation or stabilization device. A complication can occur if the bone plates are near sensory nerve distributions, especially with bone plates placed near the infraorbital nerve and the thin overlying tissues of the lower eyelid. Patients complain of sensing unpleasant thermal changes not necessarily related to actual temperature changes. The plate produces a dysesthesia or neuropraxia involving the distribution of the nerve and is usually resolved by removal of the bone plate 3 to 4 months after placement. We have tended to remove bone plates in patients who can tolerate the removal and in patients who are extremely thin and can sense thermal changes very quickly or can palpate the apparatus beneath thin skin. Many times the removal of the underlying bone plates can be performed under sedation and local anesthesia, without resorting to general anesthesia.

REFERENCES

1. Trunkey, D.D.: Trauma. Chalmer Lyons Annual Lecture, American Association of Oral and Maxillofacial Surgeons Scientific Session, 1987.
2. Trunkey, D.D.: Shock trauma. Can J Surg 27:479, 1984.
3. Ryckman, F.C., and Noseworthy, J.: Multisystem trauma. Symposium on Pediatric Surgery, Part I. Surg Clin North Am 65:1287, 1985.
4. Trunkey, D.D.: Trauma. Sci Am 249:28, 1983.
5. Freeark, R.J.: 1982 A.A.S.T. Presidential Address: The trauma centers: Its hospitals, head injuries, helicopters, and heroes. Trauma, 23:173, 1983.
6. Dolan, K.D., and Jacoby, C.G.: Facial fractures. Semin Roentgenol 13:37–51, 1978.
7. Lentrodt, J.: Maxillofacial injuries, statistics and causes of accidents. In Oral and Maxillofacial Traumatology. Vol 1. Edited by E. Kruger and W. Schilil. Chicago, Quintessence Publishing Company, 1982, p. 43.
8. Le Fort, R.: Etude experimentale sur les fractures de la machoire superieure. Rev. Chir., Paris, 23:1901.
9. Ord, R.A.: Post operative retrobulbar hemorrhage and blindness complicating trauma surgery. Br J Oral Surg 19:202, 1981.
10. Ord, R.A., Awty, M.D., and Pour, S.: Lateral retro-

bulbar haemorrhage: A short case report. Br J Oral Maxillofac Surg 24:1, 1986.

11. Rowe, N.L.: Maxillofacial injuries—current trends and techniques. Injury. Br J Accident Surg 16:513, 1985.
12. Manfredi, S.A., et al.: Computerized tomography scan findings in facial fractures associated with blindness. Plast Reconstr Surg 68:479, 1981.
13. Holt, J.E., Holt, G.R., and Blodgett, J.M.: Ocular injuries sustained during blunt facial trauma. Paper read to the American Academy of Ophthalmology, San Francisco, California, November 1, 1982.
14. Luce, E.A., Tubb, T.D., and Moore, A.M.: Review of 1,000 major facial fractures and associated injuries. Plast Reconstr Surg 63:26, 1978.
15. Jabaley, N.E., Lerman, M., and Sanders, H.J.: Ocular injuries and orbital fractures. Plast Reconstr Surg 56:410, 1975.
16. Atkinson, T., and Catone, G.A.: Personal communication.
17. Chandler, J.R., and Serrins, A.J.: Transantral ligation of the internal maxillary artery for epistaxis. Laryngoscope 75:1151, 1965.
18. Macri, D.R., and Makielski, K.H.: Intraoral ligation of the maxillary artery for posterior epistaxis. Laryngoscope 94:737, 1984.
19. Bucholz, R.W., Burkhead, W.Z., and Graham, W.: Occult cervical spine injuries in fatal traffic accidents. J. Trauma 19:768, 1979.
20. Huelke, D.F., O'Day, J., and Mendelsohn, R.A.: Cervical injuries suffered in automobile crashes. J Neurosurg 54:316, 1981.
21. Lewis, V.L., et al.: Facial injuries associated with cervical fractures: recognition, patterns, and management. J Trauma 25:90, 1985.
22. Marar, B.C.: Fracture of the axis arch: "hangman's fracture" of the cervical spine. Clin Orthop 106:155, 1975.
23. Merville, L.C., and Real, J.P.: Fronto-orbito nasal dislocations. Scand J Plast Reconstr Surg 15:287, 1981.
24. Cranin, A.N., et al.: The infraorbital rim staple—a new method of treating displaced and comminuted trimalar fractures. J Oral Surg 37:364, 1979.
25. Thoma, K.H.: Methods of fixation of jaw fractures and their indications. J Oral Surg 6:125, 1948.
26. Robinson, M., and Nyoon, C.: New onlay-inlay metal splint for immobilization of displaced condylar fractures. J Oral Surg 15:164, 1957.
27. Schilli, W.: Treatment possibilities in mandibular fractures. Therapiewotche 41:2005, 1969.
28. Spiessl, B.: Experience with ASIF instruments set in treatment of mandibular fractures. Schweiz Mschr Zahnheilk 79:112, 1969.
29. Luhr, H.G.: Stable osteosynthesis in mandibular fractures. Dtsch Zahnarztl Z 23:754, 1968.
30. Mittelmeier, H.: Compression osteosynthesis with self-tightening compression plates: technique and report of experience. Saarl. Westpfälz Ortopädentreffen Homburg/Saar, 1968.
31. Perren, S.M., et al.: A Dynamic compression plate. Acta Orthop Scand 125 (Suppl.):31, 1969.
32. Spiessl, B., Schargus, G., and Schroll, K.: Stable osteosynthesis in fractures of the edentulous jaw. Schweiz Mschr Zahnheilk 81:39, 1971.
33. Schilli, W., Niederdellmann, H., and Ewers, R.: Problems of functionally stable osteosynthesis in the mandible. Acta Traumatol 3:173, 1973.
34. Kai Tu, H., and Tenhulzen, D.: Compression osteosynthesis of mandibular fractures: a retrospective study. J Oral Maxillofac Surg 43:585, 1985.
35. Duker, J., Harle, F. and Olivier, D.: Wire suture or mini-plate: followup investigation of displaced zygomatic fractures. J Fortschr. Kiefer-u Gesichtschir., 22:49, 1977.

The tireless stenographic and word processing services of Ms. Margaret E. Zamanski and Ms. Marsha McGee of Pittsburgh, Pennsylvania, are acknowledged with great appreciation.

INDEX

Page numbers in *italics* indicate illustrations; page numbers followed by "t" indicate tables.